Current Research in Brain Function Augmentation

Current Research in Brain Function Augmentation

Editor: Max White

MURPHY & MOORE
www.murphy-moorepublishing.com

www.murphy-moorepublishing.com

MURPHY & MOORE

Cataloging-in-Publication Data

Current research in brain function augmentation / edited by Max White.
p. cm.
Includes bibliographical references and index.
ISBN 978-1-63987-142-1
1. Brain. 2. Brain--Physiology. 3. Brain--Localization of functions. 4. Neurophysiology. I. White, Max.
QP376 .C87 2022
612.82--dc23

© Murphy & Moore Publishing, 2022

Murphy & Moore Publishing,
1 Rockefeller Plaza,
New York City, NY 10020, USA

ISBN 978-1-63987-142-1 (Hardback)

This book contains information obtained from authentic and highly regarded sources. Copyright for all individual chapters remain with the respective authors as indicated. All chapters are published with permission under the Creative Commons Attribution License or equivalent. A wide variety of references are listed. Permission and sources are indicated; for detailed attributions, please refer to the permissions page and list of contributors. Reasonable efforts have been made to publish reliable data and information, but the authors, editors and publisher cannot assume any responsibility for the validity of all materials or the consequences of their use.

Trademark Notice: Registered trademark of products or corporate names are used only for explanation and identification without intent to infringe.

Contents

Preface

The human brain is a part of the human nervous system. This organ is responsible for controlling almost all the activities of the body. The augmentation of the brain refers to the different ways in which the performance of the brain can be boosted. It can also be used to repair the brain of a person who suffers from a neurological disease. This can be done through a variety of methods such as through brain implants, brain-machine interfaces (BMI), or through pharmacological or electrical stimulation. There are also non-invasive techniques which can activate specific areas of the brain. This book unfolds the innovative aspects of brain augmentation which will be crucial for the progress of this field in the future. The recent studies that are constantly contributing towards advancing technologies and evolution of this field are examined in detail. As this field is emerging at a rapid pace, the contents of this book will help the readers understand the modern concepts and applications of the subject.

This book has been the outcome of endless efforts put in by authors and researchers on various issues and topics within the field. The book is a comprehensive collection of significant researches that are addressed in a variety of chapters. It will surely enhance the knowledge of the field among readers across the globe.

It gives us an immense pleasure to thank our researchers and authors for their efforts to submit their piece of writing before the deadlines. Finally in the end, I would like to thank my family and colleagues who have been a great source of inspiration and support.

Editor

1

When is diminishment a form of enhancement? Rethinking the enhancement debate in biomedical ethics

Brian D. Earp[1,2,3]***, Anders Sandberg**[1,4]**, Guy Kahane**[1,3] **and Julian Savulescu**[1,2,3]

[1] Faculty of Philosophy, Oxford Uehiro Centre for Practical Ethics, University of Oxford, Oxford, UK
[2] Faculty of Philosophy, Institute for Science and Ethics, University of Oxford, Oxford, UK
[3] Faculty of Philosophy, Oxford Centre for Neuroethics, University of Oxford, Oxford, UK
[4] Faculty of Philosophy, Future of Humanity Institute, University of Oxford, Oxford, UK

Edited by:
Mikhail Lebedev, Duke University, USA

Reviewed by:
Mikhail Lebedev, Duke University, USA
Walter Glannon, University of Calgary, Canada
Saskia K. Nagel, University of Osnabrueck, Germany
Neil McArthur, University of Manitoba, Canada
Justin Caouette, University of Calgary, Canada

***Correspondence:**
Brian D. Earp, Faculty of Philosophy, Oxford Uehiro Centre for Practical Ethics, University of Oxford, Wellington Square, Suite 8, Littlegate House, St. Ebbes Street, Oxford OX1 1PT, UK
e-mail: brian.earp@gmail.com

The enhancement debate in neuroscience and biomedical ethics tends to focus on the *augmentation* of certain capacities or functions: memory, learning, attention, and the like. Typically, the point of contention is whether these augmentative enhancements should be considered permissible for individuals with no particular "medical" disadvantage along any of the dimensions of interest. Less frequently addressed in the literature, however, is the fact that sometimes the *diminishment* of a capacity or function, under the right set of circumstances, could plausibly contribute to an individual's overall well-being: more is not always better, and sometimes less is more. Such cases may be especially likely, we suggest, when trade-offs in our modern environment have shifted since the environment of evolutionary adaptation. In this article, we introduce the notion of "diminishment as enhancement" and go on to defend a *welfarist* conception of enhancement. We show how this conception resolves a number of definitional ambiguities in the enhancement literature, and we suggest that it can provide a useful framework for thinking about the use of emerging neurotechnologies to promote human flourishing.

Keywords: enhancement, neuroenhancement, welfare, well-being, neuroethics, bioethics, diminishment, empathy

INTRODUCTION

Advances in neuroscience and related fields have allowed for an unprecedented increase in our ability to intervene in brain-level processes, thereby influencing a wide range of higher-order functions and behaviors. As Nagel (2010) has noted, this growing and ever more finely-tuned capacity to tamper with even normally-functioning neural systems raises a number of ethical questions about the boundary between traditional research/clinical practice and outright human enhancement. "[A] societal climate of performance measurements and improvements," Nagel writes, has led to a "growing tendency to use medical and technological means beyond their applications in classical therapy" (p. 1). Hence, even though "most of these technologies are developed for medical or research purposes, their application for [human] enhancement interventions is at hand" (*ibid.*).

A burgeoning academic literature has begun to debate the moral propriety of such enhancement. This debate often centers on the use of neurotechnological, pharmacological, or other interventions to *increase* some human capacity or function (e.g., Bostrom, 2003, 2009; Bostrom and Roache, 2008; see also Daniels, 2000; Harris, 2007; and Kass, 2003a; especially pp. 12–13). What, after all, is the meaning of "enhance" if not to heighten, to augment, to intensify? Thus we see articles asking whether non-invasive brain stimulation should be used to enhance learning (e.g., Cohen Kadosh et al., 2012); whether we should be worried about university students taking Ritalin to improve focus (e.g., Outram, 2010); whether doctors have an obligation to ingest ergogenic drugs to stay awake during late-night surgery (e.g., Greely et al., 2008); and whether the use of mood brighteners is getting out of hand (e.g., Farah, 2002). The "augmentative" flavor of much of this work can be seen in a recent article by Dees (2007, p. 372):

> [Now or in the near future] drugs may be able to improve our ability to think. Amphetamines can help people to learn skilled motor tasks, like playing the piano, more rapidly. Cholinsterase inhibitors now help [patients] to improve their attention and memory, and better versions may help virtually anyone. Amphetamines, like Ritalin, improve focus, attention, and memory... Some drugs may help the formation of long-term memories and thereby facilitate learning... [Drugs can also] alter people's moods.... Soon drugs almost certainly will be developed that will "brighten" the mood of anyone who takes them.

Bostrom and Roache (2008) take a similar approach: "One important way in which the human condition could be changed is through the enhancement of basic human capacities... There are various ways in which we can currently improve [these capacities, including] stamina, strength, dexterity, flexibility, coordination, agility, and conditioning" (pages 1 and 7 [1]). In another paper, Bostrom (2009, p. 8[2]) asks us to

[1] Page numbers are from the online version available at http://www.nickbostrom.com/ethics/human-enhancement.pdf
[2] Page number is from the online version available at http://www.nickbostrom.com/ethics/dignity-enhancement.pdf

> Consider, for example, enhancements in executive function and self-control, concentration, or of our ability to cope with stressful situations; further, consider enhancements of mental energy that would make us more capable of independent initiative and that would reduce our reliance on external stimuli such as television; consider perhaps also enhancement of our ability to withstand mild pains and discomforts, and to more effectively self-regulate our consumption of food, exercise, and sleep.

Note the specific focus here on *capacities, moods,* or *functions* that might be improved by the pharmacological (or other) intervention—"improved" in the sense of facilitating *more* of whatever it is that the function normally does (see Dresler et al., 2013 for a recent review). We can summarize this sort of approach as follows:

> **The Functional-Augmentative Approach to Enhancement**: Interventions are considered enhancements insofar as they improve some capacity or function (such as cognition, vision, hearing, alertness) by increasing the ability of the function to do what it normally does.

The debate then typically turns on whether the proposed capacity-enhancement should be considered *permissible* for someone who does not suffer a "medical" disadvantage along that dimension (Daniels, 2000; Allhoff et al., 2009). In this context, a distinction is frequently drawn between "enhancement" (on the one hand) and mere "treatment" or "therapy" (on the other), with the implication often being that the former may be morally problematic in ways that the latter may not be. This consideration suggests a second approach to understanding enhancement:

> **The Not-Medicine Approach to Enhancement (Treatment vs. Enhancement)** (see, e.g., Sabin and Daniels, 1994; Juengst, 1998; Daniels, 2000; Kass, 2003b; Pellegrino, 2004): On this view, "the term *enhancement* [characterizes] interventions designed to improve human form or functioning *beyond what is necessary to sustain or restore good health*" (Juengst, 1998, emphasis added).

There are other approaches as well. In an earlier work, we identified two additional ways of understanding enhancement—the sociological-pragmatic approach and the ideological approach (see Savulescu et al., 2011, for details)—and then proceeded to outline a new account of enhancement, which we argued was preferable to the others: the welfarist approach. This approach can be defined as follows:

> **The Welfarist Approach to Enhancement:** "Enhancement" should be defined to mean any change in the biology or psychology of a person which increases the chances of leading a good life in a given set of circumstances.

In the present article, we wish to develop our defense of this welfarist account by contrasting it specifically with the "augmentative" functionalist approach [3] (i.e., enhancement of some capacity; see **Table 1** for a selective summary)—as well as the related "not-medicine" approach to enhancement—in light of recent discussions in neuroethics that seem to break the conventional mold. We introduce the notion of "diminishment as enhancement" and focus on a set of cases in which "subtractive" interventions—that is, interventions geared toward *weakening* a given capacity or function—might plausibly contribute to individual welfare enhancement in line with the definition just laid out. We conclude by discussing some of the advantages that this welfarist conception has over other common definitions.

DISCUSSION

What do we mean by "diminishment"? We can dispense with a potential red herring. We do *not* mean to draw attention to specific neural pathways or low-level mechanisms whose weakening or disruption might go on to yield some higher-order functional outcome. For instance, stimulants such as Ritalin, sometimes used to augment focus and concentration, could in principle be understood as "diminishments" since—on at least at one level of description—they actually *limit* the reuptake of neurotransmitters, ultimately producing their stimulating effects [4]. Likewise, TMS and other forms of brain stimulation may involve *disrupting*

[3] One may wonder just how common this approach is—that is, how frequently it is encountered in the literature compared to other approaches. As noted above, in addition to the work of prominent figures such as Bostrom—who define enhancement explicitly in terms of augmentation of functions or capacities (see especially Bostrom, 2009)—the most commonly referenced account is the "not-medicine" approach, which distinguishes enhancement from treatment, as in the seminal report from the President's Council on Bioethics, "Beyond Therapy" (Kass, 2003b). "Therapy" is ordinarily understood as being an attempt to address disease, which on the dominant account after Boorse (1977) is species-typical subfunctioning (see also Daniels, 1985). Therefore, on the "not-medicine" approach as well, enhancement just is the improvement of some function within (or beyond) the normal range. We do not suggest, of course, that the functional-augmentative view is the only view one encounters in the literature, nor that cases of functional diminishment are never employed in these debates. Indeed, one of the classic examples of "enhancement" from the field—the blunting of painful memories (which we discuss below)—is quite common. However, in our reading of the literature, it is examples relating to capacity augmentation that are much more frequently encountered and actually used as illustrations of enhancement; and when instances of diminishment are raised, their specific implications for the conceptual understanding of enhancement is rarely if ever addressed. In addition, the link between the intervention (whether augmentative or diminishing) and *well-being* is not commonly articulated as such, with other goals such as "self improvement" being either stated or implicitly assumed (e.g., Farah, 2013).

[4] Though note, as a reviewer points out: diminishment-as-enhancement "can work at both lower (neurobiological) and higher (mental, psychological) levels in a complementary way [depending upon the way the enhancement is described]. While methylphenidate produces its stimulating effect by limiting the reuptake of dopamine, it enhances one's capacity to be more attentive to and focused on a particular task by diminishing the content and scope of one's attention" (emphasis added). Thus we can see that it is possible to augment (via diminishment) a given capacity (here, focus), not only by interfering with some lower-order neurological process, but even by diminishing an inversely related higher-order capacity: in this example, the scope of one's attention. Therefore it is important to make clear (as we do in a subsequent paragraph) that our emphasis in this paper is on interventions that would diminish the targeted higher-order capacity itself (i.e., focus), rather than either (a) some lower-order mechanism whose diminishment would actually

Table 1 | Selective summary of "augmentative" neural enhancements, means, and references.

Function	Means	References
Attention	Nicotine, Modafinil, caffeine, glucose, aerobic exercise, rTMS, computer training, meditation	Benton et al., 1994; Hilgetag et al., 2001; Rezvani and Levin, 2001; Newhouse et al., 2004; Repantis et al., 2010; Smith et al., 2010; Chiesa et al., 2011; Zelinski et al., 2011
Empathy and mind-reading	Oxytocin, MDMA	Bartz et al., 2010; Hysek et al., 2012
Executive function	Aerobic exercise; computer training; meditation	Smith et al., 2010; Chiesa et al., 2011; Nouchi et al., 2012
Learning—including implicit learning, verbal learning, and numerical learning	Amphetamine, methylphenidate, a large number of synaptic-plasticity affecting drugs, tDCS, various memory arts and mnemonic systems	Soetens et al., 1993; Clark et al., 1999; Kincses et al., 2004; Williams and Eskandar, 2006; Lee and Silva, 2009; Cohen Kadosh et al., 2010; Repantis et al., 2010; Javadi et al., 2012; Suthana et al., 2012
Inhibitory control and self control	Modafinil, Atomoxetine, glucose	Turner et al., 2003; Galliot et al., 2007; Chamberlain et al., 2009
Memory—including working memory, memory encoding, and memory consolidation	Glucose, donepezil, physiostigmine, exercise, tDCS, Ampakines, Modafinil, methylphenidate, computer training, protein, meditation	Elliott and Sahakian, 1997; Furey et al., 2000; Lynch, 2002; Turner et al., 2003; Barch, 2004; Marshall et al., 2004; Fregni et al., 2005; Luber et al., 2007; Jaeggi et al., 2008; Ohn et al., 2008; Riby et al., 2008; Thorell et al., 2009; Smith et al., 2010; Chiesa et al., 2011; Teo et al., 2011; Jones et al., 2012
Planning	Methylphenidate	Elliott and Sahakian, 1997
Reaction speed	Glucose	Owens and Benton, 1994
Recall	tDCS	Gagnon et al., 2010; Ross et al., 2010
Wakefulness/alertness	Caffeine, Modafinil, amphetamine, other stimulants	Hartmann and Cravens, 1976; Smith, 2002; Baranski et al., 2004

activity in one region as a means to enhancing function in another (or at another level of description). For example, TMS can reduce interference between similar-sounding words in phonological memory (likely by disrupting the phonological store), thereby improving verbal recall (Kirschen et al., 2006). In these sorts of cases, it is the higher-order function itself that we take to be the target of enhancement (i.e., the capacity for focus, concentration, or recollection), whereas the lower-order "diminishment" is merely instrumental.

By contrast, we intend to highlight interventions that serve to diminish the higher-order capacities themselves. That is, we want to focus on interventions that make concentration (for example) *worse*—by virtue of *whatever* neural mechanism is involved. Consider some illustrative cases. Should soldiers be given propranolol to *reduce* the emotional intensity of wartime memories (e.g., Henry et al., 2007)? Should a battered spouse use "anti-love" neurotechnology to *sever* the emotional attachment she has with her abuser (Earp et al., 2013)? Should sex offenders have to undergo "chemical *castration*" as a condition of parole (e.g., Gupta, 2012)? Should appetite *suppressants* be developed for mass-market consumption (e.g., Farah, 2013)? These are just a few recent examples of potential interventions that might reduce or diminish a higher-order capacity.

Interventions of this kind raise many of the same patterns of ethical concern as the more conventional cases of functional enhancement typically encountered in the bioethics literature. For example: who should administer the drug or apply the technology? Should the intervention be regulated? How? Is a threat to autonomy or authenticity potentially implied? And what sort of externalities might need to be anticipated?

At the same time, however—given a functional-augmentative framework—these cases might seem puzzling or out of place. They seem puzzling because they apparently involve the very *opposite* of enhancement, namely, diminishment: i.e., *diminishment* of wartime memories; *diminishment* of harmful love; *diminishment* of ill-directed lust, and so on. How might these seemingly opposite-to-enhancement outcomes be made to square

increase the target capacity, or (b) an inversely-related higher-order capacity, whose diminishment would have a similar effect.

with the seemingly similar-to-enhancement applicability of "standard" bioethical analysis?

There is a straightforward solution to this puzzle. Sometimes, diminishment *is* enhancement—on the welfarist definition of the term (see above). That is, once we shift our focus from the particular *capacity* or *function* being modified to the overall *normative goal* of the modification itself, we begin to see that "enhancement" may be more broadly understood as having something to do with well-being—a goal that the welfarist definition makes explicit. On this account, in order for an intervention to count as an enhancement, it does not matter if the capacity itself is being modified "up" or being modified "down." Nor does it matter if the modification is being accomplished by means[5] of a drug, a biochip, an electrical brain-stimulator, or something more familiar and lower tech. Nor does it matter if the intervention is called "medicine" or "therapy" or "beyond therapy" or anything else. If it increases the person's chances of leading a good life in the relevant circumstances, then we propose that it should be considered an enhancement.

IMPLICATIONS OF THE ARGUMENT

Well... so what? What does this welfarist definition get us? How will it be *useful* for medical professionals, neuroethicists, and other stakeholders engaged in these sorts of discussions? Finally, what advantages does it have over other definitions used throughout the literature?

First, and most basically, it acknowledges that "more" is not always "better." As commonplace a maxim as this is, it is not always duly appreciated. As the neuroscientist Baron-Cohen (2011) has recently argued, even such "obviously" beneficial human capacities as the ability to empathize may have maladaptive consequences in certain cases. For example, too much empathy might drive a person to prioritize attending to others' feelings over meeting her own basic needs. Or consider "empathy fatigue"—a term used by Stebnicki (2007) to refer to the physical and emotional exhaustion that grief and trauma counselors sometimes come to face: their inability to *distance* themselves emotionally from the pain and suffering of their clients ultimately prevents them from doing their job. Likewise, Williams (1989) has hypothesized that among helping professionals, high emotional empathizers may be disposed to earlier career burnout.

The same lesson may apply to other "obviously" beneficial capacities such as intelligence or IQ. While super-intelligence might seem to be an enviable trait or disposition, being "too smart for one's own good" is not always a mere teasing admonition: for many intellectually gifted individuals, very high intelligence can come at a direct cost to their overall well-being (Harrison and Van Haneghan, 2011). Furthermore, intelligence is not sufficient for achieving the good life, but is merely instrumental, and IQ enhancement *per se* does not seem to have any clearly determinate value (Tännsjö, 2009).

Likewise, the ability to remember well would seem to be a beneficial thing: "memory makes us" (it has been said) and many elderly people are very sad to see their powers of recollection fade over time. But as any victim of rape might tell you—and as the soldiers we referred to earlier would hasten to agree—sometimes memory can be a devastating shackle. In addition, research has shown that excessive autobiographical memory (hyperthymesia) can interfere with the basic business of living one's life (Parker et al., 2006).

Finally, even romantic love—undoubtedly the most celebrated emotional capacity of all—can be dangerous or even life-threatening when the object of affection is cruel or abusive. Some victims of domestic violence, for example, find themselves unable to diminish their passionate feelings for their abuser, despite being fully aware that their long-term well-being and even basic physical safety may be under threat by remaining in the relationship (Earp et al., 2013, 2014, under review; see also Earp et al., 2012, for further discussion).

The implication in all of this is clear; and here we reaffirm our thesis to drive it home: Sometimes, diminishing a certain *capacity* or *function*—under the right set of circumstances—could quite plausibly *enhance* a person's overall well-being.[6]

SOME FINE-TUNING

Given this possibility, one might be tempted to argue that functional diminishment would only enhance well-being by bringing the individual back from a *pathological* state to a species-typical state. Yet while this direction of change could reasonably describe a number of specific cases, it is unlikely to hold as a general rule. This is because what it is that enhances well-being is not species-general, but rather context-specific. Thus, as Dees (2007) notes, "beta blockers [can be used to] decrease stress and nervousness, and so they help even normal people cope with abnormal situations" (p. 372). In the context of a public performance, for example, even a quite ordinary stress reaction could interfere with an individual's well-being, given the context-local goals of the performer: hence "[the] widespread use [of beta-blockers] among concert performers is legendary" (*ibid.*) Likewise, in the notorious "Ashley case" (Liao et al., 2007), the parents of a severely brain-impaired child wanted to stunt her growth by using estrogen therapy (as well as remove her uterus and breast buds) in order to improve her quality of life. While parts of the treatment and even the motivations behind it may certainly be called into question, it is at least plausible to think that reducing Ashley's growth, all things considered, would count in favor of her own best interests. For example, Ashley's parents suggested that her smaller size would make it easier to carry her around, thus allowing her to participate more fully in the activities of daily living. If so, then approaching the normal human size range would *not* improve well-being, whereas the proposed diminishment might.

[5]Note that the means "do not matter" only in the specific sense stated—i.e., in terms of whether some intervention should be counted as an enhancement. By contrast, the means might very well matter in terms of having different safety profiles, etc. Furthermore, there is no reason to think that all means will be normatively equivalent either, even if well-being is taken as the explicit goal of enhancement. This is because there are other normatively-relevant considerations besides well-being, such as justice or fairness, which may impact upon the evaluation of means (as well as other factors related to enhancement), as we discuss in a later section.

[6]This sort of welfare enhancement is likeliest to occur, we suggest, when the functional diminishment in question results in optimal levels of capacity functioning for successful adaptation to the demands of the environment.

But what is the more general thrust of the argument? In other words, when, or under what conditions, is (functional) diminishment likely to produce (well-being) enhancement? We have already discussed context-specific and "pathological" cases, but others suggest themselves as well. One plausible view is that we should expect promising enhancers when the trade-offs in our living conditions have shifted from the environment of evolutionary adaptation (Bostrom and Sandberg, 2008). While some changes no doubt enable well-being enhancement in the sense of getting *more* of something that was limited in the past because of its cost, there are likely other domains in which something has lost importance today. For example, fight-or-flight reactions that would have served well in an environment flush with predators might today contribute more to stress, cardiovascular disease, and problems with anxiety (Bracha and Maser, 2008). Anti-parasite immune cells can become overactive in our relatively clean environment, triggering allergies (Sironi and Clerici, 2010). And ancient hunger drives can lead to obesity in today's societies, given the unprecedented availability of low-nutrient, high-calorie foods (e.g., Serlie et al., 2011). These examples provide further potential cases in which we might judiciously *diminish* our body's natural responses in order to improve our overall well-being.

CONCLUSION

Our aim in this article has been simple. It has been to rethink, or at least to problematize, the chiefly "augmentative" flavor of discourse surrounding neurotechnological enhancement. We do not mean to imply, of course, that all or even most of the diminishments we have discussed are currently technologically feasible, nor do we suggest that they would always be the best solution to the problem at hand. As Levy (2012) has recently argued, when faced with a detrimental mismatch between our capacities and our context, it is often better to change our environmental conditions than it is to re-tool our biology, all things considered. Other times, the best course of action might be to pursue a complementary strategy that involves the use of brain-level interventions alongside other types of approaches (Savulescu and Sandberg, 2008). The answer is likely to be different for different cases.

Yet whatever position one takes on the proper balance of intervention strategies, we have tried to show that there is something to be gained by distinguishing functional enhancement from enhancement of well-being. For any disposition, trait, or function, there is likely to be a discrete range of optimal levels (of intensity, sensitivity, etc.) for the given set of conditions, and too much or too little may detract from health or happiness. Identifying diminishment as a possible form of human enhancement, therefore, invites us to ask whether we may have *too much* X for the best life, based on the relevant local circumstances and other facets of modern living.

Another advantage of the welfarist definition of enhancement is that it can handle not only cases of functional diminishment (our emphasis in this paper), but even unusual cases including *extensions* of the body, in which a new capacity is added that did not exist before. One example of such a case is the use of implanted magnets for "magnetic vision" (Larratt, 2004). While this type of intervention is clearly "augmentative" (in the sense of adding something rather than subtracting), it differs from the usual augmentative cases—which involve intensifying an existing capacity—in that it introduces a novel capacity that would not exist at all without the enhancement. Similarly other forms of body-modifications may be seen as attempts to enhance well-being through bringing the body more in line with personal ideals of self-expression. These cases, too, may not involve the "enhancement" of any existing capacity, but rather welfare enhancement more broadly construed through the employment of biotechnology.

We are careful to note that we have left untouched important questions about who would administer these new technologies, under what specific conditions; how their advisability would be decided upon (especially as compared to other, potentially less invasive, forms of intervention); how long their effects should be expected to last; what risks or side-effects might be involved; and whether any regulatory structures would have to be put in place to accommodate their existence. These types of questions are bound to overlap with analogous puzzles being worked out in the "augmentative" enhancement literature, so we will leave their discussion for another day. Here we have endeavored, not to cultivate a vast procedural forest, but rather to plant a conceptual seed.

FINAL THOUGHTS

As we have argued elsewhere (Savulescu et al., 2011), the "enhancement debates" in biomedical ethics have been needlessly encumbered by the existence of a hodge-podge of ill-defined, poorly articulated notions of enhancement—often only implicitly communicated—along with endless to-ing and fro-ing about the relationship between enhancement and the limits of medicine. Re-casting "enhancement" as being essentially related to welfare, however, provides several distinct advantages:

> It ties enhancement to the value of well-being... It offers a general framework for thinking about well-being. It offers more than a mere list of value claims. It singles out well-being as one dimension of value that is constitutive of genuine human enhancement. But it leaves open substantive and contentions questions about the nature of well-being, and important empirical questions about the impact of some treatment on well-being. [Moreover], the welfarist approach distinguishes ways in which some treatment might benefit a person from other relevant values, such as justice. It thus allows us to say that although some treatment is an enhancement (i.e., contributes to individuals' well-being), it might nevertheless be bad overall, because its employment in the current social context will lead to far greater injustice. (p. 7)

Finally, we note that people's normal brain functions will differ across time and circumstance. They will differ between people as well. We can now *control* function, at least in part, through the use of neurotechnology and biomedicine, and our ability to do so is likely to become increasingly more potent as well as more targeted in the decades to come. We suggest that we should tie this ability to a robust account of well-being (e.g., Kahane and Savulescu, 2008; Earp et al., under review), and seek to maximize function toward that end, whether the capacity itself is being augmented (as is typically emphasized in these debates) or indeed (as we emphasize here) effectively diminished.

AUTHORS' CONTRIBUTIONS

Brian D. Earp wrote the first draft of the essay, and undertook final edits to synthesize the contributions of the other authors. Anders Sandberg provided some of the scientific examples, and drafted the argument about shifting evolutionary trade-offs. Guy Kahane contributed substantial intellectual content and edited and approved the final draft. Julian Savulescu conceived the general argument and contributed substantially to the concluding paragraphs.

AUTHORS' INFORMATION

Brian D. Earp studied philosophy, psychology, and cognitive science at Yale and Oxford universities and is a Research Fellow in the Oxford Uehiro Centre for Practical Ethics as well as a Consultant with the Oxford Centre for Neuroethics. Anders Sandberg trained in computer science, neuroscience, and medical engineering, and is a James Martin Research Fellow at Oxford's Future of Humanity Institute. Guy Kahane holds two degrees in philosophy from the University of Oxford and serves as Deputy Director of both the Uehiro Centre for Practical ethics and the Oxford Centre for Neuroethics. Julian Savulescu is qualified in medicine, bioethics, and analytic philosophy, and holds the Chair in Practical Ethics at the University of Oxford.

ACKNOWLEDGMENTS

This work was supported in part by a University Award from the Wellcome Trust (#WT087208MF), by the Wellcome Trust #08604/Z/08/Z, by the Oxford Martin School, and by the Volkswagen Foundation.

REFERENCES

Allhoff, F., Lin, P., Moor, J., and Weckert, J. (2009). Ethics of human enhancement: 25 questions & answers. *Stud. Ethics Law Technol.* 4, 1–50. doi: 10.2202/1941-6008.1110

Baranski, J. V., Pigeau, R., Dinich, P., and Jacobs, I. (2004). Effects of modafinil on cognitive and meta–cognitive performance. *Hum. Psychopharmacol. Clin. Exp.* 19, 323–332 doi: 10.1002/hup.596

Barch, D. (2004). Pharmacological manipulation of human working memory. *Psychopharmacology* 174, 126–135. doi: 10.1007/s00213-003-1732-3

Baron-Cohen, S. (2011). "Autism, empathizing-systemizing (e-s) theory, and pathological altruism," in *Pathological Altruism,* eds B. Oakley, A. Knafo, G. Madhaven, and D. S. Wilson (Oxford: Oxford University Press), 344–348.

Bartz, J. A., Zaki, J., Bolger, N., Hollander, E., Ludwig, N. N., Kolevzon, A., et al. (2010). Oxytocin selectively improves empathic accuracy. *Psychol. Sci.* 21, 1426–1428. doi: 10.1177/0956797610383439

Benton, D., Owens, D. S., and Parker, P. Y. (1994). Blood glucose influences memory and attention in young adults. *Neuropsychologia* 32, 595–607. doi: 10.1016/0028-3932(94)90147-3

Boorse, C. (1977). Health as a theoretical concept. *Philos. Sci.* 44, 542–573. doi: 10.1086/288768

Bostrom, N. (2003). Human genetic enhancements: a transhumanist perspective. *J. Value Inq.* 37, 493–506. doi: 10.1023/B:INQU.0000019037.67783.d5

Bostrom, N. (2009). Dignity and enhancement. *Contemp. Read. Law Soc. Justice* 2, 84–115.

Bostrom, N., and Roache, R. (2008). "Ethical issues in human enhancement," in *New Waves in Applied Ethics*, ed J. Ryberg, (New York, NY: Palgrave Macmillan), 120–152.

Bostrom, N., and Sandberg, A. (2008). "The wisdom of nature: an evolutionary heuristic for human enhancement," in *Human Enhancement*, eds J. Savulescu and N. Bostrom (Oxford: Oxford University Press), 375–416.

Bracha, H. S., and Maser, J. D. (2008). Anxiety and posttraumatic stress disorder in the context of human brain evolution: a role for theory in DSM–V? *Clin. Psychol. Sci. Pract.* 15, 91–97. doi: 10.1111/j.1468-2850.2008.00113.x

Chamberlain, S. R., Hampshire, A., Müller, U., Rubia, K., Del Campo, N., Craig, K., et al. (2009). Atomoxetine modulates right inferior frontal activation during inhibitory control: a pharmacological functional magnetic resonance imaging study. *Biol. Psychiatry* 65, 550–555. doi: 10.1016/j.biopsych.2008.10.014

Chiesa, A., Calati, R., and Serretti, A. (2011). Does mindfulness training improve cognitive abilities? A systematic review of neuropsychological findings. *Clin. Psychol. Rev.* 31, 449–464. doi: 10.1016/j.cpr.2010.11.003

Clark, K. B., Naritoku, D. K., Smith, D. C., Browning, R. A., and Jensen, R. A. (1999). Enhanced recognition memory following vagus nerve stimulation in human subjects. *Nat. Neurosci.* 2, 94–98. doi: 10.1038/4600

Cohen Kadosh, R., Levy, N., O'Shea, J., Shea, N., and Savulescu, J. (2012). The neuroethics of non-invasive brain stimulation. *Curr. Biol.* 22, R108–R111. doi: 10.1016/j.cub.2012.01.013

Cohen Kadosh, R., Soskic, S., Iuculano, T., Kanai, R., and Walsh, V. (2010). Modulating neuronal activity produces specific and long-lasting changes in numerical competence. *Curr. Biol.* 20, 2016–2020. doi: 10.1016/j.cub.2010.10.007

Daniels, N. (1985). *Just Health Care.* Cambridge: Cambridge University Press. doi: 10.1017/CBO9780511624971

Daniels, N. (2000). Normal functioning and the treatment-enhancement distinction. *Camb. Q. Healthc. Ethics* 9, 309–322. doi: 10.1017/S0963180100903037

Dees, R. H. (2007). Better brains, better selves? The ethics of neuroenhancements. *Kennedy Inst. Ethics J.* 17, 371–395. doi: 10.1353/ken.2008.0001

Dresler, M., Sandberg, A., Ohla, K., Bublitz, C., Trenado, C., Mroczko-Wasowicz, A., et al. (2013). Non-pharmacological cognitive enhancement. *Neuropharmacology* 64, 529–543. doi: 10.1016/j.neuropharm.2012.07.002

Earp, B. D., Sandberg, A., and Savulescu, J. (2012). Natural selection, childrearing, and the ethics of marriage (and divorce): building a case for the neuroenhancement of human relationships. *Philos. Technol.* 25, 561–587. doi: 10.1007/s13347-012-0081-8

Earp, B. D., Sandberg, A., and Savulescu, J. (2014). Brave new love: the threat of high-tech "conversion" therapy and the bio-oppression of sexual minorities. *Am. J. Bioeth. Neurosci.* 5, 4–12. doi: 10.1080/21507740.2013.863242

Earp, B. D., Wudarczyk, O. A., Sandberg, A., and Savulescu, J. (2013). If I could just stop loving you: anti-love biotechnology and the ethics of a chemical breakup. *Am. J. Bioeth.* 13, 3–17. doi: 10.1080/15265161.2013.839752

Elliott, R., and Sahakian, B. J. (1997). Effects of methylphenidate on spatial working memory and planning in healthy young adults. *Psychopharmacology* 131, 196–206. doi: 10.1007/s002130050284

Farah, M. J. (2002). Emerging ethical issues in neuroscience. *Nat. Neurosci.* 5, 1123. doi: 10.1038/nn1102-1123

Farah, M. J. (2013). *Cognitive Enhancement.* Available online at: http://www.neuroethics.upenn.edu/index.php/penn-neuroethics-briefing/cognitive-enhancement

Fregni, F., Boggio, P. S., Nitsche, M., Bermpohl, F., Antal, A., Feredoes, E., et al. (2005). Anodal transcranial direct current stimulation of prefrontal cortex enhances working memory. *Exp. Brain Res.* 166, 23–30. doi: 10.1007/s00221-005-2334-6

Furey, M. L., Pietrini, P., and Haxby, J. V. (2000). Cholinergic enhancement and increased selectivity of perceptual processing during working memory. *Science* 290, 2315–2319. doi: 10.1126/science.290.5500.2315

Gagnon, G., Blanchet, S., Grondin, S., and Schneider, C. (2010). Paired-pulse transcranial magnetic stimulation over the dorsolateral prefrontal cortex interferes with episodic encoding and retrieval for both verbal and non-verbal materials. *Brain Res.* 1344, 148–158. doi: 10.1016/j.brainres.2010.04.041

Galliot, M. T., Baumeister, R. F., DeWall, C. N., Maner, J. K., Plant, E. A., Tice, D. M., et al. (2007). Self-control relies on glucose as a limited energy source: willpower is more than a metaphor. *J. Pers. Soc. Psychol.* 92, 325–336. doi: 10.1037/0022-3514.92.2.325

Greely, H., Sahakian, B., Harris, J., Kessler, R. C., Gazzaniga, M., Campbell, P., et al. (2008). Towards responsible use of cognitive-enhancing drugs by the healthy. *Nature* 456, 702–705. doi: 10.1038/456702a

Gupta, K. (2012). Protecting sexual diversity: rethinking the use of neurotechnological interventions to alter sexuality. *AJOB Neurosci.* 3, 24–28. doi: 10.1080/21507740.2012.694391

Harris, J. (2007). *Enhancing Evolution: The Ethical Case for Making Better People.* Princeton: Princeton University Press.

Harrison, G. E., and Van Haneghan, J. P. (2011). The gifted and the shadow of the night: Dabrowski's overexcitabilities and their correlation to insomnia, death anxiety, and fear of the unknown. *J. Educ. Gift.* 34, 669–697. doi: 10.1177/016235321103400407

Hartmann, E., and Cravens, J. (1976). Sleep: effects of d-and l-amphetamine in man and in rat. *Psychopharmacology* 50, 171–175. doi: 10.1007/BF00430488

Henry, M., Fishman, J. R., and Youngner, S. J. (2007). Propranolol and the prevention of post-traumatic stress disorder: is it wrong to erase the "sting" of bad memories? *Am. J. Bioeth.* 7, 12–20. doi: 10.1080/15265160701518474

Hilgetag, C. C., Theoret, H., and Pascual-Leone, A. (2001). Enhanced visual spatial attention ipsilateral to rTMS-induced 'virtual lessons' of human parietal cortex. *Nat. Neurosci.* 4, 953–957. doi: 10.1038/nn0901-953

Hysek, C. M., Domes, G., and Liechti, M. E. (2012). MDMA enhances "mind reading" of positive emotions and impairs "mind reading" of negative emotions. *Psychopharmacology* 222, 293–302. doi: 10.1007/s00213-012-2645-9

Jaeggi, S. M., Buschkuehl, M., Jonides, J., and Perrig, W. J. (2008). Improving fluid intelligence with training on working memory. *Proc. Natl. Acad. Sci. U.S.A.* 105, 6829–6833. doi: 10.1073/pnas.0801268105

Javadi, A. H., Cheng, P., and Walsh, V. (2012). Short duration transcranial direct current stimulation (tDCS) modulates verbal memory. *Brain Stimul.* 5, 468–474. doi: 10.1016/j.brs 2011.08.003

Jones, E. K., Sünram-Lea, S. I., and Wesnes, K. A. (2012). Acute ingestion of different macronutrients differentially enhances aspects of memory and attention in healthy young adults. *Biol. Psychol.* 89, 477–486. doi: 10.1016/j.biopsycho.2011.12.017

Juengst, E. T. (1998). "What does *enhancement* mean?" in *Enhancing Human Traits: Ethical and Social Implications*, ed E. Parents (Washington, DC: Georgetown University Press), 29–47.

Kahane, G., and Savulescu, J. (2008). "The welfarist account of disability," in *Disability and Disadvantage*, eds A. Cureton and K. Brownlee (Oxford: Oxford University Press), 14–53.

Kass, L. R. (2003a). Ageless bodies, happy souls. *New Atlantis* 1, 9–28. Available online at: http://www.thenewatlantis.com/publications/ageless-bodies-happy-souls

Kass, L. R. (2003b). *Beyond Therapy: Biotechnology and The Pursuit of Happiness.* Washington, DC: President's Council on Bioethics.

Kincses, T. Z., Antal, A., Nitsche, M. A., Bártfai, O., and Paulus, W. (2004). Facilitation of probabilistic classification learning by transcranial direct current stimulation of the prefrontal cortex in the human. *Neuropsychologia* 42, 113–117. doi: 10.1016/S0028-3932(03)00124-6

Kirschen, M., Davis-Ratner, M., Jerde, T. E., Schraedley-Desmond, P., and Desmond, J. (2006). Enhancement of phonological memory following transcranial magnetic stimulation (TMS). *Behav. Neurol.* 17, 187–194. doi: 10.1155/2006/469132

Larratt, S. (2004). *The Gift of Magnetic Vision. BMEzine.com.* Available online at: http://news.bme.com/2004/02/06/the-gift-of-magnetic-vision-the-publishers-ring/

Lee, Y. S., and Silva, A. J. (2009). The molecular and cellular biology of enhanced cognition. *Nat. Rev. Neurosci.* 10, 126–140. doi: 10.1038/nrn2572

Levy, N. (2012). Ecological engineering: reshaping our environments to achieve our goals. *Philos. Technol.* 25, 589–604. doi: 10.1007/s13347-012-0065-8

Liao, S. M., Savulescu, J., and Sheehan, M. (2007). The Ashley treatment: best interests, convenience, and parental decision-making. *Hastings Cent. Rep.* 37, 16–20. doi: 10.1353/hcr.2007.0027

Luber, B., Kinnunen, L. H., Rakitin, B. C., Ellsasser, R., Stern, Y., and Lisanby, S. H. (2007). Facilitation of performance in a working memory task with rTMS stimulation of the precuneus: frequency-and time-dependent effects. *Brain Res.* 1128, 120–129. doi: 10.1016/j.brainres.2006.10.011

Lynch, G. (2002). Memory enhancement: the search for mechanism-based drugs. *Nat. Neurosci.* 5, 1035–1038. doi: 10.1038/nn935

Marshall, L., Mölle, M., Hallschmid, M., and Born, J. (2004). Transcranial direct current stimulation during sleep improves declarative memory. *J. Neurosci.* 24, 9985–9992. doi: 10.1523/JNEUROSCI.2725-04.2004

Nagel, S. K. (2010). Too much of a good thing? Enhancement and the burden of self-determination. *Neuroethics* 3, 109–119. doi: 10.1007/s12152-010-9072-6

Newhouse, P. A., Potter, P., and Singh, A. (2004). Effects of nicotinic stimulation on cognitive performance. *Curr. Opin. Pharmacol.* 4, 36–46. doi: 10.1016/j.coph.2003.11.001

Nouchi, R., Taki, Y., Takeuchi, H., Hashizume, H., Akitsuki, Y., Shigemune, Y., et al. (2012). Brain training game improves executive functions and processing speed in the elderly: a randomized controlled trial. *PLoS ONE* 7:e29676. doi: 10.1371/journal.pone.0029676

Ohn, S. H., Park, C. I., Yoo, W. K., Ko, M. H., Choi, K. P., Kim, G. M., et al. (2008). Time-dependent effect of transcranial direct current stimulation on the enhancement of working memory. *Neuroreport* 19, 43–47. doi: 10.1097/WNR.0b013e3282f2adfd

Outram, S. M. (2010). The use of methylphenidate among students: the future of enhancement? *J. Med. Ethics* 36, 198–202. doi: 10.1136/jme.2009.034421

Owens, D. S., and Benton, D. (1994). The impact of raising blood glucose on reaction times. *Neuropsychobiology* 30, 106–113. doi: 10.1159/000119146

Parker, E. S., Cahill, L., and McGaugh, J. L. (2006). A case of unusual autobiographical remembering. *Neurocase* 12, 35–49. doi: 10.1080/13554790500473680

Pellegrino, E. D. (2004). *Biotechnology, Human Enhancement, and the Ends of Medicine. The Center for Bioethics and Human Dignity.* Available online at: http://www.cbhd.org/resources/biotech/pellegrino

Repantis, D., Schlattmann, P., Laisney, O., and Heuser, I. (2010). Modafinil and methylphenidate for neuroenhancement in healthy individuals: a systematic review. *Pharmacol. Res.* 62, 187–206. doi: 10.1016/j.phrs.2010.04.002

Rezvani, A. H., and Levin, E. D. (2001). Cognitive effects of nicotine. *Biol. Psychiatry* 49, 258–267. doi: 10.1016/S0006-3223(00)01094-5

Riby, L. M., McLaughlin, J., Riby, D. M., and Graham, C. (2008). Lifestyle, glucose regulation and the cognitive effects of glucose load in middle-aged adults. *Br. J. Nutr.* 100, 1128–1134. doi: 10.1017/S0007114508971324

Ross, L. A., McCoy, D., Wolk, D. A., Coslett, H., and Olson, I. R. (2010). Improved proper name recall by electrical stimulation of the anterior temporal lobes. *Neuropsychologia* 48, 3671–3674. doi: 10.1016/j.neuropsychologia.2010.07.024

Sabin, J. E., and Daniels, N. (1994). Determining "medical necessity" in mental health practice. *Hastings Cent. Rep.* 24, 5–13. doi: 10.2307/3563458

Savulescu, J., and Sandberg, A. (2008). Neuroenhancement of love and marriage: the chemicals between us. *Neuroethics* 1, 31–44. doi: 10.1007/s12152-007-9002-4

Savulescu, J., Sandberg, A., and Kahane, G. (2011). "Well-being and enhancement," in *Enhancing Human Capacities*, eds J. Savulescu, R. ter Meulen, and G. Kahane (Oxford: Wiley-Blackwell), 3–18.

Serlie, M. J., La Fleur, S. E., Fliers, E., and Pijl, H. (2011). Obesity: is evolution to blame? *Neth. J. Med.* 69, 156–158. Available online at: http://www.njmonline.nl/abstract.php?i=137&PHPSESSID=

Sironi, M., and Clerici, M. (2010). The hygiene hypothesis: an evolutionary perspective. *Microbes Infect.* 12, 421–427. doi: 10.1016/j.micinf.2010.02.002

Smith, A. (2002). Effects of caffeine on human behavior. *Food Chem. Toxicol.* 40, 1243–1255. doi: 10.1016/S0278-6915(02)00096-0

Smith, P. J., Blumenthal, J. A., Hoffman, B. M., Cooper, H., Strauman, T. A., Welsh-Bohmer, K., et al. (2010). Aerobic exercise and neurocognitive performance: a meta-analytic review of randomized controlled trials. *Psychosom. Med.* 72, 239–252. doi: 10.1097/PSY.0b013e3181d14633

Soetens, E., Hoodge, R. D., and Hueting, J. E. (1993). Amphetamine enhances human-memory consolidation. *Neurosci. Lett.* 161, 9–12. doi: 10.1016/0304-3940(93)90127-7

Stebnicki, M. (2007). Empathy fatigue: healing the mind, body, and spirit of professional counselors. *Am. J. Psychiatr. Rehabil.* 10, 317–338. doi: 10.1080/15487760701680570

Suthana, N., Haneef, Z., Stern, J., Mukamel, R., Behnke, E., Knowlton, B., et al. (2012). Memory enhancement and deep-brain stimulation of the entorhinal area. *N. Engl. J. Med.* 366, 502–510. doi: 10.1056/NEJMoa1107212

Tännsjö, T. (2009). Ought we to enhance our cognitive capacities? *Bioethics* 23, 421–432. doi: 10.1111/j.1467-8519.2008.00721.x

Teo, F., Hoy, K. E., Daskalakis, Z. J., and Fitzgerald, P. B. (2011). Investigating the role of current strength in tDCS modulation of working memory performance in healthy controls. *Front. Psychiatry* 2:45. doi: 10.3389/fpsyt.2011.00045

Thorell, L. B., Lindqvist, S., Bergman Nutley, S., Bohlin, G., and Klingberg, T. (2009). Training and transfer effects of executive functions in preschool children. *Dev. Sci.* 12, 106–113. doi: 10.1111/j.1467-7687.2008.00745.x

Turner, D. C., Robbins, T. W., Clark, L., Aron, A. R., Dowson, J., and Sahakian, B. J. (2003). Cognitive enhancing effects of modafinil in healthy volunteers. *Psychopharmacology* 165, 260–269. doi: 10.1007/s00213-002-1250-8

Williams, C. (1989). Empathy and burnout in male and female helping professionals. *Res. Nurs. Health* 12, 169–178. doi: 10.1002/nur.4770120307

Williams, Z. M., and Eskandar, E. N. (2006). Selective enhancement of associative learning by microstimulation of the anterior caudate. *Nat. Neurosci.* 9, 562–568. doi: 10.1038/nn1662

Zelinski, E. M., Spina, L. M., Yaffe, K., Ruff, R., Kennison, R. F., Mahncke, H. W., et al. (2011). Improvement in memory with plasticity-based adaptive cognitive training: results of the 3-month follow-up. *J. Am. Geriatr. Soc.* 59, 258–265. doi: 10.1111/j.1532-5415.2010.03277.x

2

Hemodynamic responses on prefrontal cortex related to meditation and attentional task

Singh Deepeshwar *, Suhas Ashok Vinchurkar, Naveen Kalkuni Visweswaraiah and Hongasandra RamaRao Nagendra

ANVESANA Research Laboratory, Department of Yoga and Life Sciences, Swami Vivekananda Yoga Research Foundation, Bangalore, Karnataka, India

Edited by:
Mikhail Lebedev, Duke University, USA

Reviewed by:
José M. Delgado-García, University Pablo de Olavide, Seville, Spain
Laura Marzetti, University "G. d'Annunzio" of Chieti-Pescara, Italy

***Correspondence:**
Singh Deepeshwar, ANVESANA Research Laboratory, Department of Yoga and Life Sciences, Swami Vivekananda Yoga Research Foundation, #19 Eknath Bhavan, Gavipuram Circle, K.G. Nagar, Bangalore – 560019, Karnataka, India
e-mail: deepeshwar.singh@gmail.com

Recent neuroimaging studies state that meditation increases regional cerebral blood flow (rCBF) in the prefrontal cortex (PFC). The present study employed functional near infrared spectroscopy (fNIRS) to evaluate the relative hemodynamic changes in PFC during a cognitive task. Twenty-two healthy male volunteers with ages between 18 and 30 years (group mean age ± SD; 22.9 ± 4.6 years) performed a color-word stroop task before and after 20 min of meditation and random thinking. Repeated measures ANOVA was performed followed by a *post hoc* analysis with Bonferroni adjustment for multiple comparisons between the mean values of "During" and "Post" with "Pre" state. During meditation there was an increased in oxy-hemoglobin (ΔHbO) and total hemoglobin (ΔTHC) concentration with reduced deoxy-hemoglobin (ΔHbR) concentration over the right prefrontal cortex (rPFC), whereas in random thinking there was increased ΔHbR with reduced total hemoglobin concentration on the rPFC. The mean reaction time (RT) was shorter during stroop color word task with concomitant reduction in ΔTHC after meditation, suggestive of improved performance and efficiency in task related to attention. Our findings demonstrated that meditation increased cerebral oxygenation and enhanced performance, which was associated with activation of the PFC.

Keywords: meditation, attention task, Stroop task, fNIRS, cerebral blood flow

INTRODUCTION

Meditation is a complex mental process that aims to calm the fluctuations of the mind and improve cognitive functions. Several meditation techniques from diverse traditions (e.g., Transcendental meditation, Buddhists, Zen, Yoga, Vipassana, Brahmakumari, Mindfulness-based stress reduction (MBSR) etc.,) demonstrated that regular practice of meditation develops awareness to the contents of subjective experience, including thoughts, sensations, intentions, and emotions (Saggar et al., 2012). It is considered as a voluntary means of mental training to achieve greater control of higher mental functions. Traditional yoga texts like Patanjali's Yoga *Sutras* (the Sage Patanjali', *Circa* 900 B.C.) and *Bhagavad Gita* (*Circa* 400–600 B.C.) very well describe the connection between meditation and mental modifications. Traditionally, two states of meditation have been described, viz., (i) focused meditation (*dharana* in Sanskrit, Patanjali's Yoga *Sutras*, Chapter III, Verse 1), and this state is supposed to lead to the next stage of effortless mental expansion i.e., (iii) meditation (*dhyana* in Sanskrit; Patanjali's Yoga *Sutras*, Chapter III, Verse 2). When not in meditation, it is said that the mind may be in two other states (Telles et al., 2012). These are (i) random thinking (*cancalata* in Sanskrit; *Bhagavad Gita*, chapter VI, *verse* 34); and (ii) non-meditative focused thinking (*ekagrata* in Sanskrit; *Bhagavad Gita*, chapter VI, *verse* 12) (Telles et al., 2014).

In recent years, there have been a number of neuroimaging studies showing that meditation improves cognitive performance as signified by behavioral and neurophysiological measures (Tang et al., 2007; Lutz et al., 2009). Previous studies have shown that the practice of meditation enhances behavioral performance viz., perceptual discrimination and sustained attention during visual discrimination task (MacLean et al., 2010). Meditation practice develops the ability to engage the attention onto an object for extended periods of time (Carter et al., 2005; Jha et al., 2007; Lutz et al., 2008). It improves the control over the distribution of limited brain resources in the temporal domain, as measured by the attentional blink task (van Leeuwen et al., 2009; Slagter et al., 2011). Long term meditation practice has been found to enhance cognitive performance (Cahn and Polich, 2006), attentional focus, alerting (Jha et al., 2007), processing speed (Lutz et al., 2009; Slagter et al., 2009), and overall information processing (van Vugt and Jha, 2011). In a study, Buddhist meditation practitioners showed mindfulness meditation was positively correlated with sustained attention, when compared to non-meditation practitioners (Moore and Malinowski, 2009). Improvements in sustained attention and attentional error monitoring demonstrated a positive correlation with increased activation in executive attention networks in meditators (Short et al., 2010). Other studies have shown that meditation is associated with improved conflict scores on the attention network test (Tang et al., 2007), reduced interference (Chan and Woollacott, 2007) and enhanced attentional performance during the stroop task compared to meditation-naïve control group (Moore and Malinowski, 2009). These studies provide significant evidence of meditation promoting the higher-order cognitive processing (Zeidan et al., 2010), particularly, the features of conflict monitoring and cognitive control processes.

The stroop task is one of the most frequently used models of the conflict processing (Szűcs et al., 2012) in cognitive neuroscience. Stroop color word task performance evaluates flexibility in the purview of cognitive processes and behavior which requires both attention and impulse control. The simultaneous presentation of the prime color and a written word stimulus will either facilitate (when the color and word stimuli are congruent, e.g., "b-l-u-e" written in the color blue) or interfere (the incongruent stroop trial, e.g., "blue" written in red) with color naming (MacLeod, 1991; Peterson et al., 1999). Previous studies on stroop test have consistently shown that responses in naming the ink color of incongruent color word are much slower than in naming the ink color of neutral (Zysset et al., 2007), and responses are often, but not always, faster when color and word are congruent than in the neutral condition. It supports the hypothesis that, both the task relevant and task irrelevant dimensions of stroop task activate the same response in the congruent condition, in contrast, these dimensions stimulate opposing response tendencies in the incongruent condition (Morton and Chambers, 1973; Posner and Snyder, 1975; Szűcs et al., 2012).

Recent studies reported that regular practice of meditation may alter brain structure and function related to attention (Lazar et al., 2005; Holzel et al., 2011; Kozasa et al., 2012). A study on 20 experienced participants of extensive Insight meditation, that involves focused attention to internal experiences, reported increased cortical thickness in prefrontal cortex (PFC) and right anterior insula associated with attention, interoception and sensory processing in meditation participants compared with matched controls (Lazar et al., 2005).

In order to examine neuronal activity and hemodynamic changes in the brain regions during meditation, the application of different neuroimaging techniques (viz., fMRI and MEG) would be beneficial. The neuronal activity during meditation has been reported in several electroencephalography (EEG) and magnetoencephalography (MEG) studies. Experienced meditators showed an increased EEG power in lower frequency bands (theta, delta and alpha) (Kubota et al., 2001; Takahashi et al., 2005) compared to controls. An EEG study on Transcendental Meditation, showed intermittent prominent bursts of frontally dominant theta activity at an average maximal amplitude of 135 μV in 21 practitioners (Hebert and Lehmann, 1977). Zen meditators showed fast theta and slow alpha power during meditation (Takahashi et al., 2005) demonstrating enhanced automatic memory and reduction in conceptual thinking following meditation (Faber et al., 2014). In a single MEG study on twelve long term Buddhist meditators were assessed in two distinct types of self-awareness, i.e., "narrative" and "minimal" in mindfulness-induced selflessness awareness (Dor-Ziderman et al., 2013). It was found that there was a reduction in gamma band (60–80 Hz) power in frontal, and medial prefrontal areas, and reduced beta band (13–25 Hz) power in ventral medial prefrontal, medial posterior and lateral parietal regions (Dor-Ziderman et al., 2013) and right inferior parietal lobules. These studies are consistent with fMRI and NIRS findings. Functional magnetic resonance imaging (fMRI) poses several challenges such as high sensitivity to participant's motion, a loud, restrictive environment, low temporal resolution, and relatively high cost (Cui et al., 2011). Some of these challenges are overcome with new optical imaging technique: NIRS measure's changes in oxy-hemoglobin and deoxy-hemoglobin (ΔHbO and ΔHbR) concentration changes from the cortical surface and less invasive and expensive than fMRI (Bunce et al., 2006). Functional near infrared spectroscopy (fNIRS) is a compact and portable optical technique to monitor hemodynamics of the brain in real time (Son and Yazici, 2006; Lin et al., 2009).

Brain hemodynamic responses during meditation, i.e., ΔHbO, ΔHbR and total hemoglobin changes (ΔTHC) are in its infancy. In fact, there is only one study that assessed deoxyhemoglobin changes with a single wavelength probe placed over the left PFC during Qigong meditation (Cheng et al., 2010). Practitioners showed decrease in deoxy-hemoglobin and increase in oxy-hemoglobin concentration that suggest, meditation lead to left prefrontal activation during meditation.

With this background, the present study was designed to assess the bilateral prefrontal hemodynamic responses in meditation and random thinking. Additionally, we investigated the hemodynamic changes and performance during a stroop color word task before and after meditation and random thinking. Since, stroop color word task is known to measure attention, interference, processing speed, and executive attention, we expected that this task to be the most sensitive to the effects of meditation.

MATERIALS AND METHODS

PARTICIPANTS

A total of 25 right handed healthy male participants with ages ranging from 19 and 30 years (Mean, SD; 23.4 ± 3.7 years) were recruited from S-VYASA (a Yoga University), South India. All participants had a minimum of 12-month experience in meditation (group average experience ± S.D., 15.6 ± 14.2 months) on the Sanskrit syllable "*OM*". Three participants were excluded from the study because of large motion artifacts in the signals due to head movements or because of failure in probe placement due to obstruction by hair (Taga et al., 2003; Minagawa-Kawai et al., 2011). Thus, only data from 22 participants (mean age 22.9 ± 4.6 years) were included in the final analysis. Participants fulfilling the following criteria were included in the study: (i) the participants with at least 12 months of meditation experience; (ii) male participants alone were studied as cognitive abilities and cerebral blood flow (Brackley et al., 1999) have been shown to fluctuate which the phases of menstrual cycle (Yadav et al., 2002); and (iii) no history of smoking; and (iv) normal health on a routine clinical examination. Participants with following criteria were excluded from the study: (i) persons on any

Table 1 | Characteristics of 22 participants.

Characteristics	
Age (in years) (group mean ± S.D.)	22.9 ± 4.6 years
Years of education	
17 years and more	6 (27.3%)
Upto 15 years	10 (45.5%)
Upto 12 years	6 (27.3%)
Type of meditation	Meditation on the Sanskrit syllable *"OM"*
Experience of meditation practice (in months)	
6–12 months	4 (18.2%)
13–24 months	3 (13.6%)
25–36 months	7 (31.8%)
37–48 months	6 (27.3%)
48–60 months	2 (9.1%)

medication or herbal remedy; (ii) participants having clinical evidence of medical, neuropsychological, or drug abuse that would potentially alter cerebral blood flow (Liddle et al., 1992; Newberg et al., 2010a,b; Goldstein and Volkow, 2011); and (iii) any visual deficit; and (iv) any cognitive impairment. None of the potential participants were involved in any other ongoing research activity. The characteristics of participants are given in **Table 1**.

The study was approved by the Institutional Ethics Committee of S-VYASA, a Yoga University (No.-RES/IEC-S-VYASA/11/2011). The study protocol, nature of the experiments and the operating mode of the instrument was explained to the subjects before obtaining signed informed consent.

DESIGN

The protocol utilized in the present study consisted of two sessions i.e., random thinking (*cancalata*) and meditation (*dhyana*), and eight States (Pre, Stroop_Pre, During (D1-D4 each of 5 min), Stroop_Post, and Post). Each participant was assessed for both the meditation and control session on two separate consecutive days. The sessions were randomized online with randomization software.[1] During the acquisition and analysis of data, researcher was blinded to the session of the individual. The total duration of the each session was 60 min: Pre (5 min), Stroop_Pre (15 min), During (20 min), Stroop_Post (15 min), and Post (5 min). The schematic presentation of the design has been given in **Figure 1**.

Apart from their prior experience of meditation on "*OM*", all participants were given a 3 month orientation, 5 days a week under the guidance of an experienced meditation teacher. The purpose of this orientation was for to ensure uniformity among all practitioners based on specific instructions.

INTERVENTIONS

Each participant sat cross-legged with eyes closed and followed pre-recorded instructions throughout meditation and random thinking sessions. An emphasis was placed on slowly, practice with awareness of physical and mental sensations, and relaxation. The duration of each session was 20 min between 06:00 to 06:30 h conducted 5 days a week. The theoretical aspects of the meditation were detailed by the meditation teacher on the first day. Following this, the practice of each session began with pre-recorded instructions. The practice of meditation was evaluated based on their self-reporting and by consultations with the meditation teacher. The two phases—random thinking (Rand) and meditative defocusing were as follows:

1. ***Random thinking:***
   Participants were asked to listen a compiled audio CD consisting of brief periods of random conversation, announcements, various advertisements and non-connected talks recorded from a local radio station transmission and allow their thoughts to wander freely. All these non-connected conversations could induce the state of random thinking.
2. ***Meditative de-focusing or effortless meditation:***
   In effortless meditation session, each participant was instructed to dwell effortlessly on thoughts of "*OM*", particularly on the subtle (rather than physical) attributes and connotations of the syllable with closed eyes. This involved combined mental chanting with effortless defocusing on syllable "*OM*". This gradually allowed the participants to experience brief periods of silence, which they reported after the session.

ASSESSMENTS PROCEDURE

Laboratory environment

All Participants were assessed in a sound and light dampening Faraday cage. Participants' were monitored using a closed circuit television outside the cabin to detect if they moved or fell asleep during a session. During the session, instructions were passed through a two-way intercom, so that participants could remain uninterrupted. The recording room temperature was maintained at 24.0 ± 1.0°C with 56 percent average humidity during the conduct of experiments. The background noise level was 26 dB of the acoustically shielded chamber. For each participant, the data acquisition session lasted 60 min.

Functional near infrared spectroscopy (fNIRS)

A 16-channel continuous wave fNIRS imager system (FNIR1000-ACK-W, BIOPAC Systems, Inc., U.S.A) was employed to map changes in ΔHbO, ΔHbR and ΔTHC over bilateral PFC. The system consisted of a flexible probe to match contour of the human forehead (see **Figure 2**). The probe embedded with four LED diodes as light sources (at λ_1 = 730 nm, λ_2 = 830 nm, λ_3 = 850 nm) and ten photodiodes as detectors that were symmetrically arranged in an area of 3.5 × 14 cm^2, conducing to 16 nearest source—detector (i.e., channels) at 2.5 cm separation displayed in **Figure 3**. A source-detector distance provides a penetration depth of 1.25 cm (León-Carrion et al., 2008; Kim et al., 2010; Leon-Dominguez et al., 2014). The description of the probe setting is detailed in earlier studies (Krawczyk, 2002; Izzetoglu et al., 2005; Leon-Dominguez et al., 2014). During the experiment, the probe was firmly held with a velcro band on the forehead, and stretched from hairline to eyebrow in a sagittal

[1] http://www.randomizer.org

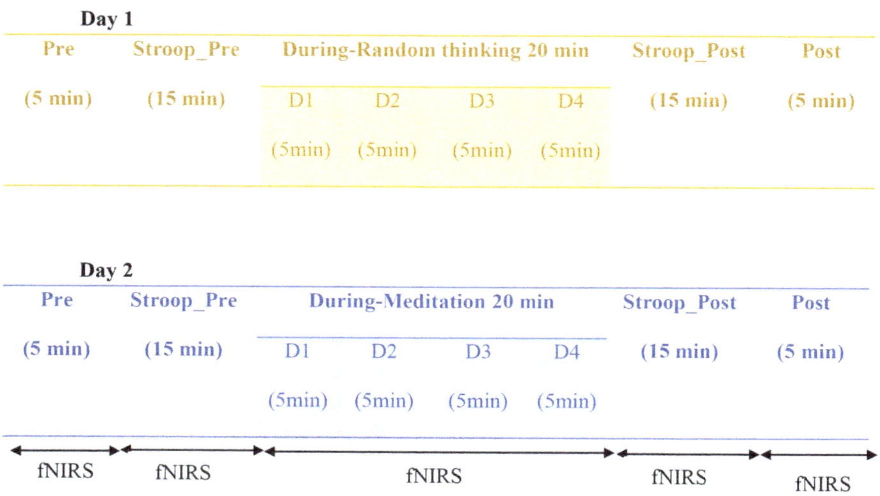

FIGURE 1 | Schematic representation of the study design. Note: Sessions were modified for each participant D1: During 1; D2: During 2; D3: During 3; D4: During 4.

direction and from ear to ear in axial direction (Tian et al., 2009). The probes were positioned bilaterally on forehead, over the left and right frontal poles, a part of dorsolateral PFC, and a portion of the ventrolateral PFC. Regional cerebral blood flow (rCBF), ΔHbO, ΔHbR, and ΔTHC for each hemisphere were updated every 0.5 s. The four LEDs flashed in sequence; the reflected light from the brain as detected with the nearest photodiodes of each LED and converted into digital signals using an analog-digital converter (ADC) card in the control box. The digital data were sent to the laptop though a serial port. The sampling rate was 3 Hz across all 16 channels. The principles of measurement were based on the modified Beer-Lambert law for highly scattering media (Plichta et al., 2006) that agrees assessing changes in ΔHbO and ΔHbR at a certain measured point (Hoshi and Tamura, 1993). Increases in ΔHbO and corresponding decrease in ΔHbR can be interpreted as a sign of functional brain activation.

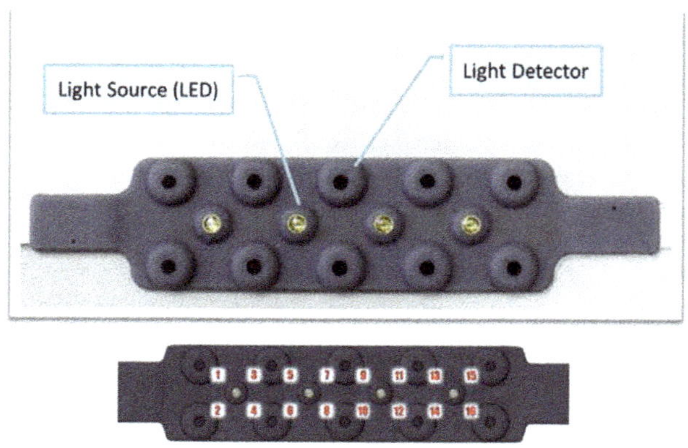

FIGURE 2 | The complete setup employed is herein presented. The fNIRS sensor is displayed with 4 light sources and 10 detectors (top) and 16 optode (channel) measurement locations registered on the sensor.

Stroop color word task

Subjects were seated comfortably on a reclining chair in a Faraday cage, facing a 21 inch LCD monitor placed at a distance of 70 cm from their eyes. Participants were required to focus on the center of the screen which was guided by a fixation object "+" followed by stimuli. Participants did a modified multiple-trial stroop task and were confronted with neutral, congruent, and incongruent stimuli on a black background using E-Prime 2.0.8.90 (Psychological Software Tools, Inc., Pittsburgh, PA, USA). The stroop color word task consisted of red, green and blue colored boxes and the corresponding written words "RED", "BLUE" and "GREEN". The color was presented as color square (4.5 × 4.5 cm) boxes on a black background. The duration of the presented square boxes and words was 500 ms each. Congruent trials comprised of square color boxes followed by words describing the color of the box written in the same color (e.g., the BLUE square box and the printed word "BLUE" in blue ink); incongruent trials comprised of words describing the color of the box written in a color other than that of the box (e.g., the RED square box and word RED written in blue ink); neutral trials comprised words written in white (e.g., the BLUE square box and word BLUE printed in white ink). Participants were instructed to reply as speedily and accurately as possible to the name of the color word (while ignoring the color itself) consistent to the color of the Box with a button press of the response key using the thumb of their right hand. To increase the potency of the conflict stimulus, 20% of trials were congruent (approximately 45 trials), 20% were incongruent (approximately 45 trials) and 50% were neutral (90 trials). The duration of the stimulus was 500 ms, with a variable interstimulus interval (ISI) of 1000–2500 ms the experimental steps are illustrated in **Figure 4**.

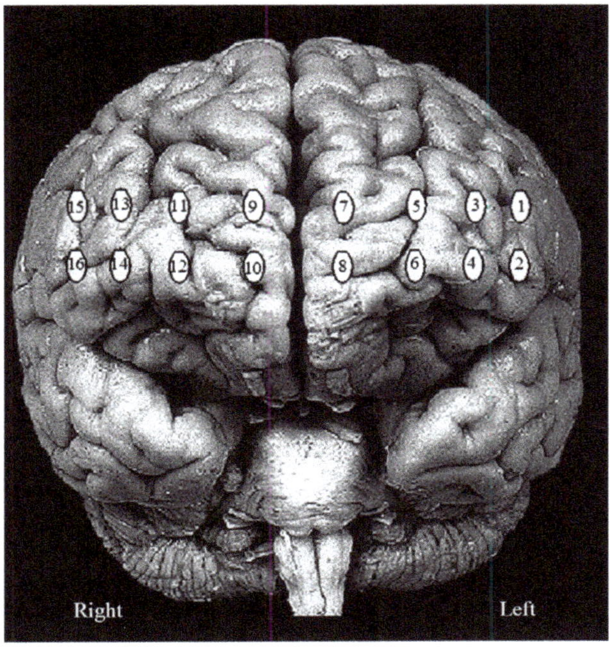

FIGURE 3 | The 16 fNIRS optode (channel) measurement locations registered on the brain surface image are presented.

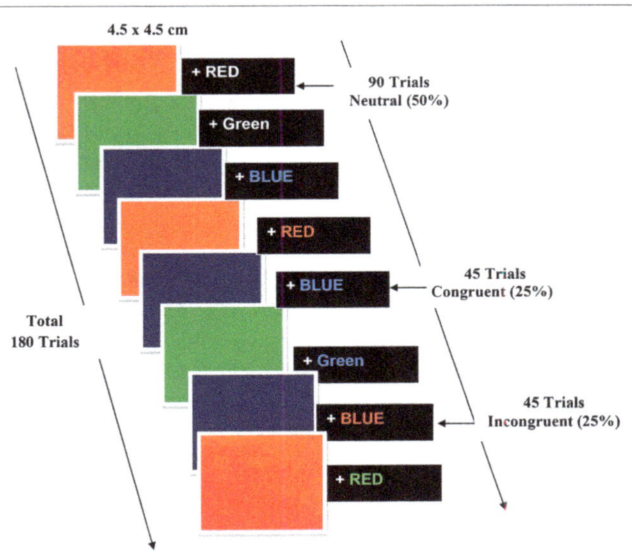

FIGURE 4 | Experimental steps of Color word Stroop Task.

Data acquisition

The participants were assessed in two separate sessions i.e., random thinking and meditation while recording hemodynamic activity on the PFC using 16-channel continuous wave fNIRS system. On the preceding day and on the day of the recording, participants were asked to avoid tea and coffee which are known to influence cognitive performance (Nehlig, 2010) and cerebral blood flow (Addicott et al., 2009). Where this was unavoidable the session was engaged on another day. The participants wore a flexible sensor pad over prefrontal region and covered with a black cloth. The probable artifacts such as heart rate pulsation, respiration and high frequency noise in raw data, which may possibly be induced by autonomic arousal caused during stroop task, was eliminated with pre designed finite impulse response (FIR) filters based on type, order, window function and cut-off frequency. For the present study, raw data were acquired from the probe, which is pre-filtered by two filters and processed in the data processing unit using COBI filter module. The first filter is a 10th order low-pass filter with cutoff frequency of 0.1 Hz with Blackman window. The second filter is a 20th order low-pass, with the normalized cut-off frequency of 0.1 Hz which uses a Hamming window. The filtered data were averaged according to the tasks and conditions for further statistical analysis.

Data analysis

The hemodynamic responses of bilateral PFC were recorded and data were averaged according to the task condition (pre, stroop_pre, during, stroop_post and post). Statistical analysis has been carried out on these differential values. Filtered data were tested with Kolmogorov-Smirnov test for normality. Repeated measures analysis of variance (RM-ANOVA) was used because the same individuals were assessed in repeated sessions on two separate days (i.e., random thinking and meditation). RM-ANOVA was performed with three "within subjects" factors, i.e., Factor 1: Sessions (random thinking and meditation); Factor 2: PFC (right and left). Factor 3: States ("Pre", "Stroop_Pre", "During" (D1 to D4), "Stroop_Post" and "Post"). The repeated measures ANOVAs were carried out for concentration changes of oxygenated and deoxygenated hemoglobin and total hemoglobin change (ΔHbO, ΔHbR and ΔTHbC) across the right and left PFC. This was followed by a *post hoc* analysis with Bonferroni adjustment for multiple comparisons between the mean values of different states ("During" and "Post") and all comparisons were made with the respective "Pre" state.

Moreover, for analysis of stroop task we compared the mean reaction time (ms) of neutral, congruent and incongruent conditions and hemodynamic responses of stroop color word task before and after the sessions (random thinking and meditation). The results were averaged for each side of PFC (right and left), parameter and subject separately to compare between different conditions and sessions. A repeated measures ANOVA was carried for multiple comparisons following Bonferroni adjustment. Statistical analyses were carried out using the Statistical software SPSS version 20.0 (SPSS Inc., Chicago, USA). The alpha level was set at $p < 0.05$. The effect size (d) defined by Cohen (1988), as the mean change score divided by the standard deviation of change, calculated for further statistical analysis.

RESULTS

BEHAVIORAL RESULTS

Reaction times (RTs) were computed solely from the correctly answered trials. With respect to RT, a repeated—measures 3 way ANOVA with Sessions (random thinking and meditation) × States ("Stroop_Pre", "Stroop_Post") × Conditions (neutral vs. congruent vs. incongruent). Repeated measures ANOVA demonstrated a significant main effect for Sessions ($F_{(1,21)}$ = 4.862, p = 0.039, η^2p = 0.188); Conditions ($F_{(2,42)}$ = 24.12, p < 0.001, η^2p = 0.535); States ($F_{(1,21)}$ = 6.696, p < 0.023, η^2p = 0.242), and the significant interaction between Sessions × States ($F_{(1,21)}$ = 45.36, p < 0.001, η^2p = 0.684).

Post hoc analysis revealed that there was a significant improvement in cognitive performance after meditation in all three conditions (neutral, congruent and incongruent) compared to random thinking session given in **Table 1**. The RTs differed in all the conditions (neutral vs. congruent vs. incongruent) in both the sessions. These findings verify that our attentional manipulation was indeed effective.

The RTs were compared using two-tailed paired sample t-test, revealed significant differences among all three conditions (neutral, congruent and incongruent) in two different sessions (meditation and random thinking). In random thinking session, there were significant differences in neutral vs. congruent: $t_{(21)}$ = −3.86, p = 0.001; congruent vs. incongruent: $t_{(21)}$ = −2.31, p = 0.031; neutral vs. incongruent: $t_{(21)}$= −5.92, p < 0.001 whereas in meditation session, there was a significant difference in neutral—congruent: $t_{(21)}$ = −4.47, p < 0.001; congruent—incongruent: $t_{(21)}$ = −1.85, p > 0.05 (NS); neutral—incongruent: $t_{(21)}$ = −6.148, p < 0.001. The mean RTs were significantly shorter in the neutral (p = 0.002), congruent (p < 001) and incongruent (p < 0.003) conditions after meditation session whereas after the random thinking session, mean RTs were delayed in the neutral (p = 0.034) and incongruent (p = 0.008) conditions. The average RTs for neutral, congruent, and incongruent trials of the stroop color word task are given in **Table 2**. Subjects made negligible errors during the color word matching stroop task. For error rates, we did not make any statistical test, since their distributions are clearly not Gaussian. However, it can be supposed that interference effect also reveals itself in error rates. In summary, behavioral results of the stroop color word task are in accordance with the literature, as demonstrated by a clear interference effect in the participants for meditation and random thinking sessions.

HEMODYNAMIC RESPONSES IN STROOP COLOR WORD TASK

In the present study, the 16 channel fNIRS device provided a set of time series recorded over the PFC. The locations of the probed regions are shown in **Figure 2**. The order of the channels is from left to right, i.e., "1" is on the left and "16" is on the right as depicted in **Figure 3**. Analysis of hemoglobin signals i.e., ΔHbO or ΔHbR is still a controversial issue, specifically which hemoglobin signal is more reliably associated with brain activity still remain unclear (Schroeter et al., 2002). In this study, we have utilized three wavelengths (i.e.,750, 803 and 850 nm). This combination is suitable only for detecting ΔHbO signal. Therefore we used ΔHbO, ΔHbR and ΔTHC signals for statistical analysis. The groups mean values ± S.D. for the ΔHbO, ΔHbR and ΔTHC in stroop task and the two sessions (random thinking and meditation) in "Pre", "During" and "Post" states are given in **Table 3**.

For ΔHbO, the repeated—measures ANOVA for Sessions (Random thinking and Meditation) × PFC (Left and Right) × States ("Stroop_Pre", "Stroop_Post") revealed no significant main effect for Sessions, States and PFC. There was a significant interaction between PFC × States ($F_{(1,175)}$ = 9.87, p < 0.01, η^2p = 0.053); Sessions × PFC × States ($F_{(1,175)}$ = 3.17, p < 0.01, η^2p = 0.040).

For ΔHbR, the repeated—measures ANOVA demonstrated significant main effect for Sessions ($F_{(1,175)}$ = 9.99, p < 0.01, η^2p = 0.054); PFC ($F_{(1,175)}$ = 4.57, p < 0.05, η^2p = 0.025). Also, there was a significant interaction between Sessions × PFC (F = 5.11, p < 0.05, η^2p = 0.028); Sessions × States ($F_{(1,175)}$ = 22.13, p < 0.001, η^2p = 0.112); Sessions × PFC × States ($F_{(1,175)}$ = 9.81, p < 0.01, η^2p = 0.053).

For total hemoglobin (ΔTHC), the repeated—measures ANOVA revealed that there was a significant main effect for PFC ($F_{(1,175)}$ = 9.71, p < 0.01, η^2p = 0.053), and the significant interaction between Sessions × PFC ($F_{(1,175)}$ = 5.33, p < 0.01, η^2p = 0.03); Sessions × States ($F_{(1,175)}$ = 19.87, p < 0.001, η^2p = 0.102); PFC × States ($F_{(1,175)}$ = 5.96, p < 0.05, η^2p = 0.033); Sessions × PFC × States ($F_{(1,175)}$ = 14.20, p < 0.001, 0.075).

The *post hoc* analysis with Bonferroni corrections demonstrated forehead hemodynamic responses during stroop task related to random thinking and meditation sessions are given in **Table 3**. The results demonstrated a significant decrease in the concentration of ΔHbO in left PFC (p = 0.016) and in the right PFC (p = 0.032) after random thinking session during stroop color word task, whereas, there was a significant improvement in ΔHbO in left PFC (p = 0.006) and right PFC (p = 0.046) following the meditation session.

From the above observations, it can be concluded that meditation enhances bilaterally activation of the anterior PFC

Table 2 | Group mean values ± S.D. of the reaction time scores (ms) of Stroop color word Task.

Sessions	States	Pre	Post	*t*-value	*P* value	% Change
Rand	Neutral	643.18 ± 130.654	660.00 ± 113.641	−2.274	**0.034***	2.62
	Congruent	783.64 ± 117.333	790.91 ± 119.440	−0.876	0.391	0.93
	Incongruent	871.41 ± 136.070	892.73 ± 136.004	−2.920	**0.008****	2.45
Med	Neutral	638.64 ± 118.615	617.73 ± 121.653	3.533	**0.002****	−3.27
	Congruent	794.55 ± 118.029	764.55 ± 112.238	6.205	**<0.001*****	−3.78
	Incongruent	865.00 ± 137.797	819.09 ± 133.627	3.302	**0.003****	−5.31

**p < 0.05; p < **0.01; ***p < 0.001; repeated measures of ANOVA with Bonferroni adjustment comparing Post values with Pre values. Values are group means ± S.D. Rand—Random Thinking; Med—Meditation.*

Table 3 | Group mean values ± S.D. of the oxyhemoglobin (ΔHbO), deoxyhemoglobin (ΔHbR) and total hemoglobin change (ΔTHC) of Stroop color word task before, during and after random thinking (rand) and meditation (Med).

Sessions	Voxels	Pre	Stroop_Pre	During				Stroop_Post	Post
				D1	D2	D3	D4		
				Oxyhemoglobin (ΔHbO)					
Rand	**Left PFC**	−0.71 ± 3.71	−0.64 ± 7.39	0.51 ± 7.58	0.15 ± 6.69	0.25 ± 7.16	0.21 ± 7.61	0.83 ± 7.41	0.80 ± 7.22
	Right PFC	−2.65 ± 5.56	0.81 ± 4.59	−2.21 ± 12.47	−1.30 ± 12.45	−1.69 ± 12.67	−1.65 ± 12.49	−1.56 ± 11.90	−1.00 ± 10.02
Med	**Left PFC**	−0.43 ± 6.53	−0.93 ± 2.55	−1.13 ± 3.17	−0.79 ± 3.22	−0.64 ± 3.54	−0.77 ± 3.98	−0.09 ± 5.15	0.44 ± 5.25
	Right PFC	−2.45 ± 7.18	−1.30 ± 2.64	**−0.71 ± 4.07***	**−0.44 ± 3.84***	**−0.19 ± 3.86****	−0.89 ± 3.70	−0.79 ± 3.89	**0.35 ± 4.41*****
				Deoxyhemoglobin (ΔHbR)					
Rand	**Left PFC**	−0.20 ± 15.36	−1.70 ± 4.23	−2.03 ± 5.27	−0.98 ± 5.94	−0.73 ± 6.45	−0.73 ± 6.57	−0.32 ± 8.80	−0.91 ± 8.10
	Right PFC	−5.18 ± 10.80	−2.86 ± 3.65	−3.22 ± 6.89	**−1.78 ± 5.75*****	**−0.48 ± 8.08*****	**0.01 ± 8.05*****	**1.22 ± 8.18*****	**0.19 ± 10.25*****
Med	**Left PFC**	−1.57 ± 6.61	−1.27 ± 8.85	−2.82 ± 18.20	−2.25 ± 18.82	−2.38 ± 19.15	−2.29 ± 18.82	−2.28 ± 19.80	−2.23 ± 17.63
	Right PFC	−3.90 ± 8.22	−3.00 ± 7.93	−7.19 ± 23.46	−8.16 ± 23.09	−8.14 ± 23.43	**−8.15 ± 22.72***	−7.28 ± 23.56	−7.04 ± 19.93
				Total hemoglobin change (ΔTHC)					
Rand	**Left PFC**	−1.70 ± 5.39	−1.83 ± 9.87	−1.58 ± 20.98	−1.39 ± 21.02	−1.73 ± 21.40	−1.66 ± 21.16	−1.71 ± 21.56	−1.02 ± 19.70
	Right PFC	−4.29 ± 6.67	−3.28 ± 9.05	−8.85 ± 28.49	**−9.07 ± 27.55***	**−10.41 ± 26.99*****	**−10.28 ± 26.52*****	**−10.26 ± 26.89****	**−8.41 ± 21.55****
Med	**Left PFC**	−0.78 ± 17.63	−2.98 ± 7.98	−3.50 ± 9.7	−2.18 ± 10.23	−1.82 ± 10.74	−1.98 ± 11.34	−1.21 ± 14.27	−1.15 ± 13.88
	Right PFC	−5.11 ± 11.97	−4.36 ± 5.29	−4.37 ± 7.48	**−2.83 ± 7.18****	**−1.94 ± 8.48*****	**−2.16 ± 9.14****	**−1.45 ± 10.11****	**−0.57 ± 11.07*****

$^{**}p < 0.01$; repeated measures of ANOVA with Bonferroni adjustment comparing During and Post values with Pre values. Values are group means ± S.D.

and consequently, a stronger increase of oxygenation and cerebral blood flow during stroop task at the right PFC due to interference reduction.

HEMODYNAMICS RESPONSES IN MEDITATION AND RANDOM THINKING

For ΔHbO, the repeated—measures ANOVA for Sessions (Random thinking and Meditation) × PFC (Left and Right) × States (Pre Stroop_Pre, D1-D4, Stroop_Post, Post) demonstrated a significant main effects for States ($F_{(7,1225)} = 5.23$, $p < 0.001$, $\eta^2 p = 0.029$). There was a significant interaction between the PFC × States ($F_{(7,1225)} = 2.42$, $p < 0.001$, $\eta^2 p = 0.014$); Sessions × Hemispheres × States ($F_{(7,1225)} = 7.32$, $p < 0.05$, $\eta^2 p = 0.040$).

For ΔHbO, the repeated—measures ANOVA showed there was a significant main effect for Sessions ($F_{(1,175)} = 12.20$, $p < 0.001$, $\eta^2 p = 0.065$); PFC ($F_{(1,175)} = 7.89$, $p < 0.01$, $\eta^2 p = 0.043$) and States ($F_{(7,1225)} = 3.55$, $p < 0.001$, $\eta^2 p = 0.019$). There was a significant interaction between the Sessions × PFC ($F_{(1,175)} = 4.13$, $p < 0.001$, $\eta^2 p = 0.023$); Sessions × States ($F_{(7,1225)} = 9.99$, $p < 0.001$, $\eta^2 p = 0.054$); Sessions × PFC × States ($F_{(7,1225)} = 10.37$, $p < 0.001$, $\eta^2 p = 0.056$).

For total hemoglobin change (ΔTHC), there was a significant main effect for Sessions ($F_{(1,175)} = 5.07$, $p < 0.05$, $\eta^2 p = 0.028$); PFC ($F_{(1,175)} = 12.20$, $p < 0.001$, $\eta^2 p = 0.065$); and States ($F_{(1,175)} = 2.79$, $p < 0.01$, $\eta^2 p = 0.016$) and a significant interaction between the Sessions × PFC ($F_{(1,175)} = 6.45$, $p < 0.05$, $\eta^2 p = 0.036$); Sessions × States ($F_{(7,1225)} = 9.06$, $p < 0.001$, $\eta^2 p = 0.049$); PFC × States ($F_{(7,1225)} = 2.34$, $p < 0.05$, $\eta^2 p = 0.036$]; Session × PFC × State ($F_{(7,1225)} = 14.51$, $p < 0.001$).

Post hoc analyses with Bonferroni corrections were performed on ΔHbO, ΔHbR and ΔTHC and all comparisons were made with respective "Pre" state. These have been summarized in **Table 3**. There was a significant increase in ΔHbR at the right PFC ($p = 0.005$) after random thinking session whereas there was a significant increase in the left PFC ($p = 0.02$) and in right PFC ($p < 0.001$) after meditation session. Similarly, in ΔTHC, there was a significant decrease in blood flow change in the right PFC ($p < 0.001$) after the random thinking session whereas there was a significant increase in blood flow change in the left ($p = 0.03$) and in right PFC ($p < 0.001$) after meditation session.

In summary, as described in **Table 3** and in Line diagrams (**Figures 5–7**), there was a positive trend to show a significant increase in the concentration of oxyhemoglobin change (ΔHbO) during meditation session at right PFC (as shown in **Figure 5**). There was a significant decrease in deoxyhemoglobin change (ΔHbR) (as shown in **Figure 6**) during meditation session whereas there was a significant increase in the concentration of deoxyhemoglobin change during random thinking session at the right PFC. Additionally, there was also a significant increase in the total hemoglobin change (ΔTHC) during and after meditation sessions (**Figure 7**) and decrease in the total hemoglobin change (ΔTHC) during and after random thinking session.

DISCUSSION

The primary goal of the present study was to ascertain whether meditation increases rCBF at bilateral PFC, measured with fNIRS, compared to random thinking. Our secondary goal was to observe the RT scores and relative changes in cerebral blood flow, and to determine if there are persistent effects following meditation session compared to random thinking session. Results as confirmed with recent studies on meditation with spectroscopy (Cheng et al., 2010), SPECT imaging (Newberg et al., 2001, 2010a,b; Cohen et al., 2009) and fMRI (Short et al., 2010; Guleria et al., 2013; Zeidan et al., 2014) have revealed that meditation program resulted in significant increases in baseline CBF ratios in the prefrontal, superior, inferior and orbital frontal cortex, dorsolateral prefrontal cortex (DLPFC), right dorsal medial frontal lobe, cingulate gyrus and right sensorimotor cortex. In present study, we found that brain activation, measured by changes in ΔHbO and ΔTHC concentration in the right prefrontal area was followed by a strong decrease in ΔHbR concentration during meditation. Additionally, the rCBF significantly increased in the right frontal lobe during stroop task after meditation, which suggest the improvement in the participant's performance (reaction time) during the task. The total blood oxygenation (ΔTHC) level in the PFC could rise with increasing task load from neutral to congruent, and then incongruent; this would demonstrate a positive correlation with performance measures. The changes in regional blood flow is mediated by changes in neural activity in a single region or in several selective regions of the brain (Lauritzen, 2001).

Earlier studies have demonstrated that the PFC is activated particularly on the right PFC and anterior cingulate cortex (ACC) in willful act and tasks that require intense focused and sustained attention (Frith et al., 1991; Pardo et al., 1991; Vogt et al., 1992; Petersen and Posner, 2012). A study on eight Tibetan Buddhist meditators demonstrated improved activity in the PFC bilaterally (though greater on the right hemisphere) and the cingulate gyrus during meditation (Newberg and Iversen, 2003). This suggests that meditation begins with activation of the PFC and anterior cingulate gyrus associated with the will or intent to clear the mind of thoughts or to focus on an object (Edwards et al., 2012).

Meditation increases CBF and decreases cerebrovascular resistance (CVR) suggesting a contributing vascular mechanism (Jevning et al., 1996) which reflect cerebral activation. The CVR reduction being associated with cognitive improvement which suggests a vascular contribution to cognitive enhancement (Nation et al., 2013). During meditation, the activation of right PFC is theoretically associated with the activity in the reticular nucleus of the thalamus. This activation may be accomplished by the PFC's production and distribution of glutamate, a known excitatory neurotransmission (Cheramy et al., 1987; Finkbeiner, 1987), which communicate with other brain structures such as lateral geniculate and lateral posterior nuclei of the thalamus (Portas et al., 1998). An early study on meditation with single photon emission computed tomography (SPECT) demonstrated a general increase in thalamic activity that was proportional to the activity levels in the PFC (Newberg et al., 2001; Edwards et al., 2012). The activation on the right PFC causes increased activity in the reticular nucleus during meditation, the results may be decreased sensory input entering into the posterior superior parietal lobule which is involved in the analysis and integration of higher order visual, auditory, and somesthetic information (Adair et al., 1995).

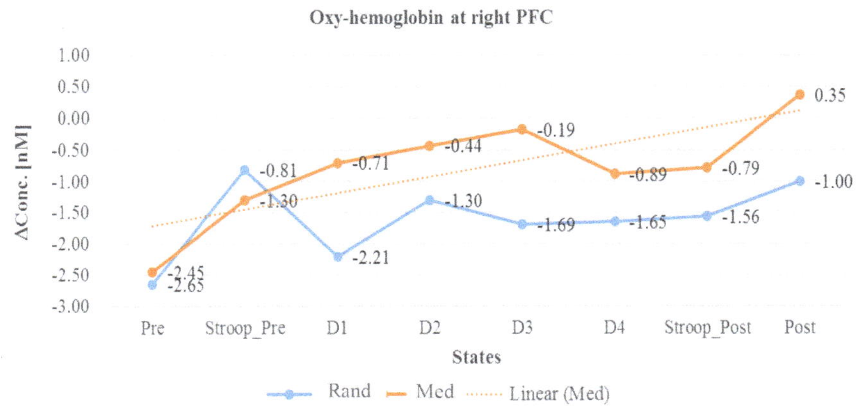

FIGURE 5 | Line graph represents averaged Oxy-hemoglobin change at right prefrontal cortex (rPFC) in two sessions i.e., random thinking and meditation and Stroop task. Note: Line graph represents comparisons between baseline, stroop_pre, during sessions (random thinking and meditation), stroop_post, and post. Stroop Pre showed higher Oxy-hemoglobin change compared to baseline. During and after meditation, the cerebral oxygenation was higher in rPFC compared to random thinking.

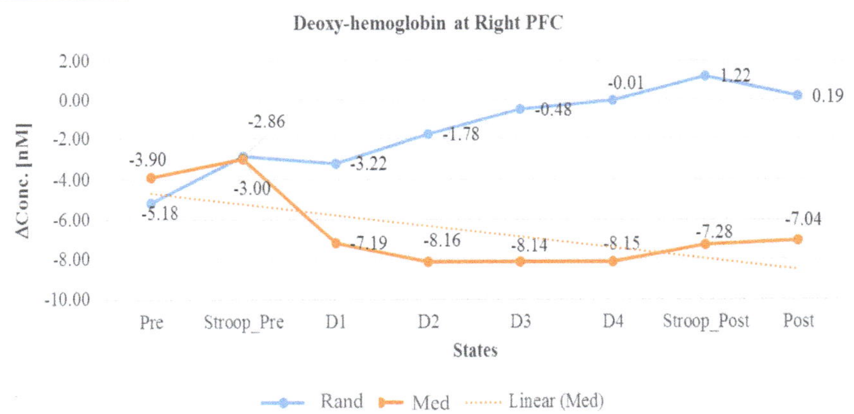

FIGURE 6 | Line graph represents averaged Deoxy-hemoglobin change at right PFC in two sessions i.e., random thinking and meditation and Stroop task. Note: Line graph represents de-oxyhemoglobin changes was higher in right PFC during random thinking (D2, D3, and D4), stroop task and after random thinking. In other hand, during meditation, there was a decrease in de-oxyhemoglobin in D3 level in rPFC.

A major strength of the present study was to examine the states of meditation and random thinking related hemodynamic responses in cerebral oxygenation during performance of the stroop color word task. It is a well established phenomenon that executive processes are facilitated by the frontal lobe and due to stroop interference brain activity may depend on increased ability to recruit frontal neural resources (Schroeter et al., 2004b). This allowed us to examine whether there is an increase in oxygenation with meditation corresponding to an ability to recruit appropriate resources for task performance or a decrease in activation corresponding to better optimization and possible reduction in task difficulty with meditation. In a study, fNIRS showed stroop interference is consistently associated with the ACC and the lateral prefrontal cortex (LPFC), especially the DLPFC, where the ACC is considered to be susceptible to conflict, and the DLPFC is purported to implement cognitive control (Carter et al., 2000; Leung et al., 2000). DLPFC may involve attentional maintenance while ACC monitors performance (MacDonald et al., 2000). Another similar study suggested meditation may enhance specific subcomponents of attention such as conflict monitoring or performance (Jha et al., 2007). Although fNIRS cannot monitor the cortical activation in the ACC because its measurement is limited to lateral cortical surfaces, it has successfully monitored the activation of the LPFC associated with stroop interference (Schroeter et al., 2002, 2003, 2004a,b; Ehlis et al., 2005).

There have been several neuroimaging studies evaluating the cerebral blood flow and performance of different meditation practices using behavioral, EEG and (Carter et al., 2005) fMRI imaging. Previous studies on meditation and EEG reported, greater midline theta power and slow alpha power in the frontal area during meditation (Takahashi et al., 2005; Chan

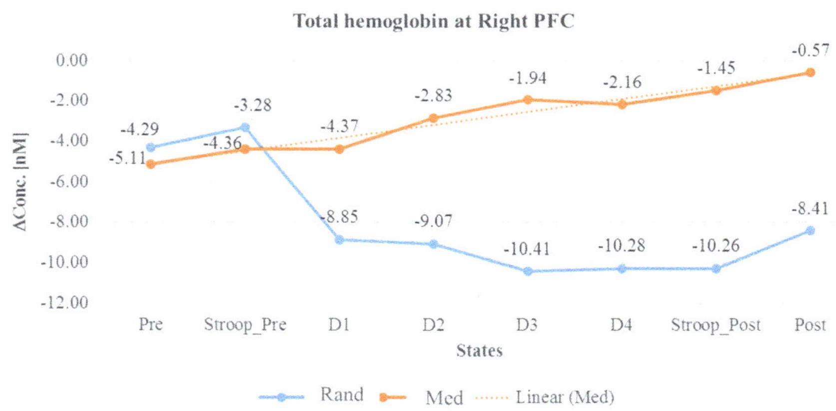

FIGURE 7 | Line graph represents averaged total hemoglobin change at rPFC in two sessions i.e., random thinking and meditation and Stroop task. Note: Line graph represents total hemoglobin change was higher in rPFC during meditation (D2, D3, and D4), in stroop task, and in post session. In other hand, there was a decrease in rPFC during random thinking (D2, D3, and D4), in stroop task and in post session.

et al., 2008). Zazen meditation showed increased alpha-1 and alpha-2 frequency activity of EEG in right prefrontal areas including insula, parts of the somatosensory, motor cortices and temporal areas (Faber et al., 2014). A subsequent study, on Satyananda Yoga meditation practice, showed greater source activity in low frequencies (particularly theta and alpha 1) during mental calculation, body-steadiness and mantra meditation (Thomas et al., 2014). Additionally, body-steadiness and mantra meditation showed greatest activity in right side of superior frontal and precentral gyri, parietal and occipital lobes. Similarly, neuroimaging studies on meditation practice, when compared to the control session showed significantly increased oxy-hemoglobin and CBF in the medial PFC which was associated with the intense focus-based component of the practice (Wang et al., 2011). Meditation involves attentional regulation and leads to increased activity in brain regions associated with attention such as DLPFC and ACC. The long-term practitioners had significantly more consistent and sustained activation in the DLPFC and the ACC during meditation vs. control in comparison to short-term practitioners (Baron Short et al., 2010). These studies suggest that willful acts and tasks that require sustained attention are initiated via activity in the PFC, particularly in the right hemisphere (Posner and Petersen, 1990; Frith et al., 1991; Pardo et al., 1991; Ingvar, 1994). Meditation requires focus of attention on objects which thereby activates PFC, particularly in the right hemisphere (Cohen et al., 2009), as well as the cingulate gyrus (Herzog et al., 1990; Lazar et al., 2000; Newberg et al., 2001). This demonstrated that during meditation there was an increased activity in the PFC bilaterally (greater on the right) and the cingulate gyrus (Newberg and Iversen, 2003). Therefore, the process of meditation seems to happen by activation of the prefrontal and cingulate cortex which are associated with the will or intent to clear one's mind of thoughts or to focus on an object.

In other imaging studies on meditation, there have been inconsistent results regarding the frontal cortex. A recent study showed decreased frontal activity during externally guided word generation compared to internal or volitional word generation (Cross et al., 2012). Thus, prefrontal and cingulate activation may be associated with the volitional aspects of meditation. Meditation with fluorodeoxyglucose (FDG) PET in eight subjects undergoing Yoga meditative relaxation (Herzog et al., 1990) reported increased rCBF in the frontal: occipital ratio of cerebral metabolism. Specifically, there was a mild increase in the frontal lobe, but marked decreases in metabolism in the occipital and superior parietal lobes. In addition to these studies, the PFC is reported to have a crucial role in social cognitive skills and along with the cingulate gyrus governs social behavior tasks related to Theory of Mind, empathy, moral reasoning, and evaluation of emotional states (Declerck et al., 2006). The PFC is essential for flexible behavior because it inhibits the habitual responses that have become inappropriate (Mesulam, 1998). But, an increase in the activity of PFC (determined by fNIRS) is not necessarily beneficial always. For example, animal experimentation has shown that the electrical activation of the medial PFC prevent the proper sequence of pressing the lever and collecting the reward (a pellet of food) in an operant condition task (Cross et al., 2012; Jurado-Parras et al., 2012) and also prevent the expression of an already acquired classically conditioned eyelid response (Leal-Campanario et al., 2007, 2013). However, in our study we infer that activation of prefrontal cortices after meditation had beneficial effects on cognition as manifested by improved performance in stroop color word task.

The present study reported increased oxy-hemoglobin concentration because of enhanced neural activity and cerebral blood flow in the prefrontal area during meditation compared to random thinking. In such studies, it is very important to understand the influences of systemic artifacts such as those from the heart, breathing, superficial perfusion, etc., which may be induced by the cognitive tasks related stress and autonomic responses. For example, a recent study performed on peripheral physiological measurements with temporal correlations of fNIRS and fMRI signals concluded that the physiological basis of the systemic artifact is a task-evoked sympathetic arterial vasoconstriction monitored by a decrease in venous volume and these artifacts are fairly common (Kirilina et al., 2012). They also suggested that the separation of fNIRS signals originating from activated brain and from scalp is a necessary precondition for unbiased fNIRS brain activation maps and pre-processing of the raw data using high definition filters is necessary.

In summary, the results of the present study provided first evidence that the oxygenation levels are increased in the PFC during meditation compared with random thinking in the same practitioners. Further event-related NIRS studies may apply well-tested fMRI paradigms in studies with children and patients, utilizing the advantages of the method.

ACKNOWLEDGMENTS

This research work was supported by the Center for Advanced Research in Yoga and Neurophysiology, Swami Vivekananda Yoga Research Foundation, Bangalore, India. We are gateful to Dr. Shirley Telles, Dr. Manjunath N.K. and Dr. Hemant Bhargav for their support and guidelines with regards to data acquisition and analysis.

REFERENCES

Adair, J. C., Gilmore, R. L., Fennell, E. B., Gold, M., and Heilman, K. M. (1995). Anosognosia during intracarotid barbiturate anesthesia: unawareness or amnesia for weakness. *Neurology* 45, 241–243. doi: 10.1212/wnl.45.2.241

Addicott, M. A., Yang, L. L., Peiffer, A. M., Burnett, L. R., Burdette, J. H., Chen, M. Y., et al. (2009). The effect of daily caffeine use on cerebral blood flow: how much caffeine can we tolerate? *Hum. Brain Mapp.* 30, 3102–3114. doi: 10.1002/hbm.20732

Baron Short, E., Kose, S., Mu, Q., Borckardt, J., Newberg, A., George, M. S., et al. (2010). Regional brain activation during meditation shows time and practice effects: an exploratory FMRI study. *Evid. Based Complement. Alternat. Med.* 7, 121–127. doi: 10.1093/ecam/nem163

Brackley, K. J., Ramsay, M. M., Broughton Pipkin, F., and Rubin, P. C. (1999). The effect of the menstrual cycle on human cerebral blood flow: studies using Doppler ultrasound. *Ultrasound Obstet. Gynecol.* 14, 52–57. doi: 10.1046/j.1469-0705.1999.14010052.x

Bunce, S., Izzetoglu, M., Izzetoglu, K., Onaral, B., and Pourrezaei, K. (2006). Functional near infrared spectroscopy: an emerging neuroimaging modality. *IEEE Eng. Med. Biol. Mag. Spec. Issue Clin. Neuroengineering* 25, 54–62. doi: 10.1109/MEMB.2006.1657788

Cahn, B. R., and Polich, J. (2006). Meditation states and traits: EEG, ERP and neuroimaging studies. *Psychol. Bull.* 132, 180–211. doi: 10.1037/0033-2909.132.2.180

Carter, C. S., Macdonald, A. M., Botvinick, M., Ross, L. L., Stenger, V. A., Noll, D., et al. (2000). Parsing executive processes: strategic vs. evaluative functions of the anterior cingulate cortex. *Proc. Natl. Acad. Sci. U S A* 97, 1944–1948. doi: 10.1073/pnas.97.4.1944

Carter, O. L., Presti, D. E., Callistemon, C., Ungerer, Y., Liu, G. B., and Pettigrew, J. D. (2005). Meditation alters perceptual rivalry in Tibetan Buddhist monks. *Curr. Biol.* 15, R412–R413. doi: 10.1016/j.cub.2005.05.043

Chan, A. S., Han, Y. M. Y., and Cheung, M.-C. (2008). Electroencephalographic (EEG) measurements of mindfulness-based Triarchic body-pathway relaxation technique: a pilot study. *Appl. Psychophysiol. Biofeedback* 33, 39–47. doi: 10.1007/s10484-008-9050-5

Chan, D., and Woollacott, M. (2007). Effects of level of meditation experience on attentional focus: is the efficiency of executive or orientation networks improved? *J. Altern. Complement. Med.* 13, 651–657. doi: 10.1089/acm.2007.7022

Cheng, R. W. F., Borrett, D. S., Cheng, W., Kwan, H. C., and Cheng, R. S. S. (2010). Human prefrontal cortical response to the meditative state: a spectroscopy study. *Int. J. Neurosci.* 120, 483–488. doi: 10.3109/00207454.2010.483650

Cheramy, A., Romo, R., and Glowinski, J. (1987). "Role of corticostriatal glutamatergic neurons in the presynaptic control of dopamine release," in *Neurotransmitter Interactions in the Basal Ganglia*, eds M. Sandler, C. Feuerstein and B. Scatton (New York: Raven), 131–133.

Cohen, J. (1988). *Statistical Power Analysis for the Behavioral Sciences.* 2nd Edn. Hillsdale, NJ: Erlbaum.

Cohen, D. L., Wintering, N., Tolles, V., Townsend, R. R., Farrar, J. T., Galantino, M. L., et al. (2009). Cerebral blood flow effects of yoga training: preliminary evaluation of 4 cases. *J. Altern. Complement. Med.* 15, 9–14. doi: 10.1089/acm.2008.0008

Cross, L., Brown, M. W., Aggleton, J. P., and Warburton, E. C. (2012). The medial dorsal thalamic nucleus and the medial prefrontal cortex of the rat function together to support associative recognition and recency but not item recognition. *Learn. Mem.* 20, 41–50. doi: 10.1101/lm.028266.112

Cui, X., Bray, S., Bryant, D. M., Glover, G. H., and Reiss, A. L. (2011). A quantitative comparison of NIRS and fMRI across multiple cognitive tasks. *Neuroimage* 54, 2808–2821. doi: 10.1016/j.neuroimage.2010.10.069

Declerck, C. H., Boone, C., and De Brabander, B. (2006). On feeling in control: a biological theory for individual differences in control perception. *Brain Cogn.* 62, 143–176. doi: 10.1016/j.bandc.2006.04.004

Dor-Ziderman, Y., Berkovich-Ohana, A., Glicksohn, J., and Goldstein, A. (2013). Mindfulness-induced selflessness: a MEG neurophenomenological study. *Front. Hum. Neurosci.* 7:582. doi: 10.3389/fnhum.2013.00582

Edwards, J., Peres, J., Monti, D., and Newberg, A. (2012). "The neurobiological correlates of meditation and mindfulness," in *Exploring Frontiers of the Mind-Brain Relationship SE - 6 Mindfulness in Behavioral Health*, eds A. Moreira-Almeida and F. Santana Santos (New York: Springer), 97–112.

Ehlis, A.-C., Herrmann, M. J., Wagener, A., and Fallgatter, A. J. (2005). Multi-channel near-infrared spectroscopy detects specific inferior-frontal activation during incongruent Stroop trials. *Biol. Psychol.* 69, 315–331. doi: 10.1016/j.biopsycho.2004.09.003

Faber, P. L., Lehmann, D., Gianotti, L. R. R., Milz, P., Pascual-Marqui, R. D., Held, M., et al. (2014). Zazen meditation and no-task resting EEG compared with LORETA intracortical source localization. *Cogn. Process.* doi: 10.1007/s10339-014-0637-x. [Epub ahead of print].

Finkbeiner, S. M. (1987). Neurotransmitter interactions in the basal ganglia. *Yale J. Biol. Med.* 60:483.

Frith, C. D., Friston, K. J., Liddle, P. F., and Frackowiak, R. S. (1991). Willed action and the prefrontal cortex in man: a study with PET. *Proc. Biol. Sci.* 244, 241–246. doi: 10.1098/rspb.1991.0077

Goldstein, R. Z., and Volkow, N. D. (2011). Dysfunction of the prefrontal cortex in addiction: neuroimaging findings and clinical implications. *Nat. Rev. Neurosci.* 12, 652–669. doi: 10.1038/nrn3119

Guleria, A., Kumar, U., Kishan, S. S. K., and Khetrapal, C. L. (2013). Effect of "SOHAM" meditation on the human brain: an fMRI study. *Psychiatry Res.* 214, 462–465. doi: 10.1016/j.pscychresns.2013.06.012

Hebert, R., and Lehmann, D. (1977). Theta bursts: an EEG pattern in normal subjects practising the transcendental meditation technique. *Electroencephalogr. Clin. Neurophysiol.* 42, 397–405. doi: 10.1016/0013-4694(77)90176-6

Herzog, H., Lele, V. R., Kuwert, T., Langen, K. J., Rota Kops, E., and Feinendegen, L. E. (1990). Changed pattern of regional glucose metabolism during yoga meditative relaxation. *Neuropsychobiology* 23, 182–187. doi: 10.1159/000119450

Holzel, B. K., Lazar, S. W., Gard, T., Schuman-Olivier, Z., Vago, D. R., and Ott, U. (2011). How does mindfulness meditation work? Proposing mechanisms of action from a conceptual and neural perspective. *Perspect. Psychol. Sci.* 6, 537–559. doi: 10.1177/1745691611419671

Hoshi, Y., and Tamura, M. (1993). Dynamic multichannel near-infrared optical imaging of human brain activity. *J. Appl. Physiol. (1985)* 75, 1842–1846.

Ingvar, D. H. (1994). The will of the brain: cerebral correlates of willful acts. *J. Theor. Biol.* 171, 7–12. doi: 10.1006/jtbi.1994.1206

Izzetoglu, M., Izzetoglu, K., Bunce, S., Ayaz, H., Devaraj, A., Onaral, B., et al. (2005). Functional near-infrared neuroimaging. *IEEE Trans. Neural Syst. Rehabil. Eng.* 13, 153–159. doi: 10.1109/TNSRE.2005.847377

Jevning, R., Anand, R., Biedebach, M., and Fernando, G. (1996). Effects on regional cerebral blood flow of transcendental meditation. *Physiol. Behav.* 59, 399–402. doi: 10.1016/0031-9384(95)02006-3

Jha, A. P., Krompinger, J., and Baime, M. J. (2007). Mindfulness training modifies subsystems of attention. *Cogn. Affect. Behav. Neurosci.* 7, 109–119. doi: 10.3758/cabn.7.2.109

Jurado-Parras, M. T., Gruart, A., and Delgado-García, J. M. (2012). Observational learning in mice can be prevented by medial prefrontal cortex stimulation and enhanced by nucleus accumbens stimulation. *Learn. Mem.* 19, 99–106. doi: 10.1101/lm.024760.111

Kim, M. N., Durduran, T., Frangos, S., Edlow, B. L., Buckley, E. M., Moss, H. E., et al. (2010). Noninvasive measurement of cerebral blood flow and blood oxygenation using near-infrared and diffuse correlation spectroscopies in critically brain-injured adults. *Neurocrit. Care* 12, 173–180. doi: 10.1007/s12028-009-9305-x

Kirilina, E., Jelzow, A., Heine, A., Niessing, M., Wabnitz, H., Brühl, R., et al. (2012). The physiological origin of task-evoked systemic artefacts in functional near infrared spectroscopy. *Neuroimage* 61, 70–81. doi: 10.1016/j.neuroimage.2012.02.074

Kozasa, E. H., Sato, J. R., Lacerda, S. S., Barreiros, M. A. M., Radvany, J., Russell, T. A., et al. (2012). Meditation training increases brain efficiency in an attention task. *Neuroimage* 59, 745–749. doi: 10.1016/j.neuroimage.2011.06.088

Krawczyk, D. C. (2002). Contributions of the prefrontal cortex to the neural basis of human decision making. *Neurosci. Biobehav. Rev.* 26, 631–664. doi: 10.1016/s0149-7634(02)00021-0

Kubota, Y., Sato, W., Toichi, M., Murai, T., Okada, T., Hayashi, A., et al. (2001). Frontal midline theta rhythm is correlated with cardiac autonomic activities during the performance of an attention demanding meditation procedure. *Brain Res. Cogn. Brain Res.* 11, 281–287. doi: 10.1016/s0926-6410(00)00086-0

Lauritzen, M. (2001). Relationship of spikes, synaptic activity and local changes of cerebral blood flow. *J. Cereb. Blood Flow Metab.* 21, 1367–1383. doi: 10.1097/00004647-200112000-00001

Lazar, S. W., Bush, G., Gollub, R. L., Fricchione, G. L., Khalsa, G., and Benson, H. (2000). Functional brain mapping of the relaxation response and meditation. *Neuroreport* 11, 1581–1585. doi: 10.1097/00001756-200005150-00041

Lazar, S. W., Kerr, C. E., Wasserman, R. H., Gray, J. R., Greve, D. N., Treadway, M. T., et al. (2005). Meditation experience is associated with increased cortical thickness. *Neuroreport* 28, 1893–1897. doi: 10.1097/01.wnr.0000186598.66243.19

Leal-Campanario, R., Delgado-García, J. M., and Gruart, A. (2013). The rostral medial prefrontal cortex regulates the expression of conditioned eyelid responses in behaving rabbits. *J. Neurosci.* 33, 4378–4386. doi: 10.1523/jneurosci.5560-12.2013

Leal-Campanario, R., Fairén, A., Delgado-García, J. M., and Gruart, A. (2007). Electrical stimulation of the rostral medial prefrontal cortex in rabbits inhibits the expression of conditioned eyelid responses but not their acquisition. *Proc. Natl. Acad. Sci. U S A* 104, 11459–11464. doi: 10.1073/pnas.0704548104

León-Carrion, J., Damas-López, J., Martín-Rodríguez, J. F., Domínguez-Roldán, J. M., Murillo-Cabezas, F., Barroso Y Martin, J. M., et al. (2008). The hemodynamics of cognitive control: the level of concentration of oxygenated hemoglobin in the superior prefrontal cortex varies as a function of performance in a modified Stroop task . *Behav. Brain Res.* 193, 248–256. doi: 10.1016/j.bbr.2008.06.013

Leon-Dominguez, U., Izzetoglu, M., Leon-Carrion, J., Solís-Marcos, I., Garcia-Torrado, F. J., Forastero-Rodríguez, A., et al. (2014). Molecular concentration of deoxyHb in human prefrontal cortex predicts the emergence and suppression of consciousness. *Neuroimage* 85(Pt. 1), 616–625. doi: 10.1016/j.neuroimage.2013.07.023

Leung, H. C., Skudlarski, P., Gatenby, J. C., Peterson, B. S., and Gore, J. C. (2000). An event-related functional MRI study of the stroop color word interference task. *Cereb. Cortex* 10, 552–560. doi: 10.1093/cercor/10.6.552

Liddle, P. F., Friston, K. J., Frith, C. D., Hirsch, S. R., Jones, T., and Frackowiak, R. S. (1992). Patterns of cerebral blood flow in schizophrenia. *Br. J. Psychiatry* 160, 179–186. doi: 10.1192/bjp.160.2.179

Lin, P. Y., Lin, S. I., Penney, T., and Chen, J. J. J. (2009). Review: applications of near infrared spectroscopy and imaging for motor rehabilitation in stroke patients. *Time* 29, 210–221.

Lutz, A., Slagter, H. A., Dunne, J. D., and Davidson, R. J. (2008). Attention regulation and monitoring in meditation. *Trends Cogn. Sci.* 12, 163–169. doi: 10.1016/j.tics.2008.01.005

Lutz, A., Slagter, H. A., Rawlings, N. B., Francis, A. D., Greischar, L. L., and Davidson, R. J. (2009). Mental training enhances attentional stability: neural and behavioral evidence. *J. Neurosci.* 29, 13418–13427. doi: 10.1523/jneurosci.1614-09.2009

MacDonald, A. W., Cohen, J. D., Stenger, V. A., and Carter, C. S. (2000). Dissociating the role of the dorsolateral prefrontal and anterior cingulate cortex in cognitive control. *Science* 288, 1835–1838. doi: 10.1126/science.288.5472.1835

MacLean, K. A., Ferrer, E., Aichele, S. R., Bridwell, D. A., Zanesco, A. P., Jacobs, T. L., et al. (2010). Intensive meditation training improves perceptual discrimination and sustained attention. *Psychol. Sci.* 21, 829–839. doi: 10.1177/0956797610371339

MacLeod, C. M. (1991). Half a century of research on the Stroop effect: an integrative review. *Psychol. Bull.* 109, 163–203. doi: 10.1037//0033-2909.109.2.163

Mesulam, M. (1998). From sensation to cognition. *Brain* 121, 1013–1052. doi: 10.1093/brain/121.6.1013

Minagawa-Kawai, Y., van der Lely, H., Ramus, F., Sato, Y., Mazuka, R., and Dupoux, E. (2011). Optical brain imaging reveals general auditory and language-specific processing in early infant development. *Cereb. Cortex* 21, 254–261. doi: 10.1093/cercor/bhq082

Moore, A., and Malinowski, P. (2009). Meditation, mindfulness and cognitive flexibility. *Conscious. Cogn.* 18, 176–186. doi: 10.1016/j.concog.2008.12.008

Morton, J., and Chambers, S. M. (1973). Selective attention to words and colours. *Q. J. Exp. Psychol.* 25, 387–397. doi: 10.1080/14640747308400360

Nation, D., Clark, L., Wierenga, C., Delano-Wood, L., Dev, S., Bangen, K., et al. (2013). Cerebrovascular resistance and cognitive decline: modulating effects of age. *Neurology* 80, P07.135.

Nehlig, A. (2010). Is caffeine a cognitive enhancer? *J. Alzheimers Dis.* 20(Suppl. 1), S85–S94. doi: 10.3233/JAD-2010-091315

Newberg, A., Alavi, A., Baime, M., Pourdehnad, M., Santanna, J., and d'Aquili, E. (2001). The measurement of regional cerebral blood flow during the complex cognitive task of meditation: a preliminary SPECT study. *Psychiatry Res.* 106, 113–122. doi: 10.1016/s0925-4927(01)00074-9

Newberg, A. B., and Iversen, J. (2003). The neural basis of the complex mental task of meditation: neurotransmitter and neurochemical considerations. *Med. Hypotheses* 61, 282–291. doi: 10.1016/s0306-9877(03)00175-0

Newberg, A. B., Wintering, N., Khalsa, D. S., Roggenkamp, H., and Waldman, M. R. (2010a). Meditation effects on cognitive function and cerebral blood flow in subjects with memory loss: a preliminary study. *J. Alzheimers Dis.* 20, 517–526. doi: 10.3233/JAD-2010-1391

Newberg, A. B., Wintering, N., Waldman, M. R., Amen, D., Khalsa, D. S., and Alavi, A. (2010b). Cerebral blood flow differences between long-term meditators and non-meditators. *Conscious. Cogn.* 19, 899–905. doi: 10.1016/j.concog.2010.05.003

Pardo, J. V., Fox, P. T., and Raichle, M. E. (1991). Localization of a human system for sustained attention by positron emission tomography. *Nature* 349, 61–64. doi: 10.1038/349061a0

Petersen, S. E., and Posner, M. I. (2012). The attention system of the human brain: 20 years after. *Annu. Rev. Neurosci.* 35, 73–89. doi: 10.1146/annurev-neuro-062111-150525

Peterson, B. S., Skudlarski, P., Gatenby, J. C., Zhang, H., Anderson, A. W., and Gore, J. C. (1999). An fMRI study of Stroop word-color interference: evidence for cingulate subregions subserving multiple distributed attentional systems. *Biol. Psychiatry* 45, 1237–1258. doi: 10.1016/s0006-3223(99)00056-6

Plichta, M. M., Herrmann, M. J., Baehne, C. G., Ehlis, A.-C., Richter, M. M., Pauli, P., et al. (2006). Event-related functional near-infrared spectroscopy (fNIRS): are the measurements reliable? *Neuroimage* 31, 116–124. doi: 10.1016/j.neuroimage.2005.12.008

Portas, C. M., Rees, G., Howseman, A. M., Josephs, O., Turner, R., and Frith, C. D. (1998). A specific role for the thalamus in mediating the interaction of attention and arousal in humans. *J. Neurosci.* 18, 8979–8989.

Posner, M. I., and Petersen, S. E. (1990). The attention system of the human brain. *Annu. Rev. Neurosci.* 13, 25–42. doi: 10.1146/annurev.ne.13.030190.000325

Posner, M. I., and Snyder, C. R. R. (1975). "Attention and cognitive control," in *Information Processing and Cognition: The Loyola Symposium*, ed R. L. SolSo (Hillsdale, NJ: Erlbaum, Lawrence Associates, Inc), 55–85.

Saggar, M., King, B. G., Zanesco, A. P., Maclean, K. A., Aichele, S. R., Jacobs, T. L., et al. (2012). Intensive training induces longitudinal changes in meditation state-related EEG oscillatory activity. *Front Hum Neurosci* 6:256. doi: 10.3389/fnhum.2012.00256

Schroeter, M. L., Zysset, S., Kruggel, F., and von Cramon, D. Y. (2003). Age dependency of the hemodynamic response as measured by functional near-infrared spectroscopy. *Neuroimage* 19, 555–564. doi: 10.1016/s1053-8119(03)00155-1

Schroeter, M. L., Zysset, S., Kupka, T., Kruggel, F., and Yves von Cramon, D. (2002). Near-infrared spectroscopy can detect brain activity during a color-word matching Stroop task in an event-related design. *Hum. Brain Mapp.* 17, 61–71. doi: 10.1002/hbm.10052

Schroeter, M. L., Zysset, S., and Von Cramon, D. Y. (2004a). Shortening intertrial intervals in event-related cognitive studies with near-infrared spectroscopy. *Neuroimage* 22, 341–346. doi: 10.1016/j.neuroimage.2003.12.041

Schroeter, M. L., Zysset, S., Wahl, M., and von Cramon, D. Y. (2004b). Prefrontal activation due to Stroop interference increases during development—an event-related fNIRS study. *Neuroimage* 23, 1317–1325. doi: 10.1016/j.neuroimage.2004.08.001

Short, E. B., Kose, S., Mu, Q., Borckardt, J., Newberg, A., George, M. S., et al. (2010). Regional brain activation during meditation shows time and practice effects: an exploratory FMRI study. *Evid Based Complement. Altern. Med.* 7, 121–127. doi: 10.1093/ecam/nem163

Slagter, H. A., Davidson, R. J., and Lutz, A. (2011). Mental training as a tool in the neuroscientific study of brain and cognitive plasticity. *Front. Hum. Neurosci.* 5:17. doi: 10.3389/fnhum.2011.00017

Slagter, H. A., Lutz, A., Greischar, L. L., Nieuwenhuis, S., and Davidson, R. J. (2009). Theta phase synchrony and conscious target perception: impact of intensive mental training. *J. Cogn. Neurosci* 21, 1536–1549. doi: 10.1162/jocn.2009.21125

Son, I.-Y., and Yazici, B. (2006). Near infrared imaging and spectroscopy for brain activity monitoring. *Adv. Sens. with Secur. Appl.* 2, 341–372. doi: 10.1007/1-4020-4295-7_15

Szűcs, D., Killikelly, C., and Cutini, S. (2012). Event-related near-infrared spectroscopy detects conflict in the motor cortex in a Stroop task. *Brain Res.* 1477, 27–36. doi: 10.1016/j.brainres.2012.08.023

Taga, G., Asakawa, K., Maki, A., Konishi, Y., and Koizumi, H. (2003). Brain imaging in awake infants by near-infrared optical topography. *Proc. Natl. Acad. Sci. U S A* 100, 10722–10727. doi: 10.1073/pnas.1932552100

Takahashi, T., Murata, T., Hamada, T., Omori, M., Kosaka, H., Kikuchi, M., et al. (2005). Changes in EEG and autonomic nervous activity during meditation and their association with personality traits. *Int. J. Psychophysiol.* 55, 199–207. doi: 10.1016/j.ijpsycho.2004.07.004

Tang, Y.-Y., Ma, Y., Wang, J., Fan, Y., Feng, S., Lu, Q., et al. (2007). Short-term meditation training improves attention and self-regulation. *Proc. Natl. Acad. Sci. U S A* 104, 17152–17156. doi: 10.1073/pnas.0707678104

Telles, S., Deepeshwar, S., Naveen, K. V., and Pailoor, S. (2014). Long latency auditory evoked potentials during meditation. *Clin. EEG Neurosci.* doi: 10.1177/1550059414544737. [Epub ahead of print].

Telles, S., Raghavendra, B. R., Naveen, K. V., Manjunath, N. K., and Subramanya, P. (2012). Mid-latency auditory evoked potentials in 2 meditative states. *Clin. EEG Neurosci.* 43, 154–160. doi: 10.1177/1550059412439963

Thomas, J., Jamieson, G., and Cohen, M. (2014). Low and then high frequency oscillations of distinct right cortical networks are progressively enhanced by medium and long term Satyananda Yoga meditation practice. *Front. Hum. Neurosci.* 8:197. doi: 10.3389/fnhum.2014.00197

Tian, F., Chance, B., and Liu, H. (2009). Investigation of the prefrontal cortex in response to duration-variable anagram tasks using functional near-infrared spectroscopy. *J. Biomed. Opt.* 14:054016. doi: 10.1117/1.3241984

van Leeuwen, S., Müller, N. G., and Melloni, L. (2009). Age effects on attentional blink performance in meditation. *Conscious. Cogn.* 18, 593–599. doi: 10.1016/j.concog.2009.05.001

van Vugt, M. K., and Jha, A. P. (2011). Investigating the impact of mindfulness meditation training on working memory: a mathematical modeling approach. *Cogn. Affect. Behav. Neurosci.* 11, 344–353. doi: 10.3758/s13415-011-0048-8

Vogt, B. A., Finch, D. M., and Olson, C. R. (1992). Functional heterogeneity in cingulate cortex: the anterior executive and posterior evaluative regions. *Cereb. Cortex* 2, 435–443. doi: 10.1093/cercor/2.6.435-a

Wang, D. J. J., Rao, H., Korczykowski, M., Wintering, N., Pluta, J., Khalsa, D. S., et al. (2011). Cerebral blood flow changes associated with different meditation practices and perceived depth of meditation. *Psychiatry Res.* 191, 60–67. doi: 10.1016/j.pscychresns.2010.09.011

Yadav, A., Tandon, O. P., and Vaney, N. (2002). Auditory evoked responses during different phases of menstrual cycle. *Indian J. Physiol. Pharmacol.* 46, 449–456.

Zeidan, F., Johnson, S. K., Diamond, B. J., David, Z., and Goolkasian, P. (2010). Mindfulness meditation improves cognition: evidence of brief mental training. *Conscious. Cogn.* 19, 597–605. doi: 10.1016/j.concog.2010.03.014

Zeidan, F., Martucci, K. T., Kraft, R. A., McHaffie, J. G., and Coghill, R. C. (2014). Neural correlates of mindfulness meditation-related anxiety relief. *Soc. Cogn. Affect. Neurosci.* 9, 751–759. doi: 10.1093/scan/nst041

Zysset, S., Schroeter, M. L., Neumann, J., and von Cramon, D. Y. (2007). Stroop interference, hemodynamic response and aging: an event-related fMRI study. *Neurobiol. Aging* 28, 937–946. doi: 10.1016/j.neurobiolaging.2006.05.008

3

Transcranial direct current stimulation: five important issues we aren't discussing (but probably should be)

Jared C. Horvath*, Olivia Carter and Jason D. Forte

Psychological Sciences, University of Melbourne, Melbourne, VIC, Australia

Edited by:
Mikhail Lebedev, Duke University, USA

Reviewed by:
Carmelo M. Vicario, University of Queensland, Australia
Nick J. Davis, Swansea University, UK

****Correspondence:***
Jared C. Horvath, Psychological Sciences, University of Melbourne, Redmond Barry Bldg. 613, Melbourne, VIC 3010, Australia
e-mail: jch155@mail.harvard.edu

Transcranial Direct Current Stimulation (tDCS) is a neuromodulatory device often publicized for its ability to enhance cognitive and behavioral performance. These enhancement claims, however, are predicated upon electrophysiological evidence and descriptions which are far from conclusive. In fact, a review of the literature reveals a number of important experimental and technical issues inherent with this device that are simply not being discussed in any meaningful manner. In this paper, we will consider five of these topics. The first, *inter-subject variability*, explores the extensive between- and within-group differences found within the tDCS literature and highlights the need to properly examine stimulatory response at the individual level. The second, *intra-subject reliability*, reviews the lack of data concerning tDCS response reliability over time and emphasizes the importance of this knowledge for appropriate stimulatory application. The third, *sham stimulation and blinding*, draws attention to the importance (yet relative lack) of proper control and blinding practices in the tDCS literature. The fourth, *motor and cognitive interference*, highlights the often overlooked body of research that suggests typical behaviors and cognitions undertaken during or following tDCS can impair or abolish the effects of stimulation. Finally, the fifth, *electric current influences*, underscores several largely ignored variables (such as hair thickness and electrode attachments methods) influential to tDCS electric current density and flow. Through this paper, we hope to increase awareness and start an ongoing dialog of these important issues which speak to the efficacy, reliability, and mechanistic foundations of tDCS.

Keywords: transcranial direct current stimulation (tDCS), variability, reliability, efficacy, mechanisms of action

INTRODUCTION

Transcranial direct current stimulation (tDCS) is currently being promoted as a cheap and effective tool to enhance cognitive and behavioral function. A recent surge of public interest in this device (evidenced by several tDCS devices appearing on the public market) has doubtless been driven by the belief that these enhancement claims are robust, reliable, and well elucidated. However, the research exploring the efficacy of tDCS is far from conclusive.

It's commonly assumed that tDCS shifts the resting membrane potential and synaptic strength of neurons in a predictable and consistent manner. More specifically, hypo-polarization of neurons under the anodal electrode is believed to increase the likelihood of their firing, whilst hyper-polarization of neurons under the cathodal electrode is believed to decrease the likelihood of their firing [for an in depth mechanistic overview, see, Stagg and Nitsche (2011)]. Similar to efficacy, however, a close inspection of the literature reveals short-comings of the anode excite/cathode inhibit model.

In response to efficacy and mechanistic uncertainties, many practitioners focus on the manipulation of three adjustable tDCS parameters: current density, electrode position, and stimulation duration. Whereas these three variables certainly play a large role in tDCS outcomes, there are a number of equally important issues relevant to both efficacy and mechanism that simply are not being discussed in any meaningful manner.

In this paper, we will explore five notable indicators and/or sources of inconsistency associated with the use of tDCS in the current literature: inter-subject variability, intra-subject reliability, lack of effective sham and blinding protocols, motor and cognitive interference, and electric current influences. Throughout this piece, we will draw examples solely from studies which explore the effects of tDCS over the motor cortex on MEP amplitude in healthy populations. We have chosen to do this for two reasons: first, MEP amplitude modulation is easily the most explored and reliably demonstrated outcome measure in the tDCS in the literature. Second, as the majority of neurophysiologic, clinical, and behavioral claims cite this work as mechanistically foundational, any issues apparent in this literature will necessarily be applicable to and concern any other outcome measure utilized.

INTER-SUBJECT VARIABILITY

tDCS must demonstrate similar (or comparable) effects across a range of people before it can be meaningfully applied in healthy and/or clinical populations. However, a survey of the literature reveals extensive between- and within-group variation suggestive of an inconsistent effect between individuals.

As an example of large between-group variation, Fricke et al. (2011) recently reported data from two different groups that underwent an identical stimulation protocol (0.0286 mA/cm^2 current density; anode M1/cathode contralateral orbit montage; 5 min duration). Whereas one group demonstrated an average MEP amplitude enhancement of 93.2% in the 5 min following tDCS, the second group demonstrated an average MEP amplitude enhancement of only 9.2%: a between-group difference of 913%. Similarly, in two different studies from 2004 using identical stimulation protocols (0.0286 mA/cm^2 current density; cathode M1/anode contralateral orbit montage; 9 min duration), Nitsche et al. reported 30 min group MEP amplitude inhibitions of 42.9% (Nitsche et al., 2004a) and 20.0% (Nitsche et al., 2004b): a difference of 110%. Even more variable, these researchers has reported group MEP amplitude enhancements following identical stimulation protocols (0.0286 mA/cm^2 current density; anode M1/cathode contralateral orbit montage; 13 min duration) ranging from 54.4% (Nitsche et al., 2003a) to 19.3% (Nitsche et al., 2009); a difference of 184%.

Specific examples of within-group variability (beyond common deviation and/or error measures) are harder to come by as very few studies include individual data with their reports. However, of the few that have, the results are illuminating. For instance, following 9 min of anodal stimulation (0.0286 mA/cm^2 current density; M1/contralateral orbit montage), Nitsche and Paulus (2001) reported one subject who demonstrated an incredible 295% increase in MEP amplitude and a second who demonstrated a weak 5% increase. More recently, following 20 min of anodal stimulation (0.06 mA/cm^2 current density; M1/Contralateral orbit montage), Tremblay et al. (2013) reported one subject who demonstrated a 251% increase in MEP amplitude and a second who demonstrated a 41% *decrease* (see also, Roche et al., 2011).

One potential explanation for this extreme between- and within-group variability is the difficulty in properly and reliably targeting TMS pulses during lengthy protocols (Herwig et al., 2001; Sparing et al., 2008; Ahdab et al., 2010). Although modern MRI guided neuronavigation systems can be used to ensure accurate coil positioning across time, many tDCS studies have not utilized (or do not report utilizing) these systems. As such, it is possible subtle variation in coil placement and orientation with time may influence response variation.

A second potential explanation for this extreme between- and within-group variability is that tDCS generates differential response at the individual level which is masked by group averaging. An individual's unique neurophysiology, anatomy, and psychology may influence his/her response to tDCS. In fact, recent modeling work suggests parameters such as skull thickness, subcutaneous fat levels, cerebrospinal fluid density, and cortical surface topography can greatly influence current flow and density patterns during stimulation (Datta et al., 2012; Truong et al., 2013). As such, elucidation of individual and environmental influences on tDCS is necessary and may only be possible by looking at response characteristics (and related correlative factors) at the individual level.

INTRA-SUBJECT RELIABILITY

Beyond individual response patterns, it must be demonstrated that people respond in a similar and predictable manner to repeated sessions of tDCS before this tool can be meaningfully applied. Unfortunately, to our knowledge, response *reliability* at the level of the individual has not been explored (or, at least, reported) in the literature to date.

Of the (only) four studies which have explored group effects of tDCS on MEP amplitude in healthy populations across multiple days, two suggest response patterns may be reliable and replicable. Alonzo et al. (2012) explored the effects of anodal stimulation (0.0571 mA/cm^2 current density; M1/contralateral orbit montage; 20 min duration) on MEP amplitude over the course of 5 days (Monday–Friday). Although these researchers reported variable baseline levels across the week, the ratio of pre- to post-stimulation group average MEP amplitudes did not significantly change from day-to-day. Using a similar protocol, Gálvez et al. (2013) reported similar findings: namely, whereas baseline levels changed throughout the week, the group averaged after-effects of daily stimulation did not significantly vary across 5 days.

Interestingly, the remaining two studies to explore group effects of tDCS on MEP amplitude in healthy populations across multiple days suggest response patterns may be unreliable and unpredictable. Monte-Silva et al. have twice looked at the effects of two sessions of tDCS on MEP amplitude with a 24 h block between sessions (Monte-Silva et al., 2010, 2012). In the first study (0.0286 mA/cm^2 current density; cathodal M1/anodal contralateral orbit montage; 9 min duration), these researchers reported significantly reduced modulation of MEP amplitude following the second session of stimulation. More concerning, in the second study (0.0286 mA/cm^2 current density; anodal M1/cathodal contralateral orbit montage; 13 min duration) these researchers reported not only a significant reduction in MEP amplitude modulation following the second session of stimulation, but also a reverse in modulation direction (inhibition rather than excitation following anodal stimulation) and unpredictable timing effects.

Considerably more data investigating effects across time is required before concluding tDCS is a reliable device. As individual response reliability is explored, however, it will be important to remember that intra-subject variability may not, in itself, suggest tDCS is unreliable. It is likely that circadian, metabolic, and hormonal cycles will differentially impact response. In fact, several researchers have already shown that stages of the menstrual cycle and cortisol levels impact plastic response to varied TMS protocols (Smith et al., 1999; Inghilleri et al., 2004; Sale et al., 2008, 2010). In addition, proper and reliable TMS coil positioning during lengthy protocols may also impact response variability (see above). With this in mind, it will certainly be informative to identify the factors that might influence unique tDCS response and whether these factor, themselves, modulate response in a reliable and predictable manner.

SHAM STIMULATION AND BLINDING

If the dichometric anode excite/cathode inhibit mechanism of tDCS is valid, then comparing the polarities to each other makes determining the true effect of each extremely difficult (as one can never be certain the exact contribution of each polarity to the overall difference). Although practitioners aware of this comparative shortcoming extol the use of various control stimulation procedures (such as *sham* or *off-target active* stimulation), these procedures have not always proven effective or reliable across varied tDCS protocols (Ambrus et al., 2012; Brunoni et al., 2013; Davis et al., 2013; Palm et al., 2013). In addition, not nearly as many researchers have utilized control conditions as one might expect. In fact, of the 80 studies published to date exploring the effect of 0.0286 mA/cm^2 tDCS current density with an M1/Orbit electrode placement on MEP modulation (the most utilized protocol in the literature), only 10 have compared results to a control condition (**Table 1**). This means 87.5% of the studies examining the foundational claim upon which the modern tDCS field is built have not utilized a proper control condition.

Comparing each polarity to its own baseline level (rather than the opposing polarity) does little to address the underlying issues inherent with sham-less protocols. It is commonly acknowledged that MEP amplitude is naturally an extremely variable measure (in fact, Valls-Sole recently pointed out, "The amplitude of MEP to single pulse TMS is not usually employed as a measure of functional relevance because of its large variability and dependence on many technical factors"; p. 9, *in press*). As such, it can be assumed there will *always* be some shift away from baseline levels, regardless of intervention (or lack thereof). Accordingly, the utilization of a control condition to differentiate between natural fluctuation and tDCS engendered effects is imperative.

As O'Connell et al. (2012) recently pointed out, tDCS blinding (especially when sham stimulation is being utilized) is of utmost importance yet incredibly difficult to achieve. In fact, these authors reported that, during stimulation using a high current density (0.0571 mA/cm^2), neither the practitioner nor participant was effectively blinded. Beyond this, observable vasodilation (typically over the right orbit) makes practitioner blinding difficult at any current density (see, Palm et al., 2013). Finally, clear sensorial differences between active and sham stimulation (primarily reported as itching, tingling, and/or burning) make blinding participants who undergo multiple conditions difficult at any current density (Davis et al., 2013). As with any scientific study, ineffective blinding may lead to a number of undesirable confounds, including expectation effects, on-the-fly protocol adjustments, and reporting/assessment biases.

In order to elucidate the effects of varied tDCS paradigms, it is essential to continue to amend current and create novel, more effective control conditions. In addition, until such time as more reliable control protocols are developed, it may be beneficial to test for and report blinding procedures and efficacy (or lack-thereof).

MOTOR AND COGNITIVE INTERFERENCE

Several lines of research suggest that any active motor and/or cognitive activity undertaken during or following tDCS can negatively interfere with or altogether abolish the effects of stimulation. The failure of many practitioners to take account of and further characterize this evidence is concerning.

Quartarone et al. (2004) were the first to report evidence of this interference effect. This group explored MEP amplitude modulation following 5 min of tDCS during motor imagery (0.0286 mA/cm^2 current density; M1/contralateral orbit montage). Whereas imagery (undertaken following stimulation) appeared to prolong the effects of cathodal stimulation, it abolished the effects of anodal stimulation. Despite this important finding (that the act of *thinking* about motor movement could potentially eliminate tDCS efficacy), this paper went largely ignored and is rarely cited.

Several additional studies have confirmed this interference effect. For instance, Antal et al. (2007) reported that a cognitive task (a combined mathematics, language, geography, and history questionnaire) undertaken during stimulation abolished the effects of both anodal and cathodal stimulation on MEP amplitude modulation (0.0286 mA/cm^2 current density; M1/contralateral orbit montage; 10 min duration). In addition, a simple motor task (pushing around a ball) undertaken during stimulation led to an equivalent decrease in MEP amplitude following both anodal and cathodal stimulation. This equivalent drop suggests the motor activity (perhaps due to fatigue of the target muscle) abolished the effect of stimulation as well. More recently, Miyaguchi et al. (2013) reported that anodal tDCS (0.0571 mA/cm^2 current density; bilateral M1 montage; 10 min duration) delivered with a concurrent non-exhaustive active or passive motor task (self initiated or machine initiated finger abduction-adduction) led to an equivalent MEP amplitude reduction as did undertaking the active motor task alone (without stimulation). Again, this suggests the motor task abolished the effect of stimulation (see also, Thirugnanasambandam et al., 2011).

Secondary evidence for an interference effect can be seen in the often reported diminished tDCS MEP amplitude modulation in voluntarily contracted muscles (common in non-hand targets) compared to resting muscles. For instance, in the 40 min following cathodal stimulation (0.0286 mA/cm^2 current density; M1/contralateral orbit montage; 15 min duration), Bradnam et al. (2010) reported an average compound MEP decrease of 15.3% in the right infraspinitus (shoulder) when the muscle was at rest, and an *increase* of 1.3% when the muscle was active. Similarly, in the 60 min following anodal stimulation (0.0571 mA/cm^2 density; M1/contralateral orbit montage; 10 min duration), Jeffery et al. (2007) reported an average MEP amplitude increase of 34.8% in the right tibialis anterior (leg) when the muscle was at rest, and an increase of only 25% when the muscle was activated. Again, these results suggest that motor activity undertaken immediately following stimulation can significantly reduce or eliminate the modulatory effects of tDCS.

These findings suggest that relatively simple and difficult to control for thoughts and/or behaviors may eliminate tDCS efficacy. Clinically, tDCS is often used as an adjunct to physical rehabilitation following stroke (for review, Johansson, 2011). If the aforementioned studies are correct, combining tDCS with motor training may eliminate any desired tDCS effect. This holds true for healthy populations as well. Oftentimes, during long-duration, off-line stimulatory protocols, participants are instructed to simply relax during tDCS. This relaxation can take

Table 1 | Studies exploring the effects of 0.0286 mA/cm^2 current density, M1/Contralateral Orbit tDCS montage on TMS elicited MEP amplitude of intrinsic hand muscles at rest in healthy participants.

Study	*N*	tDCS duration	Anode	Cathode	Control
Nitsche and Paulus, 2000 (*x4*)	10 and 9 (*x1*)/12 (*x2*)	4 s (*x1*)/5 min (*x3*)	**X** (*x4*)	**X** (*x4*)	–
Nitsche and Paulus, 2001 (*x5*)	12 (*x5*)	5, 7, 9, 11, and 13 min (*x1*)	**X** (*x5*)	–	–
Liebetanz et al., 2002	11	5 min	**X**	**X**	–
Nitsche et al., 2003a (*x3*)	12 (*x1*)/10 (*x2*)	4 s (*x1*)/9–13 min (*x2*)	**X** (*x3*)	**X** (*x3*)	–
Nitsche et al., 2003b (*x3*)	12 (*x3*)	5, 7, and 9 min (*x1*)	–	**X** (*x3*)	–
Lang et al., 2004a	8	10 min	**X**	**X**	–
Lang et al., 2004b (*x2*)	5 and 10 (*x1*)	10 min (*x2*)	**X** (*x2*)	**X** (*x2*)	**X** (*x1*)
Siebner et al., 2004 (*x2*)	5 and 8 (*x1*)	10 min (*x2*)	**X** (*x2*)	**X** (*x2*)	**X** (*x1*)
Nitsche et al., 2004a (*x4*)	6 (*x3*)/12 (*x1*)	4 s (*x1*)/7, 9–13 min (*x1*)	**X** (*x4*)	**X** (*x4*)	–
Nitsche et al., 2004b (*x3*)	12, 9, and 10 (*x1*)	4 s (*x1*)/5, 9–11 min (*x1*)	**X** (*x3*)	**X** (*x3*)	–
Nitsche et al., 2004c	12	9 min C/13 min A	**X**	**X**	–
Quartarone et al., 2004 (*x2*)	7 and 21 (*x1*)	5 min (*x2*)	**X** (*x1*)	**X** (*x1*)	–
Quartarone et al., 2005	8	10 min	**X**	**X**	**X**
Nitsche et al., 2006	12	9 min C/13 min A	**X**	**X**	–
Power et al., 2006	10	10 min	**X**	**X**	**X**
Nitsche et al., 2007a (*x8*)	12 (*x8*)	4 s (*x3*), 7 min (*x3*)10 min (*x2*)	**X** (*x8*)	**X** (*x8*)	–
Nitsche et al., 2007b	12	7 min	**X**	**X**	–
Kuo et al., 2007	7	9 min C/13 min A	**X**	**X**	–
Antal et al., 2007	12	10 min	**X**	**X**	–
Boros et al., 2008	17	13 min	**X**	–	–
Kuo et al., 2008	7	9 min C/13 min A	**X**	**X**	–
Nitsche et al., 2009	12	9 min C/13 min A	**X**	**X**	–
Monte-Silva et al., 2009 (*x4*)	12 (*x4*)	9 min C/13 min A (*x4*)	**X** (*x4*)	**X** (*x4*)	–
Monte-Silva et al., 2010 (*x2*)	12 (*x2*)	9 and 18 min (*x1*)	–	**X** (*x2*)	–
Bradnam et al., 2011	18	15 min	–	**X**	**X**
Fricke et al., 2011 (*x4*)	8–12 (*x4*)	5 min (*x2*), 7 and 10 min (*x1*)	**X** (*x4*)	**X** (*x4*)	–
List et al., 2011	12	10 min	–	**X**	–
McCambridge et al., 2011	7 Active/5 Sham	10 min	–	**X**	**X**
Munneke et al., 2011 (*x3*)	10 (*x3*)	7, 11, and 15 min (*x1*)	–	**X** (*x3*)	–
Scelzo et al., 2011	12	13 min	**X**	**X**	–
Thirugnanasambandam et al., 2011	16	20 min	**X**	**X**	–
Di Lazzaro et al., 2012	30	20 min	–	**X**	–
Hasan et al., 2012	18	9 min	–	**X**	–
Schade et al., 2012 (*x2*)	8 (*x2*)	5 min (*x2*)	**X** (*x2*)	**X** (*x2*)	–
Suzuki et al., 2012	9	10 min	**X**	**X**	**X**
Monte-Silva et al., 2012 (*x2*)	15 (*x2*)	13 and 26 min (*x1*)	**X** (*x2*)	–	–
Hasan et al., 2013	20	9 min	–	**X**	–
Batsikadze et al., 2013 (*x2*)	9 and 8 (*x1*)	20 min (*x2*)	–	**X** (*x1*)	**X** (*x1*)
Schabrun et al., 2012 (*x3*)	21 A, 9 C, 13 s	20 min (*x3*)	**X** (*x1*)	**X** (*x1*)	**X** (*x1*)
Simis et al., 2013	11	20 min	**X**	–	**X**
	TOTAL		62	67	10

A sham condition from Quartarone et al. (2004) was excluded due to reporting MEP modulation during motor imagery only (not at rest). One study from Monte-Silva et al., 2009 was excluded due to presenting replication data. A, Anode; C, Cathode; S, Sham.
Studies include the placebo condition/s in any drug or device interaction studies.

the form of reading, texting, surfing the internet, doing homework, etc. Is it possible these seemingly innocuous activities are enough to negate or otherwise interfere with the effects of tDCS as well? Additionally, in experiments utilizing MRI to explore the effects of tDCS, stimulation is often given outside the scanning room (although several tDCS devices are now MR compatible). During these protocols, participants must walk back to the scanning room and re-enter the scanner following stimulation: a series of non-trivial motor actions which may, again, interfere with or abolish any tDCS effects.

If it's possible the effects of tDCS are too weak to manifest during typical human behavior, this is important to determine before more effort and funding are expended utilizing inappropriate protocols. Until such a time as this issue is clearly resolved, it is important practitioners minimize motor and cognitive activity during and immediately following tDCS and during any proceeding procedure (including TMS and/or MRI).

ELECTRIC CURRENT INFLUENCES

There are a number of variables which may influence current density and flow to a great extent that have simply not been discussed in the literature to date. Although, as noted above, countless papers have discussed optimal electrode positioning, current density, and stimulation duration for specific outcomes (for discussion, Paulus, 2011), these discussions never seem to evolve past these three parameters.

One variable which may impact current density and flow (but which has yet to be discussed in the literature) is hair thickness. Simply put: hair is not a conductor—it is an insulator. Measurements suggest dry hair (<7% 25% H_20 content) has a resistivity of approximately $3 \times 10^{12}\Omega$/cm whilst wet hair (25% H_20 content) has a resistivity of approximately $6 \times 10^{6}\Omega$/cm (Feughelman, 1997). To put that into perspective, skin (the contact surface in many tDCS modeling studies) has a resistivity of approximately $2.15 \times 10^{-2}\Omega$/cm (see, Miranda et al., 2006; Wagner et al., 2007: Ω = Ohm: Note—lower resistivity values equate to higher conductance).

To combat this, practitioners often utilize large amounts of saline to saturate dense hair. Unfortunately, saline spread or dripping at the level of the scalp can guide current flow in undesirable and unpredictable directions. This fact can be easily demonstrated. First, place two saline soaked tDCS sponge electrodes on an easily accessible area of skin (such as the forearms or quadriceps). Next, place a piece of thick, non-conductive plastic under one of the electrodes to ensure no contact is made between the sponge and the skin. Under this set-up, you should be *un*able to complete the electric circuit. Now, cut a small hole in the plastic barrier (exposing the skin underneath), fill the small hole with saline, and run a continuous stream of saline between the hole and the sponge atop the plastic. Under this new set-up, you should be able to complete the electric circuit quite easily, regardless of how far away from the sponge you have made the small hole (if you are having trouble running a stream of saline between the electrode and the hole, you can substitute a thicker conductive gel: **Figure 1**).

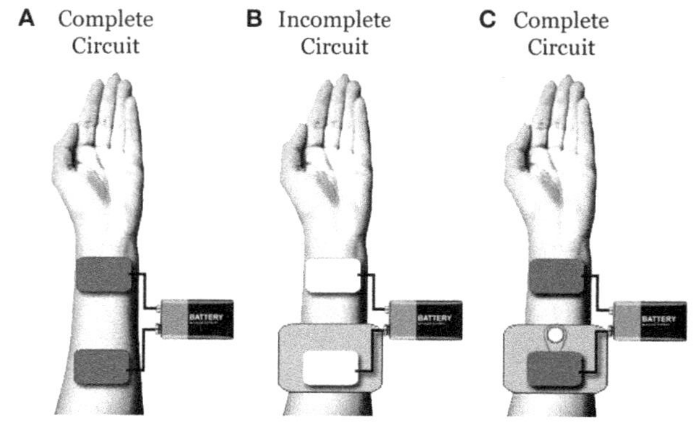

FIGURE 1 | (A) Under typical conditions, one will be able to build an electric circuit using two saline soaked tDCS sponges placed on a piece of clean skin. (B) When a piece of non-conductive plastic is placed underneath one electrode, the circuit will be broken. **(C)** When a small hole is cut in the plastic and a small stream of saline is used to connect the skin under the hole to the electrode, the circuit will be re-built. This demonstrates that, even if a tDCS electrode is not in contact with the scalp, excessive saline can be used to bridge between the electrode and the skin. Unfortunately, with excessive saline, determining the location of the circuit connection and electrical density at this point is extremely difficult.

This demonstration reveals that, even when there is no direct electrode/scalp contact (as may occur in participants with thick hair), excess saline can be used to bridge the tDCS current. However, when this is done, the precise location of the electric current entrance and/or exit points on the scalp will be largely unknown and unpredictable. In addition, when the electric current follows saline to the scalp, the current density also becomes largely unknown and unpredictable (as the number and size of contact points at the scalp becomes uncertain).

Sweat is a second often-ignored variable that may impact electric current dynamics. Because sweat increases skin conductivity (for review, Dawson et al., 2001), the amount of sweat on a participants scalp may influence current flow in important ways. It's possible that as salts, oils, and electrolytes accumulate in pores on the scalp, the skin will generate enough conductivity to ensure little or no current enters the cortex. However, aside from washing each subject's hair and ensuring a temperature controlled testing environment, how can this be accounted and/or controlled?

Finally, the means by which electrodes are held in place at the scalp may also influence electric current dynamics. For instance, several contemporary tDCS sponge electrodes include plastic rings at the corners (presumably anchor the electrode in place). Unfortunately, unless specifically manufactured, most plastics are non-conductive. Whether or not the plastic used in these electrodes has been produced to conduct electricity is uncertain, although vasodilation patterns following stimulation with these electrodes (which typically reveals no dilatory response underneath the plastic rings themselves) suggests they are not. This may impact current density and flow in unpredictable and uncontrollable ways. In addition, many practitioners hold sponge electrodes in place using rubber straps which are narrower than the electrodes themselves. With these straps, centralized pressure can cause the periphery of the electrodes to "flare" upwards reducing contact area (and, by extension, increasing current density). Given the apparent variability seen within and between individuals (outlined above), it is important to properly consider the influence these (and other) factors may be having on response characteristics.

CONCLUSION

Recently, several practitioners have noted concerns about modern tDCS conceptions and mechanistic models (Bikson, 2013; Paulus et al., 2013). In addition, a number of studies have also begun to explore response variation in response to adjustments in current density, electrode position, and/or stimulation duration (Im et al., 2008; Bikson et al., 2010; Bastani and Jaberzadeh, 2013a,b). Although doubtless important, this work does not address the larger foundational issues raised in this paper.

Although we have chosen to focus on tDCS, many of the issues examined in this paper are applicable to other non-invasive modulatory tools; such as transcranial alternating current stimulation (tACS) and transcranial random noise stimulation (tRNS). These devices are often modified tDCS devices and the protocols utilized by each are often modeled after modern tDCS protocols. Because of this, although there is not enough data in the literature to confidently discuss response variability and reliability, issues of blinding, interference, and electric current influences are highly relevant to these novel tools.

If the field of tDCS is to avoid becoming a footnote in the annals of neuroscientific research, it is time to collectively acknowledge there are shortcomings in our current understanding of this device, its functional parameters, its general efficacy, and its reliability. Rather than seeing the aforementioned issues as a detriment to the field, we should use them to guide future research and exploration. For instance, acknowledging variability can encourage us to explore individual response patterns (and correlate these with related secondary measures to tease-out possible state-dependency effects). Acknowledging the lack of effective sham and blinding techniques can encourage us to develop better more effective devices. Acknowledging the interference effect of motor and/or cognitive activity can inspire us to devise more comprehensive protocols. It is hoped that increased awareness and open discussion of these important issues will lead to a more rigorous and accurate foundation upon which tDCS can be developed into the future.

REFERENCES

Ahdab, R., Ayache, S. S., Brugieres, P., Goujon, C., and Lefaucheur, J. P. (2010). Comparison of "standard" and "navigated" procedures of TMS coil positioning over motor, premotor and prefrontal targets in patients with chronic pain and depression. *Clin. Neurophysiol.* 40, 27–36. doi: 10.1016/j.neucli.2010.01.001

Alonzo, A., Brassil, J., Taylor, J. L., Martin, D., and Loo, C. K. (2012). Daily transcranial direct current stimulation (tDCS) leads to greater increases in cortical excitability than second daily transcranial direct current stimulation. *Brain Stimul.* 5, 208–213. doi: 10.1016/j.brs.2011.04.006

Ambrus, G. G., Al-Moyed, H., Chaieb, L., Sarp, L., Antal, A., and Paulus, W. (2012). The fade-in–short stimulation–fade out approach to sham tDCS–reliable at 1 mA for naive and experienced subjects, but not investigators. *Brain Stimul.* 5, 499–504. doi: 10.1016/j.brs.2011.12.001

Antal, A., Terney, D., Poreisz, C., and Paulus, W. (2007). Towards unravelling task–related modulations of neuroplastic changes induced in the human motor cortex. *Eur. J. Neurosci.* 26, 2687–2691. doi: 10.1111/j.1460-9568.2007.05896.x

Bastani, A., and Jaberzadeh, S. (2013a). a-tDCS differential modulation of corticospinal excitability: the effects of electrode size. *Brain Stimul.* 6, 932–937. doi: 10.1016/j.brs.2013.04.005

Bastani, A., and Jaberzadeh, S. (2013b). Differential modulation of corticospinal excitability by different current densities of anodal transcranial direct current stimulation. *PLoS ONE* 8:e72254. doi: 10.1371/journal.pone.0072254

Batsikadze, G., Moliadze, V., Paulus, W., Kuo, M. F., and Nitsche, M. A. (2013). Partially non–linear stimulation intensity–dependent effects of direct current stimulation on motor cortex excitability in humans. *J. Physiol.* 591, 1987–2000. doi: 10.1113/jphysiol.2012.249730

Bikson, M. (2013). Origins of specificity during tDCS: anatomical, activity-selective, and input-bias mechanisms. *Front. Hum. Neurosci.* 7:688. doi: 10.3389/fnhum.2013.00688

Bikson, M., Datta, A., Rahman, A., and Scaturro, J. (2010). Electrode montages for tDCS and weak transcranial electrical stimulation: role of "return" electrode's position and size. *Clin. Neurophysiol.* 121, 1976. doi: 10.1016/j.clinph.2010.05.020

Boros, K., Poreisz, C., Münchau, A., Paulus, W., and Nitsche, M. A. (2008). Premotor transcranial direct current stimulation (tDCS) affects primary motor excitability in humans. *Eur. J. Neurosci.* 27, 1292–1300. doi: 10.1111/j.1460-9568.2008.06090.x

Bradnam, L. V., Stinear, C. M., and Byblow, W. D. (2011). Cathodal transcranial direct current stimulation suppresses ipsilateral projections to presumed propriospinal neurons of the proximal upper limb. *J. Neurophysiol.* 105, 2582–2589. doi: 10.1152/jn.01084.2010

Bradnam, L. V., Stinear, C. M., Lewis, G. N., and Byblow, W. D. (2010). Task-dependent modulation of inputs to proximal upper limb following transcranial direct current stimulation of primary motor cortex. *J. Neurophysiol.* 103, 2382–2389. doi: 10.1152/jn.01046.2009

Brunoni, A. R., Schestatsky, P., Lotufo, P. A., Benseñor, I. M., and Fregni, F. (2013). Comparison of blinding effectiveness between sham tDCS and placebo sertraline in a 6-week major depression randomized clinical trial. *Clin. Neurophysiol.* doi: 10.1016/j.clinph.2013.07.020. [Epub ahead of print].

Datta, A., Truong, D., Minhas, P., Parra, L. C., and Bikson, M. (2012). Inter-individual variation during transcranial direct current stimulation and normalization of dose using MRI-derived computational models. *Front. Psychiatry* 3:91. doi: 10.3389/fpsyt.2012.00091

Davis, N. J., Gold, E., Pascual-Leone, A., and Bracewell, R. M. (2013). Challenges of proper placebo control for non-invasive brain stimulation in clinical and experimental applications. *Eur. J. Neurosci.* 38, 2973–2977. doi: 10.1111/ejn.12307

Dawson, M. E., Schell, A. M., and Filion, D. L. (2001). "The electrodermal system," in *Handbook of Psycholphysiology*, eds J. T. Cacioppo, L. G. Tassinary, and G. G. Berntson (Cambridge, UK: Cambridge University Press), 159–181.

Di Lazzaro, V., Manganelli, F., Dileone, M., Notturno, F., Esposito, M., Capasso, M., et al. (2012). The effects of prolonged cathodal direct current stimulation on the excitatory and inhibitory circuits of the ipsilateral and contralateral motor cortex. *J. Neural Transm.* 119, 1499–1506. doi: 10.1007/s00702-012-0845-4

Feughelman, M. (1997). *Mechanical Properties and Structure of Alpha-Keratin Fibres: Wool, Human Hair, and Related Fibres.* Sydney, NSW: University of New South Wales Press.

Fricke, K., Seeber, A. A., Thirugnanasambandam, N., Paulus, W., Nitsche, M. A., and Rothwell, J. C. (2011). Time course of the induction of homeostatic plasticity generated by repeated transcranial direct current stimulation of the human motor cortex. *J. Neurophysiol.* 105, 1141–1149. doi: 10.1152/jn.00608.2009

Gálvez, V., Alonzo, A., Martin, D., and Loo, C. K. (2013). Transcranial direct current stimulation treatment protocols: should stimulus intensity be constant or incremental over multiple sessions. *Int. J. Neuropsychopharmacol.* 16, 13–21. doi: 10.1017/S1461145712000041

Hasan, A., Aborowa, R., Nitsche, M. A., Marshall, L., Schmitt, A., Gruber, O., et al. (2012). Abnormal bihemispheric responses in schizophrenia patients following cathodal transcranial direct stimulation. *Eur. Arch. Psychiatry Clin. Neurosci.* 262, 415–423. doi: 10.1007/s00406-012-0298-7

Hasan, A., Misewitsch, K., Nitsche, M. A., Gruber, O., Padberg, F., Falkai, P., et al. (2013). Impaired motor cortex responses in non-psychotic first-degree relatives of schizophrenia patients: a cathodal tDCS pilot study. *Brain Stimul.* 6, 821–829. doi: 10.1016/j.brs.2013.03.001

Herwig, U., Padberg, F., Unger, J., Spitzer, M., and Schönfeldt-Lecuona, C. (2001). Transcranial magnetic stimulation in therapy studies: examination of the reliability of "standard" coil positioning by neuronavigation. *Biol. Psychiatry* 50, 58–61. doi: 10.1016/S0006-3223(01)01153-2

Im, C. H., Jung, H. H., Choi, J. D., Lee, S. Y., and Jung, K. Y. (2008). Determination of optimal electrode positions for transcranial direct current stimulation (tDCS). *Phys. Med. Biol.* 53, N219. doi: 10.1088/0031-9155/53/11/N03

Inghilleri, M., Conte, A., Curra, A., Frasca, V., Lorenzano, C., and Berardelli, A. (2004). Ovarian hormones and cortical excitability. An rTMS study in humans. *Clin. Neurophysiol.* 115, 1063–1068. doi: 10.1016/j.clinph.2003.12.003

Jeffery, D. T., Norton, J. A., Roy, F. D., and Gorassini, M. A. (2007). Effects of transcranial direct current stimulation on the excitability of the leg motor cortex. *Exp. Brain Res.* 182, 281–287. doi: 10.1007/s00221-007-1093-y

Johansson, B. B. (2011). Current trends in stroke rehabilitation. A review with focus on brain plasticity. *Acta Neurol. Scand.* 123, 147–159. doi: 10.1111/j.1600-0404.2010.01417.x

Kuo, M. F., Grosch, J., Fregni, F., Paulus, W., and Nitsche, M. A. (2007). Focusing effect of acetylcholine on neuroplasticity in the human motor cortex. *J. Neurosci.* 27, 14442–14447. doi: 10.1523/JNEUROSCI.4104-07.2007

Kuo, M. F., Paulus, W., and Nitsche, M. A. (2008). Boosting focally-induced brain plasticity by dopamine. *Cereb. Cortex* 18, 648–651. doi: 10.1093/cercor/bhm098

Lang, N., Nitsche, M. A., Paulus, W., Rothwell, J. C., and Lemon, R. N. (2004a). Effects of transcranial direct current stimulation over the human motor cortex on corticospinal and transcallosal excitability. *Exp. Brain Res.* 156, 439–443. doi: 10.1007/s00221-003-1800-2

Lang, N., Siebner, H. R., Ernst, D., Nitsche, M. A., Paulus, W., Lemon, R. N., et al. (2004b). Preconditioning with transcranial direct current stimulation sensitizes the motor cortex to rapid-rate transcranial magnetic stimulation and controls the direction of after-effects. *Biol. Psychiatry* 56, 634–639. doi: 10.1016/j.biopsych.2004.07.017

Liebetanz, D., Nitsche, M. A., Tergau, F., and Paulus, W. (2002). Pharmacological approach to the mechanisms of transcranial DC–stimulation–induced after–effects of human motor cortex excitability. *Brain* 125, 2238–2247. doi: 10.1093/brain/awf238

List, J., Duning, T., Meinzer, M., Kürten, J., Schirmacher, A., Deppe, M., et al. (2011). Enhanced rapid-onset cortical plasticity in CADASIL as a possible mechanism of preserved cognition. *Cereb. Cortex* 21, 2774–2787. doi: 10.1093/cercor/bhr071

McCambridge, A. B., Bradnam, L. V., Stinear, C. M., and Byblow, W. D. (2011). Cathodal transcranial direct current stimulation of the primary motor cortex improves selective muscle activation in the ipsilateral arm. *J. Neurophysiol.* 105, 2937–2942. doi: 10.1152/jn.00171.2011

Miranda, P. C., Lomarev, M., and Hallett, M. (2006). Modeling the current distribution during transcranial direct current stimulation. *Clin. Neurophysiol.* 117, 1623–1629. doi: 10.1016/j.clinph.2006.04.009

Miyaguchi, S., Onishi, H., Kojima, S., Sugawara, K., Tsubaki, A., Kirimoto, H., et al. (2013). Corticomotor excitability induced by anodal transcranial direct current stimulation with and without non-exhaustive movement. *Brain Res.* 1529, 83–91.

Monte-Silva, K., Kuo, M. F., Hessenthaler, S., Fresnoza, S., Liebetanz, D., Paulus, W., et al. (2012). Induction of late LTP-like plasticity in the human motor cortex by repeated non-invasive brain stimulation. *Brain Stimul.* 6, 424–432. doi: 10.1016/j.brs.2012.04.011

Monte-Silva, K., Kuo, M. F., Liebetanz, D., Paulus, W., and Nitsche, M. A. (2010). Shaping the optimal repetition interval for cathodal transcranial direct current stimulation (tDCS). *J. Neurophysiol.* 103, 1735–1740. doi: 10.1152/jn.00924.2009

Monte-Silva, K., Kuo, M. F., Thirugnanasambandam, N., Liebetanz, D., Paulus, W., and Nitsche, M. A. (2009). Dose-dependent inverted U-shaped effect of dopamine (D2-like) receptor activation on focal and nonfocal plasticity in humans. *J. Neurosci.* 29, 6124–6131. doi: 10.1523/JNEUROSCI.0728-09.2009

Munneke, M. A., Stegeman, D. F., Hengeveld, Y. A., Rongen, J. J., Schelhaas, H. J., and Zwarts, M. J. (2011). Transcranial direct current stimulation does not modulate motor cortex excitability in patients with amyotrophic lateral sclerosis. *Muscle Nerve* 44, 109–114. doi: 10.1002/mus.22012

Nitsche, M. A., Doemkes, S., Karakoese, T., Antal, A., Liebetanz, D., Lang, N., et al. (2007a). Shaping the effects of transcranial direct current stimulation of the human motor cortex. *J. Neurophysiol.* 97, 3109–3117. doi: 10.1152/jn.01312.2006

Nitsche, M. A., Roth, A., Kuo, M. F., Fischer, A. K., Liebetanz, D., Lang, N., et al. (2007b). Timing-dependent modulation of associative plasticity by general network excitability in the human motor cortex. *J. Neurosci.* 27, 3807–3812. doi: 10.1523/JNEUROSCI.5348-06.2007

Nitsche, M. A., Fricke, K., Henschke, U., Schlitterlau, A., Liebetanz, D., Lang, N., et al. (2003a). Pharmacological modulation of cortical excitability shifts induced by transcranial direct current stimulation in humans. *J. Physiol.* 553, 293–301. doi: 10.1113/jphysiol.2003.049916

Nitsche, M. A., Nitsche, M. S., Klein, C. C., Tergau, F., Rothwell, J. C., and Paulus, W. (2003b). Level of action of cathodal DC polarisation induced inhibition of the human motor cortex. *Clin. Neurophysiol.* 114, 600–604. doi: 10.1016/S1388-2457(02)00412-1

Nitsche, M. A., Grundey, J., Liebetanz, D., Lang, N., Tergau, F., and Paulus, W. (2004a). Catecholaminergic consolidation of motor cortical neuroplasticity in humans. *Cereb. Cortex* 14, 1240–1245. doi: 10.1093/cercor/bhh085

Nitsche, M. A., Liebetanz, D., Schlitterlau, A., Henschke, U., Fricke, K., Frommann, K., et al. (2004b). GABAergic modulation of DC stimulation–induced motor cortex excitability shifts in humans. *Eur. J. Neurosci.* 19, 2720–2726. doi: 10.1111/j.0953-816X.2004.03398.x

Nitsche, M. A., Jaussi, W., Liebetanz, D., Lang, N., Tergau, F., and Paulus, W. (2004c). Consolidation of human motor cortical neuroplasticity by D-cycloserine. *Neuropsychopharmacology* 29, 1573. doi: 10.1038/sj.npp.1300517

Nitsche, M. A., Kuo, M. F., Karrasch, R., Wächter, B., Liebetanz, D., and Paulus, W. (2009). Serotonin affects transcranial direct current–induced neuroplasticity in humans. *Biol. Psychiatry* 66, 503–508. doi: 10.1016/j.biopsych.2009.03.022

Nitsche, M. A., Lampe, C., Antal, A., Liebetanz, D., Lang, N., Tergau, F., et al. (2006). Dopaminergic modulation of long–lasting direct current–induced cortical excitability changes in the human motor cortex. *Eur. J. Neurosci.* 23, 1651–1657. doi: 10.1111/j.1460-9568.2006.04676.x

Nitsche, M. A., and Paulus, W. (2000). Excitability changes induced in the human motor cortex by weak transcranial direct current stimulation. *J. Physiol.* 527, 633–639. doi: 10.1111/j.1469-7793.2000.t01-1-00633.x

Nitsche, M. A., and Paulus, W. (2001). Sustained excitability elevations induced by transcranial DC motor cortex stimulation in humans. *Neurology* 57, 1899–1901. doi: 10.1212/WNL.57.10.1899

O'Connell, N. E., Cossar, J., Marston, L., Wand, B. M., Bunce, D., Moseley, G. L., et al. (2012). Rethinking clinical trials of transcranial direct current stimulation: participant and assessor blinding is inadequate at intensities of 2 mA. *PLoS ONE* 7:e47514. doi: 10.1371/journal.pone.0047514

Palm, U., Reisinger, E., Keeser, D., Kuo, M. F., Pogarell, O., Leicht, G., et al. (2013). Evaluation of sham transcranial direct current stimulation for randomized, placebo-controlled clinical trials. *Brain Stimul.* 6, 690–695. doi: 10.1016/j.brs.2013.01.005

Paulus, W. (2011). Transcranial electrical stimulation (tES–tDCS; tRNS, tACS) methods. *Neuropsychol. Rehabil.* 21, 602–617. doi: 10.1080/09602011.2011.557292

Paulus, W., Peterchev, A. V., and Ridding, M. (2013). "Transcranial electric and magnetic stimulation: technique and paradigms," in *Brain Stimulation E-Book: Handbook of Clinical Neurology*, Vol. 116, Series eds M. J. Aminoff, F. Boller, and D. F. Swaab (Amsterdam, ND: Elsevier B.V.), 329.

Power, H. A., Norton, J. A., Porter, C. L., Doyle, Z., Hui, I., and Chan, K. M. (2006). Transcranial direct current stimulation of the primary motor cortex affects cortical drive to human musculature as assessed by intermuscular coherence. *J. Physiol.* 577, 795–803. doi: 10.1113/jphysiol.2006.116939

Quartarone, A., Morgante, F., Bagnato, S., Rizzo, V., Sant'Angelo, A., Aiello, E., et al. (2004). Long lasting effects of transcranial direct current stimulation on motor imagery. *Neuroreport* 15, 1287–1291. doi: 10.1097/01.wnr.0000127637.22805.7c

Quartarone, A., Rizzo, V., Bagnato, S., Morgante, F., Sant'Angelo, A., Romano, M., et al. (2005). Homeostatic-like plasticity of the primary motor hand area is impaired in focal hand dystonia. *Brain* 128, 1943–1950. doi: 10.1093/brain/awh527

Roche, N., Lackmy, A., Achache, V., Bussel, B., and Katz, R. (2011). Effects of anodal transcranial direct current stimulation over the leg motor area on lumbar spinal network excitability in healthy subjects. *J. Physiol.* 589, 2813–2826. doi: 10.1113/jphysiol.2011.205161

Sale, M. V., Ridding, M. C., and Nordstrom, M. A. (2008). Cortisol inhibits neuroplasticity induction in human motor cortex. *J. Neurosci.* 28, 8285–8293. doi: 10.1523/JNEUROSCI.1963-08.2008

Sale, M. V., Ridding, M. C., and Nordstrom, M. A. (2010). Circadian modulation off neuroplasticity in humans and potential therapeutic implications. *Rev. Neurosci.* 21, 55–66. doi: 10.1515/REVNEURO.2010.21.1.55

Scelzo, E., Giannicola, G., Rosa, M., Ciocca, M., Ardolino, G., Cogiamanian, F., et al. (2011). Increased short latency afferent inhibition after anodal transcranial direct current stimulation. *Neurosci. Lett.* 498, 167–170. doi: 10.1016/j.neulet.2011.05.007

Schabrun, S. M., Chipchase, L. S., Zipf, N., Thickbroom, G. W., and Hodges, P. W. (2012). Interaction between simultaneously applied neuromodulatory interventions in humans. *Brain Stimul.* 6, 624–630. doi: 10.1016/j.brs.2012.09.009

Schade, S., Moliadze, V., Paulus, W., and Antal, A. (2012). Modulating neuronal excitability in the motor cortex with tDCS shows moderate hemispheric asymmetry due to subjects' handedness: a pilot study. *Restor. Neurol. Neurosci.* 30, 191–198. doi: 10.3233/RNN-2012-110175

Siebner, H. R., Lang, N., Rizzo, V., Nitsche, M. A., Paulus, W., Lemon, R. N., et al. (2004). Preconditioning of low-frequency repetitive transcranial magnetic stimulation with transcranial direct current stimulation: evidence for homeostatic plasticity in the human motor cortex. *J. Neurosci.* 24, 3379–3385. doi: 10.1523/JNEUROSCI.5316-03.2004

Simis, M., Adeyemo, B. O., Medeiros, L. F., Miraval, F., Gagliardi, R. J., and Fregni, F. (2013). Motor cortex-induced plasticity by noninvasive brain stimulation: a comparison between transcranial direct current stimulation and transcranial magnetic stimulation. *Neuroreport* 24, 973–975. doi: 10.1097/WNR.0000000000000021

Smith, M. J., Keel, J. C., Greenberg, B. D., Adams, L. F., Schmidt, P. J., Rubinow, D. A., et al. (1999). Menstrual cycle effects on cortical excitability. *Neurology* 53, 2069–2069. doi: 10.1212/WNL.53.9.2069

Sparing, R., Buelte, D., Meister, I. G., Pauš, T., and Fink, G. R. (2008). Transcranial magnetic stimulation and the challenge of coil placement: a comparison of conventional and stereotaxic neuronavigational strategies. *Hum. Brain Mapp.* 29, 82–96. doi: 10.1002/hbm.20360

Stagg, C. J., and Nitsche, M. A. (2011). Physiological basis of transcranial direct current stimulation. *Neuroscientist* 17, 37–53. doi: 10.1177/1073858410386614

Suzuki, K., Fujiwara, T., Tanaka, N., Tsuji, T., Masakado, Y., Hase, K., et al. (2012). Comparison of the after-effects of transcranial direct current stimulation over the motor cortex in patients with stroke and healthy volunteers. *Int. J. Neurosci.* 122, 675–681. doi: 10.3109/00207454.2012.707715

Thirugnanasambandam, N., Sparing, R., Dafotakis, M., Meister, I. G., Paulus, W., Nitsche, M. A., et al. (2011). Isometric contraction interferes with transcranial direct current stimulation (tDCS) induced plasticity–evidence of state-dependent neuromodulation in human motor cortex. *Restor. Neurol. Neurosci.* 29, 311–320. doi: 10.3233/RNN-2011-0601

Tremblay, S., Beaulé, V., Lepage, J. F., and Théoret, H. (2013). Anodal transcranial direct current stimulation modulates GABAB-related intracortical inhibition in the M1 of healthy individuals. *Neuroreport* 24, 46–50. doi: 10.1097/WNR.0b013e32835c36b8

Truong, D. Q., Magerowski, G., Blackburn, G. L., Bikson, M., and Alonso-Alonso, M. (2013). Computational modeling of transcranial direct current stimulation (tDCS) in obesity: impact of head fat and dose guidelines. *Neuroimage Clin.* 2, 759–766. doi: 10.1016/j.nicl.2013.05.011

Wagner, T., Fregni, F., Fecteau, S., Grodzinsky, A., Zahn, M., and Pascual-Leone, A. (2007). Transcranial direct current stimulation: a computer-based human model study. *Neuroimage* 35, 1113–1124. doi: 10.1016/j.neuroimage.2007.01.027

4

Large-scale resting state network correlates of cognitive impairment in Parkinson's disease and related dopaminergic deficits

Alexander V. Lebedev[1]*, Eric Westman[2], Andrew Simmons[3,4], Aleksandra Lebedeva[2], Françoise J. Siepel[1], Joana B. Pereira[2] and Dag Aarsland[1,2]

[1] Department of Psychiatry, Centre for Age-Related Medicine, Stavanger University Hospital, Stavanger, Norway
[2] Department of Neurobiology, Care Sciences and Society, Karolinska Institutet, Stockholm, Sweden
[3] Department of Neuroimaging, Institute of Psychiatry, King's College London, London, UK
[4] NIHR Biomedical Research Centre for Mental Health and Biomedical Research Unit for Dementia, London, UK

Edited by:
Mikhail Lebedev, Duke University, USA

Reviewed by:
Nicola B. Mercuri, University of Rome, Italy
Simon J. G. Lewis, Brain and Mind Research Institute, Australia
Andrew V. Poliakov, Seattle Children's Hospital, USA

***Correspondence:**
Alexander V. Lebedev, Department of Psychiatry, Centre for Age-Related Medicine, Stavanger University Hospital, Armauer Hansens vei 20, 4011 Stavanger, Norway
e-mail: alexander.vl.lebedev@gmail.com

Cognitive impairment is a common non-motor feature of Parkinson's disease (PD). Understanding the neural mechanisms of this deficit is crucial for the development of efficient methods for treatment monitoring and augmentation of cognitive functions in PD patients. The current study aimed to investigate resting state fMRI correlates of cognitive impairment in PD from a large-scale network perspective, and to assess the impact of dopamine deficiency on these networks. Thirty PD patients with resting state fMRI were included from the Parkinson's Progression Marker Initiative (PPMI) database. Eighteen patients from this sample were also scanned with ^{123}I-FP-CIT SPECT. A standardized neuropsychological battery was administered, evaluating verbal memory, visuospatial, and executive cognitive domains. Image preprocessing was performed using an SPM8-based workflow, obtaining time-series from 90 regions-of-interest (ROIs) defined from the AAL brain atlas. The Brain Connectivity Toolbox (BCT) was used to extract nodal strength from all ROIs, and modularity of the cognitive circuitry determined using the meta-analytical software Neurosynth. Brain-behavior covariance patterns between cognitive functions and nodal strength were estimated using Partial Least Squares. Extracted latent variable (LV) scores were matched with the performances in the three cognitive domains (memory, visuospatial, and executive) and striatal dopamine transporter binding ratios (SBR) using linear modeling. Finally, influence of nigrostriatal dopaminergic deficiency on the modularity of the "cognitive network" was analyzed. For the range of deficits studied, better executive performance was associated with increased dorsal fronto-parietal cortical processing and inhibited subcortical and primary sensory involvement. This profile was also characterized by a relative preservation of nigrostriatal dopaminergic function. The profile associated with better memory performance correlated with increased prefronto-limbic processing, and was not associated with presynaptic striatal dopamine uptake. SBR ratios were negatively correlated with modularity of the "cognitive network," suggesting integrative effects of the preserved nigrostriatal dopamine system on this circuitry.

Keywords: parkinson's disease, cognition, dopamine, resting state fMRI, SPECT, graph theory, nodal strength, modularity

INTRODUCTION

Cognitive impairment is a very important and common non-motor feature of Parkinson's disease (PD) with a major impact on patients' and caregivers' quality of life, as well as healthcare costs (Muslimovic et al., 2005; Vossius et al., 2011; Svenningsson et al., 2012). Approximately one-fifth of newly diagnosed PD patients fulfill clinical criteria for mild cognitive impairment (PD-MCI) (Aarsland et al., 2009) and about one-sixth develop dementia after 5 years (Williams-Gray et al., 2009).

Although the exact role and mechanisms of the dopaminergic system in cognition are still a matter of debate, there is no doubt that its preservation is crucial for cognitive functioning of PD patients. Thus, there is strong evidence suggesting that the impairment of at least 3 major dopaminergic pathways (nigrostriatal, mesocortical, mesolimbic) originating in the brainstem play a very important role in cognitive dysfunction associated with PD (Narayanan et al., 2013).

Previous neuroimaging studies assessing brain networks *in vivo* have shown impairment of the dopaminergic pathways and related neural circuits in PD. Numerous studies on cognitive dysfunction associated with PD have revealed structural and functional abnormalities within the cortico-strio-thalamo-cortical circuits, known to be largely modulated by the dopaminergic system (Hirano et al., 2012; Christopher and Strafella, 2013).

Decreased 6-[^{18}F]-fluorodopa (^{18}F-DOPA) uptake in the anterior cingulate cortex, ventral striatum and right caudate nucleus has been found in PD patients with dementia (PDD) compared to PD (Ito et al., 2002). Studies employing Single Photon Emission Computed Tomography (SPECT) with the dopamine transporter-binding ligands (DaTSCAN) also suggest more severe striatal presynaptic dopaminergic deficiency in PDD compared to PD patients, especially in the caudate nuclei (O'Brien et al., 2004). In addition, there is also evidence suggesting an association between striatal ^{18}F-DOPA uptake and executive performance in PD patients (Bruck et al., 2001; Cheesman et al., 2005; Cropley et al., 2008).

Several ^{18}F-fludeoxyglucose Positron Emission Tomography (FDG-PET) studies analyzing brain networks in PD have identified partially overlapping patterns of brain metabolic changes associated with cognitive impairment in multiple domains, suggesting that the PD-related profile of cognitive impairment is associated with reduced glucose metabolism mainly in prefrontal, parietal, hippocampal, and striatal regions (Mentis et al., 2002; Huang et al., 2007a,b; Eidelberg, 2009). $H_2^{15}O$-PET studies have shown an impaired basal ganglia and dorsolateral prefrontal response during executive task performance in PD (Owen et al., 1998; Dagher et al., 2001; Cools et al., 2002).

Functional MRI studies have also revealed abnormalities within the frontal-subcortical circuits in patients with PD. For instance, an abnormal fronto-striatal response during executive task performance has been found in cognitively impaired PD patients compared to non-impaired ones (Lewis et al., 2003). Another fMRI study assessing working memory and motor functions in ON and OFF dopaminergic medication states in PD patients (Mattay et al., 2002) found increased prefrontal and parietal activations during the working memory task performance in the OFF state, which were positively correlated with errors during the task. Studies focusing on set-shifting paradigms have found a PD-associated pattern of prefrontal and parietal response characterized by either reduced or increased activation depending on whether the caudate nucleus was involved in the task (Monchi et al., 2004, 2007).

Notably, a pharmacological fMRI study in healthy subjects revealed a significant effect of L-dopa administration on striatal functional connectivity (Kelly et al., 2009). In addition to its effects on motor networks, L-dopa increased functional connectivity between the ventral striatum and ventrolateral prefrontal cortex, and disrupted connectivity of the striatum with components of the default mode network (Kelly et al., 2009). Impaired deactivation of the default mode network during executive task performance has been reported in several fMRI studies of PD (Tinaz et al., 2008; Van Eimeren et al., 2009). Resting state fMRI studies have reported abnormal cortico-striatal connectivity in PD (Wu et al., 2009; Helmich et al., 2010; Kwak et al., 2010), while L-DOPA administration has been shown to enhance functional connectivity in the frontal areas of the sensorimotor network (Esposito et al., 2013).

The brain is a complex biological system that demonstrates emergent network properties on different scales, even at a cellular and single-structure level (Welsh et al., 2010). At the cellular scale, neocortical neurons are organized into sets of structurally and physiologically merged modules (Mountcastle, 1997), which in turn, are grouped into functionally segregated hypercolumns, wired with inter-modular connections. At the larger scale, system-wide coordination of the brain networks give rise to the coherent dynamic states that support cognitive functions and behavior (Sporns, 2013). Large-scale network architecture of the human brain appears to combine two principles of structural and functional organization. On the one hand, densely connected network modules or communities promote specialized processing and *functional segregation*. On the other hand, these specialized communities are interconnected via long-distance pathways that ensure efficient *functional integration* across multiple functional domains. Maintaining the balance between segregation and integration is thought to be essential for establishing complex network dynamics that support cognition (Sporns, 2010).

Recent advances in neuroscience and mathematical modeling have made it possible to apply classical concepts of graph theory to the analysis of brain network structure and dynamics (Rubinov and Sporns, 2010; Sporns, 2010). Graph-theoretical studies of structural and functional networks of the brain have revealed "small-world" properties (Achard and Bullmore, 2007), i.e., the coexistence of dense local connectivity with relatively sparse long-range connections. Such small-world networks combine high clustering with a relatively short path length between any pair of the elements (e.g., brain regions). The "small-world" model may be of functional importance as it balances functional segregation (high modularity or clustering) and functional integration (short path length) and thus offers a network architecture that may be well-suited for neuronal information processing (Sporns and Zwi, 2004).

To date, there are very few studies of PD employing graph theoretical framework for fMRI data analysis. Skidmore et al. found reduced whole-brain global efficiency in PD (Skidmore et al., 2011). Compared to healthy controls, 14 PD patients included in the study demonstrated reduced local efficiency (nodal level) in the precentral regions, primary and secondary visual cortex. Another recent study found global reduction of network-level processing efficacy in PD. Analysis of network modules indicated decreased interaction of the visual network with other brain modules, but abnormally increased connectivity within the sensorimotor network. The authors interpreted the latter as a compensatory mechanism aimed at overcoming the striato-cortical functional deficit within the motor loops, which may also be associated with loss of mutual inhibition between brain networks (Gottlich et al., 2013).

To the best of our knowledge, there are no previous studies assessing brain correlates of PD-related cognitive impairment employing both dopamine transporter imaging and fMRI with graph theory metrics.

In the present study, we assessed global and local network-level correlates of cognitive dysfunction and related dopaminergic impairment in PD using the graph theory metrics of nodal strength and modularity.

We hypothesized that the PD-related profile of cognitive impairment would be associated mainly with abnormalities within the fronto-subcortical (impaired cortico-striatal connectivity) and fronto-parietal circuits, which are closely related to nigrostriatal deficiency.

METHODS

The main workflow steps are illustrated in **Figure S1**.

INCLUSION AND EXCLUSION CRITERIA

We included all 30 subjects (31 minus one subject excluded during quality control due to "cuts" of dorsal cortical areas) with rs-fMRI enrolled in the Parkinson's Progression Marker Initiative (PPMI) (in total 452 PD patients), a multicenter study launched in 2010 designed to identify progression biomarkers in newly diagnosed PD patients (www.ppmi-info.org/data).

Inclusion criteria required that subjects must have at least two of the following symptoms: resting tremor, bradykinesia, rigidity or either asymmetric resting tremor or asymmetric bradykinesia. In addition, the subjects had to be drug naïve, Hoehn and Yahr stage I or II at baseline, and a screening ^{123}I-FP-CIT SPECT scan, sensitive to the loss of striatal dopamine transporter (DaT) binding.

Exclusion criteria were atypical PD syndromes due to drugs or metabolic disorders, encephalitis, or other degenerative diseases. In addition, it was required that the subject was not taking levodopa, DA agonists, MAO-B inhibitors, amantadine, or other PD medication; or had taken levodopa or dopamine agonists prior to baseline for more than a total of 60 days.

NEUROPSYCHOLOGICAL ASSESSMENT

In addition to a cognitive screening test, the Montreal Cognitive Assessment (MoCA), all subjects underwent a neuropsychological test battery developed to assess major cognitive domains affected by PD.

Visuospatial function was evaluated using the 15-item version of the Benton's Judgment of Line Orientation Test, which examines the ability of a subject to estimate angular relationships between line segments by visually matching angled line pairs to 11 numbered radii forming a semi-circle (Benton et al., 1978).

Verbal memory was assessed using the Hopkins Verbal Learning Test-Revised (HVLT-R) (Shapiro et al., 1999), which consists of presenting a list of 12 words over three learning trials. With each repetition, subjects are expected to learn additional words on the list and increase their performance with each trial. Total immediate recall or encoding (sum of trial 1–3) and delayed recall (after 20–25 min) scores were included in this study.

Executive functions were evaluated using three semantic fluency tests (names of animals, fruits, and vegetables, in 1 min each), the MoCA subtests of phonemic fluency (words that start from the letter "F," in 1 min) and alternating trail making (drawing a line, going from a number to a letter, in ascending order; score 0–1).

Attention was assessed by the Letter-Number Sequencing Test (LNST), in which a combination of numbers and letters is read to the subject who is then asked to recall the numbers, first in ascending order and then the letters in alphabetical order. The Symbol Digit Modalities Test (SDMT) was also used to assess attention, in which specific numbers had to be paired with geometric figures based on a reference key within 90 s.

COGNITIVE DOMAINS

Three cognitive domains were calculated based on the standardized tests for memory, visuospatial, and attention/executive functioning. Raw values were converted to z-scores using the mean and standard deviation of the healthy control group. Domain composite scores were calculated by averaging z-scores of the standardized tests in each cognitive domain.

In the *memory domain*, three learning trials and the delayed recall of HVLT-R were included. The *visuospatial domain* included the Benton judgment of line orientation. The *attention/executive domain* included the LNST, SDMT, semantic fluency, and the phonemic fluency test. No corrections were performed to adjust the tests scores for age or gender given that the subsequent analyses included these variables as nuisances.

Since the calculated composite scores for cognitive domains were scaled and reflected positive cognitive performance (the higher the score, the better functioning in a corresponding domain), we defined the "motor" domain by inverting and scaling UPDRS-III raw scores in order to achieve the same variable scale and direction (higher scores correspond to better motor function) when assessing and plotting the results.

AUTOMATED META-ANALYSIS IN NEUROSYNTH

In order to support our hypotheses and to objectively identify regions that are relevant for cognitive functions, an automated search using the meta-analytical software Neurosynth (http://neurosynth.org) was undertaken. This approach utilizes text-mining and machine-learning techniques to perform probabilistic mapping between neural and cognitive states (Yarkoni et al., 2011). In the present study, the Python-based version (https://github.com/neurosynth/neurosynth) was used. The database was accessed on 24.10.13, searching for the key-words "executive" (237 studies), "visuospatial" ($n = 116$) and "memory" ($n = 1470$).

After the search overlapping patterns were found between cognitive domains. They were in line with the regions that have revealed an association with cognitive impairment in PD highlighted in the introduction. Thus, the profile of visuospatial functions included prefrontal, parietal, and occipital regions. The "executive" pattern contained prefrontal [with more extended involvement of dorsolateral prefrontal cortex (DLPFC)], cingulate, superior parietal, temporo-occipital, basal ganglia, and cerebellar regions. Finally, the "memory" profile, in addition to prefrontal and parietal regions, also included hippocampus, temporal areas, and basal ganglia.

Due to the observed overlap, the resulting statistical maps were merged and overlaid with the Automated Anatomical Labeling (AAL) atlas in order to have an unbiased definition of ROIs associated with cognitive functions for further network analysis. The main steps of the meta-analysis and the resulting maps are illustrated in **Figure S2**.

MRI

Image acquisition

A standardized MRI protocol included acquisition of whole-brain structural and functional scans on 3 Tesla Siemens Trio Tim MR system. More details can be found in the MRI technical operations manual at http://www.ppmi-info.org/.

3D T1 structural images were acquired in a sagittal orientation using a MPRAGE GRAPPA protocol with Repetition Time (TR) = 2300 ms, Echo Time (TE) = 2.98 ms, Field of View (FoV) = 256 mm, Flip Angle (FA) = 9° and 1 mm^3 isotropic voxel.

For each subject, 212 BOLD echo-planar rs-fMRI images (40 slices each, ascending direction) were acquired during a 8 min, 29 s scanning session (acquisition parameters: $TR = 2400$ ms, $TE = 25$ ms, $FoV = 222$ mm, $FA = 80°$ and 3.3 mm^3 isotropic voxels). Subjects were instructed to rest quietly, keeping their eyes open and not to fall asleep.

^{123}I-FP-CIT SPECT

In the fMRI + DaTSCAN subgroup ($n = 18$), only those PD patients who had both fMRI and DaTSCAN acquired within less than a week interval were included.

Image acquisition was performed 4 ± 0.5 h after injection of ^{123}I-FP-CIT, a time-point at which striatal specific binding ratios are stable (Booij et al., 1999) with a target dose of 185 MBq. The radiopharmaceutical was provided as a unit dose and filled to a standard volume, which was re-assayed.

Raw projection data were acquired into a 128 × 128 matrix with steps of 3 or 4 degrees for the total projections. Image preprocessing (reconstruction, attenuation correction, spatial normalization) was performed using the Hermes software (Medical Solutions, Stockholm, Sweden) at a central SPECT Core lab in New Haven (Connecticut, United States). Specific binding ratios were calculated for the left and right caudate nuclei according to specific binding ratio = (L/R Caudate)/(Occipital area) − 1 and then averaged for further analysis.

IMAGE PREPROCESSING

As a first step, a population template was generated from the bias-corrected T1 structural images using the Diffeomorphic Anatomical Registration Through Exponentiated Lie Algebra (DARTEL) algorithm (Ashburner, 2007) in order to improve normalization quality.

For the fMRI data, two initial echo-planar volumes were automatically removed by the scanner software to minimize T1 effects on the T2* echo-planar images, and the remaining 210 volumes underwent preprocessing in the SPM8-based (http://www.fil.ion.ucl.ac.uk/spm) pipeline implemented in the Data Processing Assistant for Resting-State fMRI: Advanced Edition (DPARSFA, version 2.3) (Chao-Gan and Yu-Feng, 2010), installed within the MATLAB environment (Matlab 8.0 and Statistics Toolbox, 2012).

Next, functional images underwent the following preprocessing steps: spatial realignment and slice-timing correction, co-registration with the high-resolution structural scans. Finally, the co-registered BOLD volumes were normalized into standardized Montreal Neurological Institute (MNI) space using the DARTEL template and resampled to 3 mm^3 isotropic voxels. Spurious variance was reduced by a voxel-specific head motion correction (Satterthwaite et al., 2013) and by regressing-out time-series from the white matter and cerebrospinal fluid. Next, the images were band-pass filtered to eliminate biologically non-relevant signals (Biswal et al., 1995; Lowe et al., 1998) (it was not necessary to use large smoothing kernels due to a ROI-based framework implemented in the study), and the resulting low-frequency fluctuations were extracted from 90 regions-of-interest (ROIs) defined in the AAL atlas (Tzourio-Mazoyer et al., 2002) and were used in the subsequent network analysis (Rubinov and Sporns, 2010).

DATA ANALYSIS

Network analysis

The data analysis workflow was developed in order to assess both regional and global network-level correlates of presynaptic DAT uptake and cognitive functions. To do this, two metrics were selected: *nodal strength* (local measure) and *modularity* of a network (global measure).

Generalization of nodal strength and modularity for positive and negative connections

In binarized networks, the number of edges emanating from a particular node is known as its degree. For non-binarized networks, this metric has generalization called nodal strength (weighted degree), defined as the sum of neighboring link weights (Rubinov and Sporns, 2010).

Although the source of negative correlations in rs-fMRI is still a matter of debate (Fox et al., 2009; Murphy et al., 2009), there is strong evidence supporting a biological origin (Chang and Glover, 2009). In light of this, generalizations of several weighted graph theory metrics have been developed taking into account negative correlations (Rubinov and Sporns, 2011).

Thus, nodal strength can be calculated for positive and negative connections. The corresponding definition is straightforward:

$$S_i^{\pm} = \sum_{j \in N} w_{ij}^{\pm} \tag{1}$$

[Equation (1), adopted from Rubinov and Sporns, 2011] Where:

N—set of all nodes in the network;

(i, j)—link between nodes i and j $(i, j \in N)$, associated with connection weights w_{ij} $(0 < |w| < 1)$

Nodal strength can therefore be computed for both positive and negative weights (±). In our analysis, the total strength of both positive and negative weights was used.

A widely used metric for network modularity is formally defined as the fraction of the edges that are within a given set of communities minus the expected fraction of edges if the network was randomly wired (Newman, 2006). The metric therefore serves as a global large-scale network measure that allows quantification of the community structure of the brain. Higher modularity values for a particular network are generally associated with denser within-modular connections, but sparser connections between nodes that are in different modules.

Generalization of the modularity to both positive and negative correlations is more complex than nodal strength due to the differences in significance of positive and negative weights when determining modularity-partitions. Therefore, a non-symmetric generalization of network modularity has been proposed as:

$$Q^* = Q^+ + \frac{v^-}{v^+ + v^-}Q^- \tag{2a}$$

or more complete definition:

$$Q^* = \frac{1}{v^+}\sum_{ij}\left(w_{ij}^+ - e_{ij}^+\right)\delta_{M_iM_j} - \frac{v^-}{v^+ + v^-}\sum_{ij}\left(w_{ij}^- - e_{ij}^-\right)\delta_{M_iM_j} \tag{2b}$$

Both equations are adopted from Rubinov and Sporns (2011)

Where:

$Q^{\pm}$—modularity;

$\left(w_{ij}^{\pm} - e_{ij}^{\pm}\right)$—difference between present within-module connection weights w and chance-expected within-module connection weights e;

$\delta_{M_iM_j} = 1$, when i and j are in the same module and $\delta_{M_iM_j} = 0$ otherwise.

$v^{\pm} = \sum_{i \in N} s_i^{\pm}$—total weight (the sum of all positive or negative weights)

The Brain Connectivity Toolbox (BCT, http://www.brain-connectivity-toolbox.net) (Rubinov and Sporns, 2010) was used to compute the described measures. Of note, connectivity matrices were neither thresholded nor binarized. Instead we employed a strategy that aimed to analyze weighted graphs by taking into account both positive and negative weights.

Next, the analysis proceeded in two directions with the aim of assessing local and global network-level correlates of cognitive functioning in PD and the impact of nigrostriatal dopaminergic deficiency on these networks.

All statistical analyses were performed using the R programming language, version 3.0.1 (R Core Team, 2013).

Dimensionality reduction: covariance patterns between nodal strength and cognitive functions

Partial Least Squares Regression (PLSR) was performed to reduce the dimensionality of the data, estimating latent components associated with composite scores for each domain (executive, memory, visuospatial).

PLSR is an effective data-driven method that allows high-dimensional associations between explanatory and response variables to be reduced into a small set of latent variables (LVs) (Wold et al., 1984). After decomposition, each of the LVs represents a distinct pattern of brain–behavior associations.

The following elements of these components were of particular interest in our study: (1) eigenvector (loadings) showing the degree to which a given LV contributes to the variance within the X-matrix (in our case, brain network measures), and (2) a set of scores representing a transform of a particular data-point into a latent component's space (the degree to which a given component is "represented" in a particular subject).

The models were assessed with leave-one-out cross-validation. As a result, 3 LVs minimizing total Root Mean Squared Error Prediction (RMSEP) for all 3 domains were selected. For details, see **Figure S3**. Individual LV scores were subsequently correlated with 3 cognitive domains using motor function, age, and sex as nuisance covariates.

GLM formula:

$$\begin{aligned} LV_N\text{−score} \sim {} & \text{(executive domain)} + \text{(memory domain)} \\ & + \text{(visuospatial domain)} + \text{(motor domain)} \\ & + \text{(age)} + \text{(sex)}. \end{aligned} \tag{3}$$

Finally, the scores were correlated with mean caudate DaT binding ratios in order to investigate which of them were influenced by nigrostriatal dopamine deficiency. The analysis was focused only on the caudate nuclei (without putamen), as this striatal structure is well-documented to be involved in cognition.

Due to the concerns regarding potential influence of motion artifacts, in addition to a voxel-specific correction strategy (Satterthwaite et al., 2013), analysis of motion with respect to the variables of interest (cognitive, motor domains, and age) was also performed. For this purpose, first principal component extracted from the absolute mean displacement values (x, y, and z axes) as well as relative displacements were used.

None of our variables of interest (executive, memory, and visuospatial domains) demonstrated significant association. The only significant associations were found for the motor domain ($p_{\text{mean displacement}} = 0.036$; $p_{\text{relative displacement}} = 0.035$) and age ($p_{\text{mean displacement}} = 0.026$), as expected. These variables were included in the modes as nuisance covariates.

Impact of nigrostriatal deficiency on the modularity of cognitive brain circuitry

For the second part, adjacency matrices were constructed using 60 AAL ROIs identified during the meta-analysis step (see Meta-Analysis section and **Figure S2**). Next, modularity was estimated based on both negative and positive weights [as described in Equations 2a and 2b].

Finally, an association between network modularity and mean DaT uptake in the caudate nuclei was analyzed using linear modeling.

RESULTS

DEMOGRAPHICS AND CLINICAL DATA

Demographics and clinical characteristics are shown in **Table 1**.

The data were representative of the entire DaTSCAN cohort of PD patients (results not shown). Of note, visuospatial functions were relatively less affected than executive and memory domains.

GRAPH THEORETICAL ANALYSIS

Brain-behavior covariance patterns

The analysis was performed with PLS LV-scores determined after the dimensionality reduction step (see corresponding Methods section).

Nodal strength

The first PLS LV captured global effects. Its higher scores were associated with higher strength of all 90 nodes with largest effects on motor, prefrontal cortices, and striatum. On a behavioral level,

Table 1 | Demographics and clinical data.

	Complete sample (n = 30)		Subsample* (n = 18)	
	Mean [±SD]	**Median (range)**	**Mean [±SD]**	**Median (range)**
Age	61.67 [±9.46]	62 (40–75)	60.11 [±9.04]	61 (44–75)
MoCA	26.67 [±3]	27 (15–30)	26.72 [±3.5]	27 (15–30)
ExecDom	−0.254 [±0.73]	−0.125 (−1.37–1.26)	−0.297 [±0.67]	−0.125 (−1.35–0.99)
MemDom	−0.51 [±1.2]	−0.41 (−2.81–1.47)	−0.73 [±1.26]	−0.51 (−2.81–1.25)
VspDom	0.06 [±0.78]	−0.06 (−1.57–0.95)	0.08 [±0.84]	0.44 (−1.57–0.95)
UPDRS III	20.2 [±10.6]	17 (7–47)	19.83 [±10.9]	17 (7–47)

Male/Female ratio was 2:1.

**Subsample of subjects who had both fMRI and DaTSCAN acquired within less than a week interval.*

MoCA, the Montreal Cognitive Assessment; ExecDom, "Executive" domain; MemDom, "Memory" domain; VspDom, "Visuospatial" domain; UPDRS III, part III of the Unified Parkinson's Disease Rating Scale.

Table 2 | Associations between component scores and behavioral data: nodal strength.

	Executive			Memory			Visuospatial			Motor		
	T	**DOF**	***p***	***T***	**DOF**	***p***	***T***	**DOF**	***p***	***T***	**DOF**	***p***
LV I	0.782	29	0.442	1.35	29	0.19	−0.89	29	0.383	3	29	0.006
LV II	−0.656	29	0.518	−2.45	29	0.022	−1.74	29	0.094	1.327	29	0.127
LV III	3.21	29	0.004	−1.74	29	0.096	1.65	29	0.113	−2.02	29	0.055

The table shows associations between latent variable (LV) scores extracted from the nodal strength data and performance in 3 cognitive (executive, memory, visuospatial) and motor domains. Positive significant associations are depicted in red and negative ones in blue.

In total, 3 models were fitted with component scores as dependent variables, cognitive domains as independent variables (other covariates: motor domain score [also shown here as an important confounder], age and sex).

T, t-statistics; ***DOF****, degrees of freedom.*

this component was positively associated with motor function (see **Table 2**, **Figure 1**).

The second LV was associated with higher degree of posterior (supramarginal, superior parietal, posterior cingulate, occipital regions) and striatal nodes, and lower prefronto-limbic (orbitofrontal, anterior cingulate, parahippocampal, temporopolar regions) nodal strength (except for operculo-triangular, middle frontal areas, and left hippocampus, which demonstrated positive associations). Behaviorally, this component displayed a negative association with memory function, that is to say that better memory performance was associated with reversed component pattern, favoring the involvement of prefronto-limbic nodes (see **Table 2**, **Figure 1**).

The third LV, in turn, favored cortical-subcortical segregation with positive associations found in dorsal cortical nodes (dorsolateral prefrontal, frontal and parietal areas) and negative in subcortical structures (hippocampi, striatum, globus pallidus), primary visual, middle temporal, and paralimbic (ventral prefrontal) areas. Higher scores of this component were associated with better executive performance (see **Table 2**, **Figure 1**).

Latent variable scores and caudate DaT uptake

Analysis of the effects of nigrostriatal dopaminergic deficiency on the LVs estimated from the nodal strength revealed significant positive associations of mean caudate SBR ratios with I and III LV-scores (See **Table 3**, **Figure 2**).

This means that higher caudate DaT binding is associated with global increase of nodal strength and segregation toward more active dorsal cortical processing when the subject is at rest.

Modularity of the cognitive circuitry and caudate DaT binding

The analysis revealed negative effects of the preserved dopaminergic function on modularity of the cognitive circuit ($T = -3.6$, 17 DOF, $p = 0.002$), suggesting greater integration among regions within this network (see **Figure 3**).

DISCUSSION

To the best of our knowledge, this is the first study to assess large-scale network correlates of PD-related cognitive impairment and presynaptic dopaminergic deficiency, combining rs-fMRI and DaTSCAN. Higher executive functional scores were associated with higher nodal strength of dorsal cortical nodes (predominantly in dorsolateral prefrontal, premotor, and superior parietal regions) and lower involvement of subcortical, occipital, temporal, and ventral cortical nodes, suggesting that relative preservation of executive functions in PD is linked to the dominance of dorsal cortical processing with inhibition of subcortical, paralimbic, and primary sensory circuitry when the subject is at resting state with eyes open. This pattern was positively influenced by higher nigrostriatal dopaminergic function.

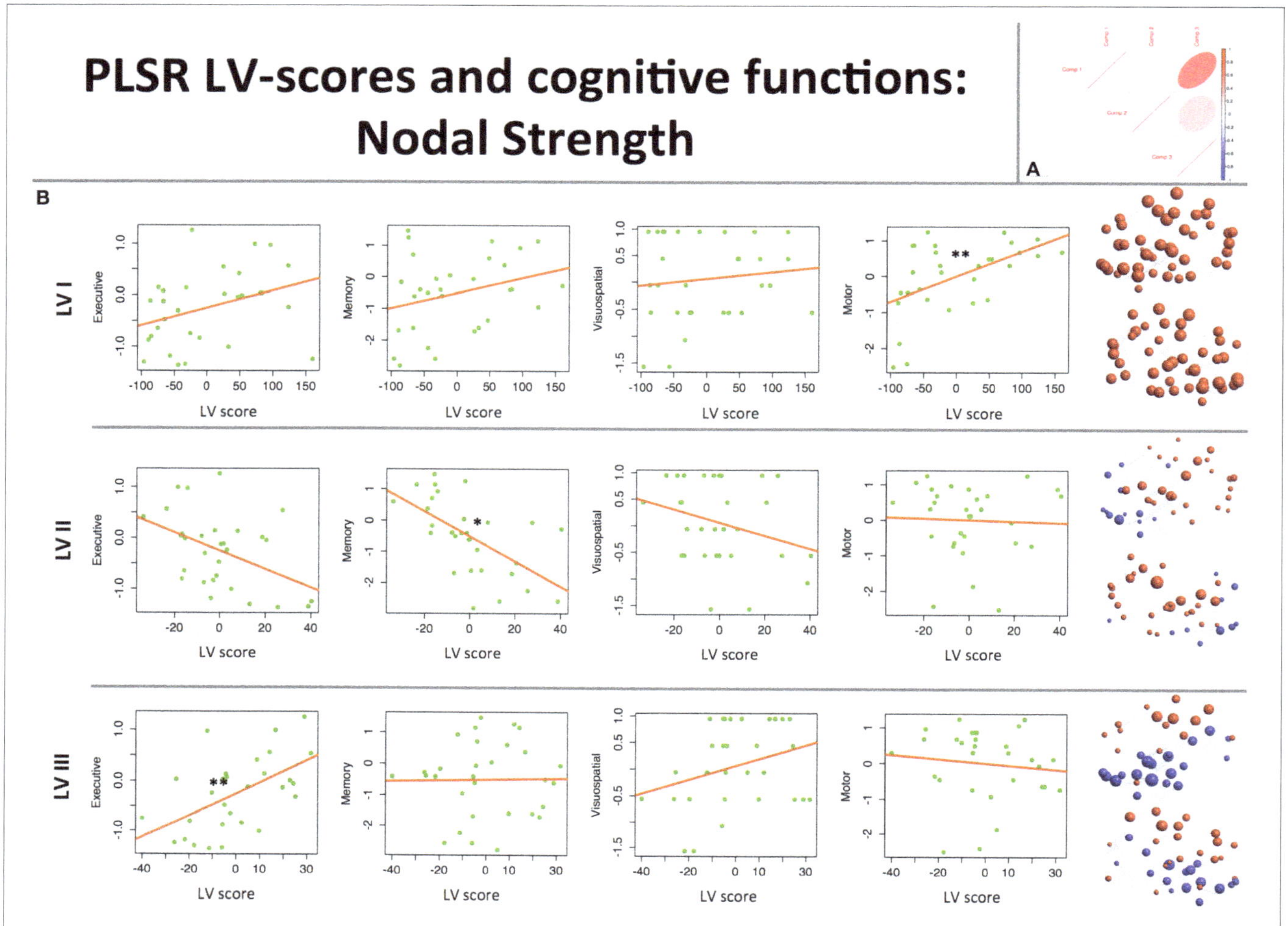

FIGURE 1 | Associations between component scores and behavioral data: nodal strength. (A) Between-component correlation plot. Positive association ($r = 0.5$) was found between latent variables (LVs) I and III. **(B)** Associations between LV scores extracted from the nodal strength data and performance in 3 cognitive (executive, memory, visuospatial) and motor domains. On the right-hand side of the graph, corresponding loading maps are depicted in brain space, reflecting the relevance of the nodes (spheres) for a particular LV, the magnitude of which is represented by nodal size. Positive loading values are depicted as red spheres, whereas negative ones are shown in blue. $^{*}p < 0.05$, $^{**}p < 0.01$.

Our results are consistent with an abnormally increased fronto-striatal connectivity found in a single-blind placebo-controlled rs-fMRI study of PD patients (Kwak et al., 2010), in which this hyperconnectivity was down-regulated by L-DOPA administration. Further analysis in this study revealed PD-related increase of power in the low-frequency band (0.02–0.05 Hz) in the striatum, which was also reduced after L-DOPA administration. Of note, this reduction correlated with L-DOPA-associated cognitive improvement. Apart from this, an increase in spontaneous oscillatory activity in the 10–35 Hz range (beta frequency band), occurring within the basal ganglia-thalamocortical networks and suppressed by dopaminergic treatment, is a well-replicated pathophysiological finding in PD (Brown et al., 2001; Levy et al., 2002; Gatev et al., 2006; Hammond et al., 2007), which provides additional support of our results converging from other imaging modalities.

The pattern associated with higher scores in the memory domain favoring prefronto-limbic processing did not reveal associations with presynaptic striatal dopamine uptake in the present study. The latter suggests that other mechanisms may be involved in the development of memory impairment associated with PD. The most likely ones are mesocortical dopaminergic deficiency (Narayanan et al., 2013) and impaired cortical cholinergic function (Bohnen et al., 2003), which in turn may at least be partly associated with concomitant cortical atrophy (Weintraub et al., 2012).

Of note, our study did not find any correlates of visuospatial impairment. However, this finding may be influenced by small sample size and due to the fact that visuospatial function was only mildly affected in the present cohort.

According to Mink's hypothesis (Mink, 1996), the basal ganglia play a crucial role in sustaining the balance between facilitation and suppression of movements. If we consider executive functions as the "movement of thoughts" a similar analogy can be drawn within this context. Indeed, cognitive frontal-subcortical loops is a widely accepted notion, where the DLPFC circuit has been documented to mediate set-shifting, complex problem-solving, retrieval abilities, organizational strategies, concept-formation, working memory (Zgaljardic et al., 2006), and other executive functions that are known to be affected in PD. Preserved nigrostriatal dopamine function therefore not only allows effective execution and termination of motor activity, but may also implement smooth switching between cognitive patterns, controlling mutual inhibition and/or facilitation of fronto-subcortical circuits. This is also supported by computational models of the basal ganglia that highlight their routing role in various cognitive functions, such as for example action-selection (Stocco et al., 2010).

Table 3 | Latent variable scores and mean caudate DaT binding.

	CN DaT binding		
	T	**DOF**	***p***
LV I	2.87	17	0.011
LV II	−0.096	17	0.925
LV III	2.281	17	0.037

The table shows associations of the PLS latent variables (LVs) extracted during the dimensionality reduction step with nigrostriatal dopaminergic function measured by ^{123}I-FP-CIT SPECT (mean caudate SBR ratios). Positive significant associations (depicted in red) were found for LVs I ("global/motor") and III ("executive").

CN, Caudate Nucleus; DaT, Dopamine Transporter; ***T****, t-statistics;* ***DOF****, degrees of freedom.*

In general, higher DaT binding values were associated with global integrative effects on the brain (global increase of nodal strength). This was also confirmed for the cognitive circuitry (defined during meta-analysis), where higher DaT SBR ratios (relative preservation of dopaminergic function) were associated with lower network-level modularity, suggesting that dopamine favors integration of the cognitive network when the subject is at rest. These results are in line with previous fMRI studies that indicated globally impaired network-level processing in PD (Skidmore et al., 2011; Gottlich et al., 2013). Negative effects of the preserved dopaminergic function on the modularity of cognitive circuitry are also in line with previous literature. Thus, a recent randomized double-blind rs-fMRI study of healthy subjects with bromocriptine administration (dopamine agonist) revealed drug-induced decreases in modularity, estimated for the whole brain (White et al., 2013). Our results also suggest that preserved nigrostriatal dopaminergic system allows supporting integrity of the cognitive network when a subject is at rest. In

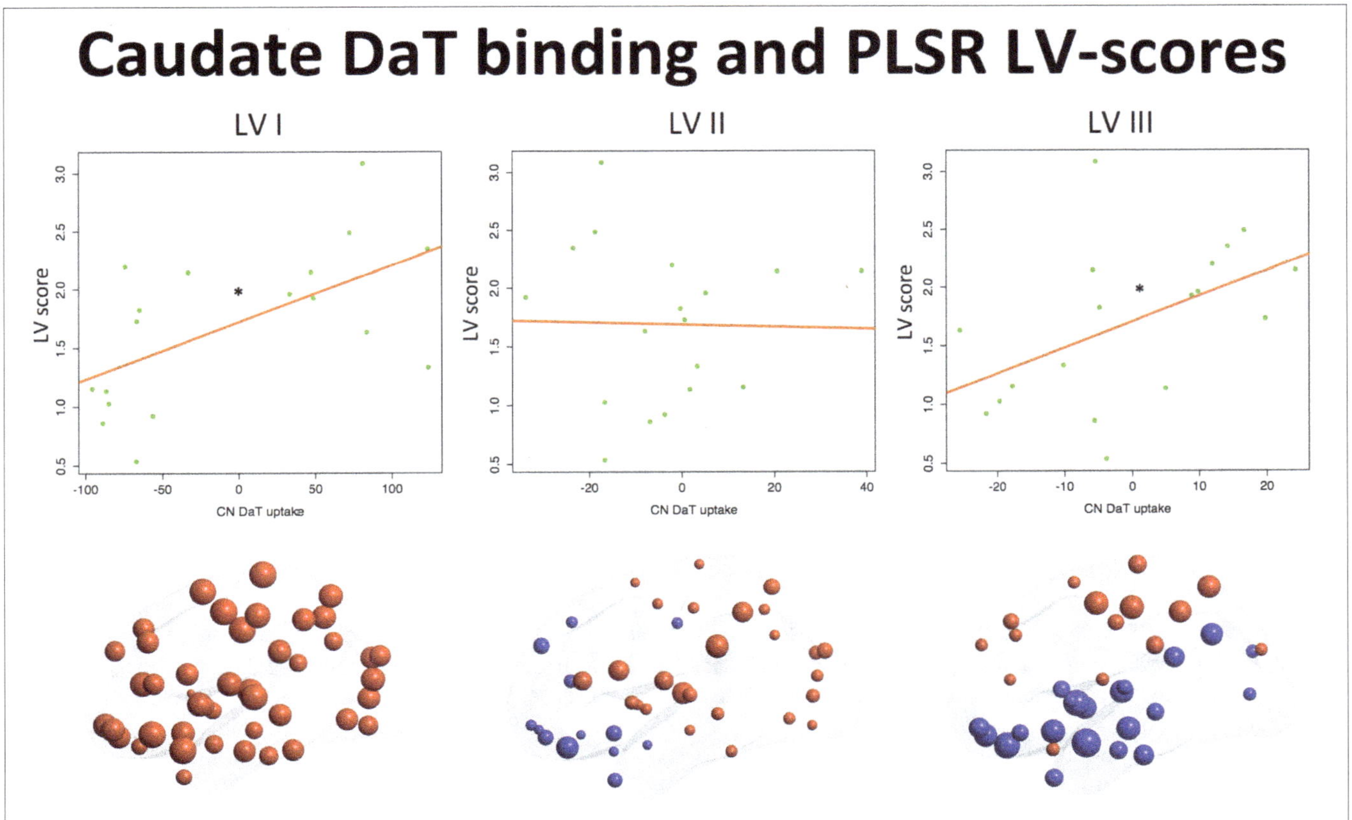

FIGURE 2 | Associations between component scores and mean caudate DaT binding. Associations of latent variable (LV) scores extracted from the nodal strength data with nigrostriatal dopaminergic function measured by ^{123}I-FP-CIT SPECT (mean caudate SBR ratios). Positive associations (*$p < 0.05$) were found for the Ist ("global/motor") and IIIrd ("executive") LVs. Corresponding loading maps are depicted in brain space, reflecting the relevance of the nodes (spheres) for a particular LV, the magnitude of which is represented by nodal size. Positive loading values are depicted as red spheres, whereas negative ones are shown in blue.

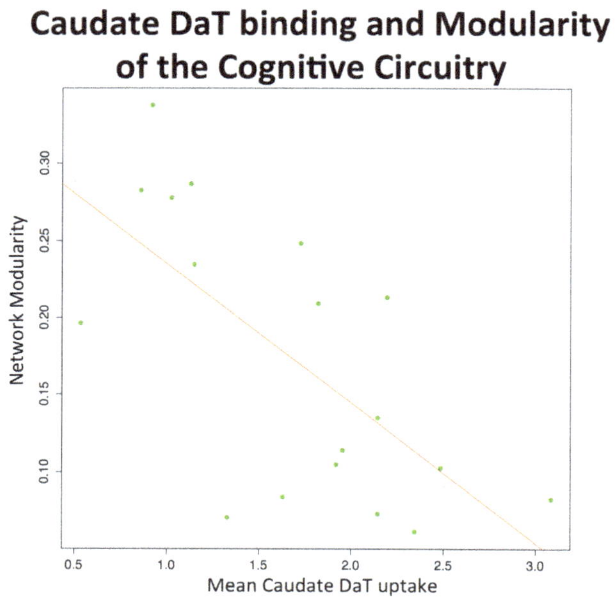

FIGURE 3 | Caudate DaT uptake and modularity of the cognitive circuitry at rest. The figure shows significant ($p < 0.01$) negative association between modularity of the cognitive circuitry (identified with automated meta-analysis) and nigrostriatal dopaminergic function measured by ^{123}I-FP-CIT SPECT (mean caudate SBR ratios).

the light of this, it would be interesting to assess the dynamics of cognitive circuitry during performance of particular executive tasks or multi-tasking, where dopamine may have different or even opposite effects on network modularity. This is supported by previous functional imaging studies of executive functions in PD, revealing that hypodopaminergic states are associated with increased prefrontal cortical responses during performance of corresponding tasks (Mattay et al., 2002), whereas L-dopa administration, in contrast, decreases it (Cools et al., 2002). In this context, it is also worth mentioning an event-related fMRI study that found PD-related brain abnormalities during performance of the set-shifting task specifically developed to elicit caudate responses (Monchi et al., 2007). Compared to the control group, patients demonstrated increased cortical activation in the condition not specifically requiring the caudate nucleus, whereas decreased cortical activation was observed in the task that involved the caudate nucleus. These studies, however, are not focused on any specific dopaminergic system, looking at general dopamine-related effects instead, and therefore do not necessarily confirm the role of exactly nigrostriatal dopaminergic system in these phenomena.

Finally, a recently published graph theoretical MEG study with longitudinal design found that progression of PD is associated with growing impairment of local integration (measured by clustering coefficient) in multiple frequency bands and loss of global brain network efficiency (based on path length) in the alpha2 frequency band. This deterioration was, in turn, correlated with cognitive and motor impairment observed during disease progression (Olde Dubbelink et al., 2014). These findings provide additional support for our results, also suggesting global positive effects of dopaminergic preservation on efficient functioning of the brain networks.

The main limitation of the present study is a relatively small sample size. In addition, the cross-sectional design complicates causal interpretation of the results. Apart from this, the resting state setting itself hampers direct interpretation of the findings with regard to the role of brain networks in cognitive task performance. Active cognitive processing is likely associated with patterns of brain dynamics that are different compared to the ones occurring when the subject is at rest. These patterns in turn may have different associations with altered dopaminergic function in PD. Therefore, this presents a need for further studies of brain dynamics underlying cognitive processing in PD and related dopaminergic deficits.

The main strengths are a multimodal approach and graph theoretical setting that have not yet been implemented together for clarifying brain mechanisms of PD-related cognitive impairment. Further strengths are a relatively broad cognitive evaluation combining multiple tests to assess three major functional domains and the drug-naïve status of the participants. Of note, although the present study specifically investigated the nigrostriatal system, the deficiency measured by ^{123}I-FP-CIT SPECT might also reflect indirect effects of neurodegeneration of dopaminergic neurons within other pathways, since the severity of dopaminergic deficits may correlate across different systems. Therefore, the results should be interpreted with caution.

To summarize, our study found that PD-related executive impairment is associated with altered balance between cortical and subcortical processing at rest, when contribution of the dorsal cortex is getting abnormally suppressed, and subcortical processing is disinhibited. This pattern (unlike brain profiles of visuospatial and memory impairment) is linked to nigrostriatal deficiency, which also has disruptive effects on cognitive circuitry at the network scale.

The results provide evidence for the contribution of the nigrostrital dopaminergic system in human cognition, and the described concept can potentially be utilized in future interventional studies to monitor the effects of treatments, including the approaches that augment cognitive functions.

ACKNOWLEDGMENTS

Data used in the preparation of this article were obtained from the Parkinson's Progression Markers Initiative (PPMI) database (www.ppmi-info.org/data). For up-to-date information on the study, visit www.ppmi-info.org. PPMI—a public-private partnership—is funded by the Michael J. Fox Foundation for Parkinson's Research and funding partners, including Abbott, Avid, Biogen Idec, Bristol-Myers Squibb, Covance, Elan, GlaxoSmithKline, Lilly, Merck, UCB, F. Hoffman-La Roche Ltd., GE Healthcare, Genentech, and Pfizer Inc. The authors are grateful to Dr. Olaf Sporns (Indiana University, USA) for the valuable discussions we had when working on the manuscript. Alexander V. Lebedev was supported by the Helse Vest Strategic Funding 2013 and MoodNet. Joana B. Pereira was funded by a Marie Curie fellowship for postdoctoral researchers (call FP7-PEOPLE-2012-IEF).

SUPPLEMENTARY MATERIAL

Figure S1 | Study Workflow. The study workflow consisted of IV main steps: (I) Selection of 30 PD subjects with fMRI data from the complete PPMI cohort and an fMRI + DaTSCAN subsample of 18 subjects; (II) Preparation of the data for further analysis that, in turn, included (IIa) calculation of composite scores for 3 cognitive domains, (IIb) automated meta-analysis to define "cognitive network," (IIc) image preprocessing and network measure extraction; (III) Dimensionality reduction with PLS followed by parametric tests evaluating associations between latent variable (LV) scores and cognitive functions; (IV) Final analysis assessing influence of caudate dopamine transporter (DaT) uptake on LV scores and modularity of the "cognitive network.

Figure S2 | Automated meta-analysis workflow. An automated search using the meta-analytical software Neurosynth (http://neurosynth.org) was undertaken in order to identify regions that are relevant for cognitive functions. The key-words "executive" (237 studies), "visuospatial" ($n = 116$) and "memory" ($n = 1470$). The profile of visuospatial functions included prefrontal, parietal, and occipital regions. The "executive" pattern contained prefrontal (with more extended involvement of DLPFC), cingulate, superior parietal, temporo-occipital, basal ganglia, and cerebellar regions. Finally, the "memory" profile, in addition to prefrontal and parietal regions, also included hippocampus, temporal areas, and basal ganglia. Due to the observed overlap, the resulting statistical maps were merged and overlaid with the Automated Anatomical Labeling (AAL) atlas defining cognitive circuitry, the modularity of which was then correlated with nigrostriatal function measured by ^{123}I-FP-CIT Single-Photon Emission Computed Tomography.

Figure S3 | Latent variable selection. The figure shows Root Mean Squared Error Prediction (RMSEP) as a function of a number of PLS latent variables (LVs). The maximum number of LVs was selected that minimized total training (red dashed line) and leave-one-out cross-validation (green solid line) errors for all the domains ($n = 3$).

REFERENCES

Aarsland, D., Bronnick, K., Larsen, J. P., Tysnes, O. B., Alves, G., and Norwegian Parkwest Study, G. (2009). Cognitive impairment in incident, untreated Parkinson disease: the Norwegian ParkWest study. *Neurology* 72, 1121–1126. doi: 10.1212/01.wnl.0000338632.00552.cb

Achard, S., and Bullmore, E. (2007). Efficiency and cost of economical brain functional networks. *PLoS Comput. Biol.* 3:e17. doi: 10.1371/journal.pcbi.0030017

Ashburner, J. (2007). A fast diffeomorphic image registration algorithm. *Neuroimage* 38, 95–113. doi: 10.1016/j.neuroimage.2007.07.007

Benton, A. L., Varney, N. R., and Hamsher, K. D. (1978). Visuospatial judgment. A clinical test. *Arch. Neurol.* 35, 364–367. doi: 10.1001/archneur.1978.00500300038006

Biswal, B., Yetkin, F. Z., Haughton, V. M., and Hyde, J. S. (1995). Functional connectivity in the motor cortex of resting human brain using echo-planar MRI. *Magn. Reson. Med.* 34, 537–541. doi: 10.1002/mrm.1910340409

Bohnen, N. I., Kaufer, D. I., Ivanco, L. S., Lopresti, B., Koeppe, R. A., Davis, J. G., et al. (2003). Cortical cholinergic function is more severely affected in parkinsonian dementia than in Alzheimer disease: an *in vivo* positron emission tomographic study. *Arch. Neurol.* 60, 1745–1748. doi: 10.1001/archneur.60.12.1745

Booij, J., Hemelaar, T. G., Speelman, J. D., De Bruin, K., Janssen, A. G., and Van Royen, E. A. (1999). One-day protocol for imaging of the nigrostriatal dopaminergic pathway in Parkinson's disease by [1231]FPCIT SPECT. *J. Nucl. Med.* 40, 753–761.

Brown, P., Oliviero, A., Mazzone, P., Insola, A., Tonali, P., and Di Lazzaro, V. (2001). Dopamine dependency of oscillations between subthalamic nucleus and pallidum in Parkinson's disease. *J. Neurosci.* 21, 1033–1038.

Bruck, A., Portin, R., Lindell, A., Laihinen, A., Bergman, J., Haaparanta, M., et al. (2001). Positron emission tomography shows that impaired frontal lobe functioning in Parkinson's disease is related to dopaminergic hypofunction in the caudate nucleus. *Neurosci. Lett.* 311, 81–84. doi: 10.1016/S0304-3940(01)02124-3

Chang, C., and Glover, G. H. (2009). Effects of model-based physiological noise correction on default mode network anti-correlations and correlations. *Neuroimage* 47, 1448–1459. doi: 10.1016/j.neuroimage.2009.05.012

Chao-Gan, Y., and Yu-Feng, Z. (2010). DPARSF: a MATLAB toolbox for "pipeline" data analysis of resting-state fMRI. *Front. Syst. Neurosci.* 4:13. doi: 10.3389/fnsys.2010.00013

Cheesman, A. L., Barker, R. A., Lewis, S. J., Robbins, T. W., Owen, A. M., and Brooks, D. J. (2005). Lateralisation of striatal function: evidence from 18F-dopa PET in Parkinson's disease. *J. Neurol. Neurosurg. Psychiatry* 76, 1204–1210. doi: 10.1136/jnnp.2004.055079

Christopher, L., and Strafella, A. P. (2013). Neuroimaging of brain changes associated with cognitive impairment in Parkinson's disease. *J. Neuropsychol.* 7, 225–240. doi: 10.1111/jnp.12015

Cools, R., Stefanova, E., Barker, R. A., Robbins, T. W., and Owen, A. M. (2002). Dopaminergic modulation of high-level cognition in Parkinson's disease: the role of the prefrontal cortex revealed by PET. *Brain* 125, 584–594. doi: 10.1093/brain/awf052

Cropley, V. L., Fujita, M., Bara-Jimenez, W., Brown, A. K., Zhang, X. Y., Sangare, J., et al. (2008). Pre- and post-synaptic dopamine imaging and its relation with frontostriatal cognitive function in Parkinson disease: PET studies with [11C]NNC 112 and [18F]FDOPA. *Psychiatry Res.* 163, 171–182. doi: 10.1016/j.pscychresns.2007.11.003

Dagher, A., Owen, A. M., Boecker, H., and Brooks, D. J. (2001). The role of the striatum and hippocampus in planning: a PET activation study in Parkinson's disease. *Brain* 124, 1020–1032. doi: 10.1093/brain/124.5.1020

Eidelberg, D. (2009). Metabolic brain networks in neurodegenerative disorders: a functional imaging approach. *Trends Neurosci.* 32, 548–557. doi: 10.1016/j.tins.2009.06.003

Esposito, F., Tessitore, A., Giordano, A., De Micco, R., Paccone, A., Conforti, R., et al. (2013). Rhythm-specific modulation of the sensorimotor network in drug-naive patients with Parkinson's disease by levodopa. *Brain* 136, 710–725. doi: 10.1093/brain/awt007

Fox, M. D., Zhang, D., Snyder, A. Z., and Raichle, M. E. (2009). The global signal and observed anticorrelated resting state brain networks. *J. Neurophysiol.* 101, 3270–3283. doi: 10.1152/jn.90777.2008

Gatev, P., Darbin, O., and Wichmann, T. (2006). Oscillations in the basal ganglia under normal conditions and in movement disorders. *Mov. Disord.* 21, 1566–1577. doi: 10.1002/mds.21033

Gottlich, M., Munte, T. F., Heldmann, M., Kasten, M., Hagenah, J., and Kramer, U. M. (2013). Altered resting state brain networks in Parkinson's disease. *PLoS ONE* 8:e77336. doi: 10.1371/journal.pone.0077336

Hammond, C., Bergman, H., and Brown, P. (2007). Pathological synchronization in Parkinson's disease: networks, models and treatments. *Trends Neurosci.* 30, 357–364. doi: 10.1016/j.tins.2007.05.004

Helmich, R. C., Derikx, L. C., Bakker, M., Scheeringa, R., Bloem, B. R., and Toni, I. (2010). Spatial remapping of cortico-striatal connectivity in Parkinson's disease. *Cereb. Cortex* 20, 1175–1186. doi: 10.1093/cercor/bhp178

Hirano, S., Shinotoh, H., and Eidelberg, D. (2012). Functional brain imaging of cognitive dysfunction in Parkinson's disease. *J. Neurol. Neurosurg. Psychiatry* 83, 963–969. doi: 10.1136/jnnp-2011-301818

Huang, C., Mattis, P., Tang, C., Perrine, K., Carbon, M., and Eidelberg, D. (2007a). Metabolic brain networks associated with cognitive function in Parkinson's disease. *Neuroimage* 34, 714–723. doi: 10.1016/j.neuroimage.2006.09.003

Huang, C., Tang, C., Feigin, A., Lesser, M., Ma, Y., Pourfar, M., et al. (2007b). Changes in network activity with the progression of Parkinson's disease. *Brain* 130, 1834–1846. doi: 10.1093/brain/awm086

Ito, K., Nagano-Saito, A., Kato, T., Arahata, Y., Nakamura, A., Kawasumi, Y., et al. (2002). Striatal and extrastriatal dysfunction in Parkinson's disease with dementia: a 6-[18F]fluoro-L-dopa PET study. *Brain* 125, 1358–1365. doi: 10.1093/brain/awf134

Kelly, C., De Zubicaray, G., Di Martino, A., Copland, D. A., Reiss, P. T., Klein, D. F., et al. (2009). L-dopa modulates functional connectivity in striatal cognitive and motor networks: a double-blind placebo-controlled study. *J. Neurosci.* 29, 7364–7378. doi: 10.1523/JNEUROSCI.0810-09.2009

Kwak, Y., Peltier, S., Bohnen, N. I., Muller, M. L., Dayalu, P., and Seidler, R. D. (2010). Altered resting state cortico-striatal connectivity in mild to moderate stage Parkinson's disease. *Front. Syst. Neurosci.* 4:143. doi: 10.3389/fnsys.2010.00143

Levy, R., Ashby, P., Hutchison, W. D., Lang, A. E., Lozano, A. M., and Dostrovsky, J. O. (2002). Dependence of subthalamic nucleus oscillations on movement and dopamine in Parkinson's disease. *Brain* 125, 1196–1209. doi: 10.1093/brain/awf128

Lewis, S. J., Dove, A., Robbins, T. W., Barker, R. A., and Owen, A. M. (2003). Cognitive impairments in early Parkinson's disease are accompanied by reductions in activity in frontostriatal neural circuitry. *J. Neurosci.* 23, 6351–6356.

Lowe, M. J., Mock, B. J., and Sorenson, J. A. (1998). Functional connectivity in single and multislice echoplanar imaging using resting-state fluctuations. *Neuroimage* 7, 119–132. doi: 10.1006/nimg.1997.0315

Matlab 8.0 and Statistics Toolbox 8.1. (2012). T. M., Inc., Natick, MA, USA.

Mattay, V. S., Tessitore, A., Callicott, J. H., Bertolino, A., Goldberg, T. E., Chase, T. N., et al. (2002). Dopaminergic modulation of cortical function in patients with Parkinson's disease. *Ann. Neurol.* 51, 156–164. doi: 10.1002/ana.10078

Mentis, M. J., McIntosh, A. R., Perrine, K., Dhawan, V., Berlin, B., Feigin, A., et al. (2002). Relationships among the metabolic patterns that correlate with mnemonic, visuospatial, and mood symptoms in Parkinson's disease. *Am. J. Psychiatry* 159, 746–754. doi: 10.1176/appi.ajp.159.5.746

Mink, J. W. (1996). The basal ganglia: focused selection and inhibition of competing motor programs. *Prog. Neurobiol.* 50, 381–425. doi: 10.1016/S0301-0082(96)00042-1

Monchi, O., Petrides, M., Doyon, J., Postuma, R. B., Worsley, K., and Dagher, A. (2004). Neural bases of set-shifting deficits in Parkinson's disease. *J. Neurosci.* 24, 702–710. doi: 10.1523/JNEUROSCI.4860-03.2004

Monchi, O., Petrides, M., Mejia-Constain, B., and Strafella, A. P. (2007). Cortical activity in Parkinson's disease during executive processing depends on striatal involvement. *Brain* 130, 233–244. doi: 10.1093/brain/awl326

Mountcastle, V. B. (1997). The columnar organization of the neocortex. *Brain* 120(Pt 4), 701–722. doi: 10.1093/brain/120.4.701

Murphy, K., Birn, R. M., Handwerker, D. A., Jones, T. B., and Bandettini, P. A. (2009). The impact of global signal regression on resting state correlations: are anti-correlated networks introduced? *Neuroimage* 44, 893–905. doi: 10.1016/j.neuroimage.2008.09.036

Muslimovic, D., Post, B., Speelman, J. D., and Schmand, B. (2005). Cognitive profile of patients with newly diagnosed Parkinson disease. *Neurology* 65, 1239–1245. doi: 10.1212/01.wnl.0000180516.69442.95

Narayanan, N. S., Rodnitzky, R. L., and Uc, E. Y. (2013). Prefrontal dopamine signaling and cognitive symptoms of Parkinson's disease. *Rev. Neurosci.* 24, 267–278. doi: 10.1515/revneuro-2013-0004

Newman, M. E. (2006). Modularity and community structure in networks. *Proc. Natl. Acad. Sci. U.S.A.* 103, 8577–8582. doi: 10.1073/pnas.0601602103

O'Brien, J. T., Colloby, S., Fenwick, J., Williams, E. D., Firbank, M., Burn, D., et al. (2004). Dopamine transporter loss visualized with FP-CIT SPECT in the differential diagnosis of dementia with Lewy bodies. *Arch. Neurol.* 61, 919–925. doi: 10.1001/archneur.61.6.919

Olde Dubbelink, K. T., Hillebrand, A., Stoffers, D., Deijen, J. B., Twisk, J. W., Stam, C. J., et al. (2014). Disrupted brain network topology in Parkinson's disease: a longitudinal magnetoencephalography study. *Brain.* 137(Pt 1), 197–207. doi: 10.1093/brain/awt316

Owen, A. M., Doyon, J., Dagher, A., Sadikot, A., and Evans, A. C. (1998). Abnormal basal ganglia outflow in Parkinson's disease identified with PET. Implications for higher cortical functions. *Brain* 121(Pt 5), 949–965. doi: 10.1093/brain/121.5.949

R Core Team. (2013). *R: A Language and Environment for Statistical Computing.* Version 3.0.1. Vienna: R Foundation for Statistical Computing. ISBN: 3-900051-07-0. Available online at: http://www.R-project.org/ [Online] [Accessed].

Rubinov, M., and Sporns, O. (2010). Complex network measures of brain connectivity: uses and interpretations. *Neuroimage* 52, 1059–1069. doi: 10.1016/j.neuroimage.2009.10.003

Rubinov, M., and Sporns, O. (2011). Weight-conserving characterization of complex functional brain networks. *Neuroimage* 56, 2068–2079. doi: 10.1016/j.neuroimage.2011.03.069

Satterthwaite, T. D., Elliott, M. A., Gerraty, R. T., Ruparel, K., Loughead, J., Calkins, M. E., et al. (2013). An improved framework for confound regression and filtering for control of motion artifact in the preprocessing of resting-state functional connectivity data. *Neuroimage* 64, 240–256. doi: 10.1016/j.neuroimage.2012.08.052

Shapiro, A. M., Benedict, R. H., Schretlen, D., and Brandt, J. (1999). Construct and concurrent validity of the Hopkins Verbal Learning Test-revised. *Clin. Neuropsychol.* 13, 348–358. doi: 10.1076/clin.13.3.348.1749

Skidmore, F., Korenkevych, D., Liu, Y., He, G., Bullmore, E., and Pardalos, P. M. (2011). Connectivity brain networks based on wavelet correlation analysis in Parkinson fMRI data. *Neurosci. Lett.* 499, 47–51. doi: 10.1016/j.neulet.2011.05.030

Sporns, O. (2010). *Networks of the Brain, 1st Edn.* Cambridge, MA: The MIT Press.

Sporns, O. (2013). Network attributes for segregation and integration in the human brain. *Curr. Opin. Neurobiol.* 23, 162–171. doi: 10.1016/j.conb.2012.11.015

Sporns, O., and Zwi, J. D. (2004). The small world of the cerebral cortex. *Neuroinformatics* 2, 145–162. doi: 10.1385/NI:2:2:145

Stocco, A., Lebiere, C., and Anderson, J. R. (2010). Conditional routing of information to the cortex: a model of the basal ganglia's role in cognitive coordination. *Psychol. Rev.* 117, 541–574. doi: 10.1037/a0019077

Svenningsson, P., Westman, E., Ballard, C., and Aarsland, D. (2012). Cognitive impairment in patients with Parkinson's disease: diagnosis, biomarkers, and treatment. *Lancet Neurol.* 11, 697–707. doi: 10.1016/S1474-4422(12)70152-7

Tinaz, S., Schendan, H. E., and Stern, C. E. (2008). Fronto-striatal deficit in Parkinson's disease during semantic event sequencing. *Neurobiol. Aging* 29, 397–407. doi: 10.1016/j.neurobiolaging.2006.10.025

Tzourio-Mazoyer, N., Landeau, B., Papathanassiou, D., Crivello, F., Etard, O., Delcroix, N., et al. (2002). Automated anatomical labeling of activations in SPM using a macroscopic anatomical parcellation of the MNI MRI single-subject brain. *Neuroimage* 15, 273–289. doi: 10.1006/nimg.2001.0978

Van Eimeren, T., Monchi, O., Ballanger, B., and Strafella, A. P. (2009). Dysfunction of the default mode network in Parkinson disease: a functional magnetic resonance imaging study. *Arch. Neurol.* 66, 877–883. doi: 10.1001/archneurol.2009.97

Vossius, C., Larsen, J. P., Janvin, C., and Aarsland, D. (2011). The economic impact of cognitive impairment in Parkinson's disease. *Mov. Disord.* 26, 1541–1544. doi: 10.1002/mds.23661

Weintraub, D., Dietz, N., Duda, J. E., Wolk, D. A., Doshi, J., Xie, S. X., et al. (2012). Alzheimer's disease pattern of brain atrophy predicts cognitive decline in Parkinson's disease. *Brain* 135, 170–180. doi: 10.1093/brain/awr277

Welsh, D. K., Takahashi, J. S., and Kay, S. A. (2010). Suprachiasmatic nucleus: cell autonomy and network properties. *Annu. Rev. Physiol.* 72, 551–577. doi: 10.1146/annurev-physiol-021909-135919

White, R., Esther Aarts, E., and D'Esposito, M. (2013). Interactions of resting state brain networks, dopamine, and working memory behavior: a resting state functional MRI study. *Neurology* 80(Meeting Abstr. 1):S54.003.

Williams-Gray, C. H., Evans, J. R., Goris, A., Foltynie, T., Ban, M., Robbins, T. W., et al. (2009). The distinct cognitive syndromes of Parkinson's disease: 5 year follow-up of the CamPaIGN cohort. *Brain* 132, 2958–2969. doi: 10.1093/brain/awp245

Wold, S., Ruhe, A., Wold, H., and Dunn, W. J. III. (1984). The collinearity problem in linear regression. The Partial Least Squares (PLS) approach to generalized inverses. *SIAM J. Sci. Stat. Comput.* 5, 735–743. doi: 10.1137/0905052

Wu, T., Wang, L., Chen, Y., Zhao, C., Li, K., and Chan, P. (2009). Changes of functional connectivity of the motor network in the resting state in

Parkinson's disease. *Neurosci. Lett.* 460, 6–10. doi: 10.1016/j.neulet.2009.05.046

Yarkoni, T., Poldrack, R. A., Nichols, T. E., Van Essen, D. C., and Wager, T. D. (2011). Large-scale automated synthesis of human functional neuroimaging data. *Nat. Methods* 8, 665–670. doi: 10.1038/nmeth.1635

Zgaljardic, D. J., Borod, J. C., Foldi, N. S., Mattis, P. J., Gordon, M. F., Feigin, A., et al. (2006). An examination of executive dysfunction associated with frontostriatal circuitry in Parkinson's disease. *J. Clin. Exp. Neuropsychol.* 28, 1127–1144. doi: 10.1080/13803390500246910

5

Activation and inhibition of posterior parietal cortex have bi-directional effects on spatial errors following interruptions

Cyrus K. Foroughi *†, Eric J. Blumberg † and Raja Parasuraman

Department of Psychology, Arch Lab, George Mason University, Fairfax, VA, USA

Edited by:
Mikhail Lebedev, Duke University, USA

Reviewed by:
Hugo Merchant, Universidad Nacional Autónoma de México, Mexico
Tal Makovski, The Open University of Israel, Israel
Vincent Clark, University of New Mexico, USA

Correspondence:
Cyrus K. Foroughi, Department of Psychology, Arch Lab, George Mason University, David King Hall 2084B, MSN 3F5, 4400 University Drive, Fairfax, VA 22030-4444, USA
e-mail: cyrus.foroughi@gmail.com

† These authors have contributed equally to this work.

Interruptions to ongoing mental activities are omnipresent in our modern digital world, but the brain networks involved in interrupted performance are not known, nor have the activation of those networks been modulated. Errors following interruptions reflect failures in spatial memory, whose maintenance is supported by a brain network including the right posterior parietal cortex (PPC). The present study therefore used bi-directional transcranial Direct Current Stimulation (tDCS) of right PPC to examine the neuromodulation of spatial errors following interruptions, as well as performance on another PPC-dependent task, mental rotation. Anodal stimulation significantly reduced the number of interruption-based errors and increased mental rotation accuracy whereas cathodal stimulation significantly increased errors and reduced mental rotation accuracy. The results provide evidence for a causal role of the PPC in the maintenance of spatial representations during interrupted task performance.

Keywords: tDCS, brain stimulation, spatial errors, interruptions, posterior parietal cortex, mental rotation, cognitive equalizing

INTRODUCTION

Interruptions to our ongoing mental activities are omnipresent in modern life—whether from cell phones, emails, navigation devices, alarms, etc. An observational study found that people are interrupted an average of 12 times per hour at work in our increasingly digital world (Cades et al., 2010), with such interruptions often leading to errors. Another study of nurses from two hospitals showed that interruptions increased both procedural (e.g., fail to check patient identification) and clinical judgment errors (e.g., give the wrong drug or wrong dose), with potentially life threatening consequences (Westbrook et al., 2010). Interruption-related errors are ubiquitous and appear to be unrelated to individual expertize (e.g., Dismukes et al., 2012; Prakash et al., 2014).

Ratwani and Trafton (2008) used eye-tracking to investigate visual search patterns of the resumption process in a simple data entry task following an interruption. The primary task required participants to place randomly generated numbers into one of fifteen different locations on a computer display following preset rules. The interruption task involved either solving math problems or performing mental rotation. Both interruption tasks impaired resumption accuracy; compared to a non-interrupted condition, individuals fixated on a location following an interruption that was further away from the correct location. However this effect was significantly larger when the interruption involved mental rotation, suggesting that the same visuo-spatial processes involved in mental rotation are important for the resumption process. Shen and Jiang (2006) also showed that an interruption involving a spatial search significantly decreased memory accuracy in a change detection search task. Both findings suggest that spatial representation may play an important role in guiding resumption after an interruption.

Despite the importance of interruptions in everyday life, the brain networks involved in interrupted performance are not known, nor have the activation of those networks been modulated. The present study used the latter strategy to better understand the neuromodulation of interruption performance. Active modulation of brain networks involved in spatial memory can provide direct evidence for the causal role of transient disruption of spatial representation in resumption performance following an interruption. There is considerable evidence that the posterior parietal cortex (PPC), and more specifically the intraparietal sulcus (IPS), is implicated in the maintenance of spatial representations (Cabeza and Nyberg, 2000; Cohen and Andersen, 2002; Jonides et al., 2005; Champod and Petrides, 2007).

These findings suggest that active stimulation or inhibition of the right PPC should respectively decrease or increase spatial errors during resumption after an interruption. We tested this hypothesis in the present study using transcranial Direct Current Stimulation (tDCS), which provides a method for non-invasive, bi-directional modulation of brain function (Nitsche and Paulus, 2000; Antal et al., 2001). The polarity of stimulation plays a critical role in how tDCS affects performance; typically anodal (positive) stimulation over a particular cortical site increases cortical excitability and can improve performance (Cohen Kadosh et al., 2010; Coffman et al., 2014; Parasuraman and McKinley, 2014), whereas cathodal (negative) stimulation over the cortical area inhibits excitability and may lead to decrements in task performance (Bikson et al., 2004; Coffman et al., 2014). We therefore hypothesized that anodal stimulation of the right PPC would reduce spatial errors following an interruption, whereas cathodal stimulation of the same brain region would increase errors. For the primary task, we used the *Financial Management Task*, a complex computer-based task (Trafton et al., 2011; see **Figure 1**) commonly used in studies of interrupted task performance and the resumption process (Trafton et al., 2003; Brumby et al., 2013). The task requires participants to store information in memory and then place that information into different locations on the computer screen, either uninterrupted or following an interruption. The interruption task required participants to solve math problems.

Our main hypothesis was that compared to a sham (placebo) group, anodal stimulation of right PPC would reduce spatial errors following an interruption, whereas cathodal stimulation would increase errors. Additionally, as a manipulation check, we also used a mental rotation task, given the causal role of the PPC in mental rotation has been previously established in a repetitive transcranial magnetic stimulation (rTMS) study (Harris and Miniussi, 2003). We hypothesized that compared to a sham (placebo) group, anodal stimulation of the right PPC would improve mental rotation accuracy, whereas cathodal stimulation would decrease accuracy. A final hypothesis, based on previous findings (e.g., Blumberg et al., in press; Tseng et al., 2012), was that lower performing individuals (those with more interruption-related errors and lower mental rotation scores) receiving anodal stimulation of the right PPC would exhibit the greatest improvements in resumption performance compared to higher performing individuals.

METHODS

PARTICIPANTS

The George Mason University Institutional Review Board (IRB) approved this study. Forty-six right-handed students (M = 19.74 years, SD = 2.2, 35 females, 11 males) from George Mason University participated for course credit. One participant was excused from the study because of problems with the stimulation delivery device and the data were excluded from all analyses. Participants were randomly assigned to one of three groups: anodal stimulation (n = 15), cathodal stimulation (n = 15), and sham stimulation (n = 15) to the PPC. Sample size was determined based on effect sizes reported in previous modulation studies using tDCS over the PPC (e.g., Sparing et al., 2009; Stone and Tesche, 2009). Thus, the group size was set *a priori* at 15 resulting in a total sample size of 45.

TDCS

An ActivaDose II Iontophoresis Delivery Unit was used to deliver constant current via two electrode pads housing saline-soaked sponges with an 11 cm^2 contact area. One electrode was placed on the scalp (directly between sites CP4 and P4, identified as CPP4 of the 10–5 EEG Scalp Recording System; Oostenveld and Praamstra, 2001)—this is the same right parietal site previously found to decrease mental rotation performance in an rTMS study (Harris and Miniussi, 2003). The reference electrode was placed on the contralateral (left) upper arm. The electrodes were attached to each participant using velcro wraps. Participants received 2 mA of current for 30 min in the active stimulation group, an amount found to be safe in a number of previous studies (Coffman et al., 2014). Participants in the sham group received a 2 mA ramp up (30 s) and then immediate ramp down (6 s) of current, receiving the full 2 mA for a very short period of time (<5 s). This short stimulation duration (applied prior to the beginning of the experimental tasks) is enough to cause similar skin sensations compared to the active stimulation group, but is generally insufficient to produce lasting causal effects on cortical excitability (Coffman et al., 2014).

FINANCIAL MANAGEMENT TASK

The goal of this task was to successfully complete a client stock order as quickly and accurately as possible. To do this, participants first selected a stock order to buy or sell and then filled in twelve pieces of information relevant to that order. This information was placed, one component at a time, in one of twelve different boxes located throughout the computer screen. Importantly, participants had to place this information in order starting with the upper left box (labeled 1 in **Figure 1**), then the upper right box (labeled 2 in **Figure 1**), and so on, until all twelve pieces of information were correctly placed. If a participant went to the wrong box (i.e., made an error), the participant was unable to fill in the information. Instead, the box that the participant was supposed to go to would turn red. This indicated that an error was made and that the participant would need to place information in the red box before moving on.

Interruptions occurred randomly throughout the duration of the financial management task. The interruption task, which replaced the primary task screen, required participants to answer multiple choice addition (math) problems that were located on the bottom, center of the computer screen for the entire duration of the 15 s interruption (see **Figure 1**). Participants answered the problems at their own pace. Immediately following the interruption, the primary task screen reappeared and participants were able to continue the primary task. Importantly, when returning to the primary task following an interruption, all of the information that was on the screen before the interruption occurred was gone. Therefore, participants needed to remember where they left off to successfully re-engage the task without making an error (see Trafton et al., 2011 for more information about the Financial Management task).

MENTAL ROTATION TASK

The Vandenberg and Kuse Mental Rotation Test, Version C (MRT-C; Peters et al., 1995; Shepard and Metzler, 1971; Vandenberg and Kuse, 1978) was used to assess mental rotation ability. This version, unlike versions A and B, and most other MRT, rotates objects around both the vertical and horizontal axes, thereby increasing the difficulty of the test. The use of

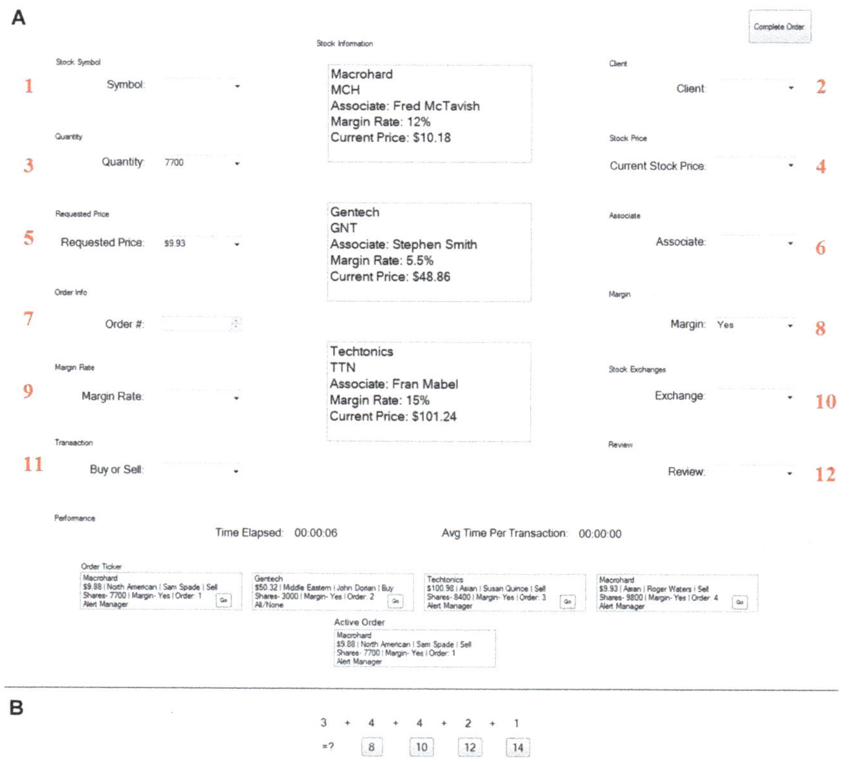

FIGURE 1 | The Financial Management Task (A) and the interruption task (B). The interruption task replaced the screen for the duration of each interruption.

this version of a mental rotation task made it less likely that individuals would be at ceiling levels of performance at baseline, thus allowing for assessment of potential improvement with anodal tDCS.

In this version, each question has one template and four possible answers (i.e., objects that when rotated match the base stimuli or objects that when rotated do not match the base stimuli). For every question, there are exactly two correct matching answers. To successfully answer the question, you must correctly identify both of the matching stimuli.

DESIGN AND PROCEDURE

Participants first signed a consent form and were then instructed on how to complete the mental rotation task (MRT-C). Each participant completed all four practice problems with the experimenter. Following practice, participants completed the first half of the test (i.e., problems 1–12). Participants were given five minutes to the complete the problems. Participants were then trained on the Financial Management task to ensure that they were familiar with the task and minimize potential learning effects. Participants were instructed to complete both tasks (primary and interruption) as quickly and accurately as possible. The trials took approximately 75 s each to complete with interruption time removed. During baseline, participants completed 9 total trials with 27 total interruptions. Interruptions occurred randomly after the successful completion of any one box. Researchers ensured the participants were actively completing the interruption task.

Following the baseline block, the tDCS unit was set up and stimulation was applied.

The DCS Sensation Questionnaire (Scheldrup et al., 2014) was administered at three time points throughout the stimulation block. This questionnaire is used to gauge the amount of itching, heat/burning, and tingling each participant felt as a result of the stimulation; participants responded by selecting their perceived sensations on a 11-point Likert scale where 0 represented no sensation at all and 10 represented the most intense sensation imaginable. This questionnaire is required by the George Mason University IRB to ensure participants safety during the experiment; thus, the data were not analyzed *post-hoc*. Once the current value reached 2.0 mA, the DCS Sensation Questionnaire was administered. Afterwards, participants completed the stimulation block of the Financial Management task, which was identical to the design of the baseline block (i.e., 9 trials with 27 random interruptions). The DCS Sensation Questionnaire was then administered a second time. Next, participants completed the second half (i.e, problems 13–24) of the mental rotation task (MRT-C). Once complete, the final DCS Sensation Questionnaire was administered. The tDCS unit was turned off and detached from the participant. They were thanked for their participation, given a short debrief about the experiment, and then left.

MEASURES

An error occurred when a participant attempted to place information in an incorrect box following an interruption; therefore, a maximum of 27 errors could be committed. Average trial completion time was computed in seconds for each participant. Performance on the interruption task was scored. Lastly, the mental rotation test (MRT-C) was scored for accuracy.

RESULTS

MANIPULATION VERIFICATION

We initially examined participants' engagement in the interruption task. Participants successfully answered 83% (SD = 5.1, range: 74–96%) of the multiple choice math problems, suggesting they were actively engaged in the interruption task and not rehearsing the primary task.

To determine if interruptions affected performance on the primary task, we compared the number of errors a participant made when completing the task without interruptions ($M = 0.47$, $SD = 0.66$) to the number of errors a participant made following an interruption ($M = 12.71$, $SD = 2.81$) in the baseline trials. A paired samples t-test confirmed that the interruptions negatively affected performance, $t_{(44)} = 27.51$, $p < 0.001$, $d = 4.10$.

Before determining if tDCS affected performance, we needed to ensure that no baseline differences existed between the three stimulation groups (anodal, cathodal, and sham). A one-way analysis of variance (ANOVA) revealed no differences existed in the number of errors made during the baseline trials between groups, $F_{(2,42)} = 0.076$, $p > 0.250$, $\eta^2_{\text{partial}} = 0.004$, see **Figure 2A**. A separate one-way ANOVA of the MRT-C revealed no differences existed in baseline scores (i.e., problems 1–12) between groups as well, $F_{(2,42)} = 0.056$, $p > 0.250$, $\eta^2_{\text{partial}} = 0.003$, see **Figure 2B**.

INTERRUPTION-RELATED ERRORS

A mixed-design ANOVA was performed to determine whether tDCS affected the number of errors participants made following an interruption. The within-subject factor was block (baseline and stimulation) and the between-subject factor was stimulation group (anodal, cathodal, and sham). Levene's test indicated equal error variances in both the baseline ($F = 0.09$, $p > 0.250$) and stimulation ($F = 0.84$, $p > 0.250$) data. There was a significant main effect of block, $F_{(1,42)} = 8.68$, $p = 0.005$, $\eta^2_{\text{partial}} = 0.17$ and a significant interaction between block and stimulation group, $F_{(2,42)} = 26.93$, $p < 0.001$, $\eta^2_{\text{partial}} = 0.56$, see **Figure 2A**.

Tests of simple main effects using a Bonferroni correction ($\alpha = 0.05$) within the anodal stimulation group revealed that significant differences existed between the number of errors in baseline ($M = 12.67$, 95% CI [11.17, 14.16]) and stimulation ($M = 9.8$, 95% CI [8.35, 11.25]), $t_{(14)} = 7.56$, $p < 0.001$, $d = 1.95$. Tests of simple main effects using a Bonferroni correction ($\alpha = 0.05$) within the cathodal stimulation group revealed that significant differences existed between the number of errors made at baseline ($M = 12.93$, 95% CI [11.44, 14.43]) and during stimulation ($M = 13.8$, 95% CI [12.35, 15.25]), $t_{(14)} = 2.29$, $p = 0.027$, $d = 0.59$. No differences existed within the sham group ($p > 0.250$). On average anodal stimulation resulted in three fewer spatial errors (i.e., 23% reduction), whereas cathodal stimulation increased spatial errors by one (i.e., 7% increase), and sham did not change performance.

Tests of simple main effects using a Bonferroni correction ($\alpha = 0.05$) within the stimulation block revealed that significant differences existed between the number of errors committed in the anodal stimulation group ($M = 9.8$, 95% CI [8.35, 11.25]) compared to both the cathodal stimulation group ($M = 13.8$, 95% CI [12.35, 15.25]), $t_{(28)} = 3.94$, $p = 0.001$, $d = 1.49$) and sham stimulation group ($M = 12.6$, 95% CI [11.15, 14.05], $t_{(28)} = 2.76$, $p = 0.026$, $d = 1.04$), but not between the cathodal and sham stimulation groups ($p > 0.250$; see **Figure 2A**). On average individuals receiving anodal stimulation made three fewer errors (i.e., 22% reduction) in the stimulation block compared to individuals in the sham stimulation group and four fewer errors (i.e., 29% reduction) compared to individuals in the cathodal stimulation group.

We also correlated the number of errors each participant in the anodal stimulation group made at baseline to their change in errors (stimulation minus baseline), revealing a significant correlation, $r_{(14)} = -0.61$, $p = 0.016$, $R^2 = 0.37$. This suggests that individuals with worse initial performance (i.e., more errors in baseline) benefitted the most from anodal stimulation, see **Figure 3A**.

MENTAL ROTATION TASK (MRT-C)

A mixed-design ANOVA was performed to determine whether tDCS affected performance on the mental rotation task. The within-subject factor was block (baseline and stimulation) and the between-subject factor was stimulation group (anodal, cathodal, and sham). Levene's test indicated equal error variances in both the baseline ($F = 0.218$, $p > 0.250$) and stimulation ($F = 0.074$, $p > 0.250$) data. There was a significant main effect of block, $F_{(1,42)}$ 8.32, $p = 0.006$, $\eta^2_{\text{partial}} = 0.17$ and a significant interaction between block and stimulation group, $F_{(2,42)} = 21.96$, $p < 0.001$, $\eta^2_{\text{partial}} = 0.51$, see **Figure 2B**.

Tests of simple main effects using a Bonferroni correction ($\alpha = 0.05$) within the anodal stimulation group revealed that significant differences existed between mental rotation accuracy during baseline ($M = 5.133$, 95% CI [4.00, 6.27]) and in stimulation ($M = 7.07$, 95% CI [5.96, 8.17]), $t_{(14)} = 6.90$, $p < 0.001$, $d = 1.78$. Tests of simple main using a Bonferroni correction ($\alpha = 0.05$) effects within the cathodal stimulation group revealed that significant differences existed between mental rotation accuracy at baseline ($M = 5.00$, 95% CI [3.86, 6.14]) and during stimulation ($M = 4.40$, 95% CI [3.29, 5.51]), $t_{(14)} = 2.14$, $p = .038$, $d = 0.55$. No differences existed within the sham group ($p > 0.250$). On average participants in the anodal stimulation group improved mental rotation score by two (i.e., 27% improvement), cathodal stimulation decreased mental rotation score by half a point (i.e., 12% reduction), and sham did not change performance.

Tests of simple main effects using a Bonferroni correction ($\alpha = 0.05$) within the stimulation block revealed that significant differences existed between MRT-C scores in the anodal stimulation group ($M = 7.07$, 95% CI [5.96, 8.17]) compared to both the cathodal stimulation group ($M = 4.40$, 95% CI [3.29, 5.51], $t_{(28)} = 3.44$, $p = 0.004$, $d = 0.89$) and sham stimulation group

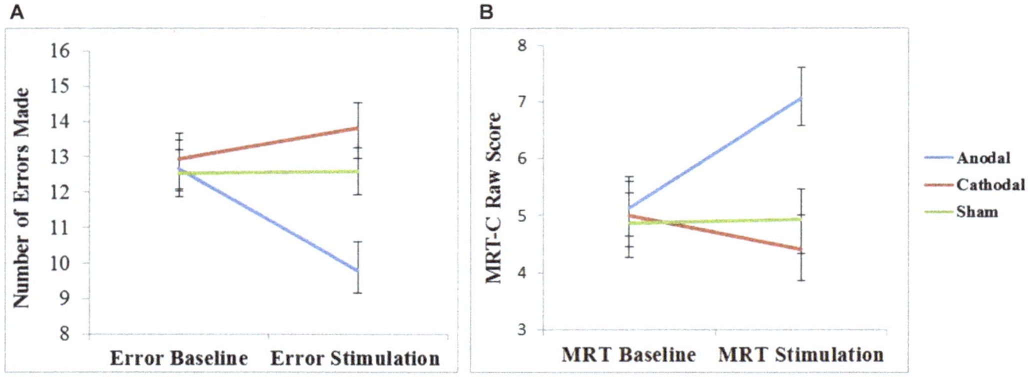

FIGURE 2 | The mean number of errors made (fewer errors represent improved performance) following an interruption (A) and the mean raw scores (higher scores represent improved performance) on the mental rotation task (B) during baseline and stimulation blocks for the three stimulation group (anodal, cathodal, and sham). Plotted with standard errors of the mean.

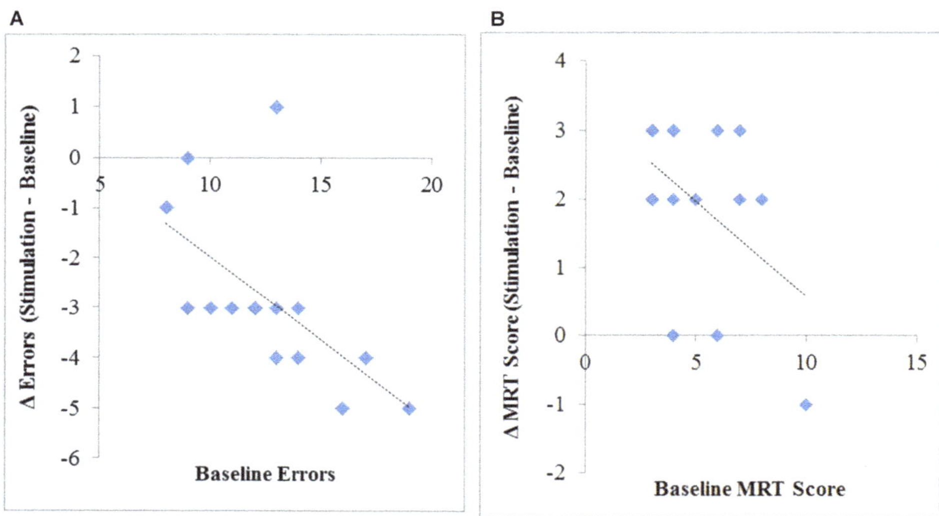

FIGURE 3 | Change (stimulation–baseline) in interruption-related errors (A) and MRT scores (B) plotted against the number of errors (A) and mean mental rotation scores (B) at baseline.

($M = 4.93$, 95% CI [3.83, 6.04], $t_{(28)} = 2.75$, $p = 0.026$, $d = 0.71$). Scores in the cathodal stimulation group were not significantly different from sham ($p > 0.250$; see **Figure 2B**). On average individuals receiving anodal stimulation scored two points higher (i.e., 30% improvement) on the mental rotation task compared to individuals in the sham stimulation group and two and a half points higher (i.e., 38% improvement) than individuals in the cathodal stimulation group.

Additionally, we correlated each participants MRT-C score in the anodal stimulation group at baseline to their change in MRT-C score (stimulation minus baseline), revealing a significant correlation, $r_{(14)} = -.47$, $p = 0.04$, $R^2 = 0.22$, however this effect is largely driven by one participant given the relatively low amount of variability ($s^2 = 4.5$) in MRT-C scores at baseline, see **Figure 3B**.

COMPLETION TIME

To determine whether tDCS affected average trial completion time, a mixed-design ANOVA was performed to determine whether tDCS affected average trial completion time across all three groups, with the within-subject factor being block (baseline and stimulation) and the between-subject factor being stimulation group (anodal, cathodal, and sham). Levene's test indicated equal error variances in both the baseline ($F = 0.859$, $p > 0.250$) and stimulation ($F = 0.331$, $p > 0.250$) data. There was a main effect of block, $F_{(1,42)} = 7.69$, $p = 0.008$, $\eta^2_{partial} = 0.16$ and a significant interaction between block and stimulation group, $F_{(2,42)} = 7.169$, $p = 0.002$, $\eta^2_{partial} = 0.25$.

Tests of simple main effects using a Bonferroni correction ($\alpha = 0.05$) within the anodal stimulation group revealed that a significant difference existed ($p < 0.001$) between average trial completion time in baseline (M = 77.07s, 95% CI [72.69, 81.45]) and average trial completion time in stimulation (M = 72.13s, 95% CI [67.93, 76.34]). No differences existed between baseline and stimulation average completion time in the cathodal or sham stimulation groups ($p > 0.250$ for both). That is, individuals in the anodal stimulation group completed the task more quickly while stimulated compared to baseline. This may not be a surprise as these same individuals made fewer errors and making an error would result in more time spent on that trial.

MENTAL ROTATION AND ERRORS

Given that the processes that guide resumption after an interruption may recruit the same neural substrates as mental rotation, it is likely that changes in one (mental rotation) may be reflected in changes in the other (resumption process, i.e., errors). To examine the extent to which they are related, we correlated the difference scores (stimulation minus baseline) for both measures, including all three stimulation groups. The analysis revealed a significant correlation, $r_{(45)} = -.72$, $p < 0.001$, $R^2 = 0.52$, see **Figure 4**. The magnitudes of the changes in performance for each measure were significantly related.

DISCUSSION

The brain networks involved in the interruption process are not known and the neuromodulation of those networks has not been previously been examined. Given that spatial representations aid in the resumption process after an interruption (Ratwani and Trafton, 2008) and that the right PPC is activated during the maintenance of spatial representations (Cabeza and Nyberg, 2000; Cohen and Andersen, 2002), we hypothesized that anodal stimulation of this region would reduce the number of errors by enhancing memory for spatial information. Additionally, we hypothesized that cathodal stimulation applied to the PPC would increase the number of errors by diminishing spatial representation ability. The results supported these hypotheses: anodal stimulation of right PPC significantly reduced the number of interruption-related errors while increasing mental rotation accuracy, whereas cathodal stimulation of the same region had the opposite effects, and sham stimulation did not affect either performance measure.

To our knowledge, this is the first demonstration of bi-directional effects of activation and inhibition of PPC on spatial errors following interruptions and on mental rotation performance. The results provide evidence for a causal role for the PPC in the maintenance of spatial representations during interrupted task performance. We also found that the magnitude of the changes in interruption-related errors with tDCS was significantly related to changes in mental rotation performance, as measured by the MRT-C. Specifically, individuals who improved in mental rotation accuracy exhibited a reduction in the number of interruption errors to a similar degree. This finding supports the idea that spatial representation ability, as assessed using the MRT-C, guides resumption after an interruption. The findings are unlikely to reflect a placebo effect given that sham stimulation did not affect performance.

Additionally, we found that lower performing individuals at baseline testing, measured by both the number of interruption errors and MRT-C, showed the greatest improvements in performance following anodal stimulation of PPC. This result suggests that individual differences in baseline ability may modulate the behavioral effects of tDCS. Such "cognitive equalizing" due to tDCS was also previously reported in a study of change detection (Tseng et al., 2012). Our finding that lower-performing individuals showed greater benefits of tDCS than higher-performing ones diminishes concerns that tDCS and other non-invasive brain stimulation techniques may widen or exacerbate ability differences in the population, thereby leading to greater social inequality (Cohen Kadosh et al., 2012).

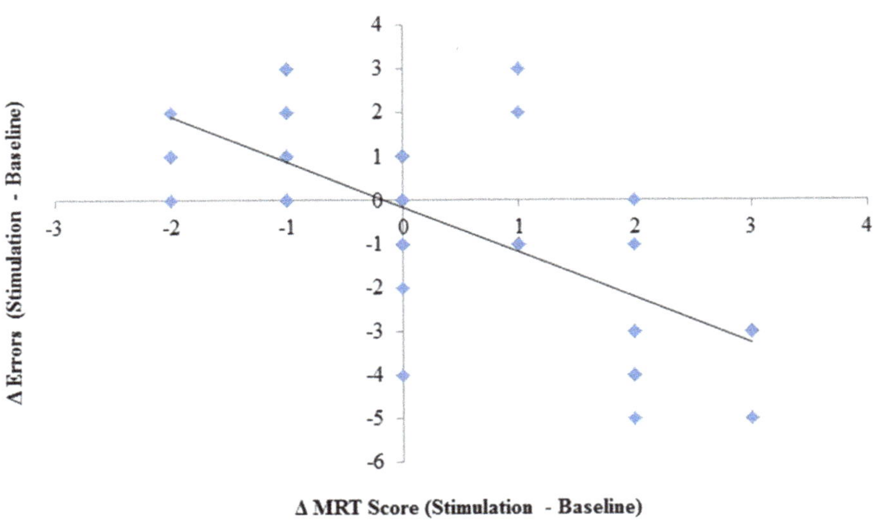

FIGURE 4 | Change (stimulation–baseline) in interruption-related errors plotted against change in mental rotation scores.

During stimulation, performance in both the interruption and mental rotation tasks was significantly greater in the anodal group than in the cathodal and sham groups. However, whereas cathodal stimulation significantly reduced performance on both tasks compared to baseline, the cathodal and sham groups did not differ significantly following stimulation. Some other previous tDCS studies have also found that effects of cathodal stimulation are often less pronounced than anodal effects (Fregni et al., 2005; Tseng et al., 2012; Coffman et al., 2014). Another limitation in the present study is that although we designed the tDCS montage to target the IPS based on current modeling (Datta et al., 2009) and previous literature (Harris and Miniussi, 2003), the relatively non-focal nature of tDCS means that other brain regions could also have been stimulated and could have played a role in the effects. In addition, each participant received only one type of stimulation; therefore it is possible that other individual differences that were not assessed in this study could have been responsible for the differential effects of anodal and cathodal stimulation on interruption errors and mental rotation performance. Additionally, math problems were included as the interruption task in the present study even though mental rotation has been shown to interfere with the resumption process to a greater extent (Ratwani and Trafton, 2008). Given that tDCS produced significant effects in resumption performance in the less interfering task (math problems), potentially greater effects may be found with mental rotation. Finally, many tasks that can be interrupted exist (e.g., giving verbal commands) that may not benefit from anodal stimulation of the PPC when interrupted because the task is not spatial in nature. Therefore, we cannot generalize our results to all tasks and forms of interruption.

This is the first study to show how noninvasive brain stimulation can reduce human error following interruptions. Interruptions are unavoidable, and while many only cause delays or reduce efficiency, they can also lead to serious errors (Westbrook et al., 2010; Prakash et al., 2014). Importantly, tDCS offers a safe, inexpensive, and easy to administer method to reduce errors during the resumption process. This study offers bi-directional causal support for the role of PPC in mental rotation ability and in the resumption process. Important issues that need to be addressed in future research include retention of tDCS-induced benefits on interruption performance and their transfer to other tasks (Parasuraman and McKinley, 2014).

ACKNOWLEDGMENTS

This research was supported by Air Force Office of Scientific Research Grant FA9550-10-1-0385 to Raja Parasuraman and the Center of Excellence in Neuroergonomics, Technology, and Cognition (CENTEC). We would like to thank Greg Trafton, Kevin Zish, and Malcolm McCurry for providing and assisting with the use of the Financial Management Task.

REFERENCES

Antal, A., Nitsche, M. A., and Paulus, W. (2001). External modulation of visual perception in humans. *Neuroreport* 12, 3553–3555. doi: 10.1097/00001756-200111160-00036

Bikson, M., Inoue, M., Akiyama, H., Deans, J. K., Fox, J. E., Miyakawa, H., et al. (2004). Effects of uniform extracellular DC electric fields on excitability in rat hippocampal slices in vitro. *J. Physiol.* 557, 175–190. doi: 10.1113/jphysiol.2003.055772

Blumberg, E. J., Foroughi, C. F., Scheldrup, M. R., Peterson, M. S., Boehm-Davis, D. A., and Parasuraman, R. (in press). Reducing the disruptive effects of interruptions with noninvasive brain stimulation. *Hum. Factors*

Brumby, D. P., Cox, A. L., Back, J., and Gould, S. J. (2013). Recovering from an interruption: investigating speed-accuracy trade-offs in task resumption behavior. *J. Exp. Psychol. Appl.* 19, 95–107. doi: 10.1037/a0032696

Cabeza, R., and Nyberg, L. (2000). Imaging cognition II: an empirical review of 275 PET and fMRI studies. *J. Cogn. Neurosci.* 12, 1–47. doi: 10.1162/08989290051137585

Cades, D. M., Werner, N. E., Boehm-Davis, D. A., and Arshad, Z. (2010). Interruptions are disruptive in the real world: evidence from an office setting. *Proc. Hum. Factors U S A* 54, 448–452. doi: 10.1177/154193121005400437

Champod, A. S., and Petrides, M. (2007). Dissociable roles of the posterior parietal and the prefrontal cortex in manipulation and monitoring processes. *Proc. Natl. Acad. Sci. U S A* 104, 14837–14842. doi: 10.1073/pnas.0607101104

Coffman, B. A., Clark, V. P., and Parasuraman, R. (2014). Battery powered thought: enhancement of attention, learning and memory in healthy adults using transcranial direct current stimulation. *Neuroimage* 85, 895–908. doi: 10.1016/j.neuroimage.2013.07.083

Cohen, Y. E., and Andersen, R. A. (2002). A common reference frame for movement plans in the posterior parietal cortex. *Nat. Rev. Neurosci.* 3, 553–562. doi: 10.1038/nrn873

Cohen Kadosh, R., Levy, N., O'Shea, J., Shea, N., and Savulescu, J. (2012). The neuroethics of non-invasive brain stimulation. *Curr. Biol.* 22, 108–111. doi: 10.1016/j.cub.2012.01.013

Cohen Kadosh, R., Soskic, S., Iuculano, T., Kanai, R., and Walsh, V. (2010). Modulating neuronal activity produces specific and long lasting changes in numerical competence. *Curr. Biol.* 20, 2016–2020. doi: 10.1016/j.cub.2010.10.007

Datta, A., Bansal, V., Diaz, J., Patel, J., Reato, D., and Bikson, M. (2009). Gyri-precise head model of transcranial direct current stimulation: improved spatial focality using a ring electrode versus conventional rectangular pad. *Brain Stimul.* 2, 201–207. doi: 10.1016/j.brs.2009.03.005

Dismukes, R. K., Loukopoulos, L. D., and Berman, B. A. (2012). *The Limits of Expertise: Rethinking Pilot Error and the Causes of Airline Accidents.* Hampshire, England: Ashgate Publishing, Ltd.

Fregni, F., Boggio, P. S., Nitsche, M., Bermpohl, F., Antal, A., Feredoes, E., et al. (2005). Anodal transcranial direct current stimulation of prefrontal cortex enhances working memory. *Exp. Brain Res.* 166, 23–30. doi: 10.1007/s00221-005-2334-6

Harris, I. M., and Miniussi, C. (2003). Parietal lobe contribution to mental rotation demonstrated with rTMS. *J. Cogn. Neurosci.* 15, 315–323. doi: 10.1162/089892903321593054

Jonides, J., Lacey, S. C., and Nee, D. E. (2005). Processes of working memory in mind and brain. *Curr. Dir. Psychol. Sci.* 14, 2–5. doi: 10.1111/j.0963-7214.2005.00323.x

Nitsche, M. A., and Paulus, W. (2000). Excitability changes induced in the human motor cortex by weak transcranial direct current stimulation. *J. Physiol.* 527, 633–639. doi: 10.1111/j.1469-7793.2000.t01-1-00633.x

Oostenveld, R., and Praamstra, P. (2001). The five percent electrode system for high-resolution EEG and ERP measurements. *Clin. Neurophysiol.* 112, 713–719. doi: 10.1016/s1388-2457(00)00527-7

Parasuraman, R., and McKinley, A. R. (2014). Using non-invasive brain stimulation to accelerate learning and enhance human performance. *Hum. Factors* 56, 816–824. doi: 10.1177/0018720814538815

Peters, M., Laeng, B., Latham, K., Jackson, M., Zaiyouna, R., and Richardson, C. (1995). A redrawn Vandenberg and Kuse mental rotations test-different versions and factors that affect performance. *Brain Cogn.* 28, 39–58. doi: 10.1006/brcg.1995.1032

Prakash, V., Koczmara, C., Savage, P., Trip, K., Stewart, J., McCurdie, T., et al. (2014). Mitigating errors caused by interruptions during medication verification and administration: interventions in a simulated ambulatory chemotherapy setting. *BMJ Qual. Saf.* 23, 884–892. doi: 10.1136/bmjqs-2013-002484

Ratwani, R. M., and Trafton, J. G. (2008). Spatial memory guides task resumption. *Vis. Cogn.* 16, 1001–1010. doi: 10.1080/13506280802025791

Scheldrup, M., Greenwood, P. M., McKendrick, R., Strohl, J., Bikson, M., Alam, M., et al. (2014). Transcranial direct current stimulation facilitates cognitive multi-task performance differentially depending on anode location and subtask. *Front. Hum. Neurosci.* 8:665. doi: 10.3389/fnhum.2014.00665

Shen, Y. J., and Jiang, Y. V. (2006). Interrupted visual searches reveal volatile search memory. *J. Exp. Psychol. Hum. Percept. Perform.* 32, 1208–1220. doi: 10.1037/0096-1523.32.5.1208

Shepard, R. N., and Metzler, J. (1971). Mental rotation of three-dimensional objects. *Science* 171, 701–703. doi: 10.1126/science.171.3972.701

Sparing, R., Thimm, M., Hesse, M. D., Küst, J., Karbe, H., and Fink, G. R. (2009). Bidirectional alterations of interhemispheric parietal balance by non-invasive cortical stimulation. *Brain* 132, 3011–3020. doi: 10.1093/brain/awp154

Stone, D. B., and Tesche, C. D. (2009). Transcranial direct current stimulation modulates shifts in global/local attention. *Neuroreport* 20, 1115–1119. doi: 10.1097/wnr.0b013e32832e9aa2

Trafton, J. G., Altmann, E. M., Brock, D. P., and Mintz, F. E. (2003). Preparing to resume an interrupted task: effects of prospective goal encoding and retrospective rehearsal. *Int. J. Hum. Comput. Stud.* 58, 583–603. doi: 10.1016/s1071-5819(03)00023-5

Trafton, J. G., Altmann, E. M., and Ratwani, R. M. (2011). A memory for goals model of sequence errors. *Cogn. Syst. Res.* 12, 134–143. doi: 10.1016/j.cogsys.2010.07.010

Tseng, P., Hsu, T. Y., Chang, C. F., Tzeng, O. J., Hung, D. L., Muggleton, N. G., et al. (2012). Unleashing potential: transcranial direct current stimulation over the right posterior parietal cortex improves change detection in low-performing individuals. *J. Neurosci.* 32, 10554–10561. doi: 10.1523/jneurosci.0362-12.2012

Vandenberg, S. G., and Kuse, A. R. (1978). Mental rotations, a group test of three-dimensional spatial visualization. *Percept. Mot. Skills* 47, 599–604. doi: 10.2466/pms.1978.47.2.599

Westbrook, J. I., Woods, A., Rob, M. I., Dunsmuir, W. T., and Day, R. O. (2010). Association of interruptions with an increased risk and severity of medication administration errors. *Arch. Intern. Med.* 170, 683–690. doi: 10.1001/archinternmed.2010.65

6

Decoding methods for neural prostheses: where have we reached?

Zheng Li[1,2]*

[1] State Key Laboratory of Cognitive Neuroscience and Learning and IDG/McGovern Institute for Brain Research, Beijing Normal University, Beijing, China
[2] Center for Collaboration and Innovation in Brain and Learning Sciences, Beijing Normal University, Beijing, China

Edited by:
Ioan Opris, Wake Forest University, USA

Reviewed by:
Gytis Baranauskas, Neuroscience Institute at Lithuanian University of Health Sciences, Lithuania
David Sussillo, Stanford University, USA

***Correspondence:**
Zheng Li, State Key Laboratory of Cognitive Neuroscience and Learning and IDG/McGovern Institute for Brain Research, Beijing Normal University, 19 Xin Jie Kou Wai Da Jie, Beijing 100875, China
e-mail: lz@bnu.edu.cn

This article reviews advances in decoding methods for brain-machine interfaces (BMIs). Recent work has focused on practical considerations for future clinical deployment of prosthetics. This review is organized by open questions in the field such as what variables to decode, how to design neural tuning models, which neurons to select, how to design models of desired actions, how to learn decoder parameters during prosthetic operation, and how to adapt to changes in neural signals and neural tuning. The concluding discussion highlights the need to design and test decoders within the context of their expected use and the need to answer the question of how much control accuracy is good enough for a prosthetic.

Keywords: brain-machine interface, brain computer interface, decoding, neural prosthetic, neural engineering, multichannel recordings, signal processing

INTRODUCTION

The field of brain-machine interfaces (BMIs) for control of motor prostheses is quickly growing (Baranauskas, 2014, for other reviews, see Tehovnik et al., 2013; Kao et al., 2014). Research in decoders, the algorithms which translate neural signals to movement commands, has largely switched focus from improving control accuracy to resolving practical considerations of future clinical deployments of prostheses. The goal of this mini-review is to briefly highlight recent (2013 to mid-2014) advances in decoding methodology for extracellular signals recorded from motor areas of the brain. The review sections are organized by main research themes, corresponding to important questions and practical considerations. At the end, the importance of developing and testing decoders in realistic contexts and the question of how much control accuracy is "good enough" for a prosthetic are discussed.

ALGORITHMS FOR DECODING

Which algorithmic framework should we use for decoding? Different algorithms offer different benefits. **Figure 1** illustrates three commonly-used methods. The Kalman filter and point process filter are state-based (modeling temporal evolution) and probabilistic (modeling and estimating uncertainty). The linear filter, in contrast, is a linear transformation of neural data to the decoded variables, with the advantages of simplicity and execution speed.

The Kalman filter's Gaussian noise model clearly does not match the data (spike counts), yet due to its accuracy and execution speed the method has remained popular since its first use by Wu et al. (2003) (Aggarwal et al., 2013; Chen et al., 2013; Dangi et al., 2013a,c; Homer et al., 2013; Ifft et al., 2013; Jarosiewicz et al., 2013; Kao et al., 2013; Merel et al., 2013; Wong et al., 2013; Zhang and Chase, 2013; Fan et al., 2014; Golub et al., 2014; Gowda et al., 2014; Homer et al., 2014). While point process filters (for a review, see Koyama et al., 2010) offer a more realistic noise model, their use in decoding is still relatively rare (Shanechi et al., 2013; Velliste et al., 2014; Xu et al., 2014), due in part to their heavier computational burden. Recently, Citi et al. (2013) extend point process methods to model refractory periods of neurons and allow for coarser time discretization by a factor of 10, which may ease this burden. However, one feature which current point process decoders lack is the ability to assign different amounts of noise or weights to different neurons.

Linear filtering, or discrete Wiener filtering, is fading in popularity. It is still used by some research groups, either because of its computational form (Badreldin et al., 2013) or when the research focuses on other aspects of decoding (Chen et al., 2013; Chhatbar and Francis, 2013; Philip et al., 2013; Suminski et al., 2013; Willett et al., 2013). A variant of the Wiener filter method, which passes the Wiener filter output through a fitted non-linear function to compute the final output, is also used (Flint et al., 2013; Scheid et al., 2013).

Several other methods have been used in the recent literature: kernel autoregressive moving average (KARMA; Wong et al., 2013), quantized kernel least mean square (Li et al., 2014), support vector machines (Cao et al., 2013; Xu et al., 2013; Wang et al., 2014), K-nearest neighbors (Brockmeier et al., 2013; Ifft et al., 2013; Xu et al., 2013), naïve Bayes (Bishop et al., 2014), and artificial neural networks (Chen et al., 2013; Mahmoudi et al., 2013; Pohlmeyer et al., 2014). All of these methods allow highly non-linear neural models.

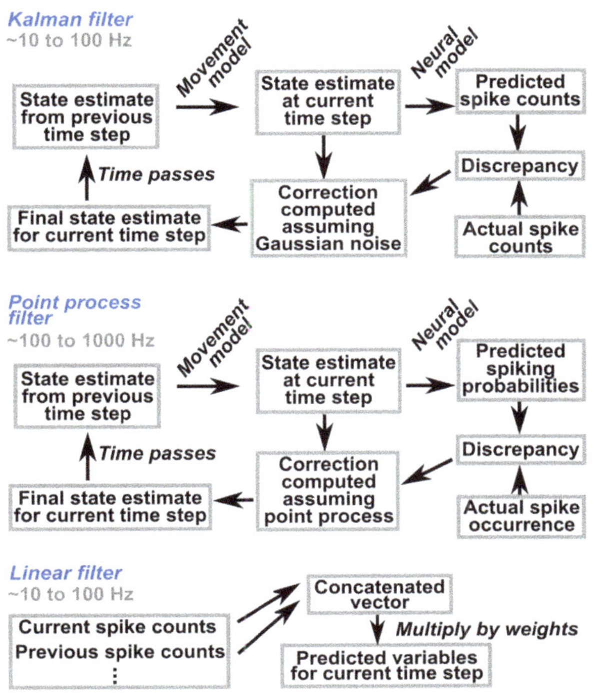

FIGURE 1 | Schematic illustration of popular decoding algorithms. The Kalman and point process filters are based on the notion of a state, which holds the current estimates of the variables of interest. The state is related to neural activity through a neural model. Bayesian computations on the neural model, assuming a distribution for noise, permit probabilistic tracking of the state based on neural activity. In contrast, the linear filter is state-less; it linearly maps the recent history of neural activity to estimates of the variables of interest.

VARIABLES TO DECODE

What values should a decoder predict? Ideally, a prosthetic should offer accurate, intuitive control that works under all likely usage contexts. In most prior work, desired positions or velocities of end-effectors were decoded. Homer et al. (2013) proposed a method for combining decoded position and velocity, to avoid choosing between the two. The method defines a quantity Δr as the difference between the decoded cursor position and the previous cursor position. The cursor position's update is a linear combination of the decoded velocity and the decoded velocity vector rotated to the direction of Δr.

Decoders aim to predict user intentions, and it is possible that intentions may be slightly different from the observed limb movements used for parameter fitting. Fan et al. (2014) showed that the heuristic for guessing user intention during online recalibration proposed by Gilja et al. (2012), and tested with human users in a study by Jarosiewicz et al. (2013), could also be applied to the initial training data for fitting decoder parameters. This method rotates the cursor's velocity vector towards the target and zeroes the velocity when the cursor is in the target. Fitting Kalman filter parameters on these estimates of intended movements, instead of actual limb movements, could achieve comparable gains in accuracy as online recalibration using the same scheme (Fan et al., 2014).

Two recent studies have explored decoding torque values, to allow a prosthetic to interact with objects with mass more naturally. Chhatbar and Francis (2013) showed that hybrid neural control by both torque and position produced more natural movements in novel dynamic environments. Decoding of position and torque was performed via a Wiener filter applied to the largest 20 principal components of neural activity. The final angular accelerations of the prosthetic joints were calculated by a weighted sum of the accelerations implied by the predicted positions and torques. Suminski et al. (2013) decoded position and velocity as well as torques of a two-link virtual arm with a Wiener filter. The kinematic variables were converted to torques using a position-derivative controller and the results were combined linearly with the directly decoded torques to produce the final torque output.

Besides kinematics and forces, the target location of a reach may be directly decoded to improve the trajectory of the reach. Shanechi et al. (2013) presented a real-time, two-stage decoder which first decoded target location during an instructed delay period and then decoded reach trajectory during the reach period. The decoded target location served as the goal position for an optimal feedback controller that acted as the movement model of the point process trajectory decoder.

To address the need for BMI control of limbs with many degrees of freedom, an important consideration for clinical deployment, Wong et al. (2013) used principal component analysis to reduce the dimensions of limb movements. They showed that decoding principal-component-space kinematic variables with KARMA or Kalman filtering was more accurate than decoding canonical-space kinematic variables. Ifft et al. (2013) decoded the kinematics of both arms during a bimanual reaching task using an unscented Kalman filter which included variables for both arms in its state.

Besides the biomimetic approach of designing a prosthetic so that it can be controlled like a natural limb, another approach is to use operant conditioning of neuron ensembles (for a review, see Sakurai et al., 2014) to let the user learn to control a new, synthetic actuator. Though more initial training may be required, greater final control accuracy may be possible using this paradigm. Balasubramanian et al. (2013) used two groups of neurons from M1 to control reach and grasp, which were simplified to one dimension each. The neuron groups were chosen based on their stability and functional connectivity, and algorithmic assistance was given during the operant conditioning process to assist neuronal learning. Badreldin et al. (2013) developed an unsupervised method for non-biomimetic linear filter initialization. The method performs an eigendecomposition of the sample covariance matrix of the neural data. The eigenvectors provide a basis for the space of all possible linear filters that could be fitted from the data. They designed a cost function to choose a particular linear filter from this space, which probably differs from the filter which would have been fitted by supervised linear regression. Their cost function optimizes for characteristics such as low jitter and evenly distributed weights among neurons.

NEURAL MODELS

How should we model neural activity? Recent studies have explored the aspects of neural models beyond movement tuning, with the hope of improving user-friendliness. Considering that a system with high latency is difficult to control, Willett et al. (2013) trained a decoder to predict intended future movements to compensate for BMI system latency and shorten the feedback loop. To predict intended future movements, they fitted a linear filter using kinematic values which were temporally offset from the neural data.

In a clinical setting, it is important that a prosthetic can be turned off when not used, to avoid undesired movements. Aggarwal et al. (2013) classified behavioral states into baseline, reaction, movement, and hold using linear discriminant analysis (LDA) on local field potentials (LFPs), and then decoded arm, hand, and finger kinematics using a Kalman filter on spike signals. The position outputs were held constant when the behavioral state decoder predicted the baseline or hold state. Similarly, Velliste et al. (2014) used LDA to detect idle (resting) arm states and set velocity to zero during idle. The baseline or idle states in these studies could serve as the "off" mode for a prosthetic.

Xu et al. (2014) included ensemble firing history, in addition to the standard tuning to kinematic variables, in the neural model. This paradigm helps model the background activity that is unrelated to movements. They used parallel computation on graphics processing units to achieve real-time execution of a point process particle filter that used this model.

NEURON SELECTION

Which neurons should we include in decoding? BMI researchers have long sought ways to reduce computational load to decoders and noise in neural data by excluding irrelevant neurons. Several recent studies have provided tools for finding relevant neurons. Chen et al. (2013) used variational Bayesian inference to fit parameters for a linear filter, a state-space model, and a non-linear echo state network. Using priors which favor small parameters, the inference procedure generated sparse parameter fits, and the zeroes in the fitted parameters can be interpreted as the absence of tuning.

Cao et al. (2013) determined which neurons modulated for reach direction versus hand configuration during grasping by using mutual information. In another study from the same group, Xu et al. (2013) proposed a supervised metric learning algorithm to optimize decoding of hand grasp configuration. Their gradient descent algorithm maximizes the difference between inter-class and intra-class distances while regularizing by the L1 norm, resulting in sparse weights which indicate relevance.

Also using a supervised approach, Brockmeier et al. (2013) proposed a method for computing a linear dimensionality reduction which maximizes the information between the class labels and the projected neural data. The low dimensional data can be used for visualization or decoding via distance-based methods such as K-nearest neighbors. Brockmeier et al. (2013) proposed an improved method that only uses inner products between inputs, allowing non-linear dimensionality reduction via the kernel trick. Their kernel metric learning algorithm aims to make data points with the same class labels lay close together in the output space.

MOVEMENT MODELS

How can we design movement models to assist decoding? Kalman and point process filters include movement models which can encode prior beliefs about how variables change over time. Cleverly engineering these models may make prostheses easier to control. Two studies examined how to improve the user's ability to stop a BMI cursor when desired. Golub et al. (2014) designed a speed-dampening Kalman filter which modifies the movement model to decrease speed when fast changes in movement direction are detected, with the goal of allowing a quick change in direction to signal the desire to stop (a "hockey stop"). Using a different approach, Velliste et al. (2014) added a separate speed variable, independent of the Cartesian velocity variables, to the state space of a point process filter. This speed term dynamically adjusts the filter's movement model error covariance so that smaller changes in position and velocity are allowed when the decoded speed is smaller.

In a general examination of movement models, Gowda et al. (2014) analyzed the linear models typically used in past studies and found that some may harbor hidden attractor points, to the detriment of controllability. They also point out that specific coefficients in movement model matrices parameterize the speed-accuracy tradeoff.

LEARNING

How can we improve decoder parameters during decoding? To handle poor initial parameter fits or changes in neural tuning after practice, continuous learning of decoder parameters may be required in a clinical device. There has been much recent work, mostly from Jose Carmena's Lab (for a review, see Carmena, 2013), on improving decoder parameter fits during BMI operation, called closed-loop decoder adaptation. They adapted Kalman filter parameters via stochastic updates based on the likelihood gradient (Dangi et al., 2013a), provided tools for analysis of adaptive methods (Dangi et al., 2013b), and applied adaptation to decoding of LFPs (Dangi et al., 2013c).

Information about the target locations of reaches can help improve the parameter learning process. Kowalski et al. (2013) proposed an algorithm which uses the joint estimation paradigm (augmenting tuning parameters into the state space), combined with the "reach state equation" (Srinivasan et al., 2006) as a way to incorporate target location in decoder recalibration. Similarly, Shanechi and Carmena (2013) designed a dual filtering method which uses the target location to assist movements towards the target. The method provides the target location, assumed known, to a linear-quadratic-Gaussian optimal feedback controller which acts as the movement model of the point process decoder. A second point process filter updates the decoder parameters.

In Suminski et al.'s (2013) study, incongruence between decoded kinematics and torques were used as an error signal for recalibration. The differences between the decoded position (and velocity) and the virtual arm's endpoint position (and velocity), as computed via the decoded torques, were used as an error signal to update torque decoder parameters via gradient descent.

Merel et al. (2013) modeled co-adaptation in BMIs as two agents (encoder and decoder) optimizing with respect to each other, under linear-quadratic-Gaussian assumptions. They derive a novel decoder update step which anticipates what the future encoder will be and updates with respect to that, instead of the current encoder. They show that this "one step ahead" update rule reduces error faster in simulations.

SIGNAL STABILITY AND ADAPTATION

Are neural signals stable over long time periods? There has been controversy as to whether updating of decoder parameters is required for long-term prosthetic usability. Recent studies have analyzed stability of signals over long time spans. Flint et al. (2013) and Scheid et al. (2013) showed that multiunit spiking activity can be stable over more than six months and LFPs can be stable for almost a year. Wang et al. (2014) found signal instability and concluded that LFPs allowed more accurate offline reconstruction than single- and multi-unit signals 1–2 years post implantation. Perge et al. (2013) found significant intra-day changes in neural firing rates and concluded that 85% of these changes were likely due to physiological mechanisms.

If decoder updates are needed, how can we improve the accuracy of updates? Recent studies have proposed heuristics to improve adaptation. Zhang and Chase (2013) used two extensions to a dual-Kalman filter. First, they updated baseline firing rates of neurons using a moving window. Second, they normalized the velocity provided to the parameter updater so that the median absolute velocity matches that of the initial training data. Kao et al. (2013) proposed a firing rate normalization that also includes a regularization term that penalizes neurons with low firing rates. They also showed that dimensionality reduction via principal component analysis improves robustness to neuron loss.

Besides updating baseline firing rates via windowed estimates, other methods for tracking baseline changes have been proposed. Bishop et al. (2014) found that most changes occur between days. They designed a classifier for movement direction using the naïve Bayes algorithm and a hierarchical model; baseline firing rates are inferred each day while the class-specific parameters and the prior distributions for the baseline firing rates are learned once on initial training data. Homer et al. (2014) designed a probabilistic algorithm for detecting infrequent, rapid changes in baseline firing rates under the Kalman filtering framework. Their method first performs a forward stepwise search for neurons which have changed in baseline firing rate and then determines the magnitude of changes.

Using a reinforcement learning approach to adaptation, two studies from the same group (Mahmoudi et al., 2013; Pohlmeyer et al., 2014) showed that an actor-critic reinforcement learning BMI that uses Hebbian learning on an artificial neural network decoder's weights could learn weights from scratch and maintain decoding accuracy despite shuffling, loss, or gain of neurons, using only a one-bit feedback signal. In another study from the same group, Prins et al. (2013) decoded a one-bit reward signal from nucleus accumbens by clustering spike counts with k-means.

DISCUSSION

As researchers focus more on practical hurdles to clinical deployment of neural prostheses, it becomes more and more important to develop and test BMI decoders in the contexts in which actual prostheses will be used, i.e., to control artificial limbs, natural limbs via functional electrical stimulation (Moritz et al., 2008; Ethier et al., 2012; Nishimura et al., 2013), or computer cursors in graphical user interfaces. By using more realistic contexts, questions such as which variables to decode or which algorithms are sufficiently fast can be answered empirically. Realistic contexts may also uncover new considerations and obstacles to overcome.

An important question which has been thus far neglected in the field is how much control accuracy is enough? Full restoration of human ability in terms of movement accuracy may come at computational and other costs, e.g., number of recording channels, which likely trade off against other figures of merit of a prosthetic system. While we should continually endeavor to improve BMI technology, from a practical standpoint, we should also answer the question of how much control is good enough, so that engineers can design systems with clear requirements in mind.

ACKNOWLEDGMENTS

The author is grateful to Joseph E. O'Doherty, Mikhail A. Lebedev, and the reviewers for their helpful comments. This work was supported by the National Key Basic Research Program of China (2014CB846101) and the Fundamental Research Funds for the Central Universities.

REFERENCES

Aggarwal, V., Mollazadeh, M., Davidson, A. G., Schieber, M. H., and Thakor, N. V. (2013). State-based decoding of hand and finger kinematics using neuronal ensemble and LFP activity during dexterous reach-to-grasp movements. *J. Neurophysiol.* 109, 3067–3081. doi: 10.1152/jn.01038.2011

Badreldin, I., Southerland, J., Vaidya, M., Eleryan, A., Balasubramanian, K., Fagg, A., et al. (2013). "Unsupervised decoder initialization for brain-machine interfaces using neural state space dynamics," in *2013 6th International IEEE/EMBS Conference on Neural Engineering (NER)* (San Diego, CA), 997–1000. doi: 10.1109/NER.2013.6696104

Balasubramanian, K., Southerland, J., Vaidya, M., Qian, K., Eleryan, A., Fagg, A. H., et al. (2013). Operant conditioning of a multiple degree-of-freedom brain-machine interface in a primate model of amputation. *Conf. Proc. IEEE Eng. Med. Biol. Soc.* 303–306. doi: 10.1109/EMBC.2013.6609497

Baranauskas, G. (2014). What limits the performance of current invasive brain machine interfaces? *Front. Syst. Neurosci.* 8:68. doi: 10.3389/fnsys.2014.00068

Bishop, W., Chestek, C. C., Gilja, V., Nuyujukian, P., Foster, J. D., Ryu, S. I., et al. (2014). Self-recalibrating classifiers for intracortical brain-computer interfaces. *J. Neural Eng.* 11:026001. doi: 10.1088/1741-2560/11/2/026001

Brockmeier, A. J., Sanchez Giraldo, L. G., Emigh, M. S., Bae, J., Choi, J. S., Francis, J. T., et al. (2013). Information-theoretic metric learning: 2-D linear projections of neural data for visualization. *Conf. Proc. IEEE Eng. Med. Biol. Soc.* 5586–5589. doi: 10.1109/EMBC.2013.6610816

Cao, Y., Hao, Y., Liao, Y., Xu, K., Wang, Y., Zhang, S., et al. (2013). Information analysis on neural tuning in dorsal premotor cortex for reaching and grasping. *Comput. Math. Methods Med.* 2013:730374. doi: 10.1155/2013/730374

Carmena, J. M. (2013). Advances in neuroprosthetic learning and control. *PLoS Biol.* 11:e1001561. doi: 10.1371/journal.pbio.1001561

Chen, Z., Takahashi, K., and Hatsopoulos, N. G. (2013). Sparse Bayesian inference methods for decoding 3D reach and grasp kinematics and joint angles with primary motor cortical ensembles. *Conf. Proc. IEEE Eng. Med. Biol. Soc.* 2013, 5930–5933. doi: 10.1109/EMBC.2013.6610902

Chhatbar, P. Y., and Francis, J. T. (2013). Towards a naturalistic brain-machine interface: hybrid torque and position control allows generalization to novel dynamics. *PLoS One* 8:e52286. doi: 10.1371/journal.pone.0052286

Citi, L., Ba, D., Brown, E. N., and Barbieri, R. (2013). Likelihood methods for point processes with refractoriness. *Neural Comput.* 26, 237–263. doi: 10.1162/NECO_a_00548

Dangi, S., Gowda, S., and Carmena, J. (2013a). Likelihood gradient ascent (LGA): a closed-loop decoder adaptation algorithm for brain-machine interfaces. *Conf. Proc. IEEE Eng. Med. Biol. Soc.* 2013, 2768–2771. doi: 10.1109/EMBC.2013.6610114

Dangi, S., Orsborn, A. L., Moorman, H. G., and Carmena, J. M. (2013b). Design and analysis of closed-loop decoder adaptation algorithms for brain-machine interfaces. *Neural Comput.* 25, 1693–1731. doi: 10.1162/NECO_a_00460

Dangi, S., So, K., Orsborn, A., Gastpar, M., and Carmena, J. (2013c). Brain-machine interface control using broadband spectral power from local field potentials. *Conf. Proc. IEEE Eng. Med. Biol. Soc.* 2013, 285–288. doi: 10.1109/EMBC.2013.6609493

Ethier, C., Oby, E. R., Bauman, M. J., and Miller, L. E. (2012). Restoration of grasp following paralysis through brain-controlled stimulation of muscles. *Nature* 485, 368–371. doi: 10.1038/nature10987

Fan, J. M., Nuyujukian, P., Kao, J. C., Chestek, C. A., Ryu, S. I., and Shenoy, K. V. (2014). Intention estimation in brain-machine interfaces. *J. Neural Eng.* 11:016004. doi: 10.1088/1741-2560/11/1/016004

Flint, R. D., Wright, Z. A., Scheid, M. R., and Slutzky, M. W. (2013). Long term, stable brain machine interface performance using local field potentials and multiunit spikes. *J. Neural Eng.* 10:056005. doi: 10.1088/1741-2560/10/5/056005

Gilja, V., Nuyujukian, P., Chestek, C. A., Cunningham, J. P., Yu, B. M., Fan, J. M., et al. (2012). A high-performance neural prosthesis enabled by control algorithm design. *Nat. Neurosci.* 15, 1752–1757. doi: 10.1038/nn.3265

Golub, M. D., Yu, B. M., Schwartz, A. B., and Chase, S. M. (2014). Motor cortical control of movement speed with implications for brain-machine interface control. *J. Neurophysiol.* doi: 10.1152/jn.00391.2013. [Epub ahead of print].

Gowda, S., Orsborn, A., Overduin, S., Moorman, H., and Carmena, J. (2014). Designing dynamical properties of brain-machine interfaces to optimize task-specific performance. *IEEE Trans. Neural Syst. Rehabil. Eng.* doi: 10.1109/tnsre.2014.2309673. [Epub ahead of print].

Homer, M., Harrison, M., Black, M., Perge, J., Cash, S., Friehs, G., et al. (2013). "Mixing decoded cursor velocity and position from an offline Kalman filter improves cursor control in people with tetraplegia," in *2013 6th International IEEE/EMBS Conference on Neural Engineering (NER)* (San Diego, CA), 715–718. doi: 10.1109/NER.2013.6696034

Homer, M., Perge, J., Black, M., Harrison, M., Cash, S., and Hochberg, L. (2014). Adaptive offset correction for intracortical brain-computer interfaces. *IEEE Trans. Neural Syst. Rehabil. Eng.* 22, 239–248. doi: 10.1109/TNSRE.2013.2287768

Ifft, P. J., Shokur, S., Li, Z., Lebedev, M. A., and Nicolelis, M. A. L. (2013). A brain-machine interface enables bimanual arm movements in monkeys. *Sci. Transl. Med.* 5:210ra154. doi: 10.1126/scitranslmed.3006159

Jarosiewicz, B., Masse, N. Y., Bacher, D., Cash, S. S., Eskandar, E., Friehs, G., et al. (2013). Advantages of closed-loop calibration in intracortical brain-computer interfaces for people with tetraplegia. *J. Neural Eng.* 10:046012. doi: 10.1088/1741-2560/10/4/046012

Kao, J., Nuyujukian, P., Stavisky, S., Ryu, S., Ganguli, S., and Shenoy, K. (2013). Investigating the role of firing-rate normalization and dimensionality reduction in brain-machine interface robustness. *Conf. Proc. IEEE Eng. Med. Biol. Soc.* 2013, 293–298. doi: 10.1109/EMBC.2013.6609495

Kao, J., Stavisky, S., Sussillo, D., Nuyujukian, P., and Shenoy, K. (2014). Information systems opportunities in brain-machine interface decoders. *Proc. IEEE* 102, 666–682. doi: 10.1109/jproc.2014.2307357

Kowalski, K. C., He, B. D., and Srinivasan, L. (2013). Dynamic analysis of naive adaptive brain-machine interfaces. *Neural Comput.* 25, 2373–2420. doi: 10.1162/NECO_a_00484

Koyama, S., Eden, U., Brown, E., and Kass, R. (2010). Bayesian decoding of neural spike trains. *Ann. Inst. Stat. Math.* 62, 37–59. doi: 10.7551/mitpress/9780262042383.003.0004

Li, L., Brockmeier, A. J., Choi, J. S., Francis, J. T., Sanchez, J. C., and Príncipe, J. C. (2014). A tensor-product-kernel framework for multiscale neural activity decoding and control. *Comput. Intell. Neurosci.* 2014:870160. doi: 10.1155/2014/870160

Mahmoudi, B., Pohlmeyer, E. A., Prins, N. W., Geng, S., and Sanchez, J. C. (2013). Towards autonomous neuroprosthetic control using Hebbian reinforcement learning. *J. Neural Eng.* 10:066005. doi: 10.1088/1741-2560/10/6/066005

Merel, J. S., Fox, R., Jebara, T., and Paninski, L. (2013). "A multi-agent control framework for co-adaptation in brain-computer interfaces," in *Advances in Neural Information Processing Systems,* (vol. 26) eds C. Burges, L. Bottou, M. Welling, Z. Ghahramani and K. Weinberger (Red Hook, NY: Curran Associates, Inc.), 2841–2849.

Moritz, C. T., Perlmutter, S. I., and Fetz, E. E. (2008). Direct control of paralysed muscles by cortical neurons. *Nature* 456, 639–642. doi: 10.1038/nature07418

Nishimura, Y., Perlmutter, S. I., and Fetz, E. E. (2013). Restoration of upper limb movement via artificial corticospinal and musculospinal connections in a monkey with spinal cord injury. *Front. Neural Circuits.* 7:57. doi: 10.3389/fncir.2013.00057

Perge, J. A., Homer, M. L., Malik, W. Q., Cash, S., Eskandar, E., Friehs, G., et al. (2013). Intra-day signal instabilities affect decoding performance in an intracortical neural interface system. *J. Neural Eng.* 10:036004. doi: 10.1088/1741-2560/10/3/036004

Philip, B., Rao, N., and Donoghue, J. (2013). Simultaneous reconstruction of continuous hand movements from primary motor and posterior parietal cortex. *Exp. Brain Res.* 225, 361–375. doi: 10.1007/s00221-012-3377-0

Pohlmeyer, E. A., Mahmoudi, B., Geng, S., Prins, N. W., and Sanchez, J. C. (2014). Using reinforcement learning to provide stable brain-machine interface control despite neural input reorganization. *PLoS One* 9:e87253. doi: 10.1371/journal.pone.0087253

Prins, N. W., Geng, S., Pohlmeyer, E. A., Mahmoudi, B., and Sanchez, J. C. (2013). Feature extraction and unsupervised classification of neural population reward signals for reinforcement based BMI. *Conf. Proc. IEEE Eng. Med. Biol. Soc.* 5250–5253. doi: 10.1109/EMBC.2013.6610733

Sakurai, Y., Song, K., Tachibana, S., and Takahashi, S. (2014). Volitional enhancement of firing synchrony and oscillation by neuronal operant conditioning: interaction with neurorehabilitation and brain-machine interface. *Front. Syst. Neurosci.* 8:11. doi: 10.3389/fnsys.2014.00011

Scheid, M., Flint, R., Wright, Z., and Slutzky, M. (2013). Long-term, stable behavior of local field potentials during brain machine interface use. *Conf. Proc. IEEE Eng. Med. Biol. Soc.* 2013, 307–310. doi: 10.1109/EMBC.2013.6609498

Shanechi, M., and Carmena, J. (2013). "Optimal feedback-controlled point process decoder for adaptation and assisted training in brain-machine interfaces," in *2013 6th International IEEE/EMBS Conference on Neural Engineering (NER)* (San Diego, USA), 653–656. doi: 10.1109/NER.2013.6696019

Shanechi, M. M., Williams, Z. M., Wornell, G. W., Hu, R. C., Powers, M., and Brown, E. N. (2013). A real-time brain-machine interface combining motor target and trajectory intent using an optimal feedback control design. *PLoS One* 8:e59049. doi: 10.1371/journal.pone.0059049

Srinivasan, L., Eden, U. T., Willsky, A. S., and Brown, E. N. (2006). A state-space analysis for reconstruction of goal-directed movements using neural signals. *Neural Comput.* 18, 2465–2494. doi: 10.1162/neco.2006.18.10.2465

Suminski, A., Fagg, A., Willett, F., Bodenhamer, M., and Hatsopoulos, N. (2013). Online adaptive decoding of intended movements with a hybrid kinetic and kinematic brain machine interface. *Conf. Proc. IEEE Eng. Med. Biol. Soc.* 2013, 1583–1586. doi: 10.1109/EMBC.2013.6609817

Tehovnik, E., Woods, L., and Slocum, W. (2013). Transfer of information by BMI. *Neuroscience* 255, 134–146. doi: 10.1016/j.neuroscience.2013.10.003

Velliste, M., Kennedy, S. D., Schwartz, A. B., Whitford, A. S., Sohn, J.-W., and McMorland, A. J. (2014). Motor cortical correlates of arm resting in the context of a reaching task and implications for prosthetic control. *J. Neurosci.* 34, 6011–6022. doi: 10.1523/JNEUROSCI.3520-13.2014

Wang, D., Zhang, Q., Li, Y., Wang, Y., Zhu, J., Zhang, S., et al. (2014). Long-term decoding stability of local field potentials from silicon arrays in primate motor cortex during a 2D center out task. *J. Neural Eng.* 11:036009. doi: 10.1088/1741-2560/11/3/036009

Willett, F. R., Suminski, A. J., Fagg, A. H., and Hatsopoulos, N. G. (2013). Improving brain-machine interface performance by decoding intended future movements. *J. Neural Eng.* 10:026011. doi: 10.1088/1741-2560/10/2/026011

Wong, Y., Putrino, D., Weiss, A., and Pesaran, B. (2013). Utilizing movement synergies to improve decoding performance for a brain machine interface. *Conf. Proc. IEEE Eng. Med. Biol. Soc.* 2013, 289–292. doi: 10.1109/EMBC.2013.6609494

Wu, W., Black, M. J., Gao, Y., Bienenstock, E., Serruya, M., Shaikhoun, A., et al. (2003). "Neural decoding of cursor motion using a Kalman filter," in *Advances in Neural Information Processing Systems* (Vol. 15), eds S. Becker, S. Thrun and K. Obermayer (Boston: MIT Press), 133–140.

Xu, K., Wang, Y., Wang, F., Liao, Y., Zhang, Q., Li, H., et al. (2014). Neural decoding using a parallel sequential Monte Carlo method on point processes with ensemble effect. *Biomed Res. Int.* 2014:685492. doi: 10.1155/2014/685492

Xu, K., Wang, Y., Wang, Y., Wang, F., Hao, Y., Zhang, S., et al. (2013). Local-learning-based neuron selection for grasping gesture prediction in motor brain machine interfaces. *J. Neural Eng.* 10:026008. doi: 10.1088/1741-2560/10/2/026008

Zhang, Y., and Chase, S. (2013). A stabilized dual Kalman filter for adaptive tracking of brain-computer interface decoding parameters. *Conf. Proc. IEEE Eng. Med. Biol. Soc.* 2013, 7100–7103. doi: 10.1109/EMBC.2013.6611194

7

Biasing neural network dynamics using non-invasive brain stimulation

Martijn E. Wokke[1,2]*, Lotte J. Talsma[1,3] and Marlies E. Vissers[1,3]

[1] Amsterdam Brain and Cognition, University of Amsterdam, Amsterdam, Netherlands
[2] Consciousness, Cognition and Computation Group, Department of Psychology, Université Libre de Bruxelles, Brussels, Belgium
[3] Department of Psychology, University of Amsterdam, Amsterdam, Netherlands

Edited by:
Mikhail Lebedev, Duke University, USA

Reviewed by:
Yoshio Sakurai, Kyoto University, Japan
Estate M. Sokhadze, University of Louisville, USA

***Correspondence:**
Martijn E. Wokke, Consciousness, Cognition and Computation Group, Department of Psychology, Université Libre de Bruxelles, Avenue Franklin Roosevelt 50, 1050 Bruxelles, Belgium
e-mail: martijnwokke@gmail.com

Recently, non-invasive brain stimulation (NBS) has been discovered as a tool to improve human performance on a wide variety of tasks. Although these observations are highly intriguing, the underlying mechanisms of such enhancements are still poorly understood. Here, we argue that in order to advance our understanding of these mechanisms it is necessary to focus on intrinsic network dynamics in the brain. Taking into account well-known network dynamics, increased excitation in one particular network or brain region may necessarily lead to inhibition of an opposing network (and vice versa). As a consequence, observed behavioral improvements due to NBS may emerge from a shift in the balance between (competing) neural networks in the brain, implicating that behavioral enhancement due to stimulation most likely comes with a cost or side effect. We conclude that more elaborate experimental designs are essential for a better understanding of the relationship between network interactions and the behavioral effects of NBS.

Keywords: performance enhancement, neural networks, neuromodulation, TMS, tDCS

INTRODUCTION

In the last decade the use of non-invasive brain stimulation (NBS) techniques in cognitive neuroscience has grown explosively. Especially transcranial magnetic stimulation (TMS) and transcranial direct current stimulation (tDCS) have proven to be fruitful tools to causally link a wide range of brain regions or neural networks to perception, motor action and higher-level cognition. Moreover, NBS has been welcomed enthusiastically as a method to improve various aspects of human behavior (Luber and Lisanby, 2014). Yet, the full scope and range of the effects of NBS are currently poorly understood. In order to gain a more thorough understanding of the effects caused by stimulation, we will advocate that the observed effects of NBS on brain functioning should be seen in the light of complex interplays between task-relevant and task-irrelevant neural networks in the brain.

Almost three decades ago, TMS was introduced by Barker and colleagues (Barker et al., 1985) as a NBS technique that was able to safely affect brain function in humans (see Rossi et al., 2009). The effect of TMS is based on the principle of electromagnetic induction, in which a rapidly changing magnetic field induces a current in an electrically conducting medium, such as neural tissue. When TMS currents meet the right requirements (e.g., amplitude, duration and frequency, see Wagner et al., 2009) neural function and behavior can be altered, even outlasting the period of stimulation. The application of tDCS in cognitive neuroscientific research was introduced several years later than TMS (Priori et al., 1998; Nitsche and Paulus 2000), but the popularity of tDCS as a neuromodulatory tool led to a rapidly growing body of research on the effects of tDCS on perception, action and cognition. tDCS can modulate cortical excitability of neural activity by the induction of weak anodal and cathodal electrical currents flowing though the cerebral cortex. The polarity is of great influence on the neuromodulatory effect of tDCS: Where anodal (positive polarization) stimulation in general facilitates cortical excitability of the underlying tissue, cathodal stimulation increases the threshold for neuronal firing (Liebetanz et al., 2002; Krause et al., 2013; however, note that the effect of polarity on neuronal firing may also depend on the state of the targeted brain region during stimulation, see e.g., Krause and Cohen Kadosh, 2014).

Initially, NBS was used to determine whether modulation of neural activity in a particular brain region was able to disrupt performance associated with normal network functioning. However, various studies began to demonstrate that tempering normal network functioning could in fact result in paradoxical improvements of performance (Luber and Lisanby, 2014). Recently, the rise of tDCS and new TMS protocols has highlighted the potential of NBS as a technique that can be used to improve brain functioning in healthy individuals or in patients suffering from neurological or psychiatric illness (Coffman et al., 2014). Although these findings are very intriguing and seem promising for both healthy and clinical populations, the underlying neural mechanisms subserving the augmentation of brain function following TMS and tDCS remains largely elusive.

In this paper we will exclusively focus on two factors that are important when considering the potential benefits and costs of neurostimulation techniques. These factors are not directly related to parameters (e.g., polarity or frequency) in *generating* a stimulation effect (for an extensive discussion of stimulation parameters in this respect, see e.g., Walsh et al., 2003; Flöel, 2014), but concern a conceptual framework for studying NBS. Firstly, there is ample evidence on facilitatory and inhibitory interactions between different functional networks in the brain (Kinsbourne, 1987; Calautti and Baron, 2003; Fox et al., 2005; Szczepanski and Kastner, 2013), stressing the importance of reckoning the brain as a complex constellation of functional networks. This notion is already widely self-evident in certain domains, such as in research on brain connectivity (e.g., Sporns, 2013) and rehabilitation (Calautti and Baron, 2003), however it currently seems to have little influence in the design and interpretation of NBS experiments and effects. Whereas it is conceivable that stimulation of one particular network or brain region may lead to cognitive benefits that come at the cost of other cognitive processes, studies reporting brain function enhancement typically focus on the effects of stimulation on the targeted process or ability, without co-assessing possible unintended effects on other functions. However, by selectively studying intended behavioral improvements, it is conceivable that cognitive enhancements are commanding the spotlights, while potential costs keep on dancing in the dark. As a consequence, current approaches obscure the value of observed enhancement effects in a broader sense. Secondly, the effects of TMS and tDCS have been shown to be dependent on the state of the probed network (Silvanto et al., 2007; Krause and Cohen Kadosh, 2014). The specific context in which stimulation is applied seems to be critical for the behavioral effect, demonstrating how observed enhancements are emerging from complex, dynamic interactions between internal and external modulations of network activity.

We will first address a small selection of studies demonstrating enhancement of performance by TMS and tDCS in the sensory and higher-level cognitive domain. We will discuss these findings in light of brain network interactions and the modulatory role of the functional state of the stimulated network, in order to illustrate the importance of taking network interactions into account when studying the effects of NBS on behavior.

ENHANCEMENT OF VISUAL PERCEPTION

One of the first studies demonstrating enhancement of sensory processing induced by TMS manipulated visual attention by applying repetitive transcranial magnetic stimulation (rTMS) to the human parietal cortex (Hilgetag et al., 2001). Previously, a great deal of what was known about the neural mechanism of visual attention stemmed from patients suffering from visual neglect. Visual neglect is typically caused by lesions to the posterior parietal (or frontal) cortex, resulting in a deficit in the ability to draw attention towards the visual space contralateral to the lesion. This pattern of findings led to a model of cross-hemispheric competition (Kinsbourne, 1987; Szczepanski and Kastner, 2013), in which the balance in interhemispheric distribution of attentional resources is maintained via mutual inhibition. Interestingly, while researchers are typically focused on contralateral attentional deficits accompanying visual neglect Hilgetag et al. (2001) demonstrated that the induction of a "virtual lesion" to the parietal cortex could actually result in increased ipsilateral visual attention. These findings demonstrate how the intrinsic balance between neural activity across hemispheres is essential for typical perceptual functioning, and how disturbance of this balance can lead to perceptual deficits such as neglect.

Disruption of more subtle network interactions than the interhemispheric interplay discussed above has also been found to affect behavioral performance. This was illustrated in a TMS experiment on visual feature processing (Walsh et al., 1998). Walsh et al. found that disruption of cortical area HMT+/V5, a key region involved in motion processing, impaired performance during a visual search task when motion was the critical target feature. In contrast, disruption of HMT+/V5 resulted in an initially unexpected enhancement of performance when color or form were the essential features of the target. The enhancement of performance caused by the disruption of HMT+/V5 was unexpected, as TMS was considered to induce neural noise, and thereby, to deteriorate normal behavior. The unexpected enhancement was interpreted to be the result of the temporarily reduced competition of (visual) brain areas for limited processing resources, such as energy and communication with other brain regions. Thus, disruption of HMT+/V5 by TMS likely shifted the balance of neural resources towards other visual areas, improving visual perception for features processed in these other brain regions. Recently, we observed additional supporting evidence for a model in which brain regions engage in a "battle for resources" (Wokke et al., 2014). In two experiments, we probed the role of area HMT+/V5 and the object sensitive lateral occipital region (LO) during a figure discrimination task that dominantly relied on HMT+/V5 processing. Disruption of activity in LO and HMT+/V5 led to opposing effects on performance, depending on the stimulation site. Disruption of HMT+/V5 resulted in decreased discriminability, whereas participants' discriminability improved when activity in LO was perturbed. Complementary to the findings by Walsh et al. (1998), we demonstrated that the workings of HMT+/V5 improved during a motion-defined figure discrimination task when we disrupted a cortical region specialized in task-irrelevant properties. These findings provide converging evidence for competitive interactions between extrastriate cortical areas. Such observations of improved performance due to reduced neural activity in task-irrelevant regions, a phenomenon that has been dubbed "addition-by-subtraction" (Luber and Lisanby, 2014), are strong examples of the notion that effects of NBS are established due to the intrinsic interactions of functional brain networks (see **Figure 1**).

IMPROVED COGNITIVE PERFORMANCE

The growing popularity of tDCS has led to a steep rise in the number of studies on enhancement of cognitive functions such as attention, (motor) learning, working memory, and even complex problem solving (Fregni et al., 2005; Cohen Kadosh et al., 2010; Chi and Snyder, 2012; Coffman et al., 2012). For example, there is evidence for a positive effect of tDCS over frontal brain regions on working memory performance. One of the first studies on the effects of tDCS on higher-order cognition used anodal tDCS over

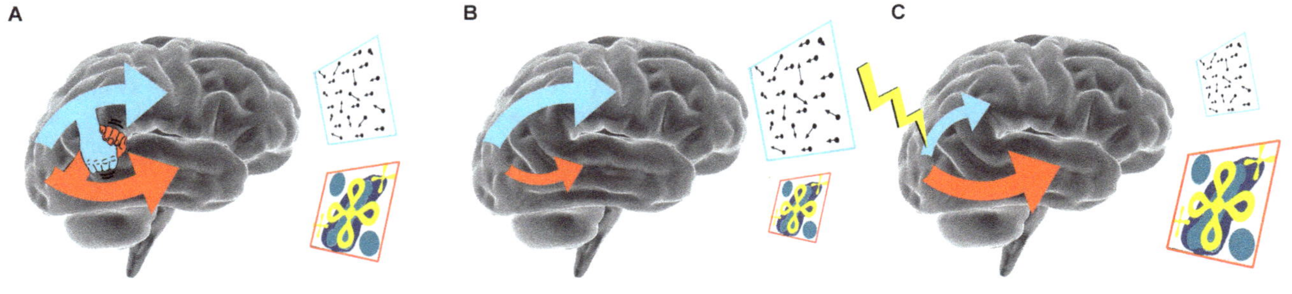

FIGURE 1 | Biasing the balance between networks with NBS. **(A)** A schematic illustration of competing network interactions in the brain during a motion discrimination (blue frame) and a shape discrimination (red frame) task, that both rely on different brain networks. **(B)** When engaging in a motion discrimination task activity in the dorsal network increases, while activity in the ventral stream decreases. **(C)** Disruption of dorsal (visual) activity results in decreased performance in motion direction discrimination while decreased dorsal competition results in enhanced performance on the shape discrimination task.

left prefrontal dorsolateral cortex (lDLPFC) to study its effects on working memory performance (e.g., Fregni et al., 2005). Anodal tDCS over lDLPFC was shown to reduce the number of errors people make on a 3-back working memory task, increasing accuracy of performance. However, there are also studies that fail to demonstrate a positive effect of tDCS on working memory functioning (for a review, see Coffman et al., 2014), complicating the interpretation of observed enhancement effects.

Recently, an elegant study by Iuculano and Cohen Kadosh (2013) revealed detrimental as well as beneficial effects of tDCS on cognition. In this study, participants performed a mathematical training during which tDCS was applied on different sites. Part of the participants received tDCS over posterior parietal cortex (PPC), whereas other participants received stimulation over DLPFC. Results showed that stimulation of the PPC led to increased speed of learning, but to impaired automaticity for the learned materials, whereas the opposite was found to be the case for stimulation over DLPFC. Thus, these findings show that stimulating the brain at different locations may have positive but also disruptive effects on cognitive performance. As suggested by the authors themselves, the eventual benefits and costs that come with a particular stimulation method may be due to corticocortical interactions, and induced shifts between metabolic prioritization. Clearly, this study illustrates the importance of broadening the scope of investigated abilities in order to detect whether behavioral improvements in one domain may come at the expense of another, emphasizing the importance of taking network configurations into account when assessing behavioral effects due to NBS. However, whereas the study by Iuculano and Cohen Kadosh (2013) was directed at comparing stimulation effects on different aspects of a targeted cognitive function (mathematical learning), it would be desirable to pursue this type of research using designs in which one single site is being stimulated, while multiple (cognitive) functions are investigated. This approach would allow one to investigate the extent to which collateral impairments in behavior arise due to intrinsic interactions between functional networks in the brain.

Another important factor to take into account is the state of a network during stimulation (Krause and Cohen Kadosh, 2014). It seems that the initial neural activation state during stimulation determines the behavioral effect of stimulation (Silvanto et al., 2008). When stimulation is applied during performance of a task, its effects have been shown to differ from stimulation during rest (Andrews et al., 2011). Another interesting finding concerning the effect of cognitive state is that application of tDCS over lateral PFC when subjects are not involved in a cognitive task, modulates activity in task-positive as well as task-negative networks (as measured with fMRI; Keeser et al., 2011). Thus, although stimulation effects depend on the currently dominant functional network, these findings show that stimulation effects are not restricted to the currently active network. Therefore, full comprehension of the potential scope of NBS requires a more complete understanding of the extent to which stimulation has an effect on targeted, as well as task-irrelevant and non-targeted networks.

OPPOSING NETWORK DYNAMICS

In the last decade a strong interest in competing network dynamics has been sparked by observed relations between opposed activity levels in task-positive (e.g., attention, fronto-parietal) and task-negative (e.g., default mode) networks and performance on a variety of tasks (Raichle et al., 2001; Fox et al., 2005; Weissman et al., 2006; Kelly et al., 2008; Hampson et al., 2010). Crucially, there seems to be a competitive balance of activity between task-positive and task-negative networks during task performance (Wojciulik and Kanwisher, 1999; McKiernan et al., 2003). During task performance activity increases in regions that are supporting task execution, whereas activity decreases in regions associated with task irrelevant (or task-opposing) processes. A growing amount of studies demonstrate the existence of strong anti-correlations between task-negative networks and task-positive networks (e.g., Fox et al., 2005). These anti-correlations have been shown to relate to performance, such that stronger anti-correlations are predictive of better cognitive performance (Kelly et al., 2008; Hampson et al., 2010). The dichotomy in activity levels observed in different networks during task performance has been suggested to be an intrinsic property of the organization of the brain (Fox et al., 2005).

It is conceivable that an external modulation of the competition between antagonistic networks in the brain could be beneficial in certain circumstances. For instance, in people with disorders such as autism spectrum disorder (ASD), anti-correlations between the default mode network and task-positive regions were found to be less pronounced than in typical subjects (Kennedy et al., 2006). In addition, decreased anti-correlations has been related to ASD symptoms (Anderson et al., 2011). These patterns demonstrate possible detrimental effects of atypical competition between different networks. Interestingly, Josipovic et al. (2012) recently demonstrated that anti-correlations between task-positive and task-negative networks could be differentially modulated depending of the cognitive style during meditation, thus disregarding them as an immutable characteristic of the organization of the brain. Further, the balance between competing networks might be adjusted dynamically to fit currently relevant behavioral goals by regulatory networks involved in top-down control (Spreng et al., 2013). Thus, whereas the interrelatedness of networks might be an inherent property of the functional organization of the brain, the balance between different network states is likely to be flexible and sensitive to top-down control. In light of these findings, NBS could be instrumental by altering the strength of competing interactions between different networks, or dichotomously increase and decrease the amount of synchrony within each network (Peña-Gómez et al., 2012).

Based on findings revealing the dynamic competition between activated and deactivated networks and their effects on behavior, it seems evident that interfering with activity in one network by applying TMS or tDCS necessarily shifts the balance between task relevant and task-irrelevant networks. Taken together with the established functional links between network anti-correlations and healthy and efficient cognitive functioning, this induced balance shift between networks is likely to have an effect on cognitive performance. Therefore, an important venue for future research employing NBS is to examine to what extent the behavioral effects of these methods can be explained by a shift in the balance of activation between different networks, rather than the current approach of solemnly focusing on altered levels of activity within one network. The notion that the balance between competing networks is an important factor may also help to explain the importance of the state of a network during application of tDCS (McKiernan et al., 2003). When taking the interconnectedness of brain networks into account, it becomes trivial that effects of brain stimulation during a state in which different functional networks are anti-correlated differs from stimulation during rest, because of the large differences in the configuration of functional networks (Silvanto et al., 2008).

Furthermore, the principle of improving one cognitive function by suppression of task-irrelevant neural processing, which was observed in TMS research described above, is possibly also at play during application of tDCS. This principle can be understood in terms of the framework proposed by Brem et al. (2014), which holds that the brain functions as a closed energy system. Under this assumption, brain stimulation would always have a “net zero-sum” effect, meaning that enhancement of one domain or function will always have costs for another domain or function. When the brain is stimulated, the distribution of resources over different brain regions or networks is externally modulated. Enhancement or suppression of activity in one neural network will necessarily lead to impairment or enhancement in another network, due to redistribution of available resources. At present we do not know whether brain stimulation exerts its effects by a temporary redistribution of resources, or whether it induces a different type of redistribution in the brain. In order to acquire more insight into the effects of NBS of distribution of neural resources, research on NBS should take the interrelatedness of different network dynamics as a central starting point.

CONCLUSIONS

In the present paper we argued that recent findings of enhancement of brain function should be seen in light of a manipulation of the balance between different functional brain networks, which can result in improved behavior when applied in the right context. However, assuming NBS is biasing the brain towards one particular functional state, this might also have detrimental effects on performance, for example, by hampering flexible transitions between functional networks. It might therefore be misleading to speak of an *enhancement* of brain function, and, alternatively, it might be more appropriate to describe the NBS effects in terms of a *bias shift*.

More research on brain-wide effects of NBS will contribute to an understanding of the way the entire brain is affected by NBS at specific sites, and may yield ways to apply these techniques in more efficient ways. In addition, with a more thorough understanding of NBS effects, brain stimulation should become more applicable outside the realm of specific lab settings. Therefore, in order to move the field of NBS and its (clinical) applications forward, it is essential to extend current studies on the effects of NBS towards investigating the effects of stimulation on task-relevant as well as task-irrelevant functional brain networks.

REFERENCES

Anderson, J. S., Nielsen, J. A., Froehlich, A. L., DuBray, M. B., Druzgal, T. J., Cariello, A. N., et al. (2011). Functional connectivity magnetic resonance imaging classification of autism. *Brain* 134, 3742–3754. doi: 10.1093/brain/awr263

Andrews, S. C., Hoy, K. E., Enticott, P. G., Daskalakis, Z. J., and Fitzgerald, P. B. (2011). Improving working memory: the effect of combining cognitive activity and anodal transcranial direct current stimulation to the left dorsolateral prefrontal cortex. *Brain Stimul.* 4, 84–89. doi: 10.1016/j.brs.2010.06.004

Barker, A. T., Jalinous, R., and Freeston, I. L. (1985). Non-invasive magnetic stimulation of human motor cortex. *The Lancet* 325, 1106–1107. doi: 10.1016/s0140-6736(85)92413-4

Brem, A. K., Fried, P. J., Horvath, J. C., Robertson, E. M., and Pascual-Leone, A. (2014). Is neuroenhancement by noninvasive brain stimulation a net zero-sum proposition?. *Neuroimage* 85, 1058–1068. doi: 10.1016/j.neuroimage.2013.07.038

Calautti, C., and Baron, J. C. (2003). Functional neuroimaging studies of motor recovery after stroke in adults a review. *Stroke* 34, 1553–1566. doi: 10.1161/01.str.0000071761.36075.a6

Chi, R. P., and Snyder, A. W. (2012). Brain stimulation enables the solution of an inherently difficult problem. *Neurosci. Lett.* 515, 121–124. doi: 10.1016/j.neulet.2012.03.012

Coffman, B. A., Clark, V. P., and Parasuraman, R. (2014). Battery powered thought: enhancement of attention, learning and memory in healthy adults using transcranial direct current stimulation. *Neuroimage* 85, 895–908. doi: 10.1016/j.neuroimage.2013.07.083

Coffman, B. A., Trumbo, M. C., and Clark, V. P. (2012). Enhancement of object detection with transcranial direct current stimulation is associated with increased attention. *BMC Neurosci.* 13:108. doi: 10.1186/1471-2202-13-108

Cohen Kadosh, R., Soskic, S., Iuculano, T., Kanai, R., and Walsh, V. (2010). Modulating neuronal activity produces specific and long-lasting changes in numerical competence. *Current Biol.* 20, 2016–2020. doi: 10.1016/j.cub.2010.10.007

Flöel, A. (2014). tDCS-enhanced motor and cognitive function in neurological diseases. *Neuroimage* 85, 934–947. doi: 10.1016/j.neuroimage.2013.05.098

Fox, M. D., Snyder, A. Z., Vincent, J. L., Corbetta, M., Van Essen, D. C., and Raichle, M. E. (2005). The human brain is intrinsically organized into dynamic, anticorrelated functional networks. *Proc. Natl. Acad. Sci. U S A* 102, 9673–9678. doi: 10.1073/pnas.0504136102

Fregni, F., Boggio, P. S., Nitsche, M., Bermpohl, F., Antal, A., Feredoes, E., et al. (2005). Anodal transcranial direct current stimulation of prefrontal cortex enhances working memory. *Exp. Brain Res.* 166, 23–30. doi: 10.1007/s00221-005-2334-6

Hampson, M., Driesen, N., Roth, J. K., Gore, J. C., and Constable, R. T. (2010). Functional connectivity between task-positive and task-negative brain areas and its relation to working memory performance. *Magn. Reson. Imaging* 28, 1051–1057. doi: 10.1016/j.mri.2010.03.021

Hilgetag, C. C., Théoret, H., and Pascual-Leone, A. (2001). Enhanced visual spatial attention ipsilateral to rTMS-induced 'virtual lesions' of human parietal cortex. *Nat. Neurosci.* 4, 953–957. doi: 10.1038/nn0901-953

Iuculano, T., and Cohen Kadosh, R. (2013). The mental cost of cognitive enhancement. *J. Neurosci.* 33, 4482–4486. doi: 10.1523/jneurosci.4927-12.2013

Josipovic, Z., Dinstein, I., Weber, J., and Heeger, D. J. (2012). Influence of meditation on anti-correlated networks in the brain. *Front. Hum. Neurosci.* 5:183. doi: 10.3389/fnhum.2011.00183

Keeser, D., Meindl, T., Bor, J., Palm, U., Pogarell, O., Mulert, C., et al. (2011). Prefrontal transcranial direct current stimulation changes connectivity of resting-state networks during fMRI. *J. Neurosci.* 31, 15284–15293. doi: 10.1523/jneurosci.0542-11.2011

Kelly, A. M., Uddin, L. Q., Biswal, B. B., Castellanos, F. X., and Milham, M. P. (2008). Competition between functional brain networks mediates behavioral variability. *Neuroimage* 39, 527–537. doi: 10.1016/j.neuroimage.2007.08.008

Kennedy, D. P., Redcay, E., and Courchesne, E. (2006). Failing to deactivate: resting functional abnormalities in autism. *Proc. Natl. Acad. Sci. U S A* 103, 8275–8280. doi: 10.1073/pnas.0600674103

Kinsbourne, M. (1987). Mechanisms of unilateral neglect. *Adv. Psychol.* 45, 69–86. doi: 10.1016/s0166-4115(08)61709-4

Krause, B., and Cohen Kadosh, R. (2014). Not all brains are created equal: the relevance of individual differences in responsiveness to transcranial electrical stimulation. *Front. Syst. Neurosci.* 8:25. doi: 10.3389/fnsys.2014.00025

Krause, B., Márquez-Ruiz, J., and Kadosh, R. C. (2013). The effect of transcranial direct current stimulation: a role for cortical excitation/inhibition balance?. *Front. Hum. Neurosci.* 7:602. doi: 10.3389/fnhum.2013.00602

Liebetanz, D., Nitsche, M. A., Tergau, F., and Paulus, W. (2002). Pharmacological approach to the mechanisms of transcranial DC-stimulation-induced after-effects of human motor cortex excitability. *Brain* 125, 2238–2247. doi: 10.1093/brain/awf238

Luber, B., and Lisanby, S. H. (2014). Enhancement of human cognitive performance using transcranial magnetic stimulation (TMS). *Neuroimage* 85, 961–970. doi: 10.1016/j.neuroimage.2013.06.007

McKiernan, K. A., Kaufman, J. N., Kucera-Thompson, J., and Binder, J. R. (2003). A parametric manipulation of factors affecting task-induced deactivation in functional neuroimaging. *J. Cogn. Neurosci.* 15, 394–408. doi: 10.1162/089892903321593117

Nitsche, M. A., and Paulus, W. (2000). Excitability changes induced in the human motor cortex by weak transcranial direct current stimulation. *J. Physiol.* 527, 633–639. doi: 10.1111/j.1469-7793.2000.t01-1-00633.x

Peña-Gómez, C., Sala-Lonch, R., Junqué, C., Clemente, I. C., Vidal, D., Bargalló, N., et al. (2012). Modulation of large-scale brain networks by transcranial direct current stimulation evidenced by resting-state functional MRI. *Brain Stimul.* 5, 252–263. doi: 10.1016/j.brs.2011.08.006

Priori, A., Berardelli, A., Rona, S., Accornero, N., and Manfredi, M. (1998). Polarization of the human motor cortex through the scalp. *Neuroreport* 9, 2257–2260.

Raichle, M. E., MacLeod, A. M., Snyder, A. Z., Powers, W. J., Gusnard, D. A., and Shulman, G. L. (2001). A default mode of brain function. *Proc. Natl. Acad. Sci. U S A* 98, 676–682. doi: 10.1073/pnas.98.2.676

Rossi, S., Hallett, M., Rossini, P. M., and Pascual-Leone, A. (2009). Safety, ethical considerations and application guidelines for the use of transcranial magnetic stimulation in clinical practice and research. *Clin. Neurophysiol.* 120, 2008–2039. doi: 10.1016/j.clinph.2009.08.016

Silvanto, J., Muggleton, N. G., Cowey, A., and Walsh, V. (2007). Neural adaptation reveals state-dependent effects of transcranial magnetic stimulation. *Eur. J. Neurosci.* 25, 1874–1881. doi: 10.1111/j.1460-9568.2007.05440.x

Silvanto, J., Muggleton, N., and Walsh, V. (2008). State-dependency in brain stimulation studies of perception and cognition. *Trends Cogn. Sci.* 12, 447–454. doi: 10.1016/j.tics.2008.09.004

Sporns, O. (2013). Network attributes for segregation and integration in the human brain. *Curr. Opin. Neurobiol.* 23, 162–171. doi: 10.1016/j.conb.2012.11.015

Spreng, R. N., Sepulcre, J., Turner, G. R., Stevens, W. D., and Schacter, D. L. (2013). Intrinsic architecture underlying the relations among the default, dorsal attention and frontoparietal control networks of the human brain. *J. Cogn. Neurosci.* 25, 74–86. doi: 10.1162/jocn_a_00281

Szczepanski, S. M., and Kastner, S. (2013). Shifting attentional priorities: control of spatial attention through hemispheric competition. *J. Neurosci.* 33, 5411–5421. doi: 10.1523/jneurosci.4089-12.2013

Wagner, T., Rushmore, J., Eden, U., and Valero-Cabre, A. (2009). Biophysical foundations underlying TMS: setting the stage for an effective use of neurostimulation in the cognitive neurosciences. *Cortex* 45, 1025–1034. doi: 10.1016/j.cortex.2008.10.002

Walsh, V., Ellison, A., Battelli, L., and Cowey, A. (1998). Task-specific impairments and enhancements induced by magnetic stimulation of human visual area V5. *Proc. Biol. Sci.* 265, 537–543. doi: 10.1098/rspb.1998.0328

Walsh, V., Pascual-Leone, A., and Kosslyn, S. M. (2003). *Transcranial Magnetic Stimulation: A Neurochronometrics of Mind.* Cambridge, MA: MIT press.

Weissman, D. H., Roberts, K. C., Visscher, K. M., and Woldorff, M. G. (2006). The neural bases of momentary lapses in attention. *Nat. Neurosci.* 9, 971–978. doi: 10.1038/nn1727

Wojciulik, E., and Kanwisher, N. (1999). The generality of parietal involvement in visual attention. *Neuron* 23, 747–764. doi: 10.1016/s0896-6273(01)80033-7

Wokke, M. E., Scholte, H. S., and Lamme, V. A. (2014). Opposing dorsal/ventral stream dynamics during figure-ground segregation. *J. Cogn. Neurosci.* 26, 365–379. doi: 10.1162/jocn_a_00497

8

Are videogame training gains specific or general?

Adam C. Oei and Michael D. Patterson*

Division of Psychology, School of Humanities and Social Sciences, Nanyang Technological University, Singapore, Singapore

Edited by:
Mikhail Lebedev, Duke University, USA

Reviewed by:
Richard Haier, University of California, USA
Kynan Eng, University of Zurich and ETH Zurich, Switzerland

***Correspondence:**
Michael D. Patterson, Division of Psychology, School of Humanities and Social Sciences, Nanyang Technological University, #04-13, 14 Nanyang Drive, Singapore 637332, Singapore
e-mail: mdpatterson@ntu.edu.sg

Many recent studies using healthy adults document enhancements in perception and cognition from playing commercial action videogames (AVGs). Playing action games (e.g., *Call of Duty, Medal of Honor*) is associated with improved bottom-up lower-level information processing skills like visual-perceptual and attentional processes. One proposal states a general improvement in the ability to interpret and gather statistical information to predict future actions which then leads to better performance across different perceptual/attentional tasks. Another proposal claims all the tasks are separately trained in the AVGs because the AVGs and laboratory tasks contain similar demands. We review studies of action and non-AVGs to show support for the latter proposal. To explain transfer in AVGs, we argue that the perceptual and attention tasks share common demands with the trained videogames (e.g., multiple object tracking (MOT), rapid attentional switches, and peripheral vision). In non-AVGs, several studies also demonstrate specific, limited transfer. One instance of specific transfer is the specific enhancement to mental rotation after training in games with a spatial emphasis (e.g., *Tetris*). In contrast, the evidence for transfer is equivocal where the game and task do not share common demands (e.g., executive functioning). Thus, the "common demands" hypothesis of transfer not only characterizes transfer effects in AVGs, but also non-action games. Furthermore, such a theory provides specific predictions, which can help in the selection of games to train human cognition as well as in the design of videogames purposed for human cognitive and perceptual enhancement. Finally this hypothesis is consistent with the cognitive training literature where most post-training gains are for tasks similar to the training rather than general, non-specific improvements.

Keywords: video games, transfer (psychology), cognition, perception, learning

INTRODUCTION

Over the last decade, effects of videogame play on human perception and cognition have been intensely studied and debated. Most studies have examined effects from action videogame (AVG) play. With a few exceptions (e.g., Boot et al., 2008; Irons et al., 2011), results from independent laboratories have shown experienced AVG players outperforming non-players in a variety of cognitive and perceptual tasks (e.g., Green and Bavelier, 2003; Colzato et al., 2010; Vallett et al., 2013).

What type of games can be considered an AVG? While the complexity and cross-fertilization across videogames makes pigeonholing each game into a distinct category difficult and somewhat arbitrary, AVGs contain many characteristics that make them unique. These include unpredictability, fast speed in presentation and response requirements, high perceptual load, the selection between multiple action plans and an emphasis on peripheral processing (Green et al., 2010a; Hubert-Wallander et al., 2011). Most of the games used in AVG studies have been first-person shooters (FPS) like *Call of Duty*, *Counterstrike*, *Unreal Tournament* and *Medal of Honor* (see also Latham et al., 2013 for more detailed descriptions of different AVGs). Although games of other genres like role-playing (e.g., *Final Fantasy*), puzzle (e.g., *Tetris*) may have one or two features in common with AVGs (e.g., speeded responses), they rarely, if ever, present these all the aforementioned demands in combination. Note that exactly what part of the AVG that leads to transfer is not yet clearly understood, and whether all or only some of the components are necessary for the transfer effects that have been observed.

Although cross-sectional comparisons suggest playing videogames leads to cognitive enhancements, they actually have little bearing on causality (Boot et al., 2011; Kristjánsson, 2013). Primary problems include issues of directionality (i.e., it is unclear whether people develop superior cognitive skills because of gaming or whether people with superior skills become gamers) and expectancy effects (people recruited for their gaming expertise are more motivated and expect to perform better) (Boot et al., 2011; Kristjánsson, 2013).

In contrast to cross-sectional studies, longitudinal-type training studies that show improved cognitive and perceptual abilities following a short bout of videogame training involving novice videogame players make stronger inferences for causality (e.g., Green and Bavelier, 2003; Wu and Spence, 2013). These games used for training are so intriguing because they were not specifically designed with the goal of training human cognition and perception (e.g., Klingberg et al., 2005; Jaeggi et al., 2011; Anguera et al., 2013). Rather, they are commercially available games designed for entertainment. Hence, learning as a result of playing these games is incidental rather than intentional.

PURPOSE AND SCOPE OF THE REVIEW

While there are many studies documenting the effects of videogame play on cognitive and perceptual skills, the mechanism of transfer is not well understood. One proposal to explain the wide range of AVG-related transfer across multiple perceptual, attentional and executive measures is that the transfer is due to a general improvement in probabilistic inference. In other words, AVG trainees become better able to use evidence from repeated presentations of a task to guide their decision-making and allocation of cognitive resources (Green et al., 2010b; Bavelier et al., 2012b). Hence, AVG experience may enhance a general capacity to control top-down attention and learning of a new task, which in turn translates to improvement across many different tasks. This process is termed "learning to learn" (Bavelier et al., 2012b). Although intriguing, this suggestion is not without problems. First, it is unclear whether this transfer to a general statistical learning ability applies only to AVG or whether it can also be used to explain transfer effects from other videogames. If only applicable to AVG-based learning, it remains unclear what is special about AVG or the exact properties that would be required in an AVG to cause transfer. Second, this hypothesis is too general such that it is not clear which tasks AVG training can and cannot transfer to. Third and most importantly, although it has been demonstrated that AVG trainees do indeed improve probabilistic inference in a visual perceptual task (Green et al., 2010b), empirical evidence is currently lacking to show that this can also account for transfer to the other tasks seen in the AVG literature.

In contrast to the view of Bavelier et al. (2012b), we argue that transfer is task-specific and limited to perceptual and cognitive skills common to both the trained videogame and laboratory transfer task. The roots of this proposal go back to the theory of identical elements (Thorndike and Woodworth, 1901). Therefore, repeated playing of a videogame allows the player to hone the shared specific demands. We argue that the tasks used to test transfer have similar demands to what is trained by AVG. To demonstrate this, we will review each task that has been improved by AVG playing and explain how demands within the AVG are similar to the task itself. The hypothesis of common demands is also consistent with evidence showing that transfer from training is more likely if training and transfer task recruited common neural regions (Dahlin et al., 2008).

The review covers both cross-sectional comparisons between experienced videogame players as well as longitudinal-type training studies. Although videogame training has been studied across the lifespan from young children (Subrahmanyam and Greenfield, 1994; Yuji, 1996) to old adults (Basak et al., 2008), Due to limited space, we limit this review to young adults, which make up the majority of the samples used in the videogame literature.

The reader should note that because of the interest generated by the groundbreaking work that emerged from the Bavelier lab (Green and Bavelier, 2003), the majority of investigations over the last decade have been focused mainly on AVGs. In contrast, non-AVGs are rarely studied. Rather, non-AVG players and non-AVG training groups are often used as control groups. Hence, inevitably a large portion of the review will document cognitive and perceptual enhancements via AVG play. Nevertheless, where available, we review evidence for transfer effects arising from non-AVGs as these studies also provide evidence to support our common demands hypothesis. We review the evidence for videogame-related transfer starting from lower level perceptual skills to higher-order cognitive control.

EVIDENCE FOR VIDEOGAME-RELATED TRANSFER

Enhancements in many visual-perceptual skills have been demonstrated empirically in many AVG-training studies and those that compared non-AVG and habitual AVG players. The different demands described above in AVGs allow predictions on what abilities are trained and the plausible transfer effects using the common demands hypothesis. Consider what is expected in a typical AVG. In these games, players often are required to detect and respond to enemies quickly as well as keeping track of them as they move around the screen. These demands are coupled with the need to attend to several items simultaneously in both central and peripheral vision. These are similar to the demands in multiple object tracking (MOT) and Useful Field of View (UFOV) tasks. Moreover, as enemies appear rapidly one after another or simultaneously, there is great emphasis on the ability to rapidly switch attention from one target to another. This is similar to an attentional blink task. In addition, players have to resist being distracted by task irrelevant stimuli no matter how salient these distractors are. This may lead to improved performance in tasks that require suppressing distractors. Failure to successfully perform any of the above may result in failure in the game mission. Because of these special properties, one can imagine that hours spent on playing action AVG play can serve to exercise many of these perceptual and attentional skills that underpin successful gameplay.

CONTRAST SENSITIVITY

An important aspect of visual perception that is enhanced by AVG playing is the ability to detect subtle contrast differences. Specifically, Li et al. (2009) showed that habitual AVG players outperformed non-videogame players in the ability to detect a low contrast Gabor patch. Additionally, videogame novices also showed enhancements in this skill following 50 h training in a fast-paced FPS relative to playing a control non-action game (*The Sims*).

At first glance, it does not appear obvious that an AVG experience demands detecting contrast differences between objects. However, note that in many action games, a strong emphasis is on distinguishing targets from non-targets to allow rapid responding. The emphasis on rapid responding thus places a demand on distinguishing a target from a non-target based on even the subtlest differences (e.g., visual characteristics such as color or contrast).

PERIPHERAL VISION

AVGs make good candidates for training peripheral vision because of their heavy emphasis on detecting targets across different central and peripheral areas. For example, in many shooter games, enemies often appear at far areas of the periphery and players must spot and dispatch them early to advance in the game. It is therefore likely that hours spent on AVG play would serve to enhance sensitivity to targets in the periphery.

One measure of peripheral vision is the UFOV, which is the total area of the visual field where useful information is captured at a glance without eye or head movements (Sanders, 1970; Ball et al., 1988). Comparisons of UFOV between regular AVG players and non-players have shown that the former exhibited superior ability to detect targets at peripheral areas of vision (10°, 20° and 30° eccentricity) (Green and Bavelier, 2003). Target detection at these eccentricities was also enhanced following AVG training for as short as 10 h relative to *Tetris* (Green and Bavelier, 2003). This enhanced target detection in regular AVG players and non-players trained to play an AVG was also found in more demanding UFOV tasks that included more distractors and a secondary task (Green and Bavelier, 2006a).

As the UFOV represents only an effective or functional field of view relevant to a particular visual task, videogame effects on peripheral vision have also been studied using clinical measures of central and peripheral visual fields. The results in Green and Bavelier (2003, 2006a), where videogame advantage extended to 30° eccentricity from fixation may have represented only the outer edges of central vision (Buckley et al., 2010). Hence, Buckley et al. (2010) tested regular AVG players and non-players on the Goldman Kinetic perimetry, a standard clinical measure of peripheral vision. Their results replicated Green and Bavelier (2003, 2006a) by showing enhanced central visual fields (30° eccentricity from fixation). Crucially, the AVG players also had, on average, a larger peripheral visual field (60° eccentricity from fixation). These results taken together provide strong evidence of AVG-related enhancements to peripheral vision, which may have ecological significance especially given that gender differences in UFOV can be reduced with AVG training (Feng et al., 2007).

Although the aforementioned studies show an AVG-related enhancement in UFOV, other studies have failed to replicate these results. Specifically, Boot et al. (2008) and Murphy and Spencer (2009) found equivalent UFOV performance in AVG and non-AVG players. Furthermore, no differences were found in UFOV improvement beyond test-retest effects in AVG trainees after 21.5 h of training relative to those trained in a strategy game and *Tetris* (Boot et al., 2008). The reason for the discrepancies in findings is unclear, but in cross-sectional comparisons, differences in selecting samples may have resulted in the null findings. For example, in Boot et al. participants in the AVG group did not exclusively play that genre but also reported playing other genres as well. As for the training study, Strobach et al. (2012) speculated that the large number of transfer tasks in their training study might have undermined any transfer effects due to test fatigue. Also, it is important to note that the transfer tasks in Boot et al. were administered three times at pre, mid and post-training. Presumably, multiple testing induced practice effects in the AVG and control groups that masked transfer effects.

DIVIDED ATTENTION

Given the nature of many fast-paced AVG, the ability to divide attention to several items confers a great advantage when playing these games. Hence, according to the common demands hypothesis playing fast-paced AVG should potentially enhance performance in tasks that require allocation of attention towards several items. Current evidence generally supports this claim (but see Boot et al., 2008).

Posner cueing

In one of the first studies that demonstrated spatial attentional advantages in videogame players, Greenfield et al. (1994) showed that expert players of the game *Robot Battle*, were superior in attending to more than one space relative to game novices using the Posner cueing task (Posner et al., 1980). Briefly, in the Posner cueing task, a cue was given to indicate the probable location of a target. There were three probabilities of the target appearing where the cue indicated—80% (high probability), 50% (neutral) or 20% (low). The speed of target detection was fastest in the high probability condition, and slowest in the low probability condition (Posner et al., 1980). In terms of overall response times, expert videogame players were faster in target detection in the high and low probability conditions compared to non-gamers. Furthermore, the videogame experts did not show an increased response time in the low probability relative to the neutral condition (Greenfield et al., 1994).

Demonstrating a causal effect, those trained to play a videogame, *Robotron*, for 5 h, where a player fended off robot attacks from many directions, showed greater improvement at the low probability condition whereas non-players showed no improvement. These results thus provided early and preliminary evidence of AVG-related advantage in attending to multiple locations in space, a demand common to many fast-paced AVG.

Flanker effects

Corroborating evidence for AVG-related superior attentional capacity to attend to more items in parallel has also been shown using different attentional tasks. In their groundbreaking work using a modified flanker task (Lavie and Cox, 1997), Green and Bavelier (2003) claimed that experienced AVG players had leftover attentional resources to attend to distractors when performing a demanding task, whereas non-gamers did not attend to them and thus were not distracted. This suggests that AVG players had greater attentional capacities to attend to multiple items in parallel. In contrast, Irons et al. (2011) failed to replicate these results. However, note that both studies were cross-sectional, not training studies. Hence, it is unclear whether the AVG advantage is causal. The discrepancy in findings may simply reflect sample differences. A training study is therefore needed to resolve this issue.

Multiple object tracking

Green and Bavelier (2006b) found that experienced AVG players were able to track on average two items more than non-gamers in an MOT task. In addition, following 30 h of training, non-players trained in an action game, *Unreal Tournament* improved accuracy rate when the number of objects to-be-tracked increased beyond four items. In contrast, accuracy rate for the control group trained in *Tetris* remained unchanged regardless of the number of targets shown. Similar enhancements were found after 20 h of training using a different measure of MOT (Oei and Patterson,

2013). Corroborating these results, Boot et al. (2008) showed that AVG players were able to track on average, at higher speeds than non-gamers.

The transfer to MOT appears confined to fast-paced FPS. In contrast, training using slower-paced AVGs or other types of AVG such as fast-paced sports game showed no such improvement (Cohen et al., 2008). Like MOT tasks, FPS have multiple fast moving objects that require simultaneous tracking. In contrast, games with multiple items on screen without requiring attention to-be-allocated to all items simultaneously (such as match-3 games) may not result in transfer after training (Oei and Patterson, 2013). However, this hypothesis remains tentative as Boot et al. (2008) failed to find evidence for enhanced MOT tracking speed in participants trained in a fast-paced FPS for 21.5 h compared to non-AVG trained participants.

Enumeration

Evidence for the enhanced ability of AVG players to attend to multiple items has also been corroborated using an enumeration task. Green and Bavelier (2006b) showed that experienced action gamers were more accurate in estimating the number of items displayed than non-action gamers. In addition, experienced action gamers were able to estimate about two items more than non-action gamers. This enhanced ability was also found after 10 h training using an FPS AVG relative to controls (*Tetris* training).

VISUAL SEARCH

FPS games are highly similar to a visual search paradigm because players must search for targets amidst distractors, such as an enemy in hiding (Wu and Spence, 2013). Indeed, converging evidence shows search advantages in habitual AVG players. First, AVG players searched faster and more efficiently overall (Hubert-Wallander et al., 2011) without sacrificing accuracy (Castel et al., 2005). Additionally, AVG players searched more accurately and faster in demanding conjunction conditions (Wu and Spence, 2013). Finally, AVG players were able to search more accurately when distracting objects were in close proximity to the target (Green and Bavelier, 2007), a condition known as crowding (Toet and Levi, 1992; Intriligator and Cavanagh, 2001).

Several longitudinal studies have corroborated the cross-sectional results. These studies used both FPS and other types of AVG training compared with non-AVG training. In a 30-h training study, Green and Bavelier (2007) found that players trained in an AVG (*Unreal Tournament*) were able to detect targets at reduced target-distractor separations compared to the non-AVG group (*Tetris*) at 0°, 10° and 25° eccentricity. Furthermore, following 10 h of training using an FPS, and a racing AVG compared to a control group (3D puzzle game, *Ballance*), Wu and Spence (2013) demonstrated greater accuracy and faster search time for both types of AVG players compared to the control game in a dual search task that involved searches in central and peripheral vision. Interestingly, the results for the FPS and racing game were equivalent. Although most racing games do not include visual search, Wu and Spence (2013) argued that for this particular racing game, the player was expected to also locate and identify several targets. Therefore, these results match the common demands hypothesis.

Demonstrating that not all AVG are alike, we failed to find an AVG-related enhancement in visual search following 20 h of FPS training (Oei and Patterson, 2013). The AVG game used in Oei and Patterson did not have search demands because enemies tended to pop out and engage the player rather than making the player search them out.

Importantly, Oei and Patterson (2013) showed that transfer is not dependent on the training game being an AVG. Instead, visual search time was significantly decreased following training in a hidden object game and a match-3 game (*Bejeweled*) that required searching a display for matching shapes. Therefore, the data in Oei and Patterson (2013) and Wu and Spence (2013) support the common demands hypothesis, such that training in games that included frequent search improved visual search performance. On the other hand, the failure to find evidence for AVG related transfer is inconsistent with a general transfer mechanism, which would lead to improvements across multiple tasks, including visual search.

CHANGE DETECTION

A fundamental requirement in any fast-paced AVG is the need to respond quickly to a sudden onset stimulus. This could be a visual anomaly such as an enemy that appears when the player is preoccupied by something else in the visual field. Given this requirement for successful gameplay, it is plausible that expert AVG players will exhibit superior ability to detect visual anomalies when they are focused on other features in their visual field.

Current evidence for enhanced change detection in AVG players remains mixed. On one hand, Murphy and Spencer (2009) showed that AVG and non-AVG players are equally as likely to miss a cross moving across their visual field while performing a counting task. On the other hand, Vallett et al. (2013), using a popular inattentional blindness task (Simons and Chabris, 1999), showed that AVG players have a significantly greater likelihood of detecting a visual anomaly (man in a gorilla suit) while performing a counting task than non-gamers. One possibility for the inconsistent finding is that the original task in Simons and Chabris presented a more salient visual anomaly than that in Murphy and Spencer. This is not unlike an AVG where a sudden-onset visual stimulus is likely to be a salient one that demands a response (e.g., enemy).

ATTENTIONAL BLINK

Attentional blink refers to a bottleneck in information processing whereby a second target (T2) presented close in time (200–500 ms) to an accurately detected first target (T1), fails to be detected (Raymond and Shapiro, 1992; Shapiro et al., 1994, 1997). Green and Bavelier (2003) reported that AVG players were less affected by attentional blink than non-gamers. Furthermore, non-gamers trained in an AVG for 10 h improved T2 detection during the intervals susceptible to the attentional blink effect (Green and Bavelier, 2003). This training-related enhancement specifically on a fast-paced FPS has generally been replicated following 12–20 h of training (Cohen et al., 2008; Oei and Patterson, 2013). Crucially, the enhancement is seen only following a fast-paced FPS, but not to other slower paced FPS, third-person shooters and sports games (Cohen et al., 2008). Compared to other

AVG, fast-paced FPS requires fast responses to rapidly presented successive targets which leads to these specific improvements (Cohen et al., 2008). This is consistent with the common demands hypothesis.

In contrast, Boot et al. (2008) and Murphy and Spencer (2009) failed to find AVG-related advantages in attentional blink performance. Importantly, no attentional blink enhancement was seen beyond test-retest effects in AVG trainees after 20 h of training (Boot et al., 2008). However, it is again important to place the findings in context of the criticisms of the study mentioned above.

SPATIAL COGNITION

Spatial cognition involves multiple components and broadly speaking refers to the skill in representing, transforming, generating and recalling symbolic, nonlinguistic information (Linn and Petersen, 1985). AVG, especially those with a first-person perspective, should be good training tools for some spatial skills due to navigation and rotation demands in 3D space (Spence and Feng, 2010; Sanchez, 2012). However, training may not transfer to other components if the relevant spatial cognitive demands are not present in the game (Okagaki and Frensch, 1994). For example, enhanced 3D mental rotation was found only following FPS training but not using games without demands to navigate in 3D space (Feng et al., 2007; Sanchez, 2012). Furthermore, the enhancement to spatial ability was specific only to mental rotation of 3D shapes but not to spatial visualization in a paper-folding task where no rotation was necessary (Sanchez, 2012).

Transfer is also seen using non-AVG training. Specifically, faster and more accurate mental rotation has been found in experienced and trained *Tetris* players (Okagaki and Frensch, 1994; Sims and Mayer, 2002; Boot et al., 2008). Unlike AVGs, *Tetris* does not involve fast responding except for the highest levels. Furthermore, new objects in *Tetris* always enter from one location (vertically from the top) and hence there is no requirement to track multiple moving objects in the periphery. There is also no requirement to construct a representation of a complex 3D environment in order to navigate. Finally, virtually no distractors appear in *Tetris*. Rather, participants must stack falling shapes efficiently using mental rotation and planning. These demands lead to different, specific effects compared to those commonly found from playing action games, indicating that *Tetris* should be classified a non-action game.

Three months of *Tetris* training was associated with decreased activation in right frontal (BA 32, 8, 9, 6, 46) as well as parietal (BA 40) areas (Haier et al., 2009). These areas have been previously been shown to be highly activated in mental rotation tasks (Cohen et al., 1996). This reduction in brain activation may suggest enhanced neural efficiency to perform mental rotation (cf. Haier et al., 1992).

Transfer effects from *Tetris* training were highly specific to mental rotation measures (Boot et al., 2008). Notably, the shapes used in the mental rotation task resembled shapes that appeared in *Tetris* (Boot et al., 2008). Conversely, no advantage was seen in skilled or trained players in mental rotation tests that did not involve *Tetris*-like shapes (Sims and Mayer, 2002; Boot et al., 2008). Furthermore, although 12 h of *Tetris* training did not result in transfer to spatial ability tests in general, examinations of the mental rotation strategies showed that *Tetris* trainees were more likely to use a Tetris-like mental rotation (clockwise rotation up to 225°) for *Tetris* shapes (Sims and Mayer, 2002).

These specific improvements thus add converging evidence to the proposal of a transfer being more likely if the game and transfer task share common demands. In contrast, a more general transfer mechanism would predict a general spatial ability or overall mental rotation enhancement. Moreover, the general learning proposal was originally proposed to explain AVG-related improvements only. Thus, the common demands theory allows explanation of more types of video-game related cognitive changes.

EXECUTIVE FUNCTIONS

Task switching

Both alternate-runs and random task switching paradigms have been employed to study the effects of videogame playing on task switching. In the former, a task-switch takes place after a fixed number of trials allowing preparation so that switching is less demanding and typically yields smaller switch costs (Monsell, 2003). In contrast, task-switches are random and unpredictable in the latter. The inability to prepare for a switch leads to greater conflicts, which in turn results in the switch cost being larger (Rogers and Monsell, 1995; Monsell, 2003).

Smaller switch costs in reaction time (RT) and accuracy have been demonstrated in regular AVG players compared to non-players in both alternate-runs and more demanding random task switches (Andrews and Murphy, 2006; Boot et al., 2008; Colzato et al., 2010; Cain et al., 2012; Green et al., 2012; Strobach et al., 2012). Greater switch cost reductions in alternate-runs task switching was found following 15 (Strobach et al., 2012) and 50 h (Green et al., 2012) of AVG training compared to controls that played non-AVGs (e.g., *Tetris* and *The Sims*).

Although task switching superiority in experienced AVG players is consistently reported, results of training studies for transfer to task switching remain equivocal. In contrast to Green et al. (2012) and Strobach et al. (2012), Boot et al. (2008) failed to find transfer effects following 21.5 h of AVG training. Different task-switching paradigms used in each study may explain the conflicting results. Specifically, while Green et al. (2012) and Strobach et al. (2012) utilized a predictable alternate-runs switch format, Boot et al. (2008) instead used a random task switching paradigm. Thus, AVG training may only improve the ability to prepare for upcoming switches but not more demanding mental flexibility measured by random task switching paradigms as these are supported by different neural and cognitive mechanisms (see Baddeley et al., 2001; Bryck and Mayr, 2005; Pereg et al., 2013).

Consistent with the argument of the common demands hypothesis, the transfer of predictable task switching may stem from the frequent practice in AVGs to switch between targets and between items during gameplay. Each activity has clear objectives with little conflict between them. Thus disengagement from a previous task to switch focus on an upcoming task is relatively easy. Take for instance switching rapidly between enemies where the switch can be planned or reactive. Either way, the action following a switch is similar. This is like a task-repeat and involves negligible response conflict. Even switching from an enemy to collecting an item (e.g., health replenishments or bonus items) is unlikely to result in any decisional or response conflicts as the actions involved with either task are distinct. These are akin to the predictable task switching condition whereby any switch is predictable and an upcoming switch or task-repeat condition can be planned in advance. In contrast, decisional conflicts like the random task switching condition are rarely, if ever, encountered in such AVGs.

Distractor suppression

Several studies indicate that AVG players are less susceptible to attentional capture by task-irrelevant stimuli than non-players. Experienced AVG players and those trained to play an AVG for 20 h were faster in responding to targets in the presence of distractors (Chisholm et al., 2010; Oei and Patterson, 2013). This advantage may stem from improved top-down suppression of attentional capture rather than a faster recovery from capture (Chisholm and Kingstone, 2012). Support for better distractor suppression in AVG players comes from neuroimaging. Relative to non-gamers, action gamers showed increased suppression of steady state visually evoked potential (SSVEP) amplitudes to unattended peripheral stimuli in a target detection task where the goal was to detect targets at central fixation or when cued, at left and right peripheries (Mishra et al., 2011). Additionally, using a visual search task with moving distractors at central or peripheral vision, action gamers showed reduced blood-oxygenated level dependent (BOLD) response in visual motion-sensitive regions (Medial Temporal/Medial Superior Temporal areas) to moving distractors compared to non-gamers (Bavelier et al., 2012a). Moreover, 10 h of AVG training has been shown to increase P2 and P3 waves at occipital and occipito-parietal sites (Wu et al., 2012) when performing an attention visual field task where one is required indicate the direction of a target amidst distractors. Increases in P2 and P3 amplitudes may reflect adaptations to task demands on attentional control in attentional selection as well as inhibition of processing of task-irrelevant stimuli (Bledowski et al., 2004; Potts et al., 2004; Sawaki and Luck, 2010; Fritzsche et al., 2011). Taken together, these findings suggest that experienced AVG players are better than their non-AVG counterparts at applying top-down control to suppress attention for task-irrelevant distractors. Longitudinal training studies further show that the advantages displayed are causal.

SPECIFIC OR GENERAL TRANSFER? THE CASE FOR SPECIFIC TRANSFER GAINS

Over the last 10 years since the seminal work of Green and Bavelier (2003), the focus of videogame training has been directed towards AVGs. The growing literature suggests that AVGs enhance lower-level information processing skills ranging from visual perception to different aspects of attention (Green and Bavelier, 2003, 2006a,b, 2007; Chisholm et al., 2010). These include expanded peripheral vision (Green and Bavelier, 2003), target discrimination, identification and contrast (Green and Bavelier, 2007; Li et al., 2009), selective attention (Wu et al., 2012) and attentional blink (Cohen et al., 2008; Green and Bavelier, 2003). In contrast, evidence for transfer to some executive functions remains equivocal (e.g., Boot et al., 2008).

Given the differing characteristics of non-action games, one would expect different types of transfer from non-action game training compared to AVG. However, unlike AVGs, not much research has been conducted to determine the range of transfer. Nevertheless, a small number of studies also suggest some benefits from non-AVGs such as *Tetris'* transfer to mental rotation (Okagaki and Frensch, 1994; Sims and Mayer, 2002; Boot et al., 2008). Importantly, like AVG, transfer effects are also quite specific to skills that are common to the trained game and transfer task (Okagaki and Frensch, 1994; Sims and Mayer, 2002; Boot et al., 2008; Oei and Patterson, 2013).

A critical question we set out to answer in this review is whether transfer gains from videogames reflect a general or more specific enhancement. One hypothesis is that a general attentional control mechanism accounts for transfer effects seen in (action) videogames. This theory suggests that (action) videogame play enhances a general learning of task statistical patterns that supports perceptual decision-making and allocation of cognitive resources (Green et al., 2010b; Bavelier et al., 2012b). However, it has not been empirically demonstrated that this mechanism can indeed account for transfer across the wide range of tasks utilized in the videogame literature. Moreover, it is unclear if such a learning mechanism is applicable to non-action games. Furthermore, the data reviewed earlier do not support this hypothesis. Specifically, if a general learning mechanism really underlies AVG-related transfer, enhancements should be seen across multiple tasks, even those that do not share overlapping demands with the trained AVG. Unfortunately, as most current studies only included transfer tasks that share common demands with the trained AVG, it is difficult to assess the validity of this hypothesis. In the few studies that included tasks that do not appear to share common demands with AVG used for training, however, AVG playing did not transfer to all tasks (e.g., Boot et al., 2008; Murphy and Spencer, 2009; Oei and Patterson, 2013).

In contrast to a general transfer mechanism, the main proposal here is that transfer effects are specific to common demands shared between the trained videogame and transfer task. This hypothesis can explain both AVG and non-AVG training effects (Oei and Patterson, 2013).

Converging evidence from neuroimaging also appears to support the current hypothesis. For instance, transfer is more likely if training and transfer tasks recruit overlapping neural regions (Dahlin et al., 2008). Evidence from the working memory training literature also supports specific over general transfer. For instance, working memory training improved performance on working memory measures but not to measures of fluid intelligence (Harrison et al., 2013; Melby-Lervåg and Hulme, 2013; Redick et al., 2013). Hence, we feel that although working memory and videogame play are different activities, they share a common principle in relation to transfer of cognitive skill in that transfer is specific to what is practiced within the training regime. In contrast, little or no transfer can be expected for skills not explicitly practiced.

We do note that although the general transfer mechanism proposed by Bavelier et al. (2012b) contrasts with the common demand specific mechanism proposal, they added a caveat that "changes in knowledge produce benefits only to the extent to which new tasks share structure with AVG. No benefits are expected in tasks that share no such structure" (Bavelier et al., 2012b). No study has yet been reported that systematically manipulates the demands contained in the AVG used for training because the definition of AVG has remained overly general, but there is some preliminary evidence that FPS AVG lead to different results than other types of AVG (Cohen et al., 2008).

CONCLUDING REMARKS AND FUTURE DIRECTIONS

Several gaps and unanswered questions still remain. First, it remains unclear how "closely-matched" the game and transfer task must be to maximize transfer. It is likely that the demands of the training game and transfer task must engage common neural networks (Dahlin et al., 2008). Nevertheless, quantitative metrics of how close a training game and the transfer tasks remains elusive and are worthy of further investigation. A quantifiable metric would be most useful especially in occupational settings in order to guide the selection of a training paradigm that maximizes transfer effects. For instance, in FPS, one could compare games with either progressively increasing speeds in which enemies appear or the number of enemies that appear simultaneously. We would predict that high-speed games would lead to a decrease in attentional blink, and faster RT, but would not have as large of an effect on MOT as the latter manipulation. To further test for the specificity of transfer effects, one could also conduct a study whereby games with different demands (or intensity) from the same genre are compared (see Cohen et al., 2008 for such an example). To determine whether general or specific transfer has occurred, it is important to include a wider variety of transfer tasks, some of which contain similar demands to the videogames and some of which measure more general learning. To test for general transfer, a videogame training regime could also target training visual attention or visual working memory and test whether improvements generalize across to the verbal or auditory modalities using material that was not trained during the games.

A second gap relates to which cognitive abilities can or cannot be improved by training. It will be important in the future to investigate which abilities are more resistant or amenable to be modified with training or whether improvement in one area will lead to worse performance in another (Takeuchi et al., 2011).

A third important issue is the durability of transfer effects. Thus far, many videogame studies have not tested whether the transfer effects remained after the laboratory tests have concluded (see Li et al., 2009; Anguera et al., 2013 for exceptions). Hence, it is unclear whether transfer effects remain after cessation of training. A main goal of a training task is the retention of skills in the long-term after the training has ceased (Schmidt and Bjork, 1992). As with any type of training, the effectiveness of videogame training should also be evaluated with this criterion.

Fourth, more research should examine individual differences in training-related transfer. It has been argued that the capacity for "cognitive modifiability" as a result of training varies from individual to individual (Calero and Navarro, 2007). It is thus unlikely that all individuals trained with a similar videogame improve similarly (see Wu et al., 2012). There are many factors that can influence plasticity and how well one responds to a training regime. Briefly, some examples of individual differences shown to influence training, cognition and transfer include age and baseline cognitive ability including intelligence (Yesavage et al., 1988, 1990; Haier et al., 1992; Verhaeghen et al., 1992; Bissig and Lustig, 2007; Calero and Navarro, 2007), gender (Feng et al., 2007) as well as lifestyle factors such as cardiovascular health and exercise (Gomez-Pinilla, 2008). Thus far, videogame training studies have not examined how these individual differences affect training-related transfer. Hence, investigating training-related transfer from an individual differences perspective is worthwhile as it can be critical for the implementation of a training regime to maximize transfer effects.

Finally, we feel that ultimately a training regime should translate to real-world applications outside of the laboratory. Thus far, the bulk of the studies have focused on laboratory tasks. Just like games have several demands in common with the cognitive tasks, we assume many everyday tasks have common demands that are trained by the videogames. Thus, we assume that playing videogames will lead to improvements in activities in everyday life. However, few studies have shown video game-related advantage in real-world activities. Videogame experience and skill has been shown to correlate with laparoscopic surgery skills (Rosser et al., 2007). Also, a short bout (10-h) of videogame training, albeit not a commercially available one, has been shown to improve flight performance in cadet pilots (Gopher et al., 1994). One potential area of future research may be to investigate whether videogame training in search skills can benefit performance in occupations that demand intense visual search skills (e.g., airport baggage scanners or air traffic controllers). Hence, the potential of videogame training advantages in real-world applications warrants further investigation.

In closing, over the last decade, we have seen considerable literature documenting the potential benefits of videogame training. With the increase in attention and effort dedicated to this area, intense debate, skepticism and scrutiny have also resulted (Boot et al., 2011, 2013; Kristjánsson, 2013). Nevertheless, such intense debate and scrutiny can only be beneficial to researchers as they strive to refine the methodology of videogame training research. Despite the increasing number of works and considerable progress, the field is still in its infancy and considerable advances are yet to be made. There are many advantages with training via a videogame. Training via videogame represents a departure from traditional learning activities in that it is highly arousing and motivating and has the potential to keep the player engaged for longer periods. With progress in computing power and artificial intelligence, there are arguably major leaps that can be made in game immersion and realism. Additionally, with input from psychologists and learning theory in videogame design, we can further tailor videogames for learning purposes. Hence, further investments in time and money to understand, research and improve transfer from videogame training to the work place, classroom and rehabilitation is surely worthwhile.

REFERENCES

Andrews, G., and Murphy, K. (2006). "Does video game playing improve executive functioning?," in *Frontiers in Cognitive Psychology*, ed M. A. Vachevsky (New York: Nova Science Publishers), 145–161.

Anguera, J. A., Boccanfuso, J., Rintoul, J. L., Al-Hashimi, O., Faraji, F., Janowich, J., et al. (2013). Video game training enhances cognitive control in older adults. *Nature* 501, 97–101. doi: 10.1038/nature12486

Baddeley, A. D., Chincotta, D., and Adlam, A. (2001). Working memory and the control of action: evidence from task switching. *J. Exp. Psychol. Gen.* 130, 641–657. doi: 10.1037/0096-3445.130.4.641

Ball, K. K., Beard, B. L., Roenker, D. L., Miller, R. L., and Griggs, D. S. (1988). Age and visual search: expanding the useful field of view. *J. Opt. Soc. Am. A* 5, 2210–2219. doi: 10.1364/josaa.5.002210

Basak, C., Boot, W. R., Voss, M. W., and Kramer, A. F. (2008). Can training in a real-time strategy video game attenuate cognitive decline in older adults? *Psychol. Aging* 23, 765–777. doi: 10.1037/a0013494

Bavelier, D., Achtman, R. L., Mani, M., and Föcker, J. (2012a). Neural bases of selective attention in action video game players. *Vision Res.* 61, 132–143. doi: 10.1016/j.visres.2011.08.007

Bavelier, D., Green, C. S., Pouget, A., and Schrater, P. (2012b). Brain plasticity through the life span: learning to learn and action video games. *Annu. Rev. Neurosci.* 35, 391–416. doi: 10.1146/annurev-neuro-060909-152832

Bissig, D., and Lustig, C. (2007). Who benefits from memory training? *Psychol. Sci.* 18, 720–726. doi: 10.1111/j.1467-9280.2007.01966.x

Bledowski, C., Prvulovic, D., Goebel, R., Zanella, F. E., and Linden, D. E. J. (2004). Attentional systems in target and distractor processing: a combined ERP and fMRI study. *Neuroimage* 22, 530–540. doi: 10.1016/j.neuroimage.2003.12.034

Boot, W. R., Blakely, D. P., and Simons, D. J. (2011). Do action video games improve perception and cognition? *Front. Psychol.* 2:226. doi: 10.3389/fpsyg.2011.00226

Boot, W. R., Kramer, A. F., Simons, D. J., Fabiani, M., and Gratton, G. (2008). The effects of video game playing on attention, memory and executive control. *Acta Psychol. (Amst)* 129, 387–398. doi: 10.1016/j.actpsy.2008.09.005

Boot, W. R., Simons, D. J., Stothart, C., and Stutts, C. (2013). The pervasive problem with placebos in psychology: why active control groups are not sufficient to rule out placebo effects. *Perspect. Psychol. Sci.* 8, 445–454. doi: 10.1177/1745691613491271

Bryck, R. L., and Mayr, U. (2005). On the role of verbalization during task set selection: switching or serial order control? *Mem. Cognit.* 33, 611–623. doi: 10.3758/bf03195328

Buckley, D., Codina, C., Bhardwaj, P., and Pascalis, O. (2010). Action video game players and deaf observers have larger Goldmann visual fields. *Vision Res.* 50, 548–556. doi: 10.1016/j.visres.2009.11.018

Cain, M. S., Landau, A. N., and Shimamura, A. P. (2012). Action video game experience reduces the cost of switching tasks. *Atten. Percept. Psychophys.* 74, 641–647. doi: 10.3758/s13414-012-0284-1

Calero, M. D., and Navarro, E. (2007). Cognitive plasticity as a modulating variable on the effects of memory training in elderly persons. *Arch. Clin. Neuropsychol.* 22, 63–72. doi: 10.1016/j.acn.2006.06.020

Castel, A. D., Pratt, J., and Drummond, E. (2005). The effects of action video game experience on the time course of inhibition of return and the efficiency of visual search. *Acta Psychol. (Amst)* 119, 217–230. doi: 10.1016/j.actpsy.2005.02.004

Chisholm, J. D., Hickey, C., Theeuwes, J., and Kingstone, A. (2010). Reduced attentional capture in action video game players. *Atten. Percept. Psychophys.* 72, 667–671. doi: 10.3758/APP.72.3.667

Chisholm, J. D., and Kingstone, A. (2012). Improved top-down control reduces oculomotor capture: the case of action video game players. *Atten. Percept. Psychophys.* 74, 257–262. doi: 10.3758/s13414-011-0253-0

Cohen, J. E., Green, C. S., and Bavelier, D. (2008). "Training visual attention with video games: not all games are created equal," in *Computer Games and Team and Individual Learning*, eds H. F. O'neil and R. S. Perez (Oxford, UK: Elsievier), 205–228.

Cohen, M. S., Kosslyn, S. M., Breiter, H. C., Digirolamo, G. J., Thompson, W. L., Anderson, A. K., et al. (1996). Changes in cortical activity during mental rotation A mapping study using functional MRI. *Brain* 119(Pt. 1), 89–100. doi: 10.1093/brain/119.1.89

Colzato, L. S., Van Leeuwen, P. J. A., Van Den Wildenberg, W. P. M., and Hommel, B. (2010). DOOM'd to switch: superior cognitive flexibility in players of first person shooter games. *Front. Psychol.* 1:8. doi: 10.3389/fpsyg.2010.00008

Dahlin, E., Neely, A. S., Larsson, A., Bäckman, L., and Nyberg, L. (2008). Transfer of learning after updating training mediated by the striatum. *Science* 320, 1510–1512. doi: 10.1126/science.1155466

Feng, J., Spence, I., and Pratt, J. (2007). Playing an action video game reduces gender differences in spatial cognition. *Psychol. Sci.* 18, 850–855. doi: 10.1111/j.1467-9280.2007.01990.x

Fritzsche, A.-S., Stahl, J., and Gibbons, H. (2011). An ERP study of target competition: individual differences in functional impulsive behavior. *Int. J. Psychophysiol.* 81, 12–21. doi: 10.1016/j.ijpsycho.2011.03.014

Gomez-Pinilla, F. (2008). The influences of diet and exercise on mental health through hormesis. *Ageing Res. Rev.* 7, 49–62. doi: 10.1016/j.arr.2007.04.003

Gopher, D., Weil, M., and Bareket, T. (1994). Transfer of skill from a computer game trainer to flight. *Hum. Factors* 36, 387–405. doi: 10.1177/001872089403600301

Green, C. S., and Bavelier, D. (2003). Action video game modifies visual selective attention. *Nature* 423, 534–537. doi: 10.1038/nature01647

Green, C. S., and Bavelier, D. (2006a). Effect of action video games on the spatial distribution of visuospatial attention. *J. Exp. Psychol. Hum. Percept. Perform.* 32, 1465–1478. doi: 10.1037/0096-1523.32.6.1465

Green, C. S., and Bavelier, D. (2006b). Enumeration versus multiple object tracking: the case of action video game players. *Cognition* 101, 217–245. doi: 10.1016/j.cognition.2005.10.004

Green, C. S., and Bavelier, D. (2007). Action-video-game experience alters the spatial resolution of vision. *Psychol. Sci.* 18, 88–94. doi: 10.1111/j.1467-9280.2007.01853.x

Green, C. S., Li, R., and Bavelier, D. (2010a). Perceptual learning during action video game playing. *Top. Cogn. Sci.* 2, 202–216. doi: 10.1111/j.1756-8765.2009.01054.x

Green, C. S., Pouget, A., and Bavelier, D. (2010b). Improved probabilistic inference as a general learning mechanism with action video games. *Curr. Biol.* 20, 1573–1579. doi: 10.1016/j.cub.2010.07.040

Green, C. S., Sugarman, M. A., Medford, K., Klobusicky, E., and Bavelier, D. (2012). The effect of action video game experience on task-switching. *Comput. Human Behav.* 28, 984–994. doi: 10.1016/j.chb.2011.12.020

Greenfield, P. M., Dewinstanley, P., Kilpatrick, H., and Kaye, D. (1994). Action video games and informal education: effects on strategies for dividing visual attention. *J. Appl. Dev. Psychol.* 15, 105–123. doi: 10.1016/0193-3973(94)90008-6

Haier, R. J., Karama, S., Leyba, L., and Jung, R. E. (2009). MRI assessment of cortical thickness and functional activity changes in adolescent girls following three months of practice on a visual-spatial task. *BMC Res. Notes* 2:174. doi: 10.1186/1756-0500-2-174

Haier, R. J., Siegel, B., Tang, C., Abel, L., and Buchsbaum, M. S. (1992). Intelligence and changes in regional cerebral glucose metabolic rate following learning. *Intelligence* 16, 415–426. doi: 10.1016/0160-2896(92)90018-m

Harrison, T. L., Shipstead, Z., Hicks, K. L., Hambrick, D. Z., Redick, T. S., and Engle, R. W. (2013). Working memory training may increase working memory capacity but not fluid intelligence. *Psychol. Sci.* 24, 2409–2419. doi: 10.1177/0956797613492984

Hubert-Wallander, B., Green, C. S., Sugarman, M., and Bavelier, D. (2011). Changes in search rate but not in the dynamics of exogenous attention in action videogame players. *Atten. Percept. Psychophys.* 73, 2399–2412. doi: 10.3758/s13414-011-0194-7

Intriligator, J., and Cavanagh, P. (2001). The spatial resolution of visual attention. *Cogn. Psychol.* 43, 171–216. doi: 10.1006/cogp.2001.0755

Irons, J. L., Remington, R. W., and Mclean, J. P. (2011). Not so fast: rethinking the effects of action video games on attentional capacity. *Aust. J. Psychol.* 63, 224–231. doi: 10.1111/j.1742-9536.2011.00001.x

Jaeggi, S. M., Buschkuehl, M., Jonides, J., and Shah, P. (2011). Short-and long-term benefits of cognitive training. *Proc. Natl. Acad. Sci. U S A* 108, 10081–10086. doi: 10.1073/pnas.1103228108

Klingberg, T., Fernell, E., Olesen, P. J., Johnson, M., Gustafsson, P., Dahlström, K., et al. (2005). Computerized training of working memory in children with ADHD–a randomized, controlled trial. *J. Am. Acad. Child Adolesc. Psychiatry* 44, 177–186. doi: 10.1097/00004583-200502000-00010

Kristjánsson, Á. (2013). The case for causal influences of action videogame play upon vision and attention. *Atten. Percept. Psychophys.* 75, 667–672. doi: 10.3758/s13414-013-0427-z

Latham, A. J., Patston, L. L. M., and Tippett, L. J. (2013). Just how expert are "expert" video-game players? Assessing the experience and expertise of video-game players across "action" video-game genres. *Front. Psychol.* 4:491. doi: 10.3389/fpsyg.2013.00941

Lavie, N., and Cox, S. (1997). On the efficiency of visual selective attention: efficient visual search leads to inefficient distractor rejection. *Psychol. Sci.* 8, 395–396. doi: 10.1111/j.1467-9280.1997.tb00432.x

Li, R., Polat, U., Makous, W., and Bavelier, D. (2009). Enhancing the contrast sensitivity function through action video game training. *Nat. Neurosci.* 12, 549–551. doi: 10.1038/nn.2296

Linn, M. C., and Petersen, A. C. (1985). Emergence and characterization of sex differences in spatial ability: a meta-analysis. *Child Dev.* 56, 1479–1498. doi: 10.2307/1130467

Melby-Lervåg, M., and Hulme, C. (2013). Is working memory training effective? A meta-analytic review. *Dev. Psychol.* 49, 270–291. doi: 10.1037/a0028228

Mishra, J., Zinni, M., Bavelier, D., and Hillyard, S. A. (2011). Neural basis of superior performance of action videogame players in an attention-demanding task. *J. Neurosci.* 31, 992–998. doi: 10.1523/jneurosci.4834-10.2011

Monsell, S. (2003). Task switching. *Trends Cogn. Sci.* 7, 134–140. doi: 10.1016/S1364-6613(03)00028-7

Murphy, K., and Spencer, A. (2009). Playing video games does not make for better visual attention skills. *J. Artic. Support Null Hypothesis* 6, 1–20.

Oei, A. C., and Patterson, M. D. (2013). Enhancing cognition with video games: a multiple game training study. *PLoS One* 8:e58546. doi: 10.1371/journal.pone.0058546

Okagaki, L., and Frensch, P. A. (1994). Effects of video game playing on measures of spatial performance: gender effects in late adolescence. *J. Appl. Dev. Psychol.* 15, 33–58. doi: 10.1016/0193-3973(94)90005-1

Pereg, M., Shahar, N., and Meiran, N. (2013). Task switching training effects are mediated by working-memory management. *Intelligence* 41, 467–478. doi: 10.1016/j.intell.2013.06.009

Posner, M. I., Snyder, C. R., and Davidson, B. J. (1980). Attention and the detection of signals. *J. Exp. Psychol.* 109, 160–174. doi: 10.1037/0096-3445.109.2.160

Potts, G. F., Patel, S. H., and Azzam, P. N. (2004). Impact of instructed relevance on the visual ERP. *Int. J. Psychophysiol.* 52, 197–209. doi: 10.1016/j.ijpsycho.2003.10.005

Raymond, J. E., and Shapiro, K. L. (1992). Temporary suppression of visual processing in an RSVP task: an attentional blink? *J. Exp. Psychol. Hum. Percept. Perform.* 18, 849–860. doi: 10.1037/0096-1523.18.3.849

Redick, T. S., Shipstead, Z., Harrison, T. L., Hicks, K. L., Fried, D. E., Hambrick, D. Z., et al. (2013). No evidence of intelligence improvement after working memory training: a randomized, placebo-controlled study. *J. Exp. Psychol. Gen.* 142, 357–379. doi: 10.1037/a0029082

Rogers, R. D., and Monsell, S. (1995). Costs of a predictable switch between simple cognitive tasks. *J. Exp. Psychol.* 124, 207–231.

Rosser, J. C., Lynch, P. J., Cuddihy, L., Gentile, D. A., Klonsky, J., and Merrell, R. (2007). The impact of video games on training surgeons in the 21st century. *Arch. Surg.* 142, 181–186. doi: 10.1001/archsurg.142.2.186

Sanchez, C. A. (2012). Enhancing visuospatial performance through video game training to increase learning in visuospatial science domains. *Psychon. Bull. Rev.* 19, 58–65. doi: 10.3758/s13423-011-0177-7

Sanders, A. F. (1970). Some aspects of the selective process in the functional visual field. *Ergonomics* 13, 101–117. doi: 10.1080/00140137008931124

Sawaki, R., and Luck, S. J. (2010). Capture versus suppression of attention by salient singletons: electrophysiological evidence for an automatic attend-to-me signal. *Atten. Percept. Psychophys.* 72, 1455–1470. doi: 10.3758/APP.72.6.1455

Schmidt, R. A., and Bjork, R. A. (1992). New conceptualizations of practice: common principles in three paradigms suggest new concepts for training. *Psychol. Sci.* 3, 207–217. doi: 10.1111/j.1467-9280.1992.tb00029.x

Shapiro, K. L., Raymond, J. E., and Arnell, K. M. (1994). Attention to visual pattern information produces the attentional blink in rapid serial visual presentation. *J. Exp. Psychol. Hum. Percept. Perform.* 20, 357–371. doi: 10.1037/0096-1523.20.2.357

Shapiro, K. L., Raymond, J. E., and Arnell, K. M. (1997). The attentional blink. *Trends Cogn. Sci.* 1, 291–296. doi: 10.1016/S1364-6613(97)01094-2

Simons, D. J., and Chabris, C. F. (1999). Gorillas in our midst: sustained inattentional blindness for dynamic events. *Perception* 28, 1059–1074. doi: 10.1068/p2952

Sims, V. K., and Mayer, R. E. (2002). Domain specificity of spatial expertise: the case of video game players. *Appl. Cogn. Psychol.* 16, 97–115. doi: 10.1002/acp.759

Spence, I., and Feng, J. (2010). Video games and spatial cognition. *Rev. Gen. Psychol.* 14, 92–104. doi: 10.1037/a0019491

Strobach, T., Frensch, P. A., and Schubert, T. (2012). Video game practice optimizes executive control skills in dual-task and task switching situations. *Acta Psychol. (Amst)* 140, 13–24. doi: 10.1016/j.actpsy.2012.02.001

Subrahmanyam, K., and Greenfield, P. M. (1994). Effect of video game practice on spatial skills in girls and boys. *J. Appl. Dev. Psychol.* 15, 13–32. doi: 10.1016/0193-3973(94)90004-3

Takeuchi, H., Taki, Y., Sassa, Y., Hashizume, H., Sekiguchi, A., Fukushima, A., et al. (2011). Working memory training using mental calculation impacts regional gray matter of the frontal and parietal regions. *PLoS One* 6:e23175. doi: 10.1371/journal.pone.0023175

Thorndike, E. L., and Woodworth, R. S. (1901). The influence of improvement in one mental function upon the efficiency of other functions. *Psychol. Rev.* 8, 247–261. doi: 10.1037/h0074898

Toet, A., and Levi, D. M. (1992). The two-dimensional shape of spatial interaction zones in the parafovea. *Vision Res.* 32, 1349–1357. doi: 10.1016/0042-6989(92)90227-a

Vallett, D. B., Lamb, R. L., and Annetta, L. A. (2013). The gorilla in the room: the impacts of video-game play on visual attention. *Comput. Human Behav.* 29, 2183–2187. doi: 10.1016/j.chb.2013.05.001

Verhaeghen, P., Marcoen, A., and Goossens, L. (1992). Improving memory performance in the aged through mnemonic training: a meta-analytic study. *Psychol. Aging* 7, 242–251. doi: 10.1037/0882-7974.7.2.242

Wu, S., Cheng, C. K., Feng, J., D'Angelo, L., Alain, C., and Spence, I. (2012). Playing a first-person shooter video game induces neuroplastic change. *J. Cogn. Neurosci.* 24, 1286–1293. doi: 10.1162/jocn_a_00192

Wu, S., and Spence, I. (2013). Playing shooter and driving videogames improves top-down guidance in visual search. *Atten. Percept. Psychophys.* 75, 673–686. doi: 10.3758/s13414-013-0440-2

Yesavage, J. A., Sheikh, J. I., Friedman, L., and Tanke, E. D. (1990). Learning mnemonics: roles of aging and subtle cognitive impairment. *Psychol. Aging* 5, 133–137. doi: 10.1037/0882-7974.5.1.133

Yesavage, J. A., Sheikh, J., Tanke, E. D., and Hill, R. (1988). Response to memory training and individual differences in verbal intelligence and state anxiety. *Am. J. Psychiatry* 145, 636–639.

Yuji, H. (1996). Computer games and information-processing skills. *Percept. Mot. Skills* 83, 643–647. doi: 10.2466/pms.1996.83.2.643

9

Transcranial direct current stimulation for memory enhancement: from clinical research to animal models

Djamila Bennabi[1†], Solène Pedron[1†], Emmanuel Haffen[1,2], Julie Monnin[1,2], Yvan Peterschmitt[1] and Vincent Van Waes[1]*

[1] EA 481 Laboratory of Integrative and Clinical Neuroscience, University of Franche-Comté/SFR FED 4234, Besançon, France
[2] INSERM CIC-IT 808 Clinical Investigation Centre for Innovative Technology, University Hospital of Besançon, Besançon, France

Edited by:
Ioan Opris, Wake Forest University, USA

Reviewed by:
Berthold Langguth, University of Regensburg, Germany
Estate M. Sokhadze, University of Louisville, USA

***Correspondence:**
Vincent Van Waes, EA 481 Laboratory of Integrative and Clinical Neuroscience, University of Franche-Comté - UFR Sciences et Techniques, 2 Place Leclerc, 25030 Besançon, France
e-mail: vincent.van_waes@univ-fcomte.fr

† Co-first authors.

There is a growing demand for new brain-enhancing technologies to improve mental performance, both for patients with cognitive disorders and for healthy individuals. Transcranial direct current stimulation (tDCS) is a non-invasive, painless, and easy to use neuromodulatory technique that can improve performance on a variety of cognitive tasks in humans despite its exact mode of action remains unclear. We have conducted a mini-review of the literature to first briefly summarize the growing amount of data from clinical trials assessing the efficacy of tDCS, focusing exclusively on learning and memory performances in healthy human subjects and in patients with depression, schizophrenia, and other neurological disorders. We then discuss these findings in the context of the strikingly few studies resulting from animal research. Finally, we highlight future directions and limitations in this field and emphasize the need to develop translational studies to better understand how tDCS improves memory, a necessary condition before it can be used as a therapeutic tool.

Keywords: tDCS, neuromodulation, prefrontal cortex, cognitive enhancement, memory

Non-invasive neuromodulatory techniques including tDCS have been shown to improve performance on a variety of cognitive domains. tDCS is a painless stimulation method that delivers subthreshold electrical currents to the brain and manipulates the resting membrane potential of cortical neurons (e.g., Stagg and Nitsche, 2011). Since the dorsolateral prefrontal cortex (DLPFC) is a crucial element in the neural network subserving executive functions (i.e., working memory, planning, goal-oriented behavior, attention, and inhibitory control; Wood and Grafman, 2003), targeting this area with neuromodulatory techniques represents a promising therapeutic option for improving cognition. In this mini-review, we summarize data obtained from clinical trials (see **Tables 1A, B**) and animal models focusing on tDCS-induced memory enhancement in healthy subjects and in subjects with psychiatric and neurological disorders known to induce mild to severe cognition impairments. Limitations and perspectives are then discussed.

HUMAN STUDIES

tDCS FOR COGNITIVE ENHANCEMENT IN HEALTHY SUBJECTS

To date, most studies conducted in healthy individuals have assessed the effect of tDCS in enhancing verbal and visuospatial components of working memory (WM) and learning processes. Fregni et al. found that online anodal tDCS at 1 mA applied over the left DLPFC enhances accuracy in a three-back letter task compared with cathodal stimulation of the same area or anodal stimulation of the primary motor cortex (Fregni et al., 2005). Based on the same paradigm, Ohn et al. investigated the time-dependency of tDCS and found an increased number of correct responses starting 20 min after the beginning of active stimulation compared to sham, whereas earlier measurements did not reveal any stimulation effects (Ohn et al., 2008). More recently, Lally et al. confirmed these results in a larger cohort, but only when subjects were tested during the stimulation session (online), without a persisting effect 48 h later (Lally et al., 2013). Mulquiney et al. obtained discordant results in a sample of 10 healthy volunteers, with no improvement in accuracy but in speed performance after anodal tDCS (Mulquiney et al., 2011). However, Marshall et al. reported increased reaction time in the same task during both anodal and cathodal bilateral intermittent stimulation over the DLPFC (Marshall et al., 2005). Andrews and collaborators investigated the impact of 1 session of anodal tDCS delivered during a WM task (n-back task) on performances on a subsequent WM task (digit span forward) (Andrews et al., 2011). Upon completion of the n-back task, they observed a significant improvement in performance on the digit span forward task. Berryhill and Jones enhanced WM by application of anodal tDCS over the left or right DLPFC in subjects with a high educational level, whereas tDCS provided no benefit in WM performance to a less educated group (Berryhill and Jones, 2012). Interestingly, Teo et al. found that WM performances are influenced by current strength of anodal tDCS (Teo et al., 2011). Gladwin et al. explored the impact of anodal left DLPFC tDCS on Sternberg task completion when distractor stimuli were presented during the retention period. tDCS improved reaction time only when the incorrect choice had been a distractor suggesting stimulation might have an effect on selective attention. In a subsequent study, they showed that tDCS improves reaction time in an implicit association test

Table 1A | Studies investigating the cognitive effects of tDCS in healthy subjects.

Study					tDCS parameters				Results
Author	**Design**	**n**	**Task**		**A/C**	**I (mA)**	**D (min)**	**E (cm^2)**	
Fregni et al., 2005	Cross over Single blind	15	n-back task	Online	F3/FP2	1	10	35	Improvement in accuracy (more correct responses) No improvement in reaction time
Ohn et al., 2008	Cross over Single blind	15	n-back task	Online Offline	F3/FP2	1	20	35	Increased number of correct responses after 30 min of stimulation with anodal stimulation
Lally et al., 2013	Cross over Double blind	21	n-back task	Online Offline	F3/cheek	1	10	35	Improvement of performance during the first stimulation phase with active stimulation
Mulquiney et al., 2011	Cross over	10	Cogstate Sternberg task	Online Offline	F3/FP2	1	10	35	2-back task: no effects of session or time in accuracy; improvement in reaction time Sternberg task: no effect of session or time
Marshall et al., 2005	Cross over Double blind	12	Modified Sternberg task	Online	F3/F4	0.26	15	64	No improvement in accuracy Slower reaction time after anodal and cathodal tDCS
Andrews et al., 2011	Cross over	10	n-back task Digit span tasks	Online Offline	F3/FP2	1	10	35	Previous application of tDCS during the n-back task resulted in increased performance on digit span forward
Berryhill and Jones, 2012	Cross over	25	n-back task	Offline	F3/cheek F4/cheek	1.5	10	35	Low education group: unchanged or impaired performance High education group: improved performance
Teo et al., 2011	Cross over Double blind	12	n-back task Sternberg task	Online Offline	F3/FP2	1 or 2	20	35	n-back task: decrease reaction time during the last 5 min of 2 mA session. Sternberg task: no difference in reaction time and accuracy between 1 mA, 2 mA, or sham stimulation
Gladwin et al., 2012a	Cross over	14	Sternberg task	Online Offline	F3/FP2	1	10	35	Improvement in reaction time, influence of interference
Gladwin et al., 2012b	Cross over	20	Modified version of the IAT	Offline	F3/FP2	1	10	35	Improvement in reaction time in the congruent rather than in the incongruent condition
Kincses et al., 2004	Cross over	14	PCL	Online	F3/Cz	1	10	35	Improvement of implicit learning by anodal but not cathodal stimulation
Hammer et al., 2011	Cross over Single blind	36	Recognition memory task	Online Offline	F3/FP2	1	30	35	Cathodal stimulation hampered memory performance after errorful learning, whereas anodal stimulation did not alter encoding and memory retrieval
Manenti et al., 2013	Cross over Single blind	64	Episodic memory task	Online	F3/F4	1.5	6	35	Improvement of verbal episodic memory with anodal tDCS applied during the retrieval phase Better performances in young subjects
Zwissler et al., 2014	Cross over Double blind	85	Episodic memory task	Online	F3/contralateral musculus deltoideus	1	15	35	Anodal tDCS increased whereas cathodal stimulation decreased the number of false alarms to lure pictures in subsequent recognition memory testing

Cz, midline central (international 10/20 EEG system); F3, left dorsolateral prefrontal cortex; F4, right dorsolateral prefrontal cortex; FP2, supraorbital right; IAT, Implicit Association Test; PCL, probabilistic classification learning; I, intensity; D, duration; E, electrodes size.

Table 1B | Studies investigating the cognitive effects of tDCS in psychiatric diseases.

Study					tDCS parameters				Results
Author	**Design**	**n**	**Task**		**A/C**	**I (mA)**	**D (min)**	**E (cm^2)**	
DEPRESSION									
Brunoni et al., 2013	Double blind RCT	28 UP	Probabilistic classification learning	Online	F3/F4	2	30	25	No improvement in implicit learning after real stimulation
Fregni et al., 2006	Double blind RCT	18 UP	Digit span forward and backward test	Online	F3/FP2	1	10	35	Improvement in working memory
Oliveira et al., 2013	Double blind RCT	28 UP	n-back task	Online	F3/F4	2	30	25	Enhancement of working memory Increase rate of correct responses Increase ability to discriminate between correct responses and false alarms
Wolkenstein and Plewnia, 2013	Double blind RCT	22 MDD	Delayed- response working memory task	Online	F3/Right upper arm	1	20	35	Enhancement of working memory performance and elimination of attentional bias
Ferrucci et al., 2009	Open label	8 MDD	Sternberg Task Word recognition task Posner paradigm	Offline	F3/F4	2	20	32	Cognitive tasks showed no significant difference between active or sham stimulation
Loo et al., 2012	Double blind RCT	64 MDD	RAVLT, Stroop Test, COWAT, Digit span, SDMT	Offline	F3/F8	2	20	35	Improvement of working memory performances, indexed by the SDMT, after 1 tDCS session No improvement in cognitive performances after 15 sessions
Palm et al., 2012	Double blind RCT	22 MDD	VLMT, RWT LNS_{WAIS}	Offline	F3/FP2	1 or 2	20	35	Cognitive tasks showed no significant difference between active or sham stimulation
SCHIZOPHRENIA									
Vercammen et al., 2011	Single blind Cross over	20	Probabilistic classification learning	Online	F3/FP2	2	20	35	Improvement in implicit learning after real stimulation in a subset of patient
Hoy et al., 2014	Double blind RCT	18	nback	Offline	F3/FP2	1 or 2	20		Improvement in working memory at 2 mA
Goder et al., 2013	Cross over	14	RAVLT	Offline	F3/F4	0–0.3	During sleep	64	Improvement in working memory
ALZHEIMER									
Boggio et al., 2009	Double blind RCT	10	Digit span test Visual recognition Memory task Stroop test	Online	F3/ FP2 T7/FP2	2	30	35	Improvement in working memory after prefrontal and temporal stimulation No effect on digit span and Stroop performance
Cotelli et al., 2014	Double blind RCT	36 (mild to moder-ate)	Face-name association memory task Memory training	Offline	F3/Right deltoid muscle	2	24		No additive effects of anodal tDCS on memory performance when combined with memory training

(Continued)

Table 1B | Continued

Study					tDCS parameters				Results
Author	**Design**	**n**	**Task**		**A/C**	**I (mA)**	**D (min)**	**E (cm^2)**	
PARKINSON									
Boggio et al., 2006	Double blind RCT	18	n-back task	Online	F3/ FP2	1 or 2	20	35	Improvement in accuracy No improvement in reaction time No effect at 1 mA
Pereira et al., 2013	Cross over	16	Semantic fluency task phonemic task	Offline	F3/FP2 P3-T5/FP2	2	20	35	Improvement in the phonemic fluency task after DLPFC tDCS
POST-STROKE									
Kang et al., 2009	Double blind RCT	10	Go/No-Go	Offline	F3/FP2	2	20	25	Improvement in response accuracy at 1 and 3 h post-stimulation
Jo et al., 2009	Double blind RCT	10	n-back task	Offline	F3/FP2	2	30	35	Improvement in the two-back task after DLPFC tDCS
Park et al., 2013	Double blind RCT	11	Seoul computerized neuropsychological test	Offline	F3/F4	2	30	25	Improvement in attention when combined with cognitive rehabilitation

COWAT, Controlled Oral Word Association Test; F3, left dorsolateral prefrontal cortex (international 10/20 EEG system); F4, right dorsolateral prefrontal cortex; FP2, supraorbital right; F8, lateral aspect of the right orbit; LNS_{WAIS}, Letter Number Sequencing Task of the Wechsler Adult Intelligence Scale; MDD, Major Depressive Disorder; RAVLT, Ray Auditory Verbal Learning Test; RCT, Randomized Controlled Trial; RWT, Regensburg Word Fluency Test; SDMT, Symbol Digit Modalities Test; UP, Unipolar Depression; I, intensity; D, duration; E, electrodes size; VLMT, Verbal Learning Memory Test, P3-T5, left temporo-parietal cortex.

without affecting the subjects' ability to overcome bias (Gladwin et al., 2012a,b).

In addition, tDCS has been recently used as an investigative tool in other memory domains. With regard to implicit memory (probabilistic classification learning), Kincses et al. first demonstrated that anodal tDCS performed over the left DLPFC at 1 mA in healthy volunteers resulted in immediate improvement in implicit learning (Kincses et al., 2004). Hammer et al. showed that cathodal stimulation hampered memory performance after errorful learning, whereas anodal stimulation did not alter encoding and memory retrieval (Hammer et al., 2011). Manenti et al. found that anodal stimulation enhances the long-term episodic memory capacities of young and older subjects with more robust effects in young participants (Manenti et al., 2013). Plewnia and collaborators also reported that tDCS shapes accuracy of episodic memory via polaritiy-specific modulation of false recognition. When applied during encoding of pictures, anodal tDCS increased whereas cathodal stimulation reduced the number of false alarms (i.e., responses to highly similar distracter images) in subsequent recognition memory testing (Zwissler et al., 2014).

tDCS FOR COGNITIVE ENHANCEMENT IN PSYCHIATRIC AND NEUROLOGICAL DISORDERS

Bifrontal tDCS has been shown to prevent procedural learning in depressive states, possibly by inducing a decrease in the activity of the right DLPFC (Brunoni et al., 2013). Beneficial effects of online stimulation applied over the left DLPFC have been reported for working memory, attentional performances, and information processing in depressed patients (Fregni et al., 2006; Oliveira et al., 2013; Wolkenstein and Plewnia, 2013). However, two randomized controlled trials and one open-label trial failed to replicate this finding with offline stimulation, suggesting that multiple tDCS sessions do not have cumulative cognitive enhancing effects (Ferrucci et al., 2009; Loo et al., 2012; Palm et al., 2012).

Only a small number of studies have examined the impact of tDCS on selective cognitive domains altered in schizophrenia. Focusing on working memory, Vercammen et al. reported that a single session of anodal tDCS to the left DLPCF improves probabilistic association learning in a specific subset of schizophrenic patients (Vercammen et al., 2011). These findings were interpreted as an enhancement of DLPFC function primarily in individuals with relatively higher neural and cognitive reserve. Hoy et al. observed the same tDCS effects on a working memory task after a 2 mA stimulation (Hoy et al., 2014). Göder et al. showed improved sleep-associated memory consolidation in patients with schizophrenia when anodal tDCS oscillating at a frequency of 0.75 Hz was applied during sleep (Goder et al., 2013).

Cognitive enhancing properties of tDCS have also been explored in a number of neurological diseases. For example, in Alzheimer disease, Boggio et al. (2009) reported short-term facilitation effects on visual recognition memory after prefrontal and temporal anodal tDCS applied 30 min at 2 mA, with no changes in attention. More recently, Cotelli et al. demonstrated that repeated sessions of anodal tDCS to the left DLFPC plus computerized memory training led to an increase in performance in a face-name association task (Cotelli et al., 2014). However, combined treatment failed to ameliorate the memory performance more than memory training alone suggesting an absence of effects of tDCS in this paradigm. It has also been shown that a single tDCS session can ameliorate memory deficits in Parkinson's disease. Boggio et al. enhanced WM by application of anodal tDCS over the left DPFC at 2 mA, whereas stimulation with intensities of 1 mA or of other area (motor cortex) provided no benefit in WM performance (Boggio et al., 2006). Pereira et al. found that anodal tDCS (at 2 mA) applied over the left DLPFC enhanced performance and functional connectivity in task-related networks in a verbal fluency task tested during fMRI (Pereira et al., 2013).

Kang et al. reported increased response accuracy in a Go/NoGo task tested 1 and 3 h after anodal stimulation at 2 mA over the DLPFC in 10 patients with post-stroke cognitive decline (MMSE ≤ 25) (Kang et al., 2009). Jo et al. also reported that 10 patients with subacute stroke achieved a significant improvement in the accuracy of verbal two-back working memory after receiving the tDCS to the left prefrontal cortex at an intensity of 2 mA for 30 min (Jo et al., 2009). Park et al. found that the concomitant use of anodal tDCS with a computer-assisted cognitive rehabilitation program had a significant effect on improving attention in post-stroke patients with mild-to-moderate cognitive dysfunction (Park et al., 2013).

In spite of the increasing number of clinical studies showing beneficial effects of prefrontal tDCS on the domains of learning and memory, its mechanism of action remains unclear. Recent clinical studies have started to tackle this question (e.g., Keeser et al., 2011a,b; Amadi et al., 2013; Dayan et al., 2013; Palm et al., 2013; Plewnia et al., 2013; Stagg and Johansen-Berg, 2013); however, the cellular mechanisms underlying tDCS will likely require the use of animal models.

ANIMAL MODELS OF tDCS

Animal models provide a powerful tool to identify the mechanisms by which tDCS modulates neural network function to support improved cognition. In rats, tDCS was first used to evaluate the safety limits of cathodal stimulations (Liebetanz et al., 2009) and to map brain activation patterns after tDCS (Takano et al., 2011). In the latter study, the authors observed significantly increased fMRI signal intensities in the frontal cortex and nucleus accumbens of rats after anodal tDCS (of the frontal lobe), suggesting that tDCS induces neuronal activation both in cortical and subcortical areas. To date, few animal studies have addressed the impact of tDCS on learning and memory processes.

tDCS FOR COGNITIVE ENHANCEMENT IN HEALTHY ANIMALS

Similar to humans, the prefrontal cortex (or more generally speaking, the frontal lobe) has been the main target of animal studies for its implication in working memory. In a recent paper, Dockery et al. performed experiments in rats using the Allothetic Place Avoidance Alternation Task (APAAT), a behavioral model of visuospatial working memory and skill learning (Dockery et al., 2011). In this paradigm, a recent memory is engaged by the necessity to remember the location of a to-be-avoided sector (punished by an electric shock), which is alternated daily. tDCS on the frontal lobe (30 min/day before the APAAT task [3 days in total], 200 μA, epicranial electrode: 3.5 mm^2 over the frontal lobe, counter electrode: 10.5 cm^2 placed between the shoulders) had no measurable short-term effect on on-going place avoidance learning. However, in a follow-up session (18 days after the last APAAT session), the rats previously treated with cathodal (but not anodal) tDCS showed significantly more efficient place avoidance and skill retention compared to controls. Other types of memory, such as associative learning processes, can also be affected by tDCS (Marquez-Ruiz et al., 2012). In this case, tDCS was applied to behaving rabbits *via* four silver-ball stimulating electrodes (1 mm in diameter, placed symmetrically above the skull 3 mm from the right S1 vibrissa area on the somatosensory cortex) with a saline-soaked sponge (35 cm^2 surface area) attached to the contralateral ear serving as the counter electrode. The authors found that the acquisition of classical eyeblink conditioning is potentiated or depressed by the simultaneous application of anodal or cathodal tDCS, respectively, when stimulation of the whisker pad was used as a conditioned stimulus. These results suggest that tDCS modulates the sensory perception processes necessary for this type of associative learning (Marquez-Ruiz et al., 2012).

Recently, we have adapted a model of tDCS in mice and tested its validity in a wide range of behavioral paradigms (Pedron et al., 2014). We applied repeated anodal tDCS over the left frontal cortex of the mouse (see, **Figures 1A,B**) and used a 2 × 20 min/day stimulation paradigm at 200 μA for 5 consecutive days. In agreement with human studies, our data suggest that repeated anodal tDCS improves long-term spatial memory (in the Morris water maze, **Figure 1C**) and working memory (object recognition, **Figure 1D**) without affecting behaviors such as locomotor activity and anxiety-related behaviors (Pedron et al., 2014).

Finally, Marshall and collaborators have investigated the interaction of tDCS with hippocampo-neocortical rhythms and reported that a transcranial slow oscillation stimulation during sleep enhances memory consolidation in rats (anodes: bilaterally over the prefrontal cortex; return electrodes: over the cerebellum; sinusoidal constant current fluctuating between 0 and 5.6 μA at a frequency of 1.5 Hz applied during non-rapid eyes movement sleep) (Binder et al., 2014a,b).

COGNITIVE ENHANCEMENT IN ANIMAL MODELS OF NEUROLOGICAL DISORDERS

To the best of our knowledge, tDCS has yet to be tested for enhancing cognition in animal models of psychiatric disorders, but it has been shown to facilitate recovery from cognitive impairments induced by stroke or status epilepticus in rats. After cerebral ischemia, Yoon et al. employed a cup-shaped anodal stimulation electrode positioned at the ischemic borderline, and a rectangular rubber cathodal electrode (80 × 60 mm) fixed on the anterior chest (Yoon et al., 2012) to inject a direct current at an intensity of 200 μA for 20 min, once a day for 5 consecutive days. Both early (1 day) and late (1 week after ischemic injury) treatment had a beneficial outcome on cognition (spatial memory evaluated in the Barnes maze test) without exacerbating ischemic volume. Interestingly, this effect was not present 1 day after tDCS, but began to appear 2 weeks after the stimulations and was maximal after 4 weeks. Therapeutic effects of tDCS on cognition were associated with an increase in the

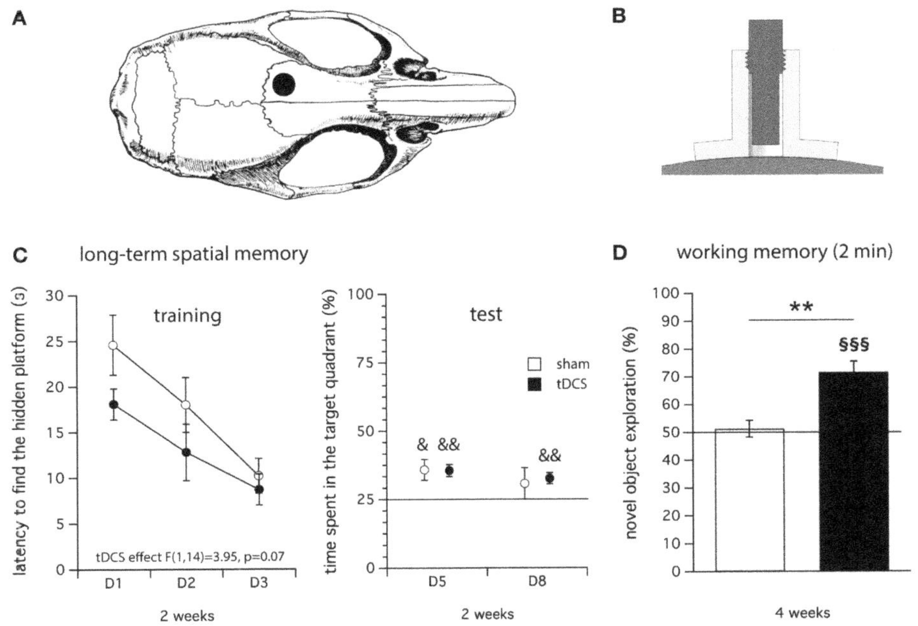

FIGURE 1 | Illustration of the tDCS device used to deliver the electrical stimulation in mice (Pedron et al., 2014) and main results obtained on cognition. (A) The center of the stimulation electrode (anode) is positioned over the left frontal cortex 1 mm anterior to the coronal fissure and 1 mm left of the sagittal fissure (Paxinos and Franklin, 2001). The cathode (rubber-plate electrode, 9.5 cm^2) is placed onto the ventral thorax (not shown). **(B)** Anode: A tubular plastic jacket (internal diameter: 2.1 mm) is surgically fixed onto the skull and filled with saline solution before the stimulation. The stimulation electrode is screwed into the tubular plastic jacket and immersed in the saline solution. Only the saline solution is in contact with the skull. **(C)** Four month-old Swiss female mice were subjected to repeated anodal tDCS for 5 consecutive days (2 × 20 min/day constant current, 0.2 mA). Long-term spatial memory was evaluated 2 weeks after the last stimulation in the Morris water navigation task (training: left; test: right). tDCS significantly improved long-term spatial memory. **(D)** Effect of repeated anodal tDCS on working memory evaluated in an object recognition task (inter-trial interval: 2 min) 4 weeks after the last stimulation. The novel object exploration (score in %) was significantly higher than 50% in the tDCS group, reflecting a better working memory performance compared to sham group for which the score was not significantly different than 50%. $^{\&}p < 0.05$ and $^{\&\&}p < 0.01$ vs. 25%, $^{**}p < 0.01$ vs. sham, $^{§§§}p < 0.001$ vs. 50%; $N = 8$ per group.

expression of Map-2 (a stabilizer of microtubules growth) and Gap-43 (a neuronal growth-promoting gene) in the early treatment group and in the late treatment group, respectively, in both peri-lesional and contra-lesional cortex. Kamida et al. used cathodal tDCS (1.5 mm to the right, 2 mm anterior from bregma; counter electrode: 1 cm needle electrode inserted into the back of the neck, 30 min per day for 2 weeks at 200 μA) to evaluate its effect on seizures and spatial memory deficits following pilocarpine-induced status epilepticus in immature rats (Kamida et al., 2011). Repeated cathodal tDCS reduced seizures, spatial memory impairments, status epilepticus-induced hippocampal cell loss, and supragranular and CA3 mossy fiber sprouting.

POTENTIAL MECHANISMS OF ACTION AND PERSPECTIVES

CANDIDATE MECHANISMS UNDERLYING tDCS ACTION ON COGNITION

To date, it is known that tDCS modifies the resting membrane potential when online and induces prolonged offline after-effects similar to long-term potentiation/depression (Paulus, 2004), considered to be the cellular mechanisms of learning and memory. For example, in humans the long-lasting effects of tDCS (both anodal and cathodal) on the primary motor cortex are suppressed after NMDA-receptor blockade indicating a dependence on glutamatergic activity (Liebetanz et al., 2002). Moreover, previous experiments in rats have shown that anodal polarization directly applied to the cortex has the ability to modulate neural plasticity (i.e., c-Fos activation) *via* activation of NMDA receptors (Islam et al., 1995).

Our team has started to investigate the role of adult neurogenesis as a mechanism involved in tDCS action. Neurogenesis in the hippocampus is of particular interest as tDCS induces both antidepressant effects and enhances cognition in humans and mice, two phenomena critically linked to the generation of new neurons in the adult dentate gyrus (Deng et al., 2010; Eisch and Petrik, 2012). In addition, the time course for the onset of long term tDCS effect on depression-related behavior and on cognition in our animal model (after several weeks, Pedron et al., 2014) is consistent with the delay necessary for newly generated cells in the hippocampus to be functionally integrated (Klempin et al., 2010). Of particular interest is the impact of tDCS on brain-derived neurotrophic factor (BDNF) levels. This growth factor is important for long-term memory (Bekinschtein et al., 2008), is involved in depressive-like behaviors and antidepressant drug action, and can modulate neurogenesis levels (Castren and Rantamaki, 2010; Vithlani et al., 2013). A recent study has shown that BDNF activation is necessary for DCS-induced long-term potentiation in mouse M1 slices

(Fritsch et al., 2010). Enhancement of motor skill acquisition by anodal tDCS also seems to be related to BDNF, as the BDNF val66met polymorphism in humans is associated with decreased proclivity to tDCS-induced benefits on skill learning (Fritsch et al., 2010). Other indirect mechanisms cannot be ruled out, such as the impact of tDCS on cortical blood perfusion (Wachter et al., 2011; Stagg et al., 2013).

LIMITATIONS AND FUTURE DIRECTIONS

One outstanding question in the above-mentioned studies is: where does the current flow? Considering that tDCS has poor spatial resolution on brain tissue, it is important to acknowledge the limitation on the precision with which tDCS is able to target specific areas of the brain. A main issue is the difference between the electrodes used in animals and those used in clinical applications, preventing direct comparisons of current density and voltage distributions between experimental models (higher current densities are often reported in animals). Because in humans the outcome of stimulation depends of the amount of current delivered, it would be necessary to test whether similar dose-response curves occur in animals and attempt stimulation parameters more closely related to clinical studies. Another limiting factor is the considerable protocol variations particularly among animal models. This lack of standardization is deleterious and could contribute to the discrepancy sometimes observed in the literature. The standardization of physical parameters, namely the current density and shape, electrodes size, shape and localization (2 epicranial electrodes vs. 1 epicranial/ 1 outside the skull), the duration and number of stimulations, and the state of animals during the stimulation (awake or anesthetized) would greatly aid in the elucidation of the mechanisms and efficacy of tDCS.

Another often overlooked point is the population on which tDCS is used. The interaction of stimulation polarity, cognitive domain and other intra- and interindividual variables such as anatomic or genetic factors (Plewnia et al., 2013; Kim et al., 2014), personality (Pena-Gomez et al., 2011; Pripfl et al., 2013), cognitive strategy (Berryhill and Jones, 2012) and baseline neuronal activation state (Jacobson et al., 2012) need to be taken into consideration. Likewise, the age at which electrical stimulation occurs (Kessler et al., 2013) might be a key determinants for the physiological and behavioral outcomes of the stimulation. tDCS effects might for example be stronger/different and possibly harmful if applied to the brain during a critical stage of development such as during adolescence when the prefrontal cortex is still not fully mature.

Finally, further basic research is needed to elucidate the duration of the effects of tDCS on memory, which require evaluations at different time-points. The eventual necessity to re-stimulate the brain to maintain the beneficial effects of tDCS has yet to be investigated.

In conclusion, the data reported here are very promising and show that electrical stimulation of the brain is able to improve cognition in humans, in both healthy and in patients with psychiatric or neurological disorders. However, before it can be applied as a therapeutic tool, there is a clear need for method standardization and for a better understanding of its mode of action through the combined use of clinical research and animal models.

ACKNOWLEDGMENT

We would like to warmly thank Adriana Caballero for proofreading and editing the manuscript.

REFERENCES

Amadi, U., Ilie, A., Johansen-Berg, H., and Stagg, C. J. (2013). Polarity-specific effects of motor transcranial direct current stimulation on fMRI resting state networks. *Neuroimage* 88C, 155–161. doi: 10.1016/j.neuroimage.2013.11.037

Andrews, S. C., Hoy, K. E., Enticott, P. G., Daskalakis, Z. J., and Fitzgerald, P. B. (2011). Improving working memory: the effect of combining cognitive activity and anodal transcranial direct current stimulation to the left dorsolateral prefrontal cortex. *Brain Stimul.* 4, 84–89. doi: 10.1016/j.brs.2010.06.004

Bekinschtein, P., Cammarota, M., Katche, C., Slipczuk, L., Rossato, J. I., Goldin, A., et al. (2008). BDNF is essential to promote persistence of long-term memory storage. *Proc. Natl. Acad. Sci. U.S.A.* 105, 2711–2716. doi: 10.1073/pnas.0711863105

Berryhill, M. E., and Jones, K. T. (2012). tDCS selectively improves working memory in older adults with more education. *Neurosci. Lett.* 521, 148–151. doi: 10.1016/j.neulet.2012.05.074

Binder, S., Berg, K., Gasca, F., Lafon, B., Parra, L. C., Born, J., et al. (2014a). Transcranial slow oscillation stimulation during sleep enhances memory consolidation in rats. *Brain Stimul.* 7, 508–515. doi: 10.1016/j.brs.2014.03.001

Binder, S., Rawohl, J., Born, J., and Marshall, L. (2014b). Transcranial slow oscillation stimulation during NREM sleep enhances acquisition of the radial maze task and modulates cortical network activity in rats. *Front. Behav. Neurosci.* 7:220. doi: 10.3389/fnbeh.2013.00220

Boggio, P. S., Ferrucci, R., Rigonatti, S. P., Covre, P., Nitsche, M., Pascual-Leone, A., et al. (2006). Effects of transcranial direct current stimulation on working memory in patients with Parkinson's disease. *J. Neurol. Sci.* 249, 31–38. doi: 10.1016/j.jns.2006.05.062

Boggio, P. S., Khoury, L. P., Martins, D. C., Martins, O. E., De Macedo, E. C., and Fregni, F. (2009). Temporal cortex direct current stimulation enhances performance on a visual recognition memory task in Alzheimer disease. *J. Neurol. Neurosurg. Psychiatr.* 80, 444–447. doi: 10.1136/jnnp.2007.141853

Brunoni, A. R., Zanao, T. A., Ferrucci, R., Priori, A., Valiengo, L., De Oliveira, J. F., et al. (2013). Bifrontal tDCS prevents implicit learning acquisition in antidepressant-free patients with major depressive disorder. *Prog. Neuropsychopharmacol. Biol. Psychiatry* 43, 146–150. doi: 10.1016/j.pnpbp.2012.12.019

Castren, E., and Rantamaki, T. (2010). The role of BDNF and its receptors in depression and antidepressant drug action: reactivation of developmental plasticity. *Dev. Neurobiol.* 70, 289–297. doi: 10.1002/dneu.20758

Cotelli, M., Manenti, R., Brambilla, M., Petesi, M., Rosini, S., Ferrari, C., et al. (2014). Anodal tDCS during face-name associations memory training in Alzheimer's patients. *Front. Aging Neurosci.* 6:38. doi: 10.3389/fnagi.2014.00038

Dayan, E., Censor, N., Buch, E. R., Sandrini, M., and Cohen, L. G. (2013). Noninvasive brain stimulation: from physiology to network dynamics and back. *Nat. Neurosci.* 16, 838–844. doi: 10.1038/nn.3422

Deng, W., Aimone, J. B., and Gage, F. H. (2010). New neurons and new memories: how does adult hippocampal neurogenesis affect learning and memory? *Nat. Rev. Neurosci.* 11, 339–350. doi: 10.1038/nrn2822

Dockery, C. A., Liebetanz, D., Birbaumer, N., Malinowska, M., and Wesierska, M. J. (2011). Cumulative benefits of frontal transcranial direct current stimulation on visuospatial working memory training and skill learning in rats. *Neurobiol. Learn. Mem.* 96, 452–460. doi: 10.1016/j.nlm.2011.06.018

Eisch, A. J., and Petrik, D. (2012). Depression and hippocampal neurogenesis: a road to remission? *Science* 338, 72–75. doi: 10.1126/science.1222941

Ferrucci, R., Bortolomasi, M., Vergari, M., Tadini, L., Salvoro, B., Giacopuzzi, M., et al. (2009). Transcranial direct current stimulation in severe, drug-resistant major depression. *J. Affect. Disord.* 118, 215–219. doi: 10.1016/j.jad.2009.02.015

Fregni, F., Boggio, P. S., Nitsche, M., Bermpohl, F., Antal, A., Feredoes, E., et al. (2005). Anodal transcranial direct current stimulation of prefrontal cortex enhances working memory. *Exp. Brain Res.* 166, 23–30. doi: 10.1007/s00221-005-2334-6

Fregni, F., Boggio, P. S., Nitsche, M. A., Marcolin, M. A., Rigonatti, S. P., and Pascual-Leone, A. (2006). Treatment of major depression with transcranial direct current stimulation. *Bipolar Disord.* 8, 203–204. doi: 10.1111/j.1399-5618.2006.00291.x

Fritsch, B., Reis, J., Martinowich, K., Schambra, H. M., Ji, Y., Cohen, L. G., et al. (2010). Direct current stimulation promotes BDNF-dependent synaptic plasticity: potential implications for motor learning. *Neuron* 66, 198–204. doi: 10.1016/j.neuron.2010.03.035

Gladwin, T. E., Den Uyl, T. E., Fregni, F. F., and Wiers, R. W. (2012a). Enhancement of selective attention by tDCS: interaction with interference in a Sternberg task. *Neurosci. Lett.* 512, 33–37. doi: 10.1016/j.neulet.2012.01.056

Gladwin, T. E., Den Uyl, T. E., and Wiers, R. W. (2012b). Anodal tDCS of dorsolateral prefontal cortex during an Implicit Association Test. *Neurosci. Lett.* 517, 82–86. doi: 10.1016/j.neulet.2012.04.025

Goder, R., Baier, P. C., Beith, B., Baecker, C., Seeck-Hirschner, M., Junghanns, K., et al. (2013). Effects of transcranial direct current stimulation during sleep on memory performance in patients with schizophrenia. *Schizophr. Res.* 144, 153–154. doi: 10.1016/j.schres.2012.12.014

Hammer, A., Mohammadi, B., Schmicker, M., Saliger, S., and Munte, T. F. (2011). Errorless and errorful learning modulated by transcranial direct current stimulation. *BMC Neurosci.* 12:72. doi: 10.1186/1471-2202-12-72

Hoy, K. E., Arnold, S. L., Emonson, M. R., Daskalakis, Z. J., and Fitzgerald, P. B. (2014). An investigation into the effects of tDCS dose on cognitive performance over time in patients with schizophrenia. *Schizophr. Res.* 155, 96–100. doi: 10.1016/j.schres.2014.03.006

Islam, N., Moriwaki, A., Hattori, Y., Hayashi, Y., Lu, Y. F., and Hori, Y. (1995). c-Fos expression mediated by N-methyl-D-aspartate receptors following anodal polarization in the rat brain. *Exp. Neurol.* 133, 25–31. doi: 10.1006/exnr.1995.1004

Jacobson, L., Koslowsky, M., and Lavidor, M. (2012). tDCS polarity effects in motor and cognitive domains: a meta-analytical review. *Exp. Brain Res.* 216, 1–10. doi: 10.1007/s00221-011-2891-9

Jo, J. M., Kim, Y. H., Ko, M. H., Ohn, S. H., Joen, B., and Lee, K. H. (2009). Enhancing the working memory of stroke patients using tDCS. *Am. J. Phys. Med. Rehabil.* 88, 404–409. doi: 10.1097/PHM.0b013e3181a0e4cb

Kamida, T., Kong, S., Eshima, N., Abe, T., Fujiki, M., and Kobayashi, H. (2011). Transcranial direct current stimulation decreases convulsions and spatial memory deficits following pilocarpine-induced status epilepticus in immature rats. *Behav. Brain Res.* 217, 99–103. doi: 10.1016/j.bbr.2010.08.050

Kang, E. K., Baek, M. J., Kim, S., and Paik, N. J. (2009). Non-invasive cortical stimulation improves post-stroke attention decline. *Restor. Neurol. Neurosci.* 27, 645–650. doi: 10.3233/RNN-2009-0514

Keeser, D., Meindl, T., Bor, J., Palm, U., Pogarell, O., Mulert, C., et al. (2011a). Prefrontal transcranial direct current stimulation changes connectivity of resting-state networks during fMRI. *J. Neurosci.* 31, 15284–15293. doi: 10.1523/JNEUROSCI.0542-11.2011

Keeser, D., Padberg, F., Reisinger, E., Pogarell, O., Kirsch, V., Palm, U., et al. (2011b). Prefrontal direct current stimulation modulates resting EEG and event-related potentials in healthy subjects: a standardized low resolution tomography (sLORETA) study. *Neuroimage* 55, 644–657. doi: 10.1016/j.neuroimage.2010.12.004

Kessler, S. K., Minhas, P., Woods, A. J., Rosen, A., Gorman, C., and Bikson, M. (2013). Dosage considerations for transcranial direct current stimulation in children: a computational modeling study. *PLoS ONE* 8:e76112. doi: 10.1371/journal.pone.0076112

Kim, J. H., Kim, D. W., Chang, W. H., Kim, Y. H., Kim, K., and Im, C. H. (2014). Inconsistent outcomes of transcranial direct current stimulation may originate from anatomical differences among individuals: electric field simulation using individual MRI data. *Neurosci. Lett.* 564, 6–10. doi: 10.1016/j.neulet.2014.01.054

Kincses, T. Z., Antal, A., Nitsche, M. A., Bartfai, O., and Paulus, W. (2004). Facilitation of probabilistic classification learning by transcranial direct current stimulation of the prefrontal cortex in the human. *Neuropsychologia* 42, 113–117. doi: 10.1016/S0028-3932(03)00124-6

Klempin, F., Babu, H., De Pietri Tonelli, D., Alarcon, E., Fabel, K., and Kempermann, G. (2010). Oppositional effects of serotonin receptors 5-HT1a, 2, and 2c in the regulation of adult hippocampal neurogenesis. *Front. Mol. Neurosci.* 3:14. doi: 10.3389/fnmol.2010.00014

Lally, N., Nord, C. L., Walsh, V., and Roiser, J. P. (2013). Does excitatory fronto-extracerebral tDCS lead to improved working memory performance? *F1000Research* 2:219. doi 10.12688/f1000research.2-219.v2

Liebetanz, D., Koch, R., Mayenfels, S., Konig, F., Paulus, W., and Nitsche, M. A. (2009). Safety limits of cathodal transcranial direct current stimulation in rats. *Clin. Neurophysiol.* 120, 1161–1167. doi: 10.1016/j.clinph.2009.01.022

Liebetanz, D., Nitsche, M. A., Tergau, F., and Paulus, W. (2002). Pharmacological approach to the mechanisms of transcranial DC-stimulation-induced after-effects of human motor cortex excitability. *Brain* 125, 2238–2247. doi: 10.1093/brain/awf238

Loo, C. K., Alonzo, A., Martin, D., Mitchell, P. B., Galvez, V., and Sachdev, P. (2012). Transcranial direct current stimulation for depression: 3-week, randomised, sham-controlled trial. *Br. J. Psychiatry* 200, 52–59. doi: 10.1192/bjp.bp.111.097634

Manenti, R., Brambilla, M., Petesi, M., Ferrari, C., and Cotelli, M. (2013). Enhancing verbal episodic memory in older and young subjects after non-invasive brain stimulation. *Front. Aging Neurosci.* 5:49. doi: 10.3389/fnagi.2013.00049

Marquez-Ruiz, J., Leal-Campanario, R., Sanchez-Campusano, R., Molaee-Ardekani, B., Wendling, F., Miranda, P. C., et al. (2012). Transcranial direct-current stimulation modulates synaptic mechanisms involved in associative learning in behaving rabbits. *Proc. Natl. Acad. Sci. U.S.A.* 109, 6710–6715. doi: 10.1073/pnas.1121147109

Marshall, L., Molle, M., Siebner, H. R., and Born, J. (2005). Bifrontal transcranial direct current stimulation slows reaction time in a working memory task. *BMC Neurosci.* 6:23. doi: 10.1186/1471-2202-6-23

Mulquiney, P. G., Hoy, K. E., Daskalakis, Z. J., and Fitzgerald, P. B. (2011). Improving working memory: exploring the effect of transcranial random noise stimulation and transcranial direct current stimulation on the dorsolateral prefrontal cortex. *Clin. Neurophysiol.* 122, 2384–2389. doi: 10.1016/j.clinph.2011.05.009

Ohn, S. H., Park, C. I., Yoo, W. K., Ko, M. H., Choi, K. P., Kim, G. M., et al. (2008). Time-dependent effect of transcranial direct current stimulation on the enhancement of working memory. *Neuroreport* 19, 43–47. doi: 10.1097/WNR.0b013e3282f2adfd

Oliveira, J. F., Zanao, T. A., Valiengo, L., Lotufo, P. A., Bensenor, I. M., Fregni, F., et al. (2013). Acute working memory improvement after tDCS in antidepressant-free patients with major depressive disorder. *Neurosci. Lett.* 537, 60–64. doi: 10.1016/j.neulet.2013.01.023

Palm, U., Fintescu, Z., Obermeier, M., Schiller, C., Reisinger, E., Keeser, D., et al. (2013). Serum levels of brain-derived neurotrophic factor are unchanged after transcranial direct current stimulation in treatment-resistant depression. *J. Affect. Disord.* 150, 659–663. doi: 10.1016/j.jad.2013.03.015

Palm, U., Schiller, C., Fintescu, Z., Obermeier, M., Keeser, D., Reisinger, E., et al. (2012). Transcranial direct current stimulation in treatment resistant depression: a randomized double-blind, placebo-controlled study. *Brain Stimul.* 5, 242–251. doi: 10.1016/j.brs.2011.08.005

Park, S. H., Koh, E. J., Choi, H. Y., and Ko, M. H. (2013). A double-blind, sham-controlled, pilot study to assess the effects of the concomitant use of transcranial direct current stimulation with the computer assisted cognitive rehabilitation to the prefrontal cortex on cognitive functions in patients with stroke. *J. Korean Neurosurg. Soc.* 54, 484–488. doi: 10.3340/jkns.2013.54.6.484

Paulus, W. (2004). Outlasting excitability shifts induced by direct current stimulation of the human brain. *Suppl. Clin. Neurophysiol.* 57, 708–714. doi: 10.1016/S1567-424X(09)70411-8

Paxinos, G., and Franklin, K. (2001). *The Mouse Brain in Stereotaxic Coordinate, 2nd Edn.* San Diego, CA; London: Academic Press.

Pedron, S., Monnin, J., Haffen, E., Sechter, D., and Van Waes, V. (2014). Repeated transcranial direct current stimulation prevents abnormal behaviors associated with abstinence from chronic nicotine consumption. *Neuropsychopharmacology* 39, 981–988. doi: 10.1038/npp.2013.298

Pena-Gomez, C., Vidal-Pineiro, D., Clemente, I. C., Pascual-Leone, A., and Bartres-Faz, D. (2011). Down-regulation of negative emotional processing by transcranial direct current stimulation: effects of personality characteristics. *PLoS ONE* 6:e22812. doi: 10.1371/journal.pone.0022812

Pereira, J. B., Junque, C., Bartres-Faz, D., Marti, M. J., Sala-Llonch, R., Compta, Y., et al. (2013). Modulation of verbal fluency networks by transcranial direct current stimulation (tDCS) in Parkinson's disease. *Brain Stimul.* 6, 16–24. doi: 10.1016/j.brs.2012.01.006

Plewnia, C., Zwissler, B., Langst, I., Maurer, B., Giel, K., and Kruger, R. (2013). Effects of transcranial direct current stimulation (tDCS) on executive functions: influence of COMT Val/Met polymorphism. *Cortex* 49, 1801–1807. doi: 10.1016/j.cortex.2012.11.002

Pripfl, J., Neumann, R., Kohler, U., and Lamm, C. (2013). Effects of transcranial direct current stimulation on risky decision making are mediated by 'hot' and 'cold' decisions, personality, and hemisphere. *Eur. J. Neurosci.* 38, 3778–3785. doi: 10.1111/ejn.12375

Stagg, C. J., and Johansen-Berg, H. (2013). Studying the effects of transcranial direct-current stimulation in stroke recovery using magnetic resonance imaging. *Front. Hum. Neurosci.* 7:857. doi: 10.3389/fnhum.2013.00857

Stagg, C. J., Lin, R. L., Mezue, M., Segerdahl, A., Kong, Y., Xie, J., et al. (2013). Widespread modulation of cerebral perfusion induced during and after transcranial direct current stimulation applied to the left dorsolateral prefrontal cortex. *J. Neurosci.* 33, 11425–11431. doi: 10.1523/JNEUROSCI.3887-12.2013

Stagg, C. J., and Nitsche, M. A. (2011). Physiological basis of transcranial direct current stimulation. *Neuroscientist* 17, 37–53. doi: 10.1177/1073858410386614

Takano, Y., Yokawa, T., Masuda, A., Niimi, J., Tanaka, S., and Hironaka, N. (2011). A rat model for measuring the effectiveness of transcranial direct current stimulation using fMRI. *Neurosci. Lett.* 491, 40–43. doi: 10.1016/j.neulet.2011.01.004

Teo, F., Hoy, K. E., Daskalakis, Z. J., and Fitzgerald, P. B. (2011). Investigating the role of current strength in tDCS modulation of working memory performance in healthy controls. *Front. Psychiatry* 2:45. doi: 10.3389/fpsyt.2011.00045

Vercammen, A., Rushby, J. A., Loo, C., Short, B., Weickert, C. S., and Weickert, T. W. (2011). Transcranial direct current stimulation influences probabilistic association learning in schizophrenia. *Schizophr. Res.* 131, 198–205. doi: 10.1016/j.schres.2011.06.021

Vithlani, M., Hines, R. M., Zhong, P., Terunuma, M., Hines, D. J., Revilla-Sanchez, R., et al. (2013). The ability of BDNF to modify neurogenesis and depressive-like behaviors is dependent upon phosphorylation of tyrosine residues 365/367 in the GABA(A)-receptor gamma2 subunit. *J. Neurosci.* 33, 15567–15577. doi: 10.1523/JNEUROSCI.1845-13.2013

Wachter, D., Wrede, A., Schulz-Schaeffer, W., Taghizadeh-Waghefi, A., Nitsche, M. A., Kutschenko, A., et al. (2011). Transcranial direct current stimulation induces polarity-specific changes of cortical blood perfusion in the rat. *Exp. Neurol.* 227, 322–327. doi: 10.1016/j.expneurol.2010.12.005

Wolkenstein, L., and Plewnia, C. (2013). Amelioration of cognitive control in depression by transcranial direct current stimulation. *Biol. Psychiatry* 73, 646–651. doi: 10.1016/j.biopsych.2012.10.010

Wood, J. N., and Grafman, J. (2003). Human prefrontal cortex: processing and representational perspectives. *Nat. Rev. Neurosci.* 4, 139–147. doi: 10.1038/nrn1033

Yoon, K. J., Oh, B. M., and Kim, D. Y. (2012). Functional improvement and neuroplastic effects of anodal transcranial direct current stimulation (tDCS) delivered 1 day vs. 1 week after cerebral ischemia in rats. *Brain Res.* 1452, 61–72. doi: 10.1016/j.brainres.2012.02.062

Zwissler, B., Sperber, C., Aigeldinger, S., Schindler, S., Kissler, J., and Plewnia, C. (2014). Shaping memory accuracy by left prefrontal transcranial direct current stimulation. *J. Neurosci.* 34, 4022–4026. doi: 10.1523/JNEUROSCI.5407-13.2014

10

rTMS neuromodulation improves electrocortical functional measures of information processing and behavioral responses in autism

Estate M. Sokhadze[1]*, Ayman S. El-Baz[2], Lonnie L. Sears[3], Ioan Opris[4] and Manuel F. Casanova[1]

[1] Department of Psychiatry and Behavioral Sciences, University of Louisville, Louisville, KY, USA
[2] Department of Bioengineering, University of Louisville, Louisville, KY, USA
[3] Department of Pediatrics, University of Louisville, Louisville, KY, USA
[4] Department of Physiology and Pharmacology, Wake Forest University, Winston-Salem, NC, USA

Edited by:
Mikhail Lebedev, Duke University, USA

Reviewed by:
Yoshio Sakurai, Kyoto University, Japan
Nivaldo Antonio Portela De Vasconcelos, Champalimaud Centre for the Unknown, Portugal
Ignacio Obeso, CNRS UMR 5229, France

***Correspondence:**
Estate M. Sokhadze, Department of Psychiatry and Behavioral Sciences, University of Louisville, 401 E Chestnut St #600, Louisville, KY 40202, USA
e-mail: tato.sokhadze@louisville.edu

Objectives: Reports in autism spectrum disorders (ASD) of a minicolumnopathy with consequent deficits of lateral inhibition help explain observed behavioral and executive dysfunctions. We propose that neuromodulation based on low frequency repetitive Transcranial Magnetic Stimulation (rTMS) will enhance lateral inhibition through activation of inhibitory double bouquet interneurons and will be accompanied by improvements in the prefrontal executive functions. In addition we proposed that rTMS will improve cortical excitation/inhibition ratio and result in changes manifested in event-related potential (ERP) recorded during cognitive tests.

Materials and Methods: Along with traditional clinical behavioral evaluations the current study used ERPs in a visual oddball task with illusory figures. We compared clinical, behavioral and electrocortical outcomes in two groups of children with autism (TMS, wait-list group). We predicted that 18 session long course in autistic patients will have better behavioral and ERP outcomes as compared to age- and IQ-matched WTL group. We used 18 sessions of 1 Hz rTMS applied over the dorso-lateral prefrontal cortex in 27 individuals with ASD diagnosis. The WTL group was comprised of 27 age-matched subjects with ASD tested twice. Both TMS and WTL groups were assessed at the baseline and after completion of 18 weekly sessions of rTMS (or wait period) using clinical behavioral questionnaires and during performance on visual oddball task with Kanizsa illusory figures.

Results: Post-TMS evaluations showed decreased irritability and hyperactivity on the Aberrant Behavior Checklist (ABC), and decreased stereotypic behaviors on the Repetitive Behavior Scale (RBS-R). Following rTMS course we found decreased amplitude and prolonged latency in the frontal and fronto-central N100, N200 and P300 (P3a) ERPs to non-targets in active TMS treatment group. TMS resulted in increase of P2d (P2a to targets minus P2a to non-targets) amplitude. These ERP changes along with increased centro-parietal P100 and P300 (P3b) to targets are indicative of more efficient processing of information post-TMS treatment. Another important finding was decrease of the latency and increase of negativity of error-related negativity (ERN) during commission errors that may reflect improvement in error monitoring and correction function. Enhanced information processing was also manifested in lower error rate. In addition we calculated normative post-error treaction time (RT) slowing response in both groups and found that rTMS treatment was accompanied by post-error RT slowing and higher accuracy of responses, whereas the WTL group kept on showing typical for ASD post-error RT speeding and higher commission and omission error rates.

Conclusion: Results from our study indicate that rTMS improves executive functioning in ASD as evidenced by normalization of ERP responses and behavioral reactions (RT, accuracy) during executive function test, and also by improvements in clinical evaluations.

Keywords: TMS, autism, ERP, motor response time, behavioral performance

INTRODUCTION

Autism Spectrum Disorders (ASD) are featured by severe deficits in social communication, social interaction, and restricted, repetitive patterns of behaviors, interests and activities (APA, 2013). Additionally, autistic individuals usually present excessive reactions to the sensory environment such as aversive reactions to visual, auditory, and tactile stimuli. These perception and sensory reactivity abnormalities are found in majority of subjects with ASD affecting their ability to effectively process information (Gomes et al., 2008). In a series of electrophysiological studies conducted by our group we explored specifics of event-related potential (i.e., ERP) reflecting information processing during performance on reaction time (RT) tasks in children with ASD (Sokhadze et al., 2009a, 2012b, 2013a; Baruth et al., 2010c; Casanova et al., 2012) Our studies were aimed to explore the manifestations of the impaired functional connectivity, excessive cortical excitation/inhibition ratio, and deficient executive functioning in ASD by analyzing behavioral performance on attention tasks with dense-array ERP recording. Analysis of ERP components is one of the most informative dynamic methods of investigation and monitoring of information processing stages in the human brain due to the high temporal resolution of this technique. Amplitude and latency of ERP waves at selected topographies reflect both early sensory perception processes and higher-level processing including attention, cortical inhibition, memory update, as well as other cognitive activity processes (Polich, 2007). ERPs provide both a method of studying chronometry of information processing stages and a tool by which to assess the neurobiology of cognitive dysfunctions present in this neurodevelopmental disorder. ERP is a very useful technique to characterize time course and amplitude of cortical responses to stimulation (Jeste and Nelson, 2009). Generally, early exogenous ERPs are believed to reflect sensory processing of a stimulus attributes (Coles and Rugg, 1995; Herrmann and Knight, 2001; Eichele et al., 2005; Folstein et al., 2008), whereas late endogenous ERPs are thought to reflect higher level cognitive processes such as attention, memory trace update, perceptual closure, etc. (Pritchard, 1981; Picton, 1992; Polich, 2003, 2007).

One of our first studies investigated ERPs that index selective attention processes in a visual novelty oddball task in children with autism and an age-matched group of typically developing children (Sokhadze et al., 2010a). The ASD group had excessive magnitude to task-irrelevant visual cues as compared to typically developing children and evidenced a lack of visual target discrimination. In a follow-up investigation we found augmented early cortical responses to novel distracters along with lower accuracy of motor response (MR) in a three-stimuli oddball task with illusory Kanizsa figures (Sokhadze et al., 2013a). We concluded that cortical responses to visual stimulation in autism might be indiscriminative during visual tasks negatively affecting selective attention. Large magnitude of electrocortical activity in response to sensory stimulation may be due to an increased ratio between excitation and inhibition in the cortex of individuals with autism (Casanova et al., 2002a,b; Rubenstein and Merzenich, 2003; Casanova, 2005, 2007). Impaired habituation and normative adaptation to repeated stimuli can be considered as an inhibitory deficit manifested in typical symptoms of autism such as stereotypy, sensory hypersensitivity, deficient social interaction skills, etc.

One of contemporary models of autism, so called "minicolumnar theory of autism" (Casanova et al., 2003, 2006a,b; Casanova, 2005, 2007) is based on neuropathological findings in our laboratory. Autism in this model is associated with cortical neurodevelopmental abnormalities. In brief, the reduced neuropil space (periphery of the minicolumn) reported in autism is the compartment where lateral inhibition sharpens the borders of minicolumns and increases their definition (Favorov and Kelly, 1994a,b; DeFelipe, 1999, 2004). The primary source of for this inhibitory effect may be derived from axon bundles of double-bouquet cells (Favorov and Kelly, 1994a). The axons of double bouquet cells arrange themselves in essentially repeatable patterns varying between 15 and 30 μm wide, depending on the cortical area examined (DeFelipe, 1999). Increases in numbers and types of inhibitory interneurons, as seen in the smaller minicolumns of autistic patients, result in greater diversity and more nuanced modulation of minicolumns. Double-bouquet cells in the peripheral neuropil space of minicolumns provide a "vertical stream of negative inhibition" (Mountcastle, 2003) surrounding the minicolumnar core. Other GABAergic cells in the minicolumn, having collateral projections extending hundreds of microns tangentially, provide lateral inhibition of surrounding minicolumns on a macrocolumnar scale.

The value of each minicolumn's output is insulated to a greater or lesser degree from the activity of its neighbors by GABAergic inhibition in its peripheral neuropil space. This allows for gradations in amplitude of excitatory activity across a minicolumnar field. Rubenstein and Merzenich (2003) have posited that reductions in GABAergic inhibitory activity may explain some symptomatology of autism, including increased incidence of seizures and auditory-tactile hypersensitivity (see also Casanova et al., 2003, 2006a,b). Oblak et al. (2010) found decreased GABA receptors in the cingulate cortex and fusiform gyrus in autism. These results may explain some symptomatology of autism, including increased incidence of seizures and sensory (e.g., auditory, tactile) hypersensitivity (Casanova et al., 2003).

This hypothesis is consistent with findings of reduced minicolumnar peripheral neuropil space in the neocortex of autistics relative to controls (Casanova et al., 2002a,b,d). In this model, a reduction in the peripheral neuropil space would result in smaller minicolumns which would coalesce into discrete, isolated islands of coordinated excitatory activity. There are considerable consequences resulting from the significant reduction of neuropil in minicolumns in autism. Reduced surround inhibition may result in an increase in the ratio of cortical excitation to inhibition and excessive amplification of sensory responses reported by autistic individuals. Several important functions of the prefrontal cortex, for instance executive functions might be affected ability of individuals with autism focus on task-relevant targets without being distracted by task-irrelevant cues (Gray et al., 2003; Folstein et al., 2008; Matzel and Kolata, 2010). There are several reviews describing consequences of increased excitation-to-inhibition (E/I) ratio both in humans and in animal models (Rubenstein and Merzenich, 2003; Renart et al., 2010; Harris and Thiele, 2011; Pinto et al., 2013). Deficits within the inhibitory elements that surround the cell minicolumn suggest a mechanistic explanation to the I/E imbalance in autism (Casanova et al., 2003). Oscillations and synchronization of pyramidal cells in and across minicolumns are maintained by networks of inhibitory GABAergic interneurons. Local I/E interactions shape neuronal representations of sensory, motor and cognitive variables, and produce local electroencephalographic (EEG) gamma oscillations. The I/E bias caused by faulty pyramidal cell-interneuronal diads provides a receptive scenario to induced gamma frequency and ERP abnormalities in autism.

TMS offers a noninvasive method for altering excitability of the neural circuits and for inducing a functional reorganization of the cortex. We reported positive effects of repetitive transcranial magnetic stimulation (rTMS) in ASD in our pilot studies using shorter (6–12 sessions) rTMS course (Sokhadze et al., 2009b, 2010a, 2012a; Baruth et al., 2010a,b, 2011; Casanova et al., 2012). TMS-based neuromodulation exerts effects on cortical excitability (Maeda et al., 2000; Pascual-Leone et al., 2000, 2002; Frye et al., 2008; Baruth et al., 2010b; Enticott et al., 2010; Sokhadze et al., 2012a; Oberman et al., 2013). It is proposed that that low-frequency (i.e., "slow"') rTMS (≤1 Hz) has inhibitory effects on stimulated cortex (Maeda et al., 2000), whereas high-frequency rTMS (>1 Hz, e.g., 5 Hz, 10 Hz etc.) increases excitability of stimulated cortex (Pascual-Leone et al., 1994, 2000, 2002; Daskalakis et al., 2002; Schutter, 2009; Wassermann and Zimmermann, 2012; Oberman et al., 2013). Probably the effect of low frequency rTMS are mediated through increases in the activation of inhibitory neurons (Hoffman and Cavus, 2002; Wagner et al., 2009). We propose that inhibitory cells such as basket and chandelier interneurons, whose projections keep no constant relation to the surface of the cortex, of the double-bouquet neurons are oriented in more geometrically exact manner and are located at the periphery of the minicolumn and therefore they are more appropriate candidate for induction by a TMS applied parallel to cortex. Low frequency rTMS in autism, may lower the cortical excitation/inhibition ratio, so called E/I ratio index.

In this study we were interested in how rTMS treatment affects specific ERP components known to index processes in sensory cortex, association cortical areas, and areas related to higher level cognitive activity. As it was mentioned above, the exogenous ERPs reflect early-stage, modality-specific, while endogenous ones reflect modality non-specific associative higher order processing of stimuli within the context of the task (Näätänen et al., 1978; Luck et al., 1990; Coles and Rugg, 1995; Hillyard and Annlo-Vento, 1998). Posterior visual P100 are generated within the fusiform gyrus with contribution from parieto-occipital and occipital cortices (Yamazaki et al., 2000). Frontal N100 ERP wave occurs within a similar time window and probably originates from more anterior frontal dipole generators (Clark et al., 1994).

The fronto-central P300 (so called P3a) reflects frontal lobe activity (Friedman et al., 1993) and in a visual oddball task with distracters is interpreted as an attentional "orienting", whereas centro-parietal and parietal P300 (P3b) is believed to reflect sustain attention and other higher level processes. This cognitive ERP component has multiple dipole sources (Townsend et al., 2001).

Negative N200 component is recorded in visual tasks over centro-parietal cortex around 200–300 ms post-stimulus (Näätänen et al., 1978, 1993) and reflects processes of stimulus categorization, perceptual closure and attention focusing signaling that a perceptual representation has been formed (Potts et al., 2004). A frontal positivity with a peak within (P2a, 180–320 ms post-stimulus) over inferior prefrontal recording sites is selectively responsive to the evaluation of the task relevance of presented stimuli, and originates from the orbito-frontal cortex (Potts et al., 1996, 1998, 2008). This frontal component may index task-relevant features of the stimulus (Kenemans et al., 1993). The fronto-central N200 according to some researchers (West, 2003; Donkers and van Boxtel, 2004; West et al., 2004) is thought to originate from the anterior cingulate cortex (ACC) and prefrontal sources and may reflect processes related to potential response conflict detection in a RT tasks and/or cortical inhibition of inappropriate MR. All ERP components have certain variability, but specific ERP measures selected for this study (frontal N100, N200 and P300, and parietal P100, N200 and P300) are less affected by variability in visual tasks and are relevant to the study goal.

We proposed that after 18 sessions of 1 Hz rTMS—administered to the dorso-lateral prefrontal cortices (DLPFC) participants with autism would demonstrate normalization of electrocortical indices of attention both at the early (P100, N100, 100–200 ms post-stimulus) and the late (i.e., P200, N200, P300, 200–600 ms) stages of sensory and cognitive processing and show improvements in MT accuracy. Mainly, we expected lower magnitude and longer latencies to visual targets (i.e., better stimulus discrimination), and attenuated reactivity to non-target illusory figures and other non-target cues. Other anticipated improvements were expected to be found in outcomes of social and behavioral functioning questionnaire and surveys. The hypothesis in this study proposed that low-frequency rTMS (i.e., inhibitory) would exert its effects through increased cortical inhibitory tone (i.e., lower E/I ratio) in the DLPFC with subsequent improvement in performance in the visual attention task. In addition we expected improvements in clinical social and behavioral evaluation outcomes.

METHODS

Participants with ASD (age range 9–21 years) were recruited through the University of Louisville Weisskopf Child Evaluation Center (WCEC). Diagnosis was made according to the Diagnostic and Statistical Manual of Mental Disorders (DSM-IV-TR) (APA, 2000) and further ascertained with the Autism Diagnostic Interview—Revised (ADI-R; Le Couteur et al., 2003). They also had a medical evaluation by a developmental pediatrician. All subjects had normal hearing based on past hearing screens. Participants with a history of seizure disorder, significant hearing or visual impairment, a brain abnormality conclusive from imaging studies or an identified genetic disorder were excluded. Fifty participants were high-functioning persons with autism diagnosis and four had Asperger Syndrome. All had full-scale IQ

>80 assessed using the Wechsler Intelligence Scale for Children, Fourth Edition (WISC-IV; Wechsler, 2003) or (for adolescents) the Wechsler Abbreviated Scale of Intelligence (WASI; Wechsler, 1999).

We enrolled 54 autistic patients, 44 males and 10 females, with a mean age of 14.5 ± 2.9 years. Twenty-seven of them were assigned to active 1.0 Hz TMS treatment (TMS group), while 27 were assigned to the WTL group. Mean age of subjects in the TMS group was 14.8 ± 3.2 years, and 14.1 ± 2.6 years in the WTL group. There was not a significant difference in either age or full-scale IQ between the TMS and WTL groups.

The study complied with all relevant national regulations and institutional policies and has been approved by the local Institutional Review Board (IRB). Participating subjects and their parents (or legal guardians) were provided with full information about the study including the purpose, requirements, responsibilities, reimbursement, risks, benefits, alternatives, and role of the local IRB. The subjects were reimbursed only for participation in two ERP tests ($25/per test). The consent and assent forms approved by the IRB were reviewed and explained to all subjects who expressed interest to participate. All questions were answered before consent signature was requested. If the individual agreed to participate, both she/he and parent/guardian signed and dated the consent or assent form and received a copy countersigned by the investigator who obtained consent.

THREE-STIMULI ODDBALL TASK WITH KANIZSA FIGURES

The stimuli employed in the test were Kanizsa square (target), Kanizsa triangle (non-target), non-Kanizsa square, and non-Kanizsa triangle (standards) (Kanizsa, 1976). The task represents a classic three-stimuli oddball with infrequent illusory Kanizsa target (square, 25%) and infrequent Kanizsa distracter (triangle, 25%) figures presented for 250 ms among frequent non-Kanizsa stimuli (so called standards, 50%) with inter-trial interval in 1,100–1,300 ms range (**Figure 1**). Totally 240 trials were presented following a brief practice block. The practice block had 20 trials only with the experimenter present in the room to make sure that subject correctly understands test conditions and recognizes target stimuli. The total time of the test including sensor application and practice was under 30 min. For better habituation and adaptation to experimental setting, the participants were encouraged to have at least one session for conditioning to brainwave sensor net (without performing task) and getting familiar with laboratory environment.

EVENT-RELATED POTENTIAL ACQUISITION AND PROCESSING

Electroencephalographic (EEG) signals from 128 sites were recorded with a dense-array EGI system (Electrical Geodesics, Inc., Eugene, Oregon). Subjects were placed in electrically and acoustically isolated camera from the Industrial Acoustics Co. (Bronx, NY). Stimulus presentation and MT collection was controlled using E-prime (PST, Inc., Pittsburg, PA). Visual stimuli were presented on a flat monitor located in 45–50 cm from the subject, and MTs were registered with a keypad (Serial Box, Inc). Sampling rate of EEG was 500 Hz, and analog Notch (60 Hz, infinite impulse response (IIR)) and analog elliptical bandpass filters were set at 0.1–200 Hz. Impedances were under 40 KΩ. Stimulus-locked EEG data were segmented off-line into 200 ms pre-stimulus baseline to 800 ms epoch post-stimulus. EEG recordings were screened for artifacts and trials with eye blinks, gross movements etc were removed using EGI software artifact rejection tools (Perrin et al., 1987; Fletcher et al., 1996; Srinivasan et al., 1998; Luu et al., 2001). The remaining artifact-free EEG data for trials with correct responses was digitally filtered using Notch filter (IIR, 5th order) and 0.3–20 Hz IIR elliptical bandpass filter. Averaged ERP data was baseline corrected (200 ms) and ERPs after averaging and baseline correction were re-referenced into an average reference frame. Response-locked EEGs were segmented into 500 ms pre-response to 500 ms post-response (i.e., commission error). More detailed account for experimental procedure and EEG data acquisition and processing can be found in our prior publications that used similar methodology (Baruth et al., 2010a,b; Casanova et al., 2012; Sokhadze et al., 2012a,b).

EVENT-RELATED POTENTIALS (ERP)

STIMULUS-LOCKED DEPENDENT ERP VARIABLES

Dependent variables for the frontal and fronto-central region-of-interest (ROI) were N100 (80–180 ms), N200 (220–350 ms), P2a (180–320 ms), and P3a (300–600 ms), and for the parietal and parieto-occipital ROI were P100 (120–180 ms), N200 (180–320 ms) and P3b (320–600 ms) ERP waves. For P2d component (i.e., differences wave of frontal P2a) we calculated difference wave (P2a to targets minus P2a to non-targets) to detect mean difference between two conditions both in amplitude and latency within 180–320 ms post-stimulus window.

RESPONSE-LOCKED EVENT-RELATED POTENTIALS (ERN/Pe)

Response locked dependent variables in this study were amplitude and latency of the Error-related Negativity (ERN peaking within 40–150 ms post-error) and Error-related Positivity (Pe, peaking within 100–300 ms post-error). The ROI for both ERN and Pe components included FCz, sites between FCz and FC3-C1, and between FCz and FC2-C2. Amplitude and latency analysis of ERN/Pe was performed with a custom-made application in Matlab (Clemans et al., 2011a). Validation of correct identification of ERN and Pe waves was further ascertained using another custom Matlab application using wavelet transformation (Clemans et al., 2011b).

TRANSCRANIAL MAGNETIC STIMULATION

Repetitive TMS was administered using a Magstim 220 device (Magstim Corp., Sheffield, UK) with a 70-mm figure-eight coil. Threshold of MT was identified for each hemisphere in all participants with autism by increasing the output of the stimulator by 5% until a 50 μV deflection or a visible twitch in the First Dorsal Interosseous (FDI) muscle was detected in at least 3 trials of stimulation over the motor cortex controlling the contralateral FDI. Electromyographic (EMG) responses were recorded with a C-2 J&J Engineering Inc multichannel physiological monitoring device with Physiodata software (J&J Engineering, Inc., Bainbridge Island, WA).

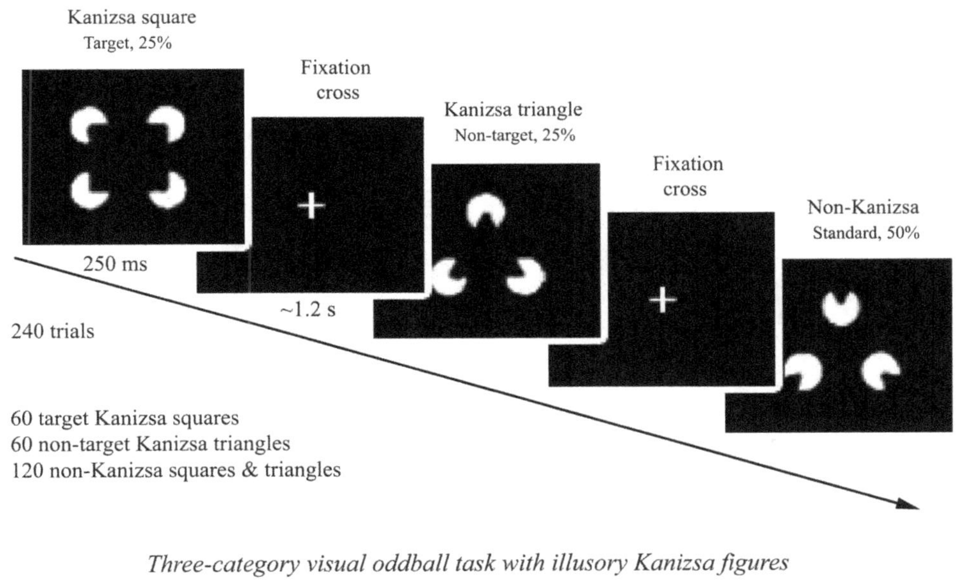

FIGURE 1 | Three-stimuli category visual oddball task with Kanizsa illusory figures. The stimulus types are: Kanizsa square (target, 25%), Kanizsa triangle (25%), non-Kanizsa square, and non-Kanizsa triangle. The non-target Kanizsa triangle is introduced to differentiate processing of Kanizsa figures and targets. The stimuli consist of either three or four inducer disks, which are considered the shape feature, and they either constitute an illusory figure (square, triangle) or not (collinearity feature).

The rTMS was administered weekly for 18 weeks with the 1st six treatments were over the left DLPFC, while the next six were over the right DLPFC, whereas remaining six treatments were done bilaterally over the DLFC (evenly at the left and right DLPFC). The DLPFC site for magnetic stimulation was found by placing the TMS coil 5 cm anterior, and in a parasagital plane, to the site of maximal FDI response. A swimming cap was used to make the TMS coil positioning easier. TMS was administered at 1.0 Hz frequency and 90% MT. There were total of 180 pulses per day session with nine trains with 20 pulses each. There were 20–30 s between the train intervals used. Decision to select 90% of the MT was based on the prior publications where rTMS was used for the stimulation of DLPFC in various neuro- and psychiatric disorders (reviewed in Pascual-Leone et al., 2000; Wassermann and Lisanby, 2001; Daskalakis et al., 2002; Gershon et al., 2003; Loo and Mitchell, 2005; Greenberg, 2007; Oberman et al., 2013).

CLINICAL SOCIAL AND BEHAVIORAL EVALUATION OUTCOMES

For the evaluation of social and behavioral functioning we utilized caregiver reports and clinician ratings of improvement. Every participant was evaluated before TMS course and within 2 weeks following TMS treatment. *Aberrant Behavior Checklist* (ABC; Aman and Singh, 1994; Aman, 2004) is a clinician administered rating scale to assess Irritability, Lethargy/Social Withdrawal, Stereotypy, Hyperactivity, and Inappropriate Speech based on parent/caregiver report. *Social Responsiveness Scale (SRS). Repetitive Behavior Scale—Revised* (RBS-R; Bodfish et al., 1999) is a caregiver completed rating scale assessing stereotyped, self-injurious, compulsive, ritualistic, sameness, and restricted range (Bodfish et al., 2000).

STATISTICAL ANALYSIS

The primary model for statistical analyses of subject-averaged ERP and MT data was the two factor repeated measure ANOVA. Dependent ERP variables were amplitude and latency of ERP at pre-determined ROIs. The within-participant factors were followings: *Stimulus* (Kanizsa target, Standard, Kanizsa Non-target), *Hemisphere* (Left, Right), and *Time* (Baseline, Post-treatment). The between-subject factor was *Group* (TMS, WTL). *Post hoc* analyses were conducted where appropriate. RT, error rate (commission, omission and total error rate), were analyzed using *Time* and *Group* factor. For clinical behavioral rating scores a *Treatment* (pre-vs. post-TMS/or waiting period) ANOVA was completed to determine changes associated with active stimulation and WTL conditions. Histograms with normal distribution curves along with skewness and kurtosis data were obtained for each dependent variables to determine normality of distribution and appropriateness of data for ANOVA and t-tests. For more reliable determination of normality of distribution residual plots (i.e., normal probability plot, histogram, vs. fits and order) were created using Minitab statistical package to indicate that treatment with ANOVA is justified. All dependent variables in the study had normal distribution. Greenhouse-Geisser corrected p-values were employed where appropriate in all ANOVAs. *A priori* hypotheses were tested with the Student's t-tests for two groups with equal variance. Confidence intervals (95% of mean, 95% CI) were calculated for each ERP data sets entered for t-tests. For the estimation of the effect size and power (Murphy and Myors, 2004) we used Partial Eta Squared (η^2) and observed power computed using $\alpha = 0.05$. SPSS 19.0 and Sigma Stat 3.1 statistical packages were used for analysis of data.

RESULTS

BEHAVIORAL RESPONSES (REACTION TIME AND ACCURACY, POST-ERROR RT)

Reaction Time (RT)

Effects of TMS on RT to targets were not significant. Comparison of RT to targets yielded no *Time* X *Group* effects.

Accuracy

Commission and omission errors analysis yielded a significant between-group difference in the commission error percentage, $F_{(1,52)} = 4.32$, $p = 0.042$. T-test showed significant decrease of commission error rate in the TMS group (mean decrease $-6.38 \pm 2.54\%$, 95% CI from -11.61 to -1.15%, $t_{(26)} = 2.50$, $p = 0.019$). We could not find between group differences in omission error rate. Total error rate (% errors) change also showed decrease only in TMS group ($-7.47 \pm 2.82\%$, 95% CI from -13.26 to -1.67%, $t_{(26)}=2.64$, $p = 0.013$).

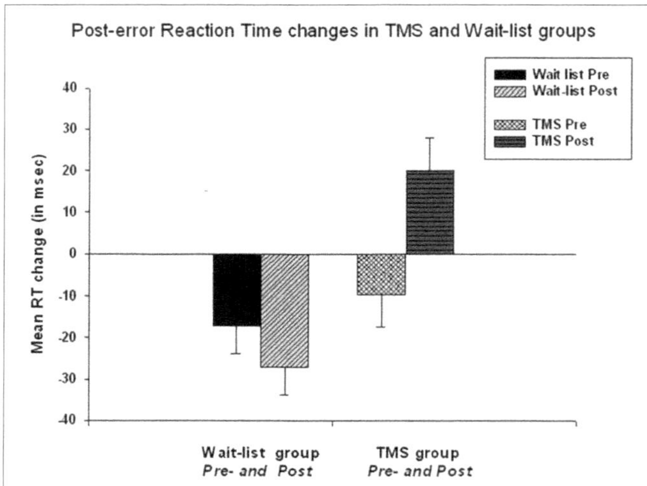

FIGURE 2 | Post-error reaction time (RT) changes in TMS and wait-list groups at the baseline and at the second test. *Time* X *Group* effect is highly significant ($F = 8.05$, $p = 0.006$). At the baseline both groups showed post-error RT speeding, while post-TMS post-error RT became positive. Change of the post-error RT in TMS group was significant ($t = 4.57$, $p < 0.001$).

Post-error RT

Main effect of *Time* (Pre, Post) on normative post-error RT slowing was highly significant ($F_{(1,50)}$=15,14, $p = 0.001$, $\eta^2 = 0.134$, observed power = 0.795 at alpha (α) = 0.05).

Repeated measure ANOVA of post-error RT slowing revealed that TMS and WTL group differences on post-error RT changes were also statistically significant, i.e., *Time* X *Group* interaction, $F_{(1,52)} = 8.05$, $p = 0.006$, $\eta^2 = 0.134$, observed power = 0.795. The TMS group showed post-error RT increase with significant positive change in post-error RT. This change was computed as post TMS post-error RT change minus pre-treatment post-error RT change (49.9 ± 55.4 ms, 95% CI from 26.42 to 69.41 ms, $t_{(26)} = 4.57$, $p < 0.001$). **Figure 2** shows that at the baseline both in WTL and TMS groups post-error RT was negative (mean post-error speeding was -23.1 ± 34.7 ms and not different between groups at pre-treatment stage), while in the TMS group post-error RT became positive (i.e., showed normative slowing), whereas it remained negative in the WTL group.

PARIETAL AND PARIETO-OCCIPITAL ERP COMPONENTS

P100

TMS course had main effects on P100 component's both amplitude ($F_{(1,52)} = 4.78$, $p = 0.033$) and latency ($F_{(1,52)} = 15.00$, $p = 0.001$). Response of this parietal and parieto-occipital P100 component (positive peak within 130–160 ms post-stimulus) to targets showed post-treatment between group difference in amplitude (2.25 ± 2.93 μV, with 95% CI from 1.14 to 3.37 μV, in TMS vs. 4.37 ± 3.89 μV, 95% CI from 2.83 to 5.91 μV, in WTL, $F_{(1,52)} = 5.31$, $p = 0.025$) and latency (153.3 ± 43.99 ms, 95% CI from 136 to 170 ms in TMS vs. 128 ± 18.42 ms, 95% CI from 121 to 135 ms in WTL, $F_{(1,52)} = 7.54$, $p = 0.008$). Group differences in response to Kanizsa targets and non-targets were more expressed in the latency of the P100 ($F_{(1,52)} = 4.91$, $p = 0.011$). The *Stimulus* (Standard, Non-target Kanizsa, Target Kanizsa) X *Time* (Pre, Post) X *Group* (TMS, WTL) effect was significant ($F_{(2,52)} = 4.34$, $p = 0.015$), and this effect was even more powerful for standard vs. target stimuli comparison ($F_{(1,52)} = 7.92$, $p = 0.007$, $\eta^2 = 0.128$, observed power = 0.789). The effect can be described as a reduced latency to non-targets and increased latency to target stimuli post-TMS but not after wait period. There were no hemispheric differences observed for P100 component.

N200

There were no group differences in amplitude of the parietal N200 component. Latency of N200 to targets showed post-treatment between group difference in latency to targets (238.72 ± 58.58 ms, 95% CI from 215 to 261 ms, in TMS vs. 201.35 ± 24.27 ms, 95% CI from 191 to 210 ms, in WTL group, $F_{(1,52)} = 9.34$, $p = 0.004$) and non-target illusory Kanizsa figures (242.31 ± 62.42 ms, 95% CI from 217 to 267 ms, in TMS vs. 208.27 ± 24.92 ms, 95% CI from 198 to 218 ms, in WTL group, $F_{(1,52)} = 6.92$, $p = 0.011$). ANOVA analysis of the latency of parietal N200 to target and non-target Kanizsa stimuli showed a *Stimulus* (Target, Non-target) X *Time* (Pre, Post) X *Group* (TMS, WTL) interaction, $F_{(2,52)} = 3.69$, $p = 0.032$. The effect was expressed as increased latency for non-target stimuli in the TMS group post-treatment. There were observed other interactions as well, for instance hemispheric one, as the effect was featured by more delayed latency at the right hemisphere in the TMS group ($F_{(1,52)} = 7.15$, $p = 0.01$, $\eta^2 = 0.121$, power = 0.747). Other notable interaction was significant *Time* X *Group* effect, $F_{(1,52)} = 4.60$, $p = 0.037$, $\eta^2 = 0.08$, observed power = 0.558, with TMS showing more prolonged N200 latency to non-target Kanizsa stimuli. *Post hoc* tests showed that in the active treatment group latency increased (e.g., to non-targets, bilaterally 24.2 ± 11.8 ms, 95% CI from 3.7 to 51.0 ms, $t_{(26)} = 2.37$, $p = 0.025$) along with attenuated amplitude (−1.39 ± 3.26μV, 95% CI from −2.63 to −0.15 μV, $t_{(26)} = 2.30$, $p = 0.029$), while changes of latency and amplitude of N200 in the WTL group were not significant (see **Figure 3**).

P300 (P3b)

We found between group differences in P3b amplitude that were expressed as more attenuated component post-treatment in TMS as compared to WTL group only to non-Kanisza standards (2.69 ± 2.96 μV, 95% CI from 0.88 to 3.61 μV, in TMS vs. 5.09 ± 3.98 μV, 95% CI from 3.21 to 6.14 μV, in WTL, $F_{(1,52)} = 5.25$, $p = 0.026$). We found no interactions of P3b amplitude using in ANOVA *Stimulus, Hemisphere, Time*, and *Group* factors. *Stimulus* (Target, Non-target Kanisza, Standard) factor had a main effect on latency of P3b ($F_{(2,53)} = 11.59$, $p < 0.001$). The latency of P3b showed significant effects of *Time* factor on each stimuli: latency of P3b to targets, 364.15 ± 63.08 ms, 95% CI from 340 to 380 ms, in TMS vs. 326.13 ± 28.27 ms, 95% CI from 314 to 337 ms, in WTL, $F_{(1,52)} = 8.16$, $p = 0.006$; non-target Kanizsa, 356.68 ± 67.26 ms, 95% CI from 333 to 384 ms, in TMS vs. 322.93 ± 21.55 ms, 95% CI from 314 to 331 ms, in WTL, $F_{(1,52)} = 6.94$, $p = 0.011$; and standards, 354.89 ± 64.68 ms, 95% CI from 330 to 379 ms, in TMS vs. 323.54 ± 20.68 ms, 95% CI from 315 to 331 ms, in WTL, ($F_{(1,52)} = 5.25$, $p = 0.026$). Repeated measure ANOVA analysis of the P3b latency also indicated a significant between groups differences for all types of illusory figures, for example, increased P3b latency as a result of rTMS (*Time* × *Group* interaction, $F_{(1,52)} = 4.32$, $p = 0.044$), that can be described as a longer post-treatment latency in TMS, shorter in WTL group.

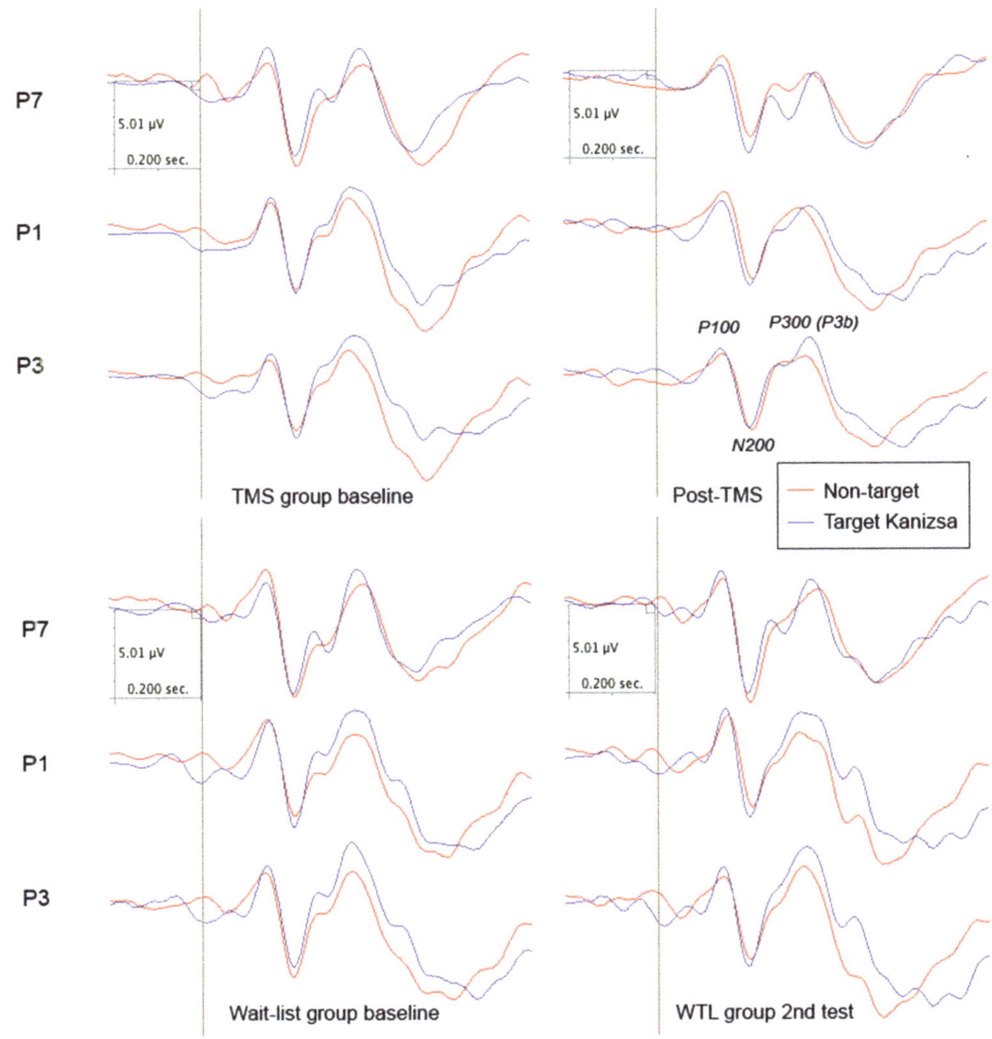

FIGURE 3 | Parietal ERPs (P1, P3, P7 sites according to 10–10 International System) to target and non-target Kanizsa figures in TMS and wait-list groups (*N* = 27/per group) before and after treatment (TMS/or wait-period).

FRONTAL AND FRONTO-CENTRAL ERP COMPONENTS

N100

Comparison of post-treatment amplitude and latency of N100 ERP component showed decreased amplitude and prolonged latency to both target and non-target Kanizsa figures in the TMS group, while N100 magnitude was practically unchanged in the WTL group. Effects of *Time* factor on amplitude and latency to targets was significant (at post-TMS test, amplitude, −1.54 ± 1.83 μV, 95% CI from −2.72 to −0.88 μV, in TMS vs. −2.91 ± 2.96 μV, 95% CI from −3.59 to −1.74 μV, in WTL, $F_{(1,52)} = 4.62$, $p = 0.036$; while latency, 140.85 ± 32.76 ms, 95% CI from 127 to 153 ms, in TMS vs. 120.83 ± 20.87 ms, 95% CI from 112 to 129 ms, in WTL group). Effects of *Time* on frontal N100 to non-targets was also statistically significant (amplitude, −1.36 ± 1.63 μV in TMS vs. −2.37 ± 2.07 μV in WTL, $F_{(1,52)} = 4.47$, $p = 0.04$; latency, 140.59 ± 23.22 ms in TMS vs. 125.4 ± 13.38 ms in WTL, $F_{(1,52)} = 8.58$, $p = 0.005$). There were no interaction of N100 amplitude and latency on *Stimulus*, *Hemisphere* and *Group* factors.

N200

There was observed significant between *Group* (TMS, WTL) difference in N200 amplitude ($F_{(1,52)} = 8.24$, $p = 0.006$, $\eta^2 = 0.119$, observed power = 0.804). A *Stimulus* (Target Kanizsa, Non-Kanizsa standard) X *Hemisphere* (Left, Right) X *Group* (TMS, WTL) interaction reached significance ($F_{(1,52)} = 4.64$, $p = 0.037$) pointing at a more negative N200 to targets with less negative N200 to non-target Kanizsa as a result of rTMS (**Figure 4**). The TMS group showed less hemispheric differences post-treatment, while the WTL group had more negative amplitude of N200 at the right hemisphere. A *Time* X *Group* effect for

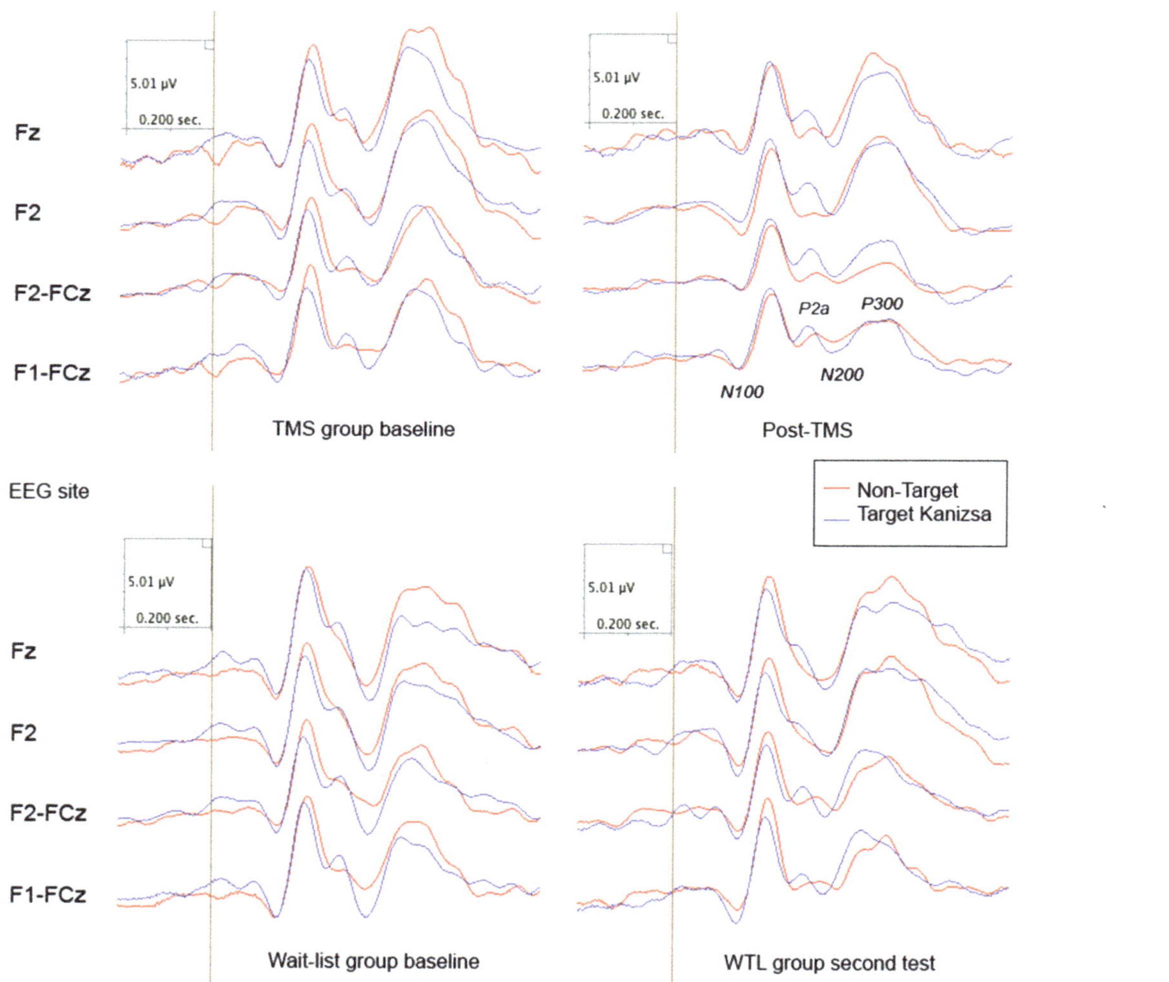

FIGURE 4 | Frontal and frono-central ERPs (Fz, F2, F2-FCz, F1-FCz) to target and non-target Kanizsa figures in TMS and wait-list groups (*N* = 27/per group) before and after treatment (TMS/ or wait-period). Frontal P2a components (280–320 ms post stimulus) is marked with a blue line.

the latency of N200 was significant ($F_{(1,52)} = 7.26$, $p = 0.009$, $\eta^2 = 0.119$, observed power = 0.754), yielding longed latency to targets post-TMS. Additionally, *post hoc* analysis using *t*-test showed that N200 latency became statistically more prolonged to target stimuli in TMS group across both hemispheres (13.31 ± 34.03 ms, 95% CI from 26.2 to 0.36 ms, $t_{(26)} = 2.10$, $p = 0.044$).

P2d

The frontal P2a calculated as a mean difference between P2a amplitude to target Kanizsa minus P2a amplitude to non-target Kanizsa stimuli. TMS had significant effect at P2d amplitude ($F_{(1,52)} = 6.56$, $p = 0.013$). The baseline values in both groups were similar (−2.35 μV in TMS vs. −2.51 μV in WTL) but showed significant difference post-treatment (1.34 ± 4.65 μV in TMS vs. −1.97 ± 3.56 in WTL group). ANOVA showed significant *Time* X *Group* interaction, $F_{(1,52)} = 4.11$, $p = 0.048$, $\eta^2 = 0.075$, observed power = 0.512. Effect can be described as P2d becoming positive post-TMS, i.e., P2a component to targets was larger than to non-targets. Paired sample *t*-test confirmed that P2d amplitude increased significantly post-TMS (3.70 ± 7.47 μV, 95% CI from 6.71 to 0.68 μV, $t_{(26)} = 2.52$, $p = 0.018$). Differences in P2d latency between groups were not significant (**Figure 5**).

P300 (P3a)

The treatment had main effect on the amplitude of the frontal P300 (P3a) component ($F_{(1,52)} = 4.27$, $p = 0.044$). The amplitude of P3a showed a *Time* X *Group* effect that was statistically significant ($F_{(1,52)} = 4.64$, $p = 0.036$). The active TMS showed post-treatment decrease of the P3a bilaterally across all stimuli, whereas WTL group showed no differences at all. Paired sample *t*-test showed that decrease of the amplitude in TMS group was significant both for non-target Kanizsa (−1.93 ± 3.09 μV, 95% CI from −0.54 to −3.33 μV, $t_{(26)} = 2.85$, $p = 0.008$) and target Kanizsa stimuli (−2.91 ± 3.84 μV, 95% CI from −0.64 to −5.18 μV, $t_{(26)} = 2.64$, $p = 0.014$). There were not detected any main effects or interactions in the latency of the frontal P3a.

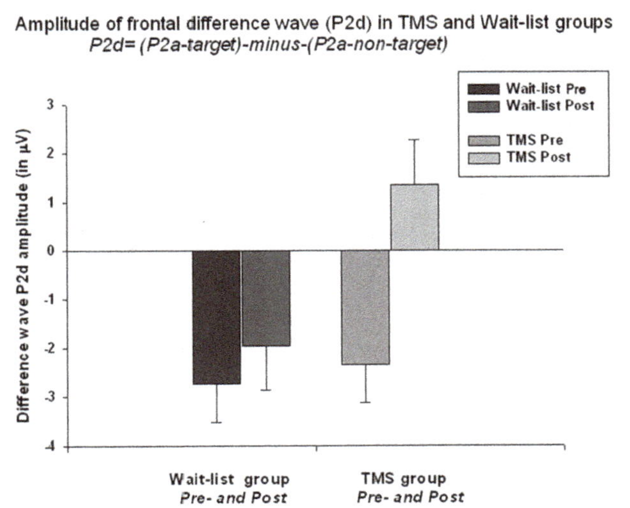

FIGURE 5 | Amplitude of the frontal P2a difference wave (so called *P2d = [P2a to targets minus P2a to non-targets]*) across both hemispheres shows *Time X Group* interactions effect ($F = 4.11$, $p = 0.048$). Difference wave (P2d) was negative at the baseline in both groups (i.e., lower amplitude to targets as compared to non-targets), but becomes positive post-TMS. Increase of P2d was significant in the TMS group ($t = 2.52$, $p = 0.018$).

RESPONSE-LOCKED FRONTAL AND FRONTO-CENTRAL ERN AND Pe

Two subjects did not show sufficient number of commission errors and were excluded from the analysis. TMS and WTL groups showed significant differences in ERN amplitude ($F_{(1,50)} = 6.20$, $p = 0.016$) and latency ($F_{(1,50)} = 5.82$, $p = 0.023$). Amplitude of ERN during commission errors across five frontal and fronto-central sites showed marginal *Time* X *Group* interaction ($F_{(1,50)} = 4.05$, $p = 0.05$), and paired-sample *t*-test showed significant increase of ERN negativity in the TMS group (by 2.97 ± 3.21 μV, 95% CI from 0.36 to 4.60 μV, $t_{(26)} = 2.40$, $p = 0.023$, see **Figure 6**). Analysis of ERN latency ANOVA yielded statistically significant *Time* X *Group* effect, ($F_{(1,50)} = 4.24$, $p = 0.041$, $\eta^2 = 0.099$, observed power = 0.55). *T*-test of the ERN latency changes in the TMS group showed significant decrease (−28.1 ± 13.8 ms, 95% CI from −4.22 to −52.1 ms, $t_{(24)} = 2.41$, $p = 0.023$). Amplitude and latency of Pe wave in both groups were not significantly changed post-treatment. **Figure 7** shows ERN and Pe waveforms in two groups at the first (baseline) and at the second test.

CLINICAL BEHAVIOR EVALUATIONS POST-TMS

We found a significant decrease in stereotype repetitive and restricted behavior patterns following 18 sessions of bilateral rTMS as measured by the RBS-R (Bodfish et al., 1999) and analyzed them using a paired sample Student's *t*-test. Total RBS-R score decreased from 23.4 to 19.1, mean decrease being

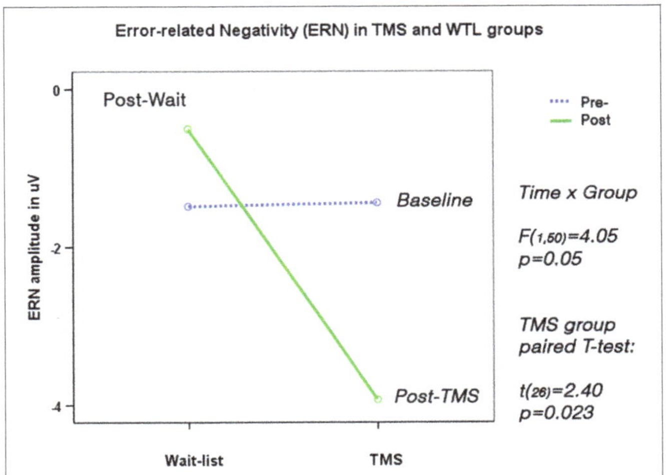

FIGURE 6 | Error-related Negativity (ERN, 40–120 ms post-error) shows *Time X Group* interaction ($F = 4.05$, $p = 0.05$). Post-TMS ERN amplitude became significantly more negative ($t = 2.40$, $p = 0.023$). $N = 26$/per group, as 2 subjects out of 54 committed no commission errors on the second test.

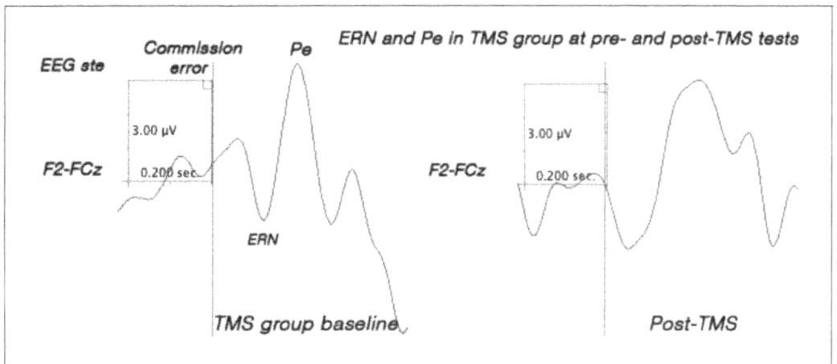

FIGURE 7 | Error-related Negativity (ERN) and Positivity (Pe) from the fronto-central midline EEG sites. Grandaverage waveforms at the fronto-central site (between F2 and FCz, N = 26 per group) show more negative amplitude and shorter latency of the ERN in the TMS group post-treatment. ERN peak occurring within 40–140 ms post-error is marked by a blue line.

-4.29 ± 5.9, 95% CI from -1.95 to -6.63, $t_{(26)} = 6.63$, $p = 0.001$. Changes in individual subscale scores is depicted at the **Figure 8**, where both Stereotypic Behavior subscale and Ritualistic/Sameness behavior subscale scores show significant decrease (accordingly -1.00 ± 1.77, 95% CI from -0.28 to -1.71, $t_{(26)} = 2.89$, $p = 0.008$ and -1.33 ± 2.21, 95% CI from -0.45 to -2.21, $t_{(26)} = 3.12$, $p = 0.004$). There was identified as well a significant reduction in Irritability subscale as measured by the ABC (Aman and Singh, 1994), i.e., -2.07 ± 5.12, 95% CI from -0.40 to -4.10, $t_{(26)} = 2.10$, $p = 0.045$. Lethargy and Hyperactivity subscales showed even more pronounced score reductions (Lethargy, -2.11 ± 3.93, 95% CI from -0.51 to -3.72, $t_{(26)} = 2.71$, $p = 0.012$; Hyperactivity, -4.03 ± 7.68, 95% from -0.99 to -7.07, $t_{(26)} = 2.72$, $p = 0.011$). Changes of individual subscale rating scores in TMS group are depicted at the **Figure 9**. The WTL group had no significant differences in any of RBS-R or ABC scale ratings as a result of the waiting period.

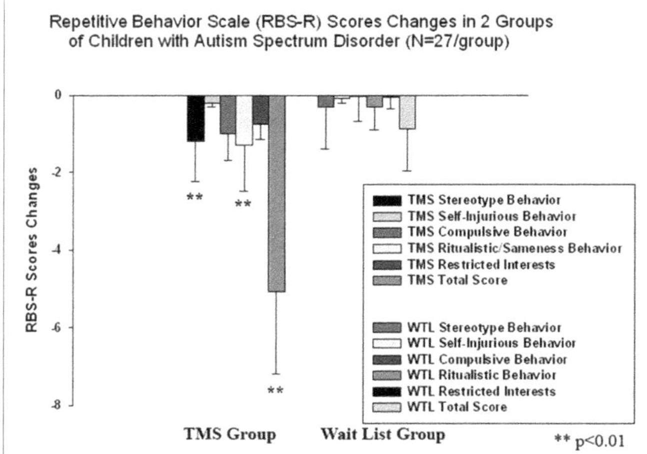

FIGURE 8 | Changes of Repetitive Behavior Scale (RBS-R) scores post-TMS/wait-list treatment as compared to baseline levels in two groups of children with ASD (N = 27/per group). Stereotype Behavior, Ritualistic Behavior and Total RBS scores decreased significantly in the TMS group.

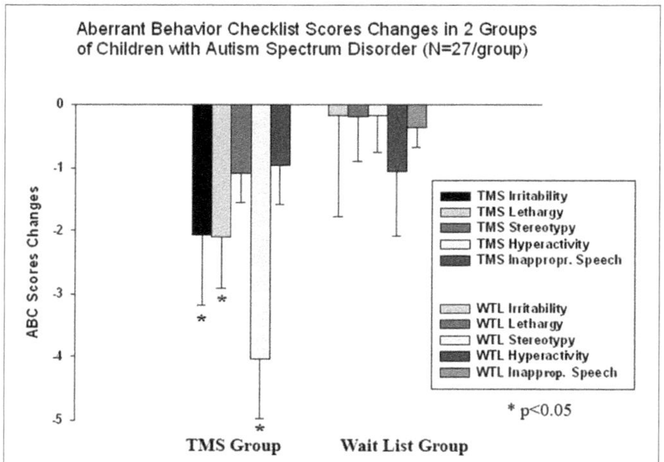

FIGURE 9 | Changes of Aberrant Behavior Checklist (ABC) scores post-TMS/wait-list treatment as compared to baseline levels in two groups of children with ASD (N = 27/per group). Irritability, Lethargy, and Hyperactivity rating scores decreased significantly post-TMS.

DISCUSSION

Our results show significant changes in behavioral responses (accuracy, post-error RT slowing) and both early and later-stage ERP indices of task-relevant signal processing as a result of 18 sessions of low frequency rTMS treatment course in children with ASD.

Participant in TMS group showed decreased amplitude and prolonged latency of parietal P100 and N200 components to all stimuli, more for non-target cues. Parietal P3b ERP component was also prolonged without amplitude change in TMS group. In our prior study (Sokhadze et al., 2009b, 2010a, 2013b) at the parietal and parieto-occipital cortices the autism group showed significantly prolonged latency of N100 and reduced amplitude of N200 to targets as compared to neurotypical controls. Latency of the P3b was longer to distracters, without any amplitude group difference to targets and novels. The ASD group had prolonged latencies to novels but not to targets, with effect being better expressed in the right hemisphere. The results indicate the excess of efforts needed for the differentiation of targets from non-target novels in individuals with ASD. TMS treatment enhanced the process of target recognition during performance on task. Especially informative in this regard was positive change of the frontal P2d difference wave that indicates increase of P2a component to target Kanizsa stimuli vs. non-target Kanizsa stimuli, thus reflecting easier discrimination of target features of the stimuli (illusory square vs. illusory triangle).

In addition, at the same frontal topography N200 component was more negative to targets as compared to non-target illusory figures and had longer latency resulting in globally higher magnitude of N200 to targets. Following TMS course the N200 component at the frontal sites became more negative to targets, and at the same time significantly less negative to both types of non-target stimuli. The positive frontal P2a component followed by the negative ERP N200 component (both of them peaking within 280–320 post-stimulus) in visual oddball tests tasks are associated with categorization, perceptual closure and attention focusing ultimately signaling that a perceptual representation has been formed (Potts et al., 2004). This wave is enhanced if the presented stimulus contains a feature or attribute defining the target in the task according to Potts et al. (2004). It was previous reported (Sokhadze et al., 2009a; Baruth et al., 2010c) that individuals with ASD as compared to typical controls showed enhanced N200 to task irrelevant as compared to task relevant stimuli, and the finding that N200 became more negative to target Kanizsa figures and less negative to non-target distracters post-rTMS treatment indicates a trend to normalization of the response pattern pointing at an improved visual signal processing and a more effective discrimination of the target.

The results indicate a reduction of the frontal P3a both to target and non-target stimuli post-TMS in our ASD patients. In our earlier studies comparing ASD and typical controls we reported that the ASD group showed prolonged N100, P100, and P3b to targets stimuli, emphasizing a change indicative of abnormalities of sustained attention compared to controls. At the same time, the ASD group exhibited a prolonged P3a to novels, and this can be considered as a marker of impaired orientation to novelty, and ultimately decreased frontal associative and integrative functioning. In the current study our results show no differences in amplitude, though the latency of the P3a was still delayed.

Over-activation in the parietal cortex at the early stages of processing of non-targets, either standards or infrequent distracters, and at the same time under-activation of integrative frontal regions at the late stages of target processing was found to occur in autism in a similar visual task that was using three-stimuli paradigm with rare novel distracters (Sokhadze et al., 2009b, 2010a). Our results in a series of visual oddball tasks indicated enhanced and prolonged early frontal ERPs and a delayed late P3a to non-target stimuli, which would suggest low selectivity in pre-processing and at a later stage under-activation of integrative regions. Overall, this is an indication of an over-connected network where sensory inputs evoke abnormally large evoked potentials for unattended stimuli such as frequent standards and rare novel distracters at all stages of visual signal processing with signs of a reduced selectivity of the activation.

The results of the current study indicate that rTMS may have facilitated attention and target discrimination by improving conflict resolutions during processing task-relevant and task-irrelevant stimuli. The latency of posterior P3b was prolonged to targets but reduced to both non-target Kanzisa and non-Kanizsa stimuli following rTMS. The P3b has been linked to task-relevance and the decision- related character of the stimulus as it indicates memory-updating and individual trial processing closure (Picton, 1992). Earlier we (Sokhadze et al., 2009a,b, 2012b) noted that individuals with autism showed prolonged P300 peak to irrelevant distracters as compared to typical controls, which was similar to effects reported by other groups (Courchesne et al., 1989; Townsend et al., 2001). The auditory and visual sensory information processing abnormalities been described in ASD by different researchers (Kemner et al., 1994, 1999; Bomba and Pang, 2004). However, most of these studies analyzed and reported outcomes of late cognitive potentials such as centro-parietal P3b (Courchesne et al., 1989; Ciesielski et al., 1990) and frontal P3a (Townsend et al., 2001). There are only a few papers reporting short latency ERP components' differences in individuals with autism. Majority of these studies emphasize over-activation as well as an abnormal pattern of basic perceptual processes such as low selectivity regardless of modality, abnormal top-down attentional control including delayed attentional orienting to novel stimuli, and deficits in information integration processes (Belmonte and Yurgelun-Todd, 2003). In typically developing children the fronto-central P3a occurs earlier in time as compared to parietal P300 (P3b), but in autistic subjects the P3a and P3b components were found to peak almost simultaneously over the frontal and parietal sites in a spatial attention test (Townsend et al., 2001). The latency of P3a is thought to be associated with the speed of attentional orienting to significant novel stimulus and reflects working memory processes in the prefrontal cortex. Centro-parietal P3b is usually described as a cognitive component that indexes context update and closure. This cognitive potential was found to be delayed but was not significantly attenuated in the group of children with autism as compared to typical controls (Sokhadze et al., 2009a,b, 2010a, 2012b).

The results of the study may indicate facilitation of visual target discrimination processes and enhanced habituation to task-irrelevant distracters post-TMS. We report significant improvement in the accuracy of MTs, lower total error rate and improved normative post-error RT slowing following 18 session long rTMS course. These result support our earlier findings outlining improvement in attention, executive control, and irrelevant response inhibition post-TMS treatment in autism.

In our initial rTMS pilot studies (Sokhadze et al., 2009b, 2010a) we used only six sessions of low frequency rTMS applied only to the left DLPFC and assessed behavioral performance in a visual attention task in children with autism. In a very similar manner, our current study also found a notable reduction in the frontal N200 and altered latency of the parietal P3b to task-irrelevant stimuli. Additionally, similar to the present investigation we also found a significant reduction in the response errors rate following a shorter courses of the prefrontal rTMS (Sokhadze et al., 2009b, 2012a; Baruth et al., 2010a). It might be stated that we found even more pronounced changes in cognitive ERPs such as P2d, N200and P3b in this study that had the greater number of rTMS treatments (18 sessions). In another study using this time 12 sessions of rTMS we found a significant reduction in repetitive and restricted behavior patterns as well as a significant reduction in irritability according to clinical and behavioral questionnaires (Casanova et al., 2012).The results of current 18 session-long rTMS treatment confirm and expand our prior findings of reduced repetitive behaviors (Sokhadze et al., 2009a,b, 2010a,b; Baruth et al., 2010b) and irritability (Baruth et al., 2010a,b) following low-frequency rTMS course. It should be noted that we found significant reductions in irritability only as a result of 12 sessions of bilateral stimulation (Baruth et al., 2010a), whereas reductions in repetitive behavior have been significant after six sessions of stimulation to the left DLPFC (Sokhadze et al., 2009b, 2010a).

It was a very reasonable decision to select DLPFC as a site for rTMS stimulation. The DLPFC processes components of working memory, decision making process, and regulates the ability to focus attention on task-relevant goals while inhibiting responses to distracters (Gray et al., 2003; Enriquez-Geppert et al., 2010; Matzel and Kolata, 2010). Suggested disruption in the ratio between cortical excitation and inhibition especially within the prefrontal cortex in individuals with autism (Casanova et al., 2002a, 2006a,b) was confirmed in individuals with Asperger syndrome (Casanova et al., 2002c). Reduced cortical inhibitory tone and an increased E/I ratio could adversely affect patterns of cortical activation, possibly resulting in isolated islands of coordinated excitatory activity and in a high comorbidity rate of ASD and epilepsy (Tuchman and Rapin, 1997). We believe that a course of 18 neuromodulatory sessions of low frequency rTMS may restore the cortical E/I balance by selective activation of double-bouquet cells at the periphery of cortical minicolumns (Casanova et al., 2006a,b; Casanova, 2007). It was shown that minicolumnar abnormalities in autism are most significant within the prefrontal cortex, more specifically, the DLPFC and the ACC (Fernandez-Duque et al., 2000; Mesulam, 2000; Casanova et al., 2002b, 2006a,b).

Rubenstein and Merzenich (2003) put forward a hypothesis that at some forms of autism could be caused by a disproportionate high level of excitation (E) or disproportionately weak inhibition (I) resulting in a high E/I ratio. Cortical circuits with such enhanced E/I level are proposed to be featured by poor functional differentiation which may lead to broad-ranging abnormalities in perception, memory and cognition, and motor control. Among other defects, individuals with autism have well known perceptual processing abnormalities, including a hypersensitivity to auditory, visual and tactile stimulation (Gomot et al., 2002; Plaisted et al., 2003). Studies of perceptual systems in animal models may provide useful insights into mechanisms underlying sensory disturbances in autism. In particular, investigations of auditory development in rats using modulated noise manipulation showed that the representation of sound inputs in the cortex remains poorly differentiated when the cortex is undergoing development under very poor signal-to-noise conditions (Chang and Merzenich, 2003). The E/I balance in the cortex is controlled by the relative numbers and functional activity of glutamatergic and GABA-ergic neurons. Neurodevelopmental abnormalities may lead to increased number, morphology or functional balance of excitatory vs. inhibitory neurons and can lead to a hyper-excitable state typical for autism. Excessive noise in cortical structures processing information also negatively affects development of normally differentiated representations. Relatively undifferentiated representations of orienting signals or significant stimuli would result in larger and less selective response. Such over-representation by non-differentiated responses could account for the strong aversive reactions to auditory, tactile and visual stimuli that are common in autism.

Casanova et al. (2003) study indicated that minicolumns in the brains of individuals with autism are narrow and have altered internal organization. More specifically, their minicolumns have less peripheral neuropil space, which is the conduit for inhibitory local circuit projections. A defect in these GABAergic interneurons may correlate with the increased E/I balance and prevalence of seizures among autistic patients. The authors concluded that GABAergic interneurons are vital for sensory signal processing (e.g., filtering capacity, proper signal discrimination, etc.), thus providing a putative correlate to autistic symptomatology. As it was noted in a recent review on use of TMS in ASD (Oberman et al., 2013), TMS could be particularly informative in detecting abnormalities in E/I ratios in ASD given theoretical studies regarding role of GABAergic interneurons in autism etiology (Hussman, 2001) and specifically role of high E/I balance in autism (Casanova et al., 2003; Rubenstein and Merzenich, 2003). Our current study is supportive of idea that rTMS is capable to improve E/I ratio as manifested in electrocortical responses to sensory stimulus processing in visual selective attention test.

This TMS study was guided by the "minicolumnar" theory of autism. The hierarchical basis of the modular organization of the cerebral cortex is well recognized in the literature. The cerebral cortex originates during brain development as germinal cells from the ventricular and later on the subventricular zones divide asymmetrically and the resulting neuroblasts migrate towards the pial surface (for review see Casanova and Trippe, 2006). The migrating neuroblasts split the preplate to form the incipient cortex wherein arriving cells acquire an orderly inside-out configuration by using either somal translocation or radial glia projections as a scaffold (Marín-Padilla, 1998). The resulting vertical arrangement of cells within this dynamic system serves as an attractor for satellite interneurons to populate its peripheral neuropil space. Radially migrating neurons provide for future pyramidal cells while those that follow a tangential path, primarily from the ganglionic eminences, are destined to be interneurons. Different types of interneurons form dyadic units with pyramidal cells and the resulting ensemble of cells, along with their afferent/efferent projections, constitute information processing units better known as minicolumns (Marin-Padilla, 2010). Recent studies indicate that higher cognitive functions including our executive functions derive from the workings of these modules or minicolumns (Opris et al., 2013).

Topographical studies of minicolumnar morphometry in ASD have shown the greatest deviance from neurotypicals within the prefrontal cortex (Casanova et al., 2002d, 2006a, 2010). Some investigators have explained this fact as resulting from the prolonged maturation time of this structure which thus provides a larger time window of opportunity for exogenous factors to alter its development (Opris and Casanova, 2014). Within the rostral brain region abnormalities within the DLPFC could serve as a pathological correlate to observed executive function deficits in autism (Opris and Casanova, 2014). Given the vertical orientation of inhibitory elements within the periphery of the minicolumns (e.g., double bouquet cells) it has been proposed that rTMS in ASD could preferentially help build the inhibitory surround of these modular structures. Since the dorsolateral prefrontal cortex has been a source of significant minicolumnopathy in published postmortem studies it could be viewed as a target for stimulation using rTMS (Casanova et al., 2002b, 2012). Furthermore, considering the trans-synaptic effects of rTMS, the large number of DLPFC connections could provide a therapeutic cascading effect in other parts of the brain. In autism computerized image analysis suggests the presence of a minicolumnopathy characterized by an increased density of modules and a diminution in their peripheral neuropil space (Casanova et al., 2002a). The deficits previously described by our group have been corroborated using a variety of neuronomorphometric techniques (e.g., Euclidean minimum spanning tree, gray level index), in an independent sample conducted by an international study where the investigators were blind to the study variables, and in the published results of other investigators (Casanova et al., 2002d, 2006a; Buxhoeveden et al., 2006). The diminished width of the minicolumnar peripheral neuropil space is seen throughout laminae II-VI, suggesting a deficit of an anatomical element in-common to all layers (Casanova et al., 2010). Since inhibitory elements populate all layers of the lateral compartment of the minicolumn pathology involving these elements could contribute to a deficit in the lateral or peripheral inhibitory surround of these modules. These findings gain credence from EEG recordings using lateral masking paradigms and threshold studies using flutter stimuli that sustain the presence of a lateral inhibitory deficit in autism (Kéïta et al., 2011; Puts et al., 2014). It is plausible to propose that low frequency rTMS is increasing inhibitory tone and improving lateral inhibition, and this may result in an enhancement of executive functions.

Executive function deficits were always in the center of attention in autism research. Executive function of behavioral performance monitoring comprises error detection and response conflict monitoring, functions that can be measured using response-locked ERPs such as ERN and Pe (Gehring et al., 1993; Carter et al., 1998; Van Veen and Carter, 2002; Mars et al., 2005; Arbel and Donchin, 2009, 2011). The ERN is a well-studied component whose parameters were investigated under different experimental task conditions, and its ties to error processing have been well established (Carter et al., 1998; Falkenstein et al., 2000; Gehring and Knight, 2000; Van Veen and Carter, 2002). There is an increased number of research studies examining ERN during commission errors in children (Davies et al., 2004). It is established that executive functions normally improve with age (Huizinga et al., 2006) along with demonstration that the ACC, which is now associated with executive performance monitoring, undergoes important maturation changes from childhood into adolescence, and then into adulthood (Arbel and Donchin, 2009, 2011). Furthermore, the studying error processing maturation can be used to understand mechanisms of various neurodevelopmental disorders, such as ADHD and ASD, which feature impairments in execute control (Liotti et al., 2005; Vlamings et al., 2008; Zhang et al., 2009; Sokhadze et al., 2010b). The ERN abnormalities are interpreted as reflecting early error processing impairments. A number of studies have investigated the functional relationship between the ERN and the fronto-central stimulus-locked N200, while some suggest that they represent distinct neurophysiological processes (Ridderinkhof et al., 2004), others suggest they represent different time points of the same process of response conflict monitoring (Yeung and Cohen, 2006).

One of the most important findings of current study was replication of the increase of ERN amplitude and shortened latency post-TMS reported in previous study using 12 sessions of rTMS (Sokhadze et al., 2012a). In accord with our previous study (Sokhadze et al., 2012a), the Pe component did not change post-TMS. This component has a more posterior topography and is expressed as a positivity elicited after the ERN (Falkenstein et al., 2000; Nieuwenhuis et al., 2001; Overbeek et al., 2005). In our earlier study with rTMS application in ASD (Sokhadze et al., 2009a,b, 2010a; Baruth et al., 2010c) we found that most of EEG changes such as ERP and evoked EEG gamma frequency oscillations occurred at the early stages of visual stimulus processing (e.g., less than 200 ms post-stimulus), and resulted in a better discrimination of target from non-target stimuli. Facilitation of target recognition following TMS treatment and more effective early inhibition of non-target distracters leads to less pronounced carryover of non-target over-processing. We suggested earlier that more expressed positive neuromodulation effects in the early ERPs rather than in the late ERPs might be due to enhanced suppression of task- irrelevant stimuli and less effortful discrimination of targets from non-targets during attention task performance.

One more critical methodological issue to be considered in absence of significant TMS effects on Pe in autism might be related to the number of commission errors as this measure depends on the actual number of committed errors (Franken et al., 2007). It is feasible to suggest that the magnitude of the Pe was affected by the reduced number of commission errors in active TMS group. Our prior investigation of ERN/Pe complex in autism (Sokhadze et al., 2010b) also did show Pe differences between ASD and typical children on the similar visual oddball task, but these differences were found only in a form of a significantly prolonged latency of the Pe in ASD group. There is a possibility of a dissociation of ERN and Pe effects since generation of Pe wave might be affected by the absence of feedback about the accuracy of the MR resulting in that lower awareness of error (Hewig et al., 2011).

In general, our findings are in concordance with a recent review of rTMS applications in autism research and treatment (Oberman et al., 2010, 2013). In that review the authors concluded that, though results of published studies are promising suggesting that specific rTMS protocols (Enticott et al., 2010, 2012, 2013; Fecteau et al., 2011) targeting selected regions of cortex may lead to improvement in behavioral deficits in some individuals with ASD, the therapeutic results have been still of preliminary character and additionally, the large-scale, controlled trials necessary to establish the safety and efficacy these neuromodulation protocols have to be conducted (Oberman et al., 2010, 2013).

Some limitations to the study should be taken into account. It is often reported in rTMS studies that effects of magnetic stimulation usually do not wash out in approximately one week. We believe that switching to once per week session regimen, (e.g., Casanova et al., 2012; Sokhadze et al., 2012a) improved our protocol and resulted in better clinical outcome measures. Probably the length of staying in the rTMS treatment rather than intensity is one of the main keys of behavioral and electrocrtical improvements that we observe in our later rTMS trials in ASD (Baruth et al., 2010b, 2011; Sokhadze et al., 2010a, 2012a; Casanova et al., 2012). It should be recognized that the power (90%) and schedule (number of magnetic pulses delivered per each session, 10–20 s break between trains, etc.) of our rTMS is relatively lower than those used by other TMS treatment protocols. However, it must be mentioned that other known TMS protocols were targeting psychopathologies such as treatment-resistant major depression, or neurological disorders such as for instance Parkinson disease in adults. One more limitation of the study is the use a waiting-list group as a control group rather than using a randomized clinical trial (RCT) design with a sham rTMS condition. Even though our group has a custom-made sham Magstim TMS coil and interface enabling blinding of TMS delivery, we considered this study as a preliminary pilot with a WTL group design, and plan to consider progression to a RCT design on the future stages. It is possible to consider as a limitation also the difficulty of proving in non-invasive human brain research that low frequency rTMS is activating primarily double-bouquet inter-neurons. We hope that future neurophysiological studies on animal models would be able to find support for our hypothesis.

In conclusion, the study showed that treatment with "slow" rTMS improved ERP indices of attention to targets, reduced over-reactivity to non-targets, significantly reduced MT errors to target stimuli, and enhanced response-locked potentials reflective of error monitoring and correction (e.g., ERN to commission errors, post-error RT slowing, etc). We also found significant reductions in both repetitive and stereotypic behaviors, reduced repetitive behaviors, hyperactivity and irritability scores according to social and behavioral clinical evaluations post-TMS. We consider that it is possible to conclude that neuromodulation using low frequency, inhibitory rTMS improved executive functioning and behavior in autism. This study provides further support to the statement that TMS can be regarded as a perspective treatment targeting core symptoms of ASD such as executive function deficits.

ACKNOWLEDGMENTS

The study was partially supported by National Institutes of Health Eureka R01 grant MH86784 to Manuel F. Casanova.

REFERENCES

Aman, M. G. (2004). Management of hyperactivity and other acting out problems in patients with autism spectrum disorder. *Semin. Pediatr. Neurol.* 11, 225–228. doi: 10.1016/j.spen.2004.07.006

Aman, M. G., and Singh, N. N. (1994). *Aberrant Behavior Checklist—Community. Supplementary Manual.* East Aurora, NY: Slosson Educational Publications.

American Psychiatric Association. (2000). *Diagnostic and Statistical Manual of Mental Disorders (DSM-IV TR).* 4th Edn. Washington, DC: American Psychiatric Association.

American Psychiatric Association. (2013). *Diagnostic and Statistical Manual of Mental Disorders (DSM-V).* 5th Edn. Washington, DC: American Psychiatric Association.

Arbel, Y., and Donchin, E. (2009). Parsing the componential structure of post-error ERPs: a principal component analysis of ERPs following errors. *Psychophysiology* 46, 1179–1189. doi: 10.1111/j.1469-8986.2009.00857.x

Arbel, Y., and Donchin, E. (2011). When a child errs: the ERN and the Pe complex. *Psychophysiology* 48, 55–63. doi: 10.1111/j.1469-8986.2010.01042.x

Baruth, J., Casanova, M. F., El-Baz, A., Horrell, T., Mathai, G., Sears, L., et al. (2010a). Low-frequency repetitive transcranial magnetic stimulation modulates evoked-gamma frequency oscillations in autism spectrum disorders. *J. Neurother.* 14, 179–194. doi: 10.1080/10874208.2010.501500

Baruth, J., Casanova, M. F., Sears, L., and Sokhadze, E. (2010c). Early-stage visual processing abnormalities in high-functioning autism spectrum disorder (ASD). *Transl. Neurosci.* 1, 177–187. doi: 10.2478/v10134-010-0024-9

Baruth, J., Williams, E., Sokhadze, E., El-Baz, A., Sears, L., and Casanova, M. F. (2011). Repetitive transcranial stimulation (rTMS) improves electroencephalographic and behavioral outcome measures in autism spectrum disorders (ASD). *Autism Sci. Digest.* 1, 52–57.

Baruth, J., Sokhadze, E., El-Baz, A., Mathai, G., Sears, L., and Casanova, M. F. (2010b). "Transcaranial magentic stimulation as a treatment for autism," in *Cutting Edge Therapies for Autism*, eds K. Siri and T. Lyons (New York: Skyhorse Publishing), 388–397.

Belmonte, M. K., and Yurgelun-Todd, D. A. (2003). Functional anatomy of impaired selective attention and compensatory processing in autism. *Brain Res. Cogn. Brain Res.* 17, 651–664. doi: 10.1016/s0926-6410(03)00189-7

Bodfish, J. W., Symons, F. J., and Lewis, M. H. (1999). *Repetitive Behavior Scale.* Morganton, NC: Western Carolina Center Research Reports.

Bodfish, J. W., Symons, F. S., Parker, D. E., and Lewis, M. H. (2000). Varieties of repetitive behavior in autism: comparisons to mental retardation. *J. Autism Dev. Disord.* 30, 237–243. doi: 10.1023/A:1005596502855

Bomba, M. D., and Pang, E. W. (2004). Cortical auditory evoked potentials in autism: a review. *Int. J. Psychophysiol.* 53, 161–169. doi: 10.1016/j.ijpsycho.2004.04.001

Buxhoeveden, D. P., Semendeferi, K., Buckwalter, J., Schenker, N., Switser, R., and Courchesne, E. (2006). Reduced minicolumns in the frontal cortex of patients with autism. *Neuropathol. Appl. Neurobiol.* 32, 483–491. doi: 10.1111/j.1365-2990.2006.00745.x

Carter, C. S., Braver, T. S., Barch, D. M., Botvinick, M. M., Noll, D., and Cohen, J. D. (1998). Anterior cingulate cortex, error detection and the online monitoring of performance. *Science* 280, 747–749. doi: 10.1126/science.280.5364.747

Casanova, M. F. (2005). "Minicolumnar pathology in autism," in *Recent Developments in Autism Research*, ed M. F. Casanova (New York: Nova Biomedical Books), 133–144.

Casanova, M. F. (2007). The neuropathology of autism. *Brain Pathol.* 17, 422–433. doi: 10.1111/j.1750-3639.2007.00100.x

Casanova, M. F., Baruth, J., El-Baz, A., Tasman, A., Sears, L., and Sokhadze, E. (2012). Repetitive transcranial magnetic stimulation (rTMS) modulates event-related potential (ERP) indices of attention in autism. *Transl. Neurosci.* 3, 170–180. doi: 10.2478/s13380-012-0022-0

Casanova, M. F., Buxhoeveden, D. P., and Brown, C. (2002a). Clinical and macroscopic correlates of minicolumnar pathology in autism. *J. Child Neurol.* 17, 692–695. doi: 10.1177/088307380201700908

Casanova, M. F., Buxhoeveden, D. P., Switala, A. E., and Roy, E. (2002b). Minicolumnar pathology in autism. *Neurology* 58, 428–432. doi: 10.1212/wnl.58.3.428

Casanova, M. F., Buxhoeveden, D. P., Switala, A. E., and Roy, E. (2002c). Asperger's syndrome and cortical neuropathology. *J. Child Neurol.* 17, 142–145. doi: 10.1177/088307380201700211

Casanova, M. F., Buxhoeveden, D. P., Switala, A. E., and Roy, E. (2002d). Neuronal density and architecture (Gray Level Index) in the brains of autistic patients. *J. Child Neurol.* 17, 515–521. doi: 10.1177/088307380201700708

Casanova, M. F., Buxhoeveden, D., and Gomez, J. (2003). Disruption in the inhibitory architecture of the cell minicolumn: implications for autism. *Neuroscientist* 9, 496–507. doi: 10.1177/1073858403253552

Casanova, M. F., El-Baz, A. S., Kamat, S. S., Dombroski, B. A., Khalifa, F., Elnakib, A., et al. (2013). Focal cortical displasias in autism spectrum disorders. *Acta Neuropathol. Commun.* 1:67. doi: 10.1186/2051-5960-1-67

Casanova, M. F., El-Baz, A. S., Vanbogaert, E., Narahari, P., and Switala, A. (2010). A topographical study of minicolumnar core width by lamina comparison between autistic subjects and controls: posible minicolumnar disruption due to an anatomical element in-common to multiple laminae. *Brain Pathol.* 20, 451–458. doi: 10.1111/j.1750-3639.2009.00319.x

Casanova, M. F., and Trippe, J. (2006). Regulatory mechanisms of cortical laminar development. *Brain Res. Rev.* 51, 72–84. doi: 10.1016/j.brainresrev.2005.10.002

Casanova, M. F., van Kooten, I., Switala, A. E., van England, H., Heinsen, H., Steinbuch, H. W. M., et al. (2006a). Abnormalities of cortical minicolumnar organization in the prefrontal lobes of autistic patients. *Clin. Neurosci. Res.* 6, 127–133. doi: 10.1016/j.cnr.2006.06.003

Casanova, M. F., van Kooten, I. A., van Engeland, H., Heinsen, H., Steinbursch, H. W. M., Hof, P. R., et al. (2006b). Minicolumnar abnormalities in autism. *Acta Neuropathol.* 112, 287–303. doi: 10.1007/s00401-006-0085-5

Chang, E., and Merzenich, M. M. (2003). Environmental noise retards auditory cortical development. *Science* 300, 498–502. doi: 10.1126/science.1082163

Ciesielski, K. T., Courchesne, E., and Elmasian, R. (1990). Effects of focused attention tasks on event-related potentials in autistic and normal individuals. *Electroencephalogr. Clin. Neurophysiol.* 75, 207–220. doi: 10.1016/0013-4694(90)90174-i

Clark, V. P., Fan, S., and Hillyard, S. A. (1994). Identification of early visual evoked potential generators by retinotopic and topographic analyses. *Hum. Brain Mapp.* 2, 170–187. doi: 10.1002/hbm.460020306

Clemans, Z., Sokhadze, E., and El-Baz, A. S. (2011b). "A custom-made Matlab program for ERP feature detection in psychological and physiological disorders using wavelet," in Presented at Research Louisville (Louisville, KY).

Clemans, Z., Sokhadze, T., and El-Baz, A. (2011a). "Custom program for extraction of event-related potential peaks in attention tasks," in Presented at Research Louisville (Louisville, KY).

Coles, M. G. H., and Rugg, M. D. (1995). "Event-related brain potentials: an introduction," in *Electrophysiology of Mind. Event-Related Brain Potentials and Cognition*, ed M. D. Rugg and M. G. H. Coles (Oxford: Oxford University Press), 1–26.

Courchesne, E., Lincoln, A. J., Yeung-Courchesne, R., Elmasian, R., and Grillon, C. (1989). Pathophysiologic findings in nonretarded autism and receptive developmental disorder. *J. Autism Dev. Disord.* 19, 1–17. doi: 10.1007/bf02212714

Daskalakis, Z. J., Christensen, B. K., Fitzgerald, P. B., and Chen, R. (2002). Transcranial magnetic stimulation: a new investigational and treatment tool in psychiatry. *J. Neuropsychiatry Clin. Neurosci.* 14, 406–415. doi: 10.1176/appi.neuropsych.14.4.406

Davies, P. L., Segalowitz, S. J., and Gavin, W. J. (2004). Development of response-monitoring ERPs in 7- to 25-year-olds. *Dev. Neuropsychol.* 25, 355–376. doi: 10.1207/s15326942dn2503_6

DeFelipe, J. (1999). Chandelier cells and epilepsy. *Brain* 122, 1807–1822. doi: 10.1093/brain/122.10.1807

DeFelipe, J. (2004). Cortical microanatomy and human brain disorders: epilepsy. *Cortex* 40, 232–233. doi: 10.1016/s0010-9452(08)70952-6

Donkers, F. C. L., and van Boxtel, G. J. M. (2004). The N2 in go/no-go tasks reflects conflict monitoring not response inhibition. *Brain Cogn.* 56, 165–176. doi: 10.1016/j.bandc.2004.04.005

Eichele, T., Specht, K., Moosmann, M., Jongsma, M. L., Quiroga, R. Q., Nordby, H., et al. (2005). Assessing the spatiotemporal evolution of neuronal activation with single-trial event-related potentials and functional MRI. *Proc. Natl. Acad. Sci. U S A* 102, 17798–17803. doi: 10.1073/pnas.0505508102

Enriquez-Geppert, S., Konrad, C., Pantev, C., and Huster, R. J. (2010). Conflict and inhibition differentially affect the N200/P300 complex in a combined go/nogo and stop-signal task. *Neuroimage* 51, 877–887. doi: 10.1016/j.neuroimage.2010.02.043

Enticott, P. G., Kennedy, H. A., Rinehart, N. J., Tonge, B. J., Bradshaw, J. L., and Fitzgerald, P. B. (2013). GABAergic activity in autism spectrum disorders: an investigation of cortical inhibition via transcranial magnetic stimulation. *Neuropharmacology* 68, 202–209. doi: 10.1016/j.neuropharm.2012.06.017

Enticott, P. G., Rinehart, N. J., Tonge, B. J., Bradshaw, J. L., and Fitzgerald, P. B. (2010). A preliminary transcranial magnetic stimulation study of cortical inhibition and excitability in high-functioning autism and Asperger disorder. *Dev. Med. Child Neurol.* 52, e179–e183. doi: 10.1111/j.1469-8749.2010.03665.x

Enticott, P. G., Rinehart, N. J., Tonge, B. J., Bradshaw, J. L., and Fitzgerald, P. B. (2012). Repetitive transcranial magnetic stimulation (rTMS) improves movement-related cortical potentials in autism spectrum disorders. *Brain Stimul.* 5, 30–37. doi: 10 1016/j.brs.2011.02.001

Falkenstein, M., Hoormann, J., Christ, S., and Hohnsbein, J. (2000). ERP components on reaction errors and their functional significance: a tutorial. *Biol. Psychol.* 51, 87–107. doi: 10.1016/s0301-0511(99)00031-9

Favorov, O. V., and Kelly, D. G. (1994a). Minicolumnar organization within somatosensory cortical segregates, I: development of afferent connections. *Cereb. Cortex* 4, 408–427. doi: 10.1093/cercor/4.4.408

Favorov, O. V., and Kelly, D. G. (1994b). Minicolumnar organization within somatosensory cortical segregates, II: emergent functional properties. *Cereb. Cortex* 4, 428–442. doi: 10.1093/cercor/4.4.428

Fecteau, S., Agosta, S., Oberman, L., and Pascual-Leone, A. (2011). Brain stimulation over Broca's area differentially modulates naming skills in neurotypical adults and individuals with Asperger's syndrome. *Eur. J. Neurosci.* 34, 158–164. doi: 10.1111/j.1460-9568.2011.07726.x

Fernandez-Duque, D., Baird, J. A., and Posner, M. I. (2000). Executive attention and metacognitive regulation. *Conscious. Cogn.* 9, 288–307. doi: 10.1006/ccog.2000.0447

Fletcher, E. M., Kussmaul, C. L., and Mangun, G. R. (1996). Estimation of interpolation errors in scalp topographic mapping. *Electroctoencephalogr. Clin. Neurophysiol.* 98, 422–434. doi: 10.1016/0013-4694(96)95135-4

Folstein, J. R., van Petten, C., and Rose, S. A. (2008). Novelty and conflict in the categorization of complex stimuli. *Psychophysiology* 45, 467–479. doi: 10.1111/j.1469-8986.2007.00628.x

Franken, I. H., van Strien, J. W., Franzek, E. J., and van de Wetering, B. J. (2007). Error-processing deficits in patients with cocaine dependence. *Biol. Psychol.* 75, 45–51. doi: 10.1016/j.biopsycho.2006.11.003

Friedman, D., Simpson, G. V., and Hamberger, M. (1993). Age-related changes in scalp topography to novel and target stimuli. *Psychophysiology* 30, 383–396. doi: 10.1111/j.1469-8986.1993.tb02060.x

Frye, R. E., Rotenberg, A., Ousley, M., and Pascual-Leone, A. (2008). Transcranial magnetic stimulation in child neurology: current and future direction. *J. Child Neurol.* 23, 79–96. doi: 10.1177/0883073807307972

Gehring, W. J., Goss, B., Coles, M. G. H., Meyer, D. E., and Donchin, E. (1993). A neural system for error detection and compensation. *Psychol. Sci.* 4, 385–390. doi: 10.1111/j.1467-9280.1993.tb00586.x

Gehring, W. J., and Knight, R. T. (2000). Prefrontal-cingulate interactions in action monitoring. *Nat. Neurosci.* 3, 516–520. doi: 10.1038/74899

Gershon, A. A., Dannon, P. N., and Grunhaus, L. (2003). Transcranial magnetic stimulation in the treatment of depression. *Am. J. Psychiatry* 160, 835–845. doi: 10.1176/appi.ajp.160.5.835

Gomes, E., Pedroso, F. S., and Wagner, M. B. (2008). Auditory hypersensitivity in the autistic spectrum disorder. *Pro Fono* 20, 279–284. doi: 10.1590/s0104-56872008000400013

Gomot, M., Giard, M. H., Adrien, J. L., Barthelemy, C., and Bruneau, N. (2002). Hypersensitivity to acoustic change in children with autism: electrophysiological evidence of left frontal cortex dysfunctioning. *Psychophysiology* 39, 577–584. doi: 10.1111/1469-8986.3950577

Gray, J. R., Chabris, C. F., and Braver, T. S. (2003). Neural mechanisms of general fluid intelligence. *Nat. Neurosci.* 6, 316–322. doi: 10.1038/nn1014

Greenberg, B. D. (2007). "Transcranial magnetic stimulation in anxiety disorders," in *Transcranial Magnetic Stimulation in Clinical Psychiatry*, ed M. S. George and R. H. Belmaker (Washington, DC: American Psychiatric Publishing, Inc.), 165–178.

Harris, K. D., and Thiele, A. (2011). Cortical state and attention. *Nat. Rev. Neurosci.* 12, 509–523. doi: 10.1038/nrn3084

Herrmann, C. S., and Knight, R. T. (2001). Mechanisms of human attention: event related potentials and oscillations. *Neurosci. Biobehav. Rev.* 25, 465–476. doi: 10.1016/s0149-7634(01)00027-6

Hewig, J., Coles, M. G. H., Trippe, R. H., Hecht, H., and Miltner, W. H. R. (2011). Dissociation of Pe and ERN/Ne in the conscious recognition of an error. *Psychophysiology* 48, 1390–1396. doi: 10.1111/j.1469-8986.2011.01209.x

Hillyard, S. A., and Annlo-Vento, L. (1998). Event-related brain potentials in the study of visual selective attention. *Proc. Natl. Acad. Sci. U S A* 95, 781–787. doi: 10.1073/pnas.95.3.781

Hoffman, R. E., and Cavus, I. (2002). Slow transcranial magnetic stimulation, long-term depotentiation and brain hyperexcitability disorders. *Am. J. Psychiatry* 159, 1093–1102. doi: 10.1176/appi.ajp.159.7.1093

Huizinga, M., Dolan, C. V., and Van Der Molen, M. W. (2006). Age-related change in executive function: developmental trends and a latent variable analysis. *Neuropsychologia* 44, 2017–2036. doi: 10.1016/j.neuropsychologia.2006.01.010

Hussman, J. P. (2001). Suppressed GABAergic inhibition as a common factor in suspected etiologies of autism. *J. Autism Dev. Disord.* 31, 247–248. doi: 10.1023/A:1010715619091

Jeste, S. S., and Nelson, C. A. 3rd. (2009). Event related potentials in the understanding of autism spectrum disorders: an analytical review. *J. Autism Dev. Disord.* 39, 495–510. doi: 10.1007/s10803-008-0652-9

Kanizsa, G. (1976). Subjective contours. *Sci. Am.* 235, 48–52. doi: 10.1038/scientificamerican0476-48

Kéïta, L., Mottron, L., Dawson, M., and Bertone, A. (2011). Atypical lateral connectivity: a neural basis for altered visuospatial processing in autism. *Biol. Psychiatry* 70, 806–811. doi: 10.1016/j.biopsych.2011.07.031

Kemner, C., van der Gaag, R. J., Verbaten, M., and van Engeland, H. (1999). ERP differences among subtypes of pervasive developmental disorders. *Biol. Psychiatry* 46, 781–789. doi: 10.1016/s0006-3223(99)00003-7

Kemner, C., Verbaten, M. N., Cuperus, J. M., Camfferman, G., and Van Engeland, H. (1994). Visual and somatosensory event-related brain potentials in autistic children and three different control groups. *Electroencephalogr. Clin. Neurophysiol.* 92, 225–237. doi: 10.1016/0168-5597(94)90066-3

Kenemans, J. L., Kok, A., and Smulders, F. T. (1993). Event-related potentials to conjunctions of spatial frequency and orientation as a function of stimulus parameters and response requirements. *Electroencephalogr. Clin. Neurophysiol.* 88, 51–63. doi: 10.1016/0168-5597(93)90028-n

Le Couteur, A., Lord, C., and Rutter, M. (2003). *The Autism Diagnostic Interview—Revised (ADI-R).* Los Angeles, CA: Western Psychological Services.

Liotti, M., Pliszka, S., Perez, R., Kothmann, D., and Woldorff, M. (2005). Abnormal brain activity related to performance monitoring and error detection in children with ADHD. *Cortex* 41, 377–388. doi: 10.1016/s0010-9452(08)70274-0

Loo, C. K., and Mitchell, P. B. (2005). A review of the efficacy of transcranial magnetic stimulation (TMS) treatment for depression and current and future strategies to optimize efficacy. *J. Affect. Disord.* 88, 255–267. doi: 10.1016/j.jad.2005.08.001

Luck, S. J., Heinze, H. J., Mangun, G. R., and Hillyard, S. A. (1990). Visual event-related potentials index focused attention within bilateral stimulus arrays. ii. Functional dissociation of P1 and N1 components. *Electroencephalogr. Clin. Neurophysiol.* 75, 528–542. doi: 10.1016/0013-4694(90)90139-b

Luu, P., Tucker, D. M., Englander, R., Lockfeld, A., Lutsep, H., and Oken, B. (2001). Localizing acute stroke-related EEC changes: assessing the effects of spatial undersampling. *J. Clin. Neurophysiol.* 18, 302–317. doi: 10.1097/00004691-200107000-00002

Maeda, F., Keenan, J. P., Tormos, J. M., Topka, H., and Pascual-Leone, A. (2000). Modulation of corticospinal excitability by repetitive transcranial magnetic stimulation. *Clin. Neurophysiol.* 111, 800–805. doi: 10.1016/s1388-2457(99)00323-5

Marín-Padilla, M. (1998). Cajal-Retzius cells and the development of the neocortex. *Trends Neurosci.* 21, 64–71. doi: 10.1016/s0166-2236(97)01164-8

Marin-Padilla, M. (2010). *The Human Brain: Prenatal Development and Structure.* New York: Springer.

Mars, R. B., Coles, M. G. H., Grol, M. J., Holroyd, C. B., Nieuwenhuis, S., Hulstijn, W., et al. (2005). Neural dynamics of error processing in medial frontal cortex. *Neuroimage* 28, 1007–1013. doi: 10.1016/j.neuroimage.2005.06.041

Matzel, L. D., and Kolata, S. (2010). Selective attention, working memory and animal intelligence. *Neurosci. Biobehav. Rev.* 34, 23–30. doi: 10.1016/j.neubiorev.2009.07.002

Mesulam, M. M. (2000). "Behavioral neuroanatomy: large-networks, association cortex, frontal syndromes, the limbic system and hemispheric specializations," in *Principles of Behavioral and Cognitive Neurology*, ed M. M. Mesulam 2nd Edn. (New York: Oxford University Press), 1–120.

Mountcastle, V. B. (2003). Introduction. Computation in cortical columns. *Cereb. Cortex* 13, 2–4.

Murphy, K. R., and Myors, B. (2004). *Statistical Power Analysis. A Simple and General Model for Traditional and Modern Hypothesis Tests.* 2nd Edn. Mahwah, NJ: Lawrence Erlbaum Associates.

Näätänen, R., Gaillard, A. W. K., and Mäntysalo, S. (1978). Early selective attention effect on evoked potential reinterpreted. *Acta Psychol.(Amst)* 42, 313–329. doi: 10.1016/0001-6918(78)90006-9

Näätänen, R., Schröge, E., Karakas, S., Tervaniemi, M., and Paavilainen, P. (1993). Development of a memory trace for a complex sound in the human brain. *Neuroreport* 4, 503–506. doi: 10.1097/00001756-199305000-00010

Nieuwenhuis, S., Ridderinkhof, K. R., Blom, J., Band, G. P., and Kok, A. (2001). Error-related brain potentials are differentially related to awareness of response errors: evidence from an antisaccade task. *Psychophysiology* 38, 752–760. doi: 10.1111/1469-8986.3850752

Oberman, L., Ifert-Miller, F., Najib, U., Bashir, S., Woollacott, I., Gonzalez-Heydrich, J., et al. (2010). Transcranial magnetic stimulation provides means to assess cortical plasticity and excitability in humans with fragile X syndrome and autism spectrum disorder. *Front. Sys. Neurosci.* 2:26. doi: 10.3389/fnsyn.2010.00026

Oberman, L., Rotenberg, A., and Pascual-Leone, A. (2013). Use of transcranial magnetic stimulation in autism spectrum disorders. *J. Autism Dev. Disord.* doi: 10.1007/s10803-013-1960-2. [Epub ahead of print].

Oblak, A. L., Gibbs, T. T., and Blatt, G. L. (2010). Decreased GABA(B) receptors in the cingulate cortex and fusiform gyrus in autism. *J. Neurochem.* 114, 1414–1423. doi: 10.1111/j.1471-4159.2010.06858.x

Opris, I., and Casanova, M. F. (2014). Prefrontal cortical minicolumn: from executive control to disrupted cognitive processing. *Brain* 137, 1863–1875. doi: 10.1093/brain/awt359

Opris, I., Santos, L., Gerhardt, G. A., Song, D., Berger, T. W., Hampson, R. E., et al. (2013). Prefrontal cortical microcircuits bind perception to executive control. *Sci. Rep.* 3:2285. doi: 10.1038/srep02285

Overbeek, T. J. M., Nieuwenhuis, S., and Ridderinkhof, K. R. (2005). Dissociable components of error processing. *J. Psychophysiol.* 19, 319–329. doi: 10.1027/0269-8803.19.4.319

Pascual-Leone, A., Davey, N. J., Rothwell, J., Wasserman, E. M., and Puri, B. K. (2002). *Handbook of Transcranial Magnetic Stimulation.* New York: Oxford University Press.

Pascual-Leone, A., Valls-Sole, J., Wasserman, E. M., and Hallett, M. (1994). Responses to rapid-rate transcranial magnetic stimulation of the human cortex. *Brain* 117, 847–858. doi: 10.1093/brain/117.4.847

Pascual-Leone, A., Walsh, V., and Rothwell, J. (2000). Transcranial magnetic stimulation in cognitive neuroscience—virtual lesion, chronometry and functional connectivity. *Curr. Opin. Neurobiol.* 10, 232–237. doi: 10.1016/s0959-4388(00)00081-7

Perrin, E., Pernier, J., Bertrand, O., Giard, M., and Echallier, J. F. (1987). Mapping of scalp potentials by surface spline interpolation. *Electroencephalogr. Clin. Neurophysiol.* 66, 75–81. doi: 10.1016/0013-4694(87)90141-6

Picton, T. W. (1992). The P300 wave of the human event-related potential. *J. Clin. Neurophysiol.* 9, 456–479. doi: 10.1097/00004691-199210000-00002

Pinto, L., Goard, M. J., Estandian, D., Xu, M., Kwan, A. C., Lee, S. H., et al. (2013). Fast modulation of visual perception by basal forebrain cholinergic neurons. *Nat. Neurosci.* 16, 1857–1863. doi: 10.1038/nn.3552

Plaisted, K., Saksida, L., Alcantara, J., and Weisblatt, E. (2003). Towards an understanding of the mechanisms of weak central coherence effects: experiments in visual configural learning and auditory perception. *Philos. Trans. R. Soc. Lond. B Biol. Sci.* 358, 375–386. doi: 10.1098/rstb.2002.1211

Polich, J. (2003). "Theoretical overview of P3a and P3b," in *Detection of Change. Event-Related Potential and fMRI Findings*, ed J. Polich (Boston: Kluwer Academic Press), 83–98.

Polich, J. (2007). Updating P300: an integrative theory of P3a and P3b. *J. Clin. Neurophysiol.* 118, 2128–2148. doi: 10.1016/j.clinph.2007.04.019

Potts, G. F., Dien, J., Harty-Speiser, A., McDougl, L. M., and Tucker, D. M. (1998). Dense sensor array topography of the event-related potential to task-relevant auditory stimuli. *Electroencephalogr. Clin. Neurophysiol.* 106, 444–456. doi: 10.1016/s0013-4694(97)00160-0

Potts, G. F., Liotti, M., Tucker, D. M., and Posner, M. I. (1996). Frontal and inferior temporal cortical activity in visual target detection: evidence from high spatially sampled event-related potentials. *Brain Topogr.* 9, 3–14. doi: 10.1007/bf01191637

Potts, G. F., Patel, S. H., and Azzam, P. N. (2004). Impact of instructed relevance on the visual ERP. *Int. J. Psychophysiol.* 52, 197–209. doi: 10.1016/j.ijpsycho.2003.10.005

Potts, G. F., Wood, S. M., Kothmann, D., and Martin, L. E. (2008). Parallel perceptual enhancement and hierarchic relevance evaluation in an audio-visual conjunction task. *Brain Res.* 1236, 126–139. doi: 10.1016/j.brainres.2008.07.104

Pritchard, W. S. (1981). Psychophysiology of P300. *Psychol. Bull.* 89, 506–540. doi: 10.1037/0033-2909.89.3.506

Puts, N. A., Wodka, E. L., Tommerdahl, M., Mostofsky, S. H., and Edden, R. A. (2014). Impaired tactile processing in children with autism spectrum disorder. *J. Neurophysiol.* 111, 1803–1811. doi: 10.1152/jn.00890.2013

Renart, A., de la Rocha, J., Bartho, P., Hollender, L., Parga, N., Reyes, A., et al. (2010). The asynchronous state in cortical circuits. *Science* 327, 587–590. doi: 10.1126/science.1179850

Ridderinkhof, K. R., Ullsperger, M., Crone, E. A., and Nieuwenhuis, S. (2004). The role of the medial frontal cortex in cognitive control. *Science* 306, 443–447. doi: 10.1126/science.1100301

Rubenstein, J. L. R., and Merzenich, M. M. (2003). Model of autism: increased ratio of excitation/inhibition in key neural systems. *Genes Brain Behav.* 2, 255–267. doi: 10.1034/j.1601-183x.2003.00037.x

Schutter, D. J. (2009). Antidepressant efficacy of high-frequency transcranial magnetic stimulation over the left dorsolateral prefrontal cortex in double-blind sham-controlled designs: a meta-analysis. *Psychol. Med.* 39, 65–75. doi: 10.1017/S0033291708003462

Sokhadze, E. M., Baruth, J., Tasman, A., and Casanova, M. F. (2013a). "Event-related potential studies of cognitive processing abnormalities in autism," in *Imaging Methods in Autism*, eds M. F. Casanova, A. El-Baz and J. S. Suri (New York: Springer), 61–86.

Sokhadze, E. M., Casanova, M. F., and Baruth, J. (2013b). "Transcranial magnetic stimulation in autism spectrum disorders," in *Transcranial Magnetic Stimulation: Methods, Clinical Uses and Effect on the Brain*, ed L. Alba-Ferrara (New York: NOVA Publishers), 219–231.

Sokhadze, E., Baruth, J. M., Sears, L., Sokhadze, G. E., El-Baz, A. S., and Casanova, M. F. (2012a). Prefrontal neuromodulation using rTMS improves error monitoring and correction functions in autism. *Appl. Psychophysiol. Biofeedback* 37, 91–102. doi: 10.1007/s10484-012-9182-5

Sokhadze, E., Baruth, J. M., Sears, L., Sokhadze, G. E., El-Baz, A. S., Williams, E. L., et al. (2012b). Event-related potential study of attention regulation during illusory figure categorization task in ADHD, autism spectrum disorder and typical children. *J. Neurother.* 16, 12–31. doi: 10.1080/10874208.2012.650119

Sokhadze, E., Baruth, J., El-Baz, A., Horrell, T., Sokhadze, G., Carroll, T., et al. (2010b). Impaired error monitoring and correction function in autism. *J. Neurother.* 14, 79–95. doi: 10.1080/10874201003771561

Sokhadze, E., Baruth, J., Tasman, A., Mansoor, M., Ramaswamy, R., Sears, L., et al. (2010a). Low-frequency repetitive transcranial magnetic stimulation (rTMS) affects event-related potential measures of novelty processing in autism. *Appl. Psychophysiol. Biofeedback* 35, 147–161. doi: 10.1007/s10484-009-9121-2

Sokhadze, E., Baruth, J., Tasman, A., Sears, L., Mathai, G., El-Baz, A., et al. (2009a). Event-related potential study of novelty processing abnormalities in autism. *Appl. Psychophysiol. Biofeedback* 34, 37–51. doi: 10.1007/s10484-009-9074-5

Sokhadze, E., El-Baz, A., Baruth, J., Mathai, G., Sears, L., and Casanova, M. F. (2009b). Effect of a low-frequency repetitive transcranial magnetic stimulation (rTMS) on induced gamma frequency oscillations and event-related potentials during processing of illusory figures in autism spectrum disorders. *J. Autism Dev. Disord.* 39, 619–634. doi: 10.1007/s10803-008-0662-7

Srinivasan, R., Tucker, D. M., and Murias, M. (1998). Estimating the spatial Nyquist of the human EEG. *Behav. Res. Meth. Instrum. Comput.* 30, 8–19. doi: 10.3758/bf03209412

Townsend, J., Westerfield, M., Leaver, E., Makeig, S., Jung, T., Pierce, K., et al. (2001). Event-related brain response abnormalities in autism: evidence for impaired cerebello-frontal spatial attention networks. *Brain Res. Cogn. Brain Res.* 11, 127–145. doi: 10.1016/s0926-6410(00)00072-0

Tuchman, R. F., and Rapin, I. (1997). Regression in pervasive developmental disorders: seizures and epileptiform electroencephalogram correlates. *Pediatrics* 99, 560–566. doi: 10.1542/peds.99.4.560

Van Veen, V., and Carter, C. S. (2002). The timing of action-monitoring process in the anterior cingulate cortex. *J. Cogn. Neurosci.* 14, 593–602. doi: 10.1162/08989290260045837

Vlamings, P. H., Jonkman, L. M., Hoeksma, M. R., van Engeland, H., and Kemner, C. (2008). Reduced error monitoring in children with autism spectrum disorder: an ERP study. *Eur. J. Neurosci.* 28, 399–406. doi: 10.1111/j.1460-9568.2008.06336.x

Wagner, T., Rushmore, J., Eden, U., and Valero-Cabre, A. (2009). Biophysical foundations underlying TMS: setting the stage for an effective use of neurostimulation in the cognitive neurosciences. *Cortex* 45, 1025–1034. doi: 10.1016/j.cortex.2008.10.002

Wassermann, E. M., and Lisanby, S. H. (2001). Therapeutic application of repetitive transcranial magnetic stimulation: a review. *Clin. Neurophysiol.* 112, 1367–1377. doi: 10.1016/s1388-2457(01)00585-5

Wassermann, E. M., and Zimmermann, T. (2012). Transcranial magnetic stimulation: therapeutic promises and scientific gaps. *Pharmacol. Ther.* 133, 98–107. doi: 10.1016/j.pharmthera.2011.09.003

Wechsler, D. (1999). *Wechsler Abbreviated Scale of Intelligence.* San Antonio, TX: Harcourt Assessment, Inc.

Wechsler, D. (2003). *Wechsler Intelligence Scale for Children.* 4th Edn. San Antonio, TX: Harcourt Assessment, Inc.

West, R. (2003). Neural correlates of cognitive control and conflict detection in the stroop and digit-location tasks. *Neuropsychologia* 41, 1122–1135. doi: 10.1016/s0028-3932(02)00297-x

West, R., Bowry, R., and McConville, C. (2004). Sensitivity of medial frontal cortex to response and nonresponse conflict. *Psychophysiology* 41, 739–748. doi: 10.1111/j.1469-8986.2004.00205.x

Yamazaki, T., Kamijo, K., Kenmochi, A., Fukuzumi, S., Kiyuna, T., and Kuroiwa, Y. (2000). Multiple equivalent current dipole source localization of visual event-related potentials during oddball paradigm with motor response. *Brain Topogr.* 12, 159–175. doi: 10.1023/A:1023467806268

Yeung, N., and Cohen, J. D. (2006). The impact of cognitive deficits on conflict monitoring. Predictable dissociations between the error-related negativity and N2. *Psychol. Sci.* 17, 164–171. doi: 10.1111/j.1467-9280.2006.01680.x

Zhang, J. S., Wang, Y., Cai, R. G., and Yan, C. H. (2009). The brain regulation mechanism of error monitoring in impulsive children with ADHD–an analysis of error related potentials. *Neurosci. Lett.* 460, 11–15. doi: 10.1016/j.neulet.2009.05.027

11

Pharmacological enhancement of memory or cognition in normal subjects

Gary Lynch[1,2]*, Conor D. Cox[2] and Christine M. Gall[2]

[1] *Department of Psychiatry and Human Behavior, University of California, Irvine, CA, USA*
[2] *Department of Anatomy and Neurobiology, University of California, Irvine, CA, USA*

Edited by:
Mikhail Lebedev, Duke University, USA

Reviewed by:
Ioan Opris, Wake Forest University, USA
Rafael Roesler, Federal University of Rio Grande do Sul, Brazil
Sam Deadwyler, Wake Forest University Health Sciences, USA
Maryam Farahmandfar, Tehran University of Medical Sciences, Iran

***Correspondence:**
Gary Lynch, Department of Psychiatry and Human Behavior, Gillespie Neuroscience Research Facility, University of California, 837 Health Science Road, Irvine, CA, 92697-1275, USA
e-mail: glynch@uci.edu

The possibility of expanding memory or cognitive capabilities above the levels in high functioning individuals is a topic of intense discussion among scientists and in society at large. The majority of animal studies use behavioral endpoint measures; this has produced valuable information but limited predictability for human outcomes. Accordingly, several groups are pursuing a complementary strategy with treatments targeting synaptic events associated with memory encoding or forebrain network operations. Transcription and translation figure prominently in substrate work directed at enhancement. Notably, the question of why new proteins would be needed for a now-forming memory given that learning-driven synthesis presumably occurred throughout the immediate past has been largely ignored. Despite this conceptual problem, and some controversy, recent studies have reinvigorated the idea that selective gene manipulation is a plausible route to enhancement. Efforts to improve memory by facilitating synaptic encoding of information have also progressed, in part due of breakthroughs on mechanisms that stabilize learning-related, long-term potentiation (LTP). These advances point to a reductionistic hypothesis for a diversity of experimental results on enhancement, and identify under-explored possibilities. Cognitive enhancement remains an elusive goal, in part due to the difficulty of defining the target. The popular view of cognition as a collection of definable computations seems to miss the fluid, integrative process experienced by high functioning individuals. The neurobiological approach obviates these psychological issues to directly test the consequences of improving throughput in networks underlying higher order behaviors. The few relevant studies testing drugs that selectively promote excitatory transmission indicate that it is possible to expand cortical networks engaged by complex tasks and that this is accompanied by capabilities not found in normal animals.

Keywords: cognitive enhancement, learning, long term potentiation, ampakine, synaptic plasticity, BDNF, F-actin, positive AMPA receptor modulators

INTRODUCTION

The present review concerns three topics, two of which involve terms—enhancement and cognition—that are not sharply defined. Usage of the former seems straightforward when applied to memory, although it is often unclear whether accelerated acquisition or an increase in encoding strength is intended. But applied to cognition, claims for enhancement face the great problem of how to quantify something for which there is no consensus measurement system. The difficulty can be reduced by focusing on cognitive activities of a type that can be described in computational terms. This, however, raises questions about the extent to which the sampled process is representative, or a major component, of cognition as the term is typically used. In response, it could reasonably be argued that cognition is a collection of semi-independent operations (e.g., categorization, value assignment) (Sugrue et al., 2005; Tsunada and Sawaguchi, 2012) but this seems unsatisfactory because the phenomenon is experienced as being, if not unitary, then at least strongly coherent. Electrophysiological and brain imaging results showing coordinated activity across broad stretches of neocortex provide some support for the idea of a system that, while capable of periodically focusing on specific tasks, usually works by integrating a vast amount of disparate material into a product accessible to consciousness. A true cognitive enhancer might therefore take the form of a treatment that increases the speed or capacity of this assembly process.

Memory enhancement, as suggested, appears to be a much more tractable problem. Retention is easily measured as is the amount of training needed to produce a given score in a test subsequent to learning. But a curious problem emerges here: few of the many pharmacological agents that produce robust enhancement of memory in animals are found to have positive effects in humans. This observation has become the subject of intense public discussion, perhaps with growing skepticism about the utility of animal studies on memory enhancement. Some neuroscientists have argued that the "failure to predict" problem reflects the widespread use of paradigms that have little relevance to human learning. These workers have devised ingenious protocols that can be used in rodents and with minor modifications in humans (e.g., Bari et al., 2008; Demeter et al., 2008; Eichenbaum and Robitsek, 2009; Zeeb et al., 2009; Demeter and Sarter, 2013). There is every reason to assume that these efforts will ultimately narrow the gap in cross-species comparisons. But there is a more fundamental issue from comparative biology that could underlie the failure-to-predict problem: humans are enormously encephalized animals and rodents aren't (neocortex makes up at least 77% of brain volume in human and just 31% in rat; Stephan et al., 1981; Swanson, 1995). Encephalization is hypothesized to result in a shift of functions from lower brain to cortex; from this perspective, humans may be using networks of a very different kind than those employed by rodents to solve similar problems.

An alternative to behaviorally based approaches to developing enhancers would be to focus on the neurobiological substrates of memory and cognition. This seems feasible in the case of memory because of the tremendous progress that has been made in identifying synaptic mechanisms that encode information. There is no good reason to think that these processes differ significantly between mammalian species and indeed comparative studies suggest that certain essential elements are evolutionarily ancient (Crystal and Glanzman, 2013). It follows from this that treatments acting on memory substrates in rodents are likely to have similar actions in human brain. Cognition again represents a much more challenging problem. However, the universally held assumption that cognitive operations arise from the transient formation of telencephalic networks points to a relatively simple idea for enhancement. Communication within and between cortical regions is mediated by glutamatergic transmission; if so, then agents that augment the release of glutamate, or the post-synaptic response to it, should facilitate the formation of cognition's substrates.

The following sections consider attempts to develop enhancers via actions on (i) different aspects of the complex machinery underlying learning-related synaptic modifications, or (ii) communication within and between cortical networks.

MEMORY ENHANCEMENT

Most research on memory enhancement deals with psychological events that precede the actual encoding of information. There is for example a very large literature describing attempts, typically using chemical agents, to increase the speed of learning by modulating arousal and attention (Lynch et al., 2011). It has become common to refer to resultant improvements as cognitive enhancement, presumably because key elements of cognition are being manipulated, but there are reasons to question this assumption (see below). There is a smaller, but rapidly growing, body of work directed at the machinery responsible for converting patterns of afferent activity into the long lasting increases in synaptic strength assumed to encode specific information. This section evaluates the latter material.

GENE EXPRESSION AND PROTEIN SYNTHESIS

Work in this area begins with the hypothesis that learning triggers the transcription or local translation of proteins that serve to consolidate the newly acquired memories, something that can take anywhere from many minutes to hours. Compounds that facilitate production of the pertinent RNAs or proteins could accordingly increase the likelihood that recent learning will lead to stable memory, and there are many reports of such effects (Guzowski et al., 2001; Plath et al., 2006; Katche et al., 2010, 2012). However, the basic idea that new protein synthesis is critical to memory formation has been controversial since its introduction more than 50 years ago (Abraham and Williams, 2008; Gold, 2008). Much of the dispute revolves around the necessary prediction that protein synthesis inhibitors will selectively block recently acquired memory; most papers report this result but others do not, or argue that observed disruptions to encoding are due to factors unrelated to synthesis (Routtenberg, 2008; Gold and Wrenn, 2012).

Beyond this, the protein synthesis argument faces certain conceptual problems. Learning is a continuous process in humans, and likely other mammals, with new encoding occurring many times a minute, as is evident with episodic memory. People recognize or recall a remarkable number of serial events when queried after a 90 min movie. Unless we make the very unlikely assumption that each item of information is encoded on a different neuron, it is difficult to see why, after hours of producing proteins needed for consolidation, a given cell would need further synthesis to stabilize a now forming memory. Along this line, it has been argued that animals exposed to an enriched environment which would entail constitutively elevated basal activity, and thus activity-driven protein synthesis, may not require additional synthesis to support LTP (Abraham and Williams, 2008) and the related encoding of hippocampus-dependent memories. There is, however, a special case in which transcription and/or broadly distributed translation could be required to securely encode a specific memory; namely, a circumstance in which continuous learning of similar material does *not* precede the new instance. Under these conditions, consolidation could depend upon proteins generated by the isolated learning episode. Note that this scenario loosely describes the great majority of animal studies testing for the contributions of protein synthesis. Certain of these arguments make relatively straightforward, readily tested predictions. For example, animals with a well-developed learning set could be given protein synthesis inhibitors after learning a single problem with or without having dealt with many such problems in the preceding hours. Such a paradigm can be achieved for rats using two-odor discriminations. If continual learning obviates the need for problem-specific synthesis, then the blockers should have no effect in a group given many trials prior to being introduced to the new test items.

There is a variant of the translation hypothesis that addresses the problem of why prior synthesis doesn't provide a sufficient supply of proteins for current learning. This involves the ample evidence for dendritic (local) translation from already in place mRNAs. One could posit a set of conditions in which new synthesis, even after recent experience, needs to occur post-acquisition for transfer into long-term storage; e.g., (1) translation occurs within very small dendritic compartments; (2) such active regions are only found in the immediate vicinity of recently modified synapses; and (3) newly formed proteins do not diffuse to any great degree. These circumstances would reduce the probability that proteins from earlier learning would be present at the large majority of current sites. But "synaptic tagging" experiments, conducted for instances where LTP in hippocampal slices is blocked by protein synthesis inhibitors, describe results that are not consistent with these postulates. Specifically, LTP induction at one input protects subsequently induced potentiation at a second input to the same region from the effects of the inhibitor (Frey and Morris, 1997; Shires et al., 2012). Given the small number of synapses that generate EPSPs of conventional amplitudes, it is extremely likely that connections from the two inputs are, for the most part, located on different dendritic segments. It follows then that proteins from the first episode must have been synthesized, or traveled, throughout much of the dendritic arborization, a point that is reinforced by evidence for tagging in the apical dendrites after stimulation of basal afferents (Alarcon et al., 2006). It will be noted that these findings align with the broad idea that continual learning maintains relevant proteins at levels sufficient for LTP-related plasticity, obviating the need for synthesis after individual learning events.

The above discussion concerns interpretative issues rather than the likelihood of achieving enhancement using the transcription / translation strategy. It may well be the case that increasing within-cell levels of proteins that support consolidation reduces the requirements for encoding persistent memories and/or increases their stability. Signaling from synapses to the nucleus or to local protein synthesis machinery involves many steps and so is likely to be a variable and somewhat uncertain process. It would not be surprising, then, if the ongoing production of memory-related elements operates at a less than optimal rate even in high performing, normal subjects. In line with this, there are multiple demonstrations that treatment with compounds that inhibit particular histone deacetylases, leading to increased transcription of select gene families, can markedly enhance memory after single training sessions (Stefanko et al., 2009; McQuown et al., 2011). Also of interest are the numerous studies showing that selective phosphodiesterase-4 inhibitors have potent enhancing effects on memory. Inhibitors of this class (e.g., Rolipram), drive the protein kinase A—CREB transcription pathway implicated in learning in a broad array of animals (including invertebrates), and so is argued to be a very ancient, evolutionarily conserved memory substrate (Tully et al., 2003; Normann and Berger, 2008). Evidence that the same results obtain after extensive experience with similar problems in the recent past, and presumably a great deal of learning-driven transcription, would constitute support for there being less than optimal production of proteins needed for encoding under normal circumstances. This would certainly encourage the idea that enhanced protein synthesis is a viable route to augmented memory.

SYNAPTIC PLASTICITY AND MEMORY ENHANCEMENT

Most mechanism-based efforts directed at improving memory have focused on synaptic plasticity and in particular the long term potentiation (LTP) effect. Researchers since the late 19th century have argued that the enormous capacity of memory is best explained by assuming that physical encoding of new information occurs at small numbers of connections between neurons. The discovery of LTP demonstrated that individual synapses in the cortical telencephalon do in fact possess the properties expected for a memory substrate (Bliss and Collingridge, 1993; Lynch, 1998, 2004b; Morris, 2003). The increase in transmission strength (magnitude of EPSCs) develops quickly, persists for a remarkable period (weeks at least) (Staubli and Lynch, 1987; Abraham, 2003), and does not disturb already potentiated contacts as likely required for a high capacity memory system. A very large body of experimental work has confirmed the tight connection between LTP and diverse instances of memory (e.g., Roman et al., 1987; Rioult-Pedotti et al., 2000; Whitlock et al., 2006). Moreover, LTP is intimately related to the theta rhythm, an oscillation long associated with learning (Buzsaki, 2005; Vertes, 2005; Snider et al., 2013); i.e., five brief (30 ms) bursts of high frequency stimulation pulses (a pattern that mimics "theta bursting" during learning) prove to be near optimal for inducing extremely stable LTP but only when separated by the period of the theta wave (Larson et al., 1986; Capocchi et al., 1992). The reasons for this have been identified (**Figure 1**).

These observations suggest the possibility of enhancing learning with drugs that promote theta activity and correlated bursts of high frequency discharges. Agents such as physostigmine, that facilitate central cholinergic transmission, promote the theta rhythm (Olpe et al., 1987; Hasselmo, 2006) and are reported to improve learning scores in certain experimental situations. Notably, drugs of this type are among the few treatments approved for Alzheimer's Disease (Clarke and Francis, 2005; Noetzli and Eap, 2013). However, cholinergic systems perform varied functions in brain, some of which are homeostatic in nature. This likely explains why drugs targeting cholinergic mechanisms have not gained widespread acceptance as plausible enhancers. Another approach based on theta activity involves the large hyperpolarizing potentials triggered within target neurons by the short train of theta bursts used to induce LTP. These after-hyperpolarizing potentials (AHPs), set in motion by cell discharges, persist throughout the duration of the theta train and serve to counteract the depolarization needed to unblock the voltage dependent, synaptic NMDA receptors. Influx of calcium through these receptors, followed by release of the cation from intracellular stores, triggers the chain of events leading to potentiation (**Figure 1**). AHPs are mediated by a set of voltage- and calcium-sensitive potassium channels, prominent among which is the SK3 channel (Hosseini et al., 2001). The bee toxin apamin blocks this channel with some selectivity and, as predicted, augments post-synaptic responses to theta burst trains; this results in a striking increase in the magnitude of LTP (Kramar et al., 2004). While a number of studies have found substantial improvements in rodent learning with apamin treatment (Ikonen and Riekkinen, 1999; Brennan et al., 2008; Vick et al., 2010), this is not a likely enhancer because of toxicology issues. But given increasing interest in applications of channel blockers for diverse clinical problems, the apamin results suggest an intriguing mechanistic target for the development of enhancers. It is of note in this regard that Brain Derived Neurotrophic Factor (BDNF), which appears to be released from terminals by theta bursts (Balkowiec and Katz, 2000; Chen et al., 2010b), also reduces AHPs at least in rats (Kramar et al., 2004). Elevating endogenous levels of this neurotrophin, which can be achieved by pharmacological manipulations described later, thus provides another avenue for enhancement.

Identification of the initial triggers for LTP, as schematized in **Figure 1**, pointed to NMDA receptor-mediated calcium influxes as a logical target for enhancement. The existence of multiple

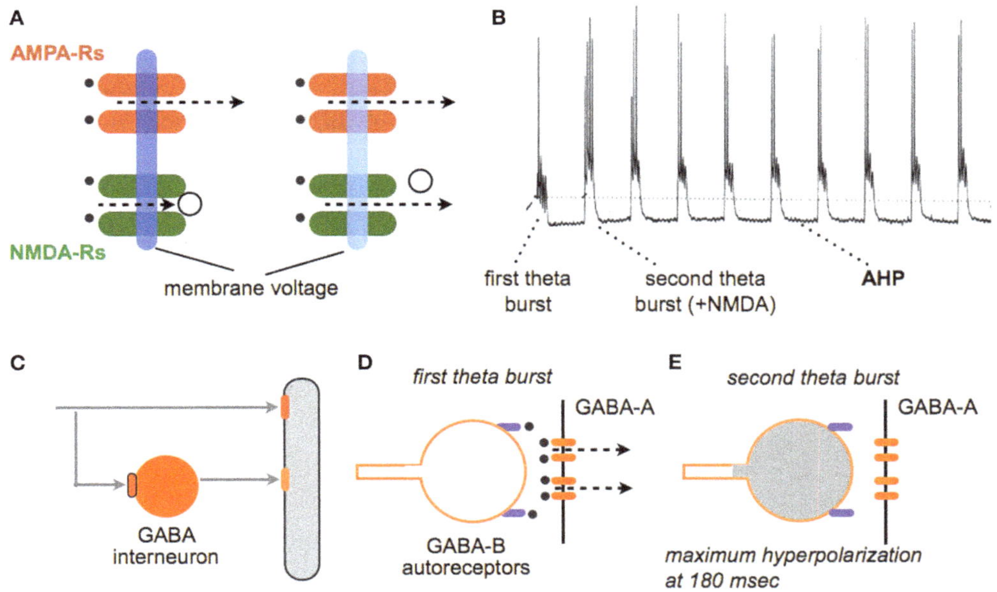

FIGURE 1 | Why theta burst stimulation (TBS) is so effective at inducing LTP. TBS (Larson et al., 1986) mimics a firing pattern found in cortical neurons during learning (Otto et al., 1991) and elicits a robust, non-decremental LTP that persists for weeks (at least). **(A)** (left side). A single stimulation pulse releases glutamate (black dots) and a partial membrane depolarization via current flux through AMPA receptors (dotted line). NMDA receptors do not open because of voltage dependent block of the ion channel (open circle). (right side) Trains of high frequency stimulation cause a greater depolarization (light blue) that removes the channel block and thereby allows current flow through calcium permeant NMDA receptors. Calcium is the initial trigger for LTP. **(B)** Intracellular recording shows that the first theta burst (four pulses at 100 Hz) in a train causes a relatively modest depolarization accompanied by a single spike; NMDA receptors make a very small contribution to this response. A second burst administered after a delay corresponding to the period of the theta wave produces a more profound depolarization with multiple spikes; this burst response contains a large NMDA receptor mediated component. Note that each theta burst in the train is followed by a large after-hyperpolarization (AHP). The AHP, which is largely mediated by calcium and voltage dependent potassium channels, tends to counteract the depolarization produced by the burst, thus capping the magnitude of NMDA receptor responses. **(C–E)** How the second and subsequent bursts generate large depolarization and unblock NMDA receptors. **(C)** A glutamatergic axon innervates a pyramidal cell dendrite (gray) and a feedforward, GABAergic interneuron (orange); note that *both* contacts use AMPA receptors (red). **(D)** A first theta burst triggers GABA release from the interneuron onto the pyramidal neuron thereby producing a di-synaptic (slightly delayed) IPSC via post-synaptic GABA-A receptors (orange ellipses); this shunts the EPSCs produced at neighboring glutamatergic synapses. The released GABA also binds to pre-synaptic, metabotrophic GABA-B auto-receptors on the releasing interneuron terminal (purple). **(E)** The auto-receptors hyperpolarize the GABAergic terminal and block release, an effect that reaches its maximum at the period of the theta wave. A theta burst arriving at this time point generates an excitatory response that is only weakly counteracted by the opening of post-synaptic GABA-A receptors (see **B**).

modulatory sites (e.g., for glycine and polyamine) on the receptors suggested a plausible route for building positive allosteric drugs (Monaghan et al., 2012). Most of this effort has been directed toward treatments for neuropathology and psychiatric disorders, most notably schizophrenia and depression (Labrie and Roder, 2010; Dang et al., 2014), rather than memory enhancement. Perhaps the most widely studied agent of this type is D-cycloserine, a compound that targets the glycine binding pocket on the receptor and facilitates channel opening (Sheinin et al., 2001; Dravid et al., 2010). It has been known for some time that the site is important for induction of LTP (Oliver et al., 1990) and, as expected from this, D-cycloserine enhances various forms of memory in animals (Flood et al., 1992; Baxter et al., 1994; Tsai et al., 1999; Normann and Berger, 2008; Peters and De Vries, 2013). There is also evidence that the endogenous neurosteroid pregnenolone sulfate (Wu et al., 1991), and other steroid-like substances (Madau et al., 2009), promote the opening of NMDA receptors and facilitate both LTP and memory. Also of note, recent work led to discovery of a naturally occurring cholesterol metabolite that facilitates NMDA receptor currents through a novel oxysterol modulatory site and markedly increases the magnitude of LTP (Paul et al., 2013). The development of positive NMDA receptor modulators is clearly a promising area with regard to enhancement.

Increasing current flux through AMPA receptors results in greater post-synaptic depolarization and thereby promotes removal of the voltage block on NMDA receptors. This suggests that increasing AMPA receptor currents should facilitate the induction of LTP. Tests of this became possible with the invention of AMPA receptor modulators that freely enter the brain and increase fast glutamatergic transmission (Lynch, 2004a). The initial positive modulators were small benzamide compounds but subsequent work from many laboratories resulted in diverse families of compounds that slow deactivation or desensitization (or both) of ligand bound AMPA receptors. Here we will refer to all agents of this type by the term, "ampakines," used for the original compounds. Through a series of electrophysiological and X-ray crystallography studies, the mechanism of ampakine action is now fairly well understood. As illustrated in **Figure 2**, each subunit of the tetrameric AMPA receptor has two large extracellular domains that form a "clamshell" that closes upon glutamate binding (Sun et al., 2002). Relaxation to the resting state, and transmitter release, terminates current flow; this process is referred to as "deactivation." The four subunits form two dimers, an arrangement that can be disrupted by ligand binding; under these conditions the channel closes but the transmitter is retained. This interesting, high affinity (slow dissociation constant) state constitutes the desensitized condition of the receptor (Hall et al., 1993). It was originally thought that desensitization is the normal route for terminating the EPSC but it now appears that deactivation is responsible for the decay rate of the synaptic response. The ampakine binding pocket is located at the dimer interface near the hinge of the clamshell (Jin et al., 2005); this strategic position explains how ampakines can affect both deactivation and desensitization (Arai et al., 1996) (**Figure 2**). Apparently, the orientation of the compounds within the pocket determines which of the two processes is most affected. There is overlap between AMPA and NMDA receptor pharmacology: compounds widely used to block the former also exhibit high affinity antagonism of the glycine modulatory site on the latter (Kessler et al., 1989). However, the ampakine pocket is distant to the extracellular domain of AMPA receptor antagonist binding and there is no evidence that these drugs affect NMDA receptor-gated currents.

Early work established that ampakines enhance both LTP and memory (Granger et al., 1993; Staubli et al., 1994), results that have been multiply replicated by different groups (Lynch, 2004a; Lynch and Gall, 2013). Versions of the drugs that simply slow deactivation lower the threshold for inducing LTP whereas those that affect both deactivation and desensitization also raise the ceiling on the degree of potentiation produced by theta bursts (Arai et al., 2002). By changing rate constants for both receptor inactivation processes, the latter compounds lead to much longer EPSCs and thus prolonged NMDA receptor-mediated calcium influxes. This presumably explains their greater potency. Surprisingly, there appear to have been no studies testing for

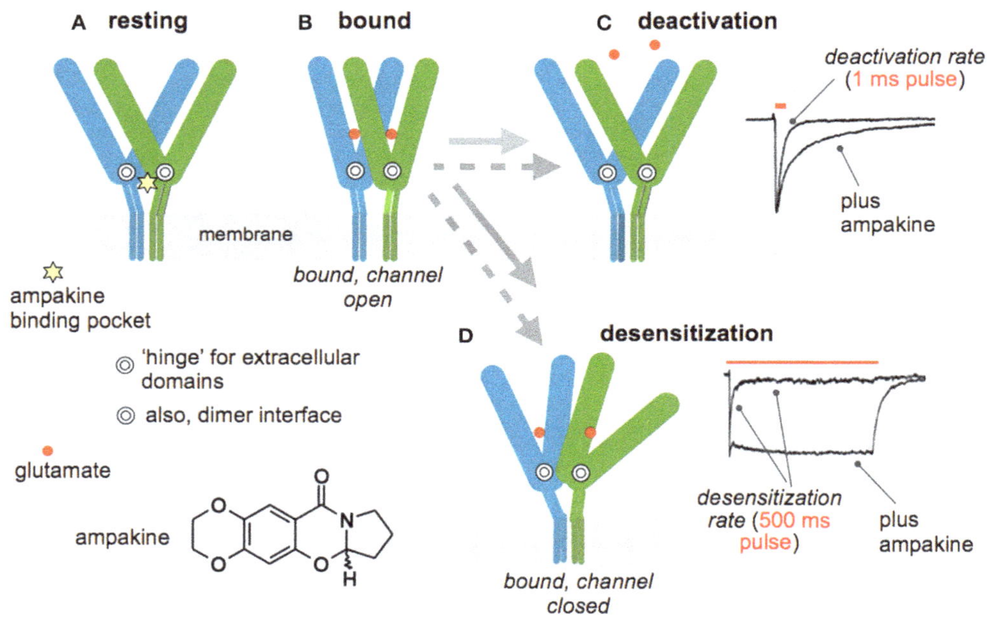

FIGURE 2 | Mode of action for positive allosteric modulators of AMPA receptors (ampakines). (A) Schematic shows two of the four subunits that comprise the AMPA receptor tetramer in the resting state; the C-tails are not included. Each subunit has two large extracellular domains that form a "clamshell" containing the glutamate binding site. The hinge of the structure is indicated by the double circle. The subunits dimerize at a zone close to the hinge. The ampakine pocket (star) is strategically located at the dimer interface adjacent to the two hinges. There are thus four neurotransmitter, and two ampakine, sites on the full AMPA receptor. **(B)** Glutamate binding is accompanied by a closing of each subunits' clamshell, resulting in opening of the ion channel and inward flux of current. The receptor then shifts into one of two configurations; the gray arrows denote the time required for the transitions in the presence (dotted) and absence (solid line) of an ampakine. **(C)** Normally, single transmission events are followed by opening of the extracellular domains and release of the transmitter, a process referred to as "deactivation." The upper trace to the right describes deactivation after a one ms pulse of glutamate to an excised patch: delivery of the ligand causes a sharp influx of current that decays after rapid washout. Bound ampakines slow reopening, resulting in a significant retardation of deactivation (bottom trace). **(D)** Prolonged stimulation of the receptor can disrupt the dimer configuration, leading to a condition in which transmitter remains bound but the ion channel returns to the closed state (desensitization). The upper trace to the right describes an instance of this in which glutamate was applied for 500 msec. An initial influx of current was followed by decay, despite continuing presence of the transmitter, to a steady state value about 1/10 of the peak flux. Ampakines stabilize the dimer configuration and, as predicted, greatly slow desensitization—current flow continues throughout the 500 ms application of glutamate. The receptor structural dynamics, including interactions with an ampakine, illustrated here are based on X-ray crystallography studies (Sun et al., 2002; Jin et al., 2005); physiological data are from patches taken from hippocampal slices (Arai et al., 1996, 2002; Arai and Lynch, 1998).

differential actions of the two functional classes of ampakine on learning.

Notably, the positive influence of acutely administered ampakines on memory are reported for aged and young animals (Granger et al., 1993, 1996; Shors et al., 1995) as well as for a broad array of species and learning tasks (Lynch, 2004a; Bernard et al., 2010). Very few effects in human have been published although one study using a short half-life, deactivation-only drug obtained evidence for memory enhancement in different tasks including ones involving complex processing (Ingvar et al., 1997).

LEARNING-RELATED SYNAPTIC MODIFICATIONS AS A TARGET FOR ENHANCEMENT STRATEGIES

The discovery of LTP (Bliss and Lomo, 1973) greatly simplified what had already been an extended search for the substrates of memory. An early and critical clue came with electron microscopic evidence that stable potentiation is accompanied by changes in the morphology of dendritic spines (Lee et al., 1979, 1980; Chang and Greenough, 1984), an observation recently and convincingly confirmed by live imaging experiments (Matsuzaki et al., 2004; Harvey and Svoboda, 2007; Kramar et al., 2012b). The initial studies also described results suggestive of an increase in synapse size and there are now data pointing to a similar effect after LTP (Chen et al., 2007) and learning (Fedulov et al., 2007). The observed anatomical restructuring implied that induction events for LTP or memory result in substantial alterations to the actin cytoskeleton. Tests of this, using a newly developed *in situ* method for labeling F-actin in hippocampal slices, found that theta bursts cause a dramatic increase in the number of spines with high concentrations of polymerized actin (Lin et al., 2005; Kramar et al., 2006). The newly formed filaments proved to be unstable for a period of 5–10 min, after which they were unaffected by depolymerizing agents (Rex et al., 2009, 2010). The experimental question then became one of how the very brief AMPA and NMDA receptor events that induce LTP lead to the formation of new actin cytoskeleton. Work using Fluorescence Deconvolution Tomography for assessing concentrations of activated signaling proteins at individual synapses, along with the use of selective inhibitors, identified multiple, GTPase-initiated signaling pathways involved in the assembly and stabilization of actin filament networks following theta burst stimulation (Kramar et al., 2009; Rex et al., 2009, 2010; Seese et al., 2012). Particularly relevant to the present topic, these studies also described membrane receptors that modulate the activity of cascades leading to the cytoskeletal reorganization required for consolidation of LTP (**Figure 3**).

Brief treatments with BDNF partially activate at least two of the signaling pathways shown in **Figure 3** and potently facilitate

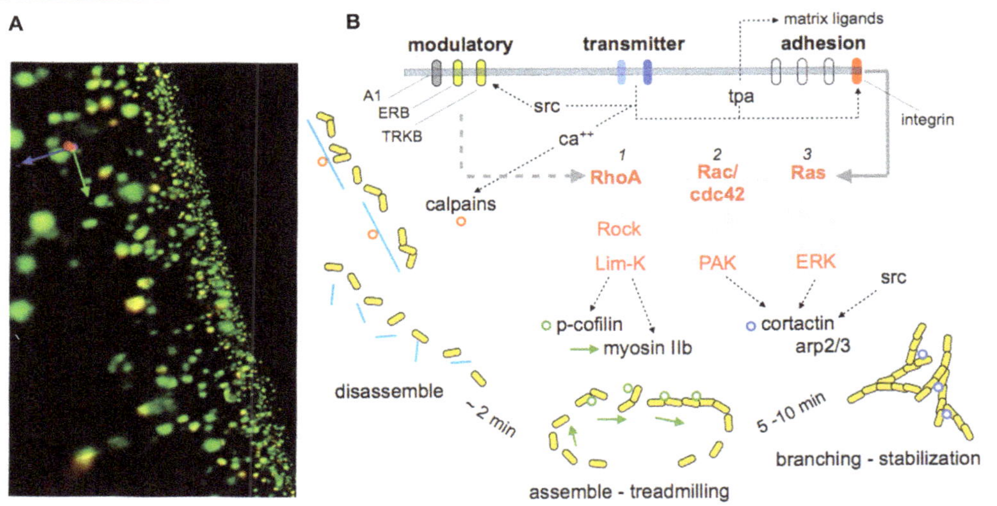

FIGURE 3 | Signaling events responsible for reorganizing the synaptic cytoskeleton and consolidating LTP. The substrate map for LTP stabilization is largely based on work using hippocampal slices, although some of the steps have been observed in learning studies. **(A)** Immunolabeled synapses surrounding the LTP site as reconstructed using Fluorescence Deconvolution Tomography (Seese et al., 2013): The green elements reflect immunostaining for PSD95, a protein that is evenly distributed within post-synaptic densities at excitatory (glutamatergic) synapses. Phosphorylated (inactivated) cofilin was immunolabeled with red fluorescence. Co-localization (p-Cofilin/PSD95) results in yellow labeling. The technique supports counts and size-measures for about 40,000 synapses per image z-stack and 160,000 synapses per slice, and calculates the number of these synaptic elements that are co-localized with the signaling protein of interest (p-Cofilin in this instance). These values are then compared for slices that did or did not receive theta burst simulation. **(B)** Schematic shows signaling pathways activated at excitatory synapses by theta burst stimulation. Transmitter receptors i) increase calcium which stimulates calpain, a spine protease (Perlmutter et al., 1988) that cleaves cross-linking proteins (blue lines) for the subsynaptic cytoskeleton, and ii) activates synaptic adhesion receptors belonging to the integrin family (Babayan et al., 2012). Integrins then engage at least two Rho family GTPases that promote the assembly of dynamic actin filaments (RhoA to cofilin and myosin) (Rex et al., 2009) and, over a period of several minutes, branching and stabilization of the reorganized cytoskeleton. The latter processes involve Rac/Cdc42 signaling to cortactin and ARP2/3. The synaptic membrane also contains receptors for the releasable factors adenosine, estrogen, and BDNF (A1, ERB, TrkB, respectively). These receptors positively and negatively (A1) influence the signaling pathways, probably at the level of the GTPases. Studies using neutralizing antisera, genetic manipulations, toxins, and enzyme blockers confirm certain key links in the model and show that disrupting these specific actin regulatory pathways blocks the consolidation, but not initial expression, of LTP.

both theta burst-driven actin polymerization and LTP (Chen et al., 2006; Rex et al., 2007). It seems likely that the LTP effects reflect both direct actions on the actin regulatory pathways and the above noted influence on AHPs generated during the theta stimulation trains (see above). Notably, scavenging extracellular BDNF blocks the stabilization of LTP produced by theta burst stimulation (Kovalchuk et al., 2002; Rex et al., 2007) as well as the associated activation of actin regulatory signaling and increases in spine F-actin (**Figure 4**); activity-induced release of the neurotrophic factor thus emerges as a key ingredient in the normal production of learning-related synaptic changes. In all, increases in BDNF signaling appear to be a biologically plausible means for enhancing memory. Peripheral administration of the protein is unlikely to have robust central effects but brain permeant agonists for its synaptic TrkB receptor have been developed and shown to improve function in varied conditions of impairment (Andero et al., 2012; Schmid et al., 2012; Ding et al., 2013; Jiang et al., 2013). Reports on how these compounds affect memory in normals have only begun to appear but initial studies indicate that acute systemic treatment can improve object recognition, object location and fear memory when given just before training (Andero et al., 2011; Bollen et al., 2013); for object location memory administration 3 h after training was also effective. These results encourage the expectation that acute systemic treatment with a TrkB agonist can facilitate both initial encoding and mechanisms of consolidation for at least some forms of memory. Further work is needed to determine the range of learning and cognitive functions that respond to this strategy and if this occurs without deleterious side effects.

Another route for utilizing BDNF in memory studies is suggested by the observation that transcription of the factor is positively regulated by neuronal activity (Isackson et al., 1991; Gall, 1992). It follows from this that increases in excitatory drive to neurons, as for example produced by ampakines, should upregulate the neurotrophin. A sizable number of studies using individual or a series of daily injections of the positive modulators have confirmed this basic idea (Lauterborn et al., 2000; Rex et al., 2006; Simmons et al., 2009; Bernard et al., 2010; Haditsch et al., 2013). The treatments rescue theta burst-induced actin polymerization and LTP in a number of animal models of human conditions in which memory loss and/or intellectual disabilities are prominent, including those for normal aging, low estrogen

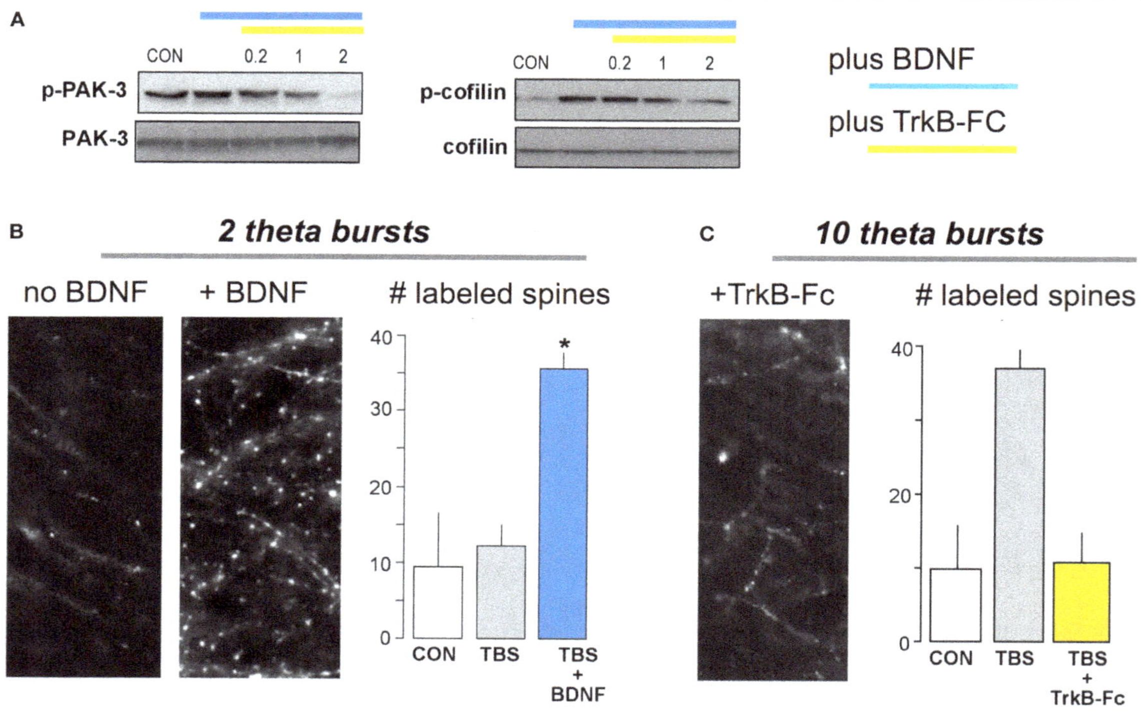

FIGURE 4 | BDNF enhances theta burst induced actin signaling and cytoskeletal assembly at hippocampal synapses. **(A)** Brief infusion of BDNF (60 ng/ml) into adult hippocampal slices increases phosphorylation of PAK and cofilin (immunoblots), two of the signaling proteins included in the schematic for LTP consolidation (**Figure 3**). Phosphorylation was blocked by addition of the extracellular BDNF scavenger TrkB-Fc (applied at 0.2–2 μg/ml). There were no evident effects of either treatment on levels of total PAK or cofilin. **(B)** Labeling of filamentous (F-) actin with fluorescence-tagged phalloidin applied to slices 10 min after delivery of two theta bursts (TBS), a number too small to generate LTP if applied alone. Pretreatment with BDNF (right image) caused a marked increase in TBS-induced labeling of dendritic spines relative to labeling in ACSF-bathed slices receiving similar stimulation. Graph: Summary of the number of spines with intense concentrations of F-actin, as assessed using automated counting for a fixed sampling field, confirmed these observations (CON, slices received low frequency stimulation only; $^{*}p < 0.01$ vs. CON). **(C)** Similar to **(B)** except that ten theta bursts were used. Pretreatment with TrkB-Fc completely blocked the otherwise robust increase in F-actin positive spines seen with ten burst TBS. Modified from Rex et al. (2007).

levels, early stage Huntington Disease, and Angelman syndrome (Rex et al., 2006; Simmons et al., 2009; Baudry et al., 2012; Kramar et al., 2012a). When tested, daily injections also reduced or eliminated memory impairments (Simmons et al., 2009; Baudry et al., 2012). Several weeks of daily ampakine treatment were shown to be well tolerated. They also markedly reduced pathology and improved motor functioning in a mouse model of early onset Huntington Disease (Simmons et al., 2011); subsequent work with systemic administration of a TrkB agonist obtained similar results (Simmons et al., 2013).

Although it is apparent that semi-chronic ampakine treatment increases BDNF protein levels, and has potent brain effects predicted from this, there appear to be no studies testing for influences of up-regulating BDNF on learning in normal, high functioning animals. This likely reflects an assignment of greater importance to treatment than to enhancement with regard to drug development. But the exciting results obtained with up-regulation and receptor agonists with regard to brain disorders make BDNF-based strategies one of the more promising mechanism-grounded approaches to achieving memory enhancement.

The substrate map for LTP consolidation includes estrogen receptor beta as a second membrane agent that exerts a powerful modulatory influence over the actin signaling leading to LTP consolidation. Thirty minute infusions of estrogen, at physiological concentrations, cause a modest increase in baseline transmission in hippocampus but a striking facilitation of LTP (Cordoba Montoya and Carrer, 1997; Foy et al., 1999; Bi et al., 2000; Kramar et al., 2009). Recent work showed that these effects are due to activation of one of the actin regulatory cascades initiated by theta bursts (i.e., RhoA>ROCK>LIMK>cofilin—see **Figure 3**) and the assembly of new filamentous actin in spine heads (Kramar et al., 2009). Unlike the case for BDNF, there are several reports that estrogen improves memory scores in high functioning subjects across tasks and species (Frye et al., 2007; Liu et al., 2008; Hara et al., 2014). Evidence for similar effects in humans appears to be lacking (Grodstein, 2013) although several studies describe a decline in verbal memory with surgical menopause and improvements with hormone replacement (Brinton, 2009). Beyond needing further evidence for effects in cognitively normal individuals, a primary barrier to development of an estrogen-based enhancement strategy lies in the fact that the steroid affects many fundamental cellular processes in brain and the periphery, and is known to facilitate certain types of cancer. More restricted actions can be had using agonists selective for the hormone's beta receptor which is, to a degree, concentrated in brain; such agonists are highly effective in LTP studies (Kramar et al., 2009). Evidence that estrogen is synthesized by hippocampal neurons and that hormone of local origin contributes significantly to hippocampal synaptic plasticity (Ooishi et al., 2012; Vierk et al., 2012) should also be noted here. Thus, it may be possible to find means to promote normal, likely activity-dependent, estrogen actions in a regionally restricted manner.

INTEGRATION: MANY PATHS TO THE SAME END

Brain scientists had proposed increases in the strength of connections between neurons as the substrate of memory before the introduction of the word "synapse" (Cajal, 1894). The idea is intuitively attractive since such increases would clearly alter the operation of cortical networks and thus behavior. In essence, it describes microscopic events that, when implemented at many sites, could be the physical instantiation of the macroscopic phenomenon of memory. From this perspective, the most direct route to memory enhancement would involve facilitating physiologically produced, long lasting increases in synaptic responses. Developing what is still only an outline of the machinery that induces, expresses, and consolidates LTP then shaped ideas about how to produce facilitation. To some extent, it also led to a unification that is perhaps under-appreciated: an unrelated array of enhancement candidates such as steroids, trophic factors, positive modulators of glutamate receptors, and channel blockers can now be seen to operate at specific levels within the same cell biological framework (Lynch et al., 2013). Optimistically, we may be approaching a reductionistic (simplifying) conceptual event with regard to enhancing encoding of specific pieces of information. Notably, something of this kind may also be going on for appreciating shared mechanistic impairments present in quite different disorders that interfere with learning: work with a sizable number of rodent models suggests that conditions with disparate etiologies result in a common endpoint failure in cytoskeletal reorganization (Lynch and Gall, 2013).

But there are warning signs with regard to the possibility that the current substrate model may be overly tailored to a specific instance of learning-related plasticity, and in particular to that found in a particular dendritic lamina (stratum radiatum) of a particular hippocampal subfield (CA1). Even within that subfield, there is good evidence that the basal dendritic field exhibits a different form of LTP (Arai et al., 1994; Kramar and Lynch, 2003). And it is now well established that the peculiar mossy fiber connections between dentate gyrus and field CA3 use a form of long lasting potentiation that bears little resemblance to that found in apical field CA1 (Staubli, 1992; Schmitz et al., 2003). It is not unreasonable to expect that additional plasticity variants will be discovered as parametric studies are carried out for other telencephalic connections; e.g., the cortico-striatal glutamatergic synapses (Jia et al., 2010) or the olfactory and associational afferents to piriform cortex (Jung et al., 1990). While these observations greatly complicate predictions about the behavioral effects of putative enhancers, they also offer intriguing possibilities concerning specificity of action. That is, there are reasons to think that different forms of synaptic potentiation may underlie different types, or aspects, of memory. An explicit proposal of this type has been advanced for the basal and apical dendrites of field CA1 (Arai et al., 1994; Kramar and Lynch, 2003): The easily induced, readily erased LTP in the basal dendritic field seems well suited for transient encoding while the higher threshold and more rapidly stabilized form in the apical field is more appropriate for long term memory. An arrangement of this type would be useful in addressing the problem of how to accomplish, through repeated sampling, low noise extraction of constancies from a novel environment (apical dendrites) while at the same time transiently storing a great deal of information much of which can be discarded as being irrelevant (basal dendrites). In any event, testing experimental compounds on various forms of plasticity could lead to agents that target particular forms of memory.

COGNITIVE ENHANCEMENT

DOES AUGMENTING MEMORY ENHANCE COGNITION?

Memory is such a prominent part of cognition that it seems obvious that enhancing the one will improve the other. However, there may be good computational reasons that cognitive benefit is gained when acquisition is less than optimal in terms of speed and strength. Animals faced with new and complex circumstances need to encode regular features without storing variable, low information elements. Otherwise, as noted earlier, the resultant memories will be noisy and less predictive of future encounters. The spaced trials effect—wherein, temporally separated training trials more efficiently support encoding than does a single "massed" session—can be seen as one adaptation toward better capture of regularities in the learning environment (Hintzman, 1976; Commins et al., 2003; Cepeda et al., 2006). That is, spacing ensures that only elements that are regularly present will be incorporated into memory while transient features will not. An enhancer could obviate the need for spacing by producing strong memory on an initial trial but would be expected to result in a noisy representation.

Tests of the above point are lacking but LTP experiments have produced what may be pertinent results. The original descriptions of links between theta burst afferent stimulation and LTP showed that, absent other manipulations, trains of ten bursts produced near maximal potentiation (Larson et al., 1986), a result that led to what has become a standard paradigm. Recently, however, it was found that a second theta train doubles the level of potentiation but only if it is delayed by about 60 min (**Figure 5**); a third stimulation train produces still more potentiation but only if it is applied at least 60 min after the second. Additional work suggested that this LTP "spaced trials effect" reflects the presence of a large population of synapses with high plasticity thresholds that are "primed" by the first theta episode and then shifted into the potentiated state by the second (Kramar et al., 2012b). These effects fit naturally within the above described substrate map for LTP: activation of synaptic integrins by a first theta burst train was followed by an approximately one hour period before these receptors could be re-engaged by additional stimulation (Babayan et al., 2012). They also set the stage for a first test of how a drug that enhances memory affects a physiological analogue of the spaced trials effect. The results were clear: infusion of an ampakine prior to theta train #1 produced the expected enhancement in the amplitude of LTP1 but also occluded further increases in the level of potentiation following a second, delayed theta train administered in the absence of the drug (Kramar et al., 2012b). Thus, the ampakine enhanced initial encoding (as multiply reported) but did so at the expense of effects of spaced stimulation, and presumably the computational advantages associated with spacing (Lynch and Gall, 2013 for a discussion).

The preceding example describes a situation in which pharmacologically augmenting memory would likely not result in enhanced cognition, at least in complex environments lacking explicit guidelines for effective performance. These are routine circumstances in which demands on cognition are high. But a great deal of cognition involves instances in which significant cues and appropriate responses are salient and predetermined, and irrelevant information is minimized. Under these conditions, enhanced encoding could be of great use in building or expanding

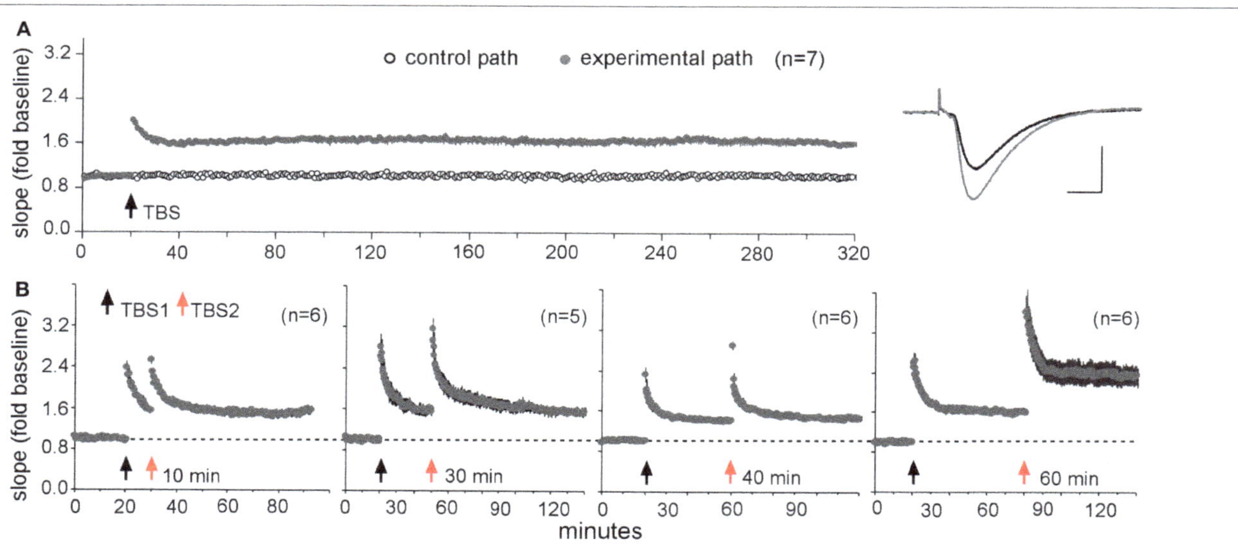

FIGURE 5 | A "spaced trials effect" for LTP. (A) Theta burst stimulation (TBS) produces stable LTP. A single train of ten bursts was delivered to one input to the CA1b recording field after 20 min of collecting baseline synaptic responses to 3/min stimulation pulses in adult rat hippocampal slices. A second input to the same dendritic region received 3/min pulses throughout the session. Note that the potentiation of the experimental input did not decay over 5 h of recording (means ± s.e.m.s for seven slices); traces at right show representative baseline (black) and potentiated (gray) responses. **(B)** Effect of a second theta train (TBS2) applied at various times after TBS1. TBS2 produced no further increases in the slopes of the responses when delayed by 10, 30, or 40 min after TBS1, but doubled the magnitude of LTP when applied after a 60 min interval. Modified from Kramar et al. (2012b).

cognitive structures. Thus, the effects of memory enhancement on cognition could prove to be situationally dependent with clear benefits in some cases and neutral or even negative influence in others.

NETWORKS AND COGNITIVE ENHANCEMENT

Discussions of neurobiological processes underlying cognition inevitably begin with the immensely complicated networks formed by cortical neurons, if for no other reason than a lack of realistic alternatives. This fundamental idea suggests two paths to *acute* enhancement. First, improving throughput within established networks should lead to faster computation and better utilization of cognitive time. Second, augmented synaptic communication could allow for the transient assembly of larger than normal networks (e.g., incorporation of additional cortical regions) to deal with a particular problem, and thus the opportunity to execute more complex or even entirely novel computations. In this sense better throughput would add capabilities, perhaps the surest measure of cognitive enhancement. Increased plasticity might add a third route to enhanced cognition by allowing for construction of functional networks that would not likely emerge under normal conditions; however, as noted in the preceding section, positive versions of such effects may be limited to particular circumstances.

There are multiple manipulations that should result in improved throughput. Communication between collections of neurons is greatly improved by synchronizing their activity, something that is accomplished in the cortical telencephalon by system-wide rhythms. These patterns are induced by diffuse ascending projections from the lower brain and drugs that affect these have predictable strong effects on rhythmic activity (Staubli and Xu, 1995; Kowalczyk et al., 2013). But, as mentioned in the discussion of memory, the diffuse systems influence a broad range of brain functions including ones that are vital to survival. And so, as in the case of memory, they do not represent a promising avenue toward enhancement in high functioning individuals. A more likely approach would be to increase transmitter release or post-synaptic responses to transmitter binding at the glutamatergic connections used for the great bulk of intra-cortical communication.

Adenosine, which depresses glutamate release via presynaptic A1 receptors (Dunwiddie and Haas, 1985), is increased in the extracellular environment during repetitive firing by two mechanisms: rapid release from post-synaptic neurons followed by slower release of ATP from glia which is then converted to adenosine by ecto-5′-nucleotidase, an enzyme located on glial membranes (Klyuch et al., 2012; Wall and Dale, 2013). These observations represent a significant part of the tripartite model (terminal bouton, spine, astrocyte) of fast, excitatory transmission (Araque et al., 1999). Selective antagonists of the A1 receptor increase glutamate release in slices and these compounds do indeed reverse impairments in LTP in slices of middle-aged rat hippocampus (Rex et al., 2005). However, despite evidence that the compounds enter the brain (Wall and Dale, 2013), there has been surprisingly little work on *in vivo* effects after peripheral administration. Perhaps the lack of interest with regard to network operations reflects understandable concern about the important roles played by adenosine in the periphery, including actions on the heart and lungs.

Nicotinic receptors for acetylcholine are also found on glutamatergic terminals where they promote release (Wonnacott, 1997) and there is evidence that this increases network throughput (Gioanni et al., 1999). Alpha7-containing and alpha4/beta2 subtypes of the receptors both appear to be effective in this regard (Dickinson et al., 2008). However, the situation is complicated by the likelihood that compounds targeting nicotinic receptors act on cholinergic and GABAergic neurons as well (Wonnacott, 1997; Alkondon and Albuquerque, 2001); moreover, it is not clear that these receptors are present throughout glutamatergic networks. In all, nicotinic receptor agonists and positive allosteric modulators can be assumed to affect portions of excitatory circuitry in the telencephalon while at the same time modifying local processing—via modulation of cholinergic input, interneurons, and glutamatergic collaterals—at individual relays. Net effects will be complex but there is good evidence that the compounds acting on frontal networks enhance "top-down" mechanisms for focusing attention (Sarter et al., 2009). Since pertinent drugs are already in clinical trials (Holmes et al., 2011; Demeter and Sarter, 2013), nicotinic compounds, and especially those targeting the alpha4/beta2 receptor subtype concentrated in brain, have to be seen as one of the most promising of current approaches to cognitive enhancement.

The ampakine compounds described in the earlier section on memory enhancement seem particularly appropriate for improving communication within and between cortical regions. Their mode of action has the virtue of relative simplicity: an extensive body of research from many laboratories has not uncovered any evidence for effects on targets other than AMPA receptors. And they produce the same facilitation of fast, excitatory transmission after peripheral administration as seen with infusions into brain slices. Indeed, ampakines appear to be the only agents so far shown to cause comparable *in vitro*/*in vivo* facilitation of EPSPs. These points lead to two critical experimental questions. First, does increasing monosynaptic transmission result in greater output from a polysynaptic network? This might seem to be a foregone conclusion but each step in a series of neuronal stations has local processing mechanisms (relays are not passive transferal points) dominated by an impressive collection of different types of inhibitory interneurons. These inhibitory elements respond both to inputs directly and to discharges from principle (glutamatergic) neurons; they also form complex local networks among themselves. It is therefore possible that strong inputs are dampened and normalized to a degree such that the second stage of a network may not pass on a larger than normal signal in the presence of an ampakine. Second, assuming augmentation of the signal does occur, what are the functional consequences of enhanced network throughput?

Brain slices provide for the simplest and most compelling tests for circuit behavior because anatomically precise stimulation and recording is possible and extrinsic modulatory (cholinergic, etc.) inputs (cholinergic, serotonergic, etc.) that might influence downstream responses are excluded. Work of this kind has established that weak facilitation of monosynaptic transmission with an ampakine results in a greatly amplified response from the output stage of the trisynaptic intra-hippocampal circuit (Sirvio et al., 1996). These observations accord with the broad idea that facilitated transmission at one connection will lead to a greater number of cells transmitting to the next. Repeated across many stages, each responding to the ampakine, this will produce a multiplier effect for drug action. This argument points to the conclusion that ampakine-type drugs will exert much greater effects in the long chains of glutamatergic neurons that constitute cortical networks than in the much simpler circuits found at lower levels of the neuraxis. Why the multiplier effect doesn't ultimately result in abnormal discharges likely reflects the above mentioned inhibitory interneurons whose influence on projection neurons also grows with increasing glutamatergic drive, as seen in input / output measurements in conventional hippocampal slice experiments. Since inhibition generated by arrival of a glutamatergic input is di- (and multi-) synaptic, there is brief widow in which network facilitation is operative. Sophisticated multi-scale (biophysics, synapses, neurons, and connectivity) computational work indicates the manner in which enhanced throughput can produce useful effects in complex cortical circuits (Bouteiller et al., 2011). However, the effects of increased EPSPs on network responses to rhythmic or complex stimulation are a critical and as yet unstudied issue.

Evidence for enhanced throughput has also been obtained in studies using *in vivo* analyses of hippocampal projections to frontal cortex (Baumbarger et al., 2001) and chronic recordings from the output stage of hippocampus (Hampson et al., 1998b). The latter rat study showed that the number of cells discharging during key steps in performing a complex task was substantially increased by systemic treatment with an ampakine (**Figure 6**). Given that the recording site was the terminus of the primary intra-hippocampal circuit, one can reasonably assume that the observed results reflected an augmentation of drug action through a polysynaptic network similar to those described for ampakines infused into hippocampal slices (Sirvio et al., 1996). But the possibility that augmented excitatory drive on ascending biogenic amine systems, whether from the drugs or the behavioral activity they produce, results in generalized increases

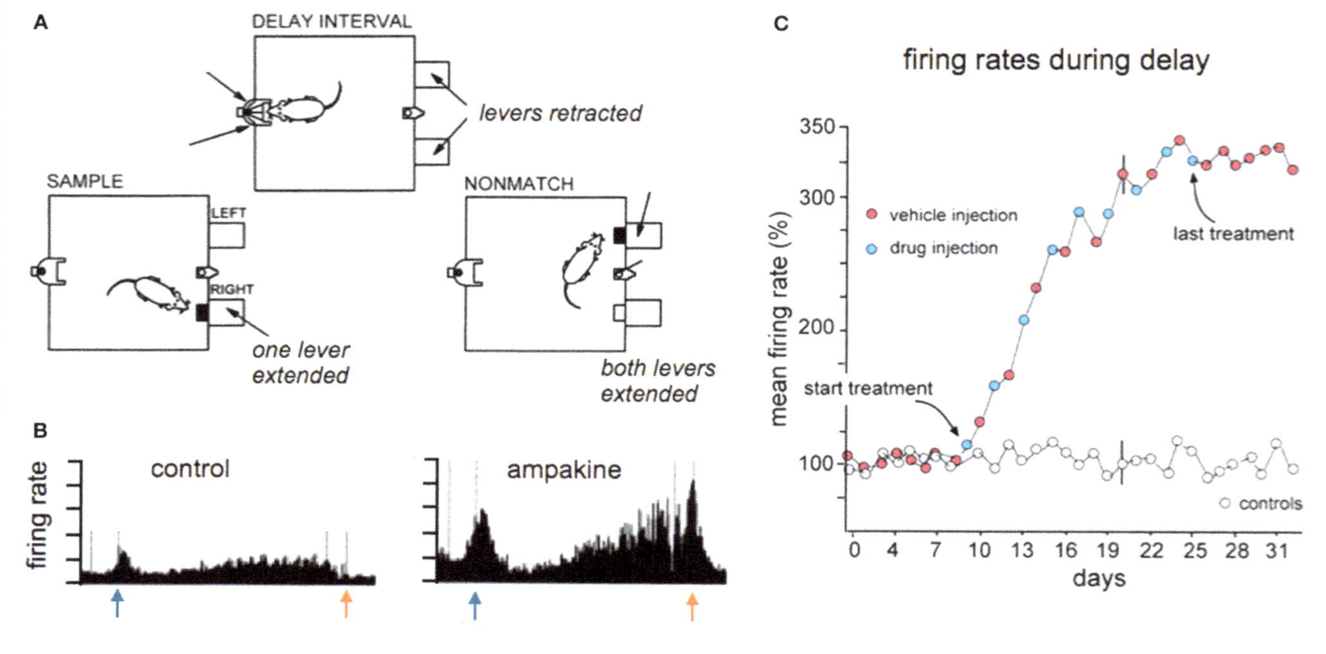

FIGURE 6 | Ampakine treatment increases neuronal activity in the terminal stage of the intra-hippocampal network and this is accompanied by supra-normal performance on a complex task. (A) Adult rats were extensively trained in the delayed non-match to sample (DNMS) task, illustrated here, wherein they were required to sequentially (i) press a bar to receive a reward (sample phase; left) at which time a light appeared on the opposite wall of the arena, (ii) move to the wall with the light during the "delay phase" (top) and perform a nose poke for random intervals until the light extinguished, and then (iii) return to the original side of the arena and press the bar that had not been originally selected (non-match phase; right). The level of success in executing the task reached asymptote after weeks of training, after which the animals were separated into vehicle or drug treated groups. Injections were given every other day. Animals given the ampakine prior to individual training sessions showed a progressive increase in correct responses over the next 2+ weeks of daily testing, ultimately reaching levels far higher than the asymptotic level maintained by vehicle-only rats (not shown; see Hampson et al., 1998b). **(B)** Chronic recordings from the same hippocampal neuron collected during task performance prior to and after the start of drug treatment. As shown, the ampakine dramatically increased the firing rate most particularly after the initial response to the sample (blue arrow) and in the delay phase leading up to the non-match choice (red arrow); this pattern and ampakine-related change was typical of field CA1 cells. **(C)** Plot shows the mean firing rate of all units recorded during the delay phase expressed as a percent of the baseline firing rate (prior to ampakine treatment): the progressive increase in firing rate in the experimental rats paralleled the increase in successful trials in the same rats. Rats given vehicle only (open circles) exhibited no change in cell firing or successful task execution over the full period of testing. Note that the increased firing in the drug group was still present on vehicle days (red dots), and indeed for the week following cessation of treatment, an effect that is interpreted as being due to facilitation of LTP-type plasticity on drug days. Adapted from Hampson et al. (1998b).

in neuronal excitability cannot be excluded in these *in vivo* studies.

FUNCTIONAL EFFECTS OF ENHANCED NETWORKS

There are relatively straightforward results showing the effects of increasing throughput in cortical networks in simple experimental paradigms. For example, unilateral lesions of the nigro-striatal projections result in a circling response to dopamine agonists; ampakines significantly expand activation of the motor cortex on the side of the lesion and this is associated with a suppression of rotations (Hess et al., 2003). Note that in this case circuits are selectively brought into play that are directly germane to the problem faced by the animal. The expectation of a more subtle version of this effect under conditions in which cortex is performing complex calculations constitutes one basis for hypothesizing that improved network throughput will result in acute enhancement of cognition. It should be noted here that the development of very fast algorithms for extracting core spatio-temporal activity patterns from multi-electrode recordings has made it possible to insert, via stimulation at many sites, information rich patterns to networks in behaving animals. These advances have opened the way to experimental testing of fundamental, long-standing assumptions about how cortical circuits process complex signals from the environment. One recent study of this kind that is particularly germane to the present discussion showed that delivery to CA1 of a "correct" pattern of activation predicted from CA3 recordings during the sample phase of a match to sample problem markedly enhanced performance of monkeys on the subsequent decision phase in difficult versions of the task (Hampson et al., 2013). These dramatic findings encourage the idea that facilitating partial or "weak" network patterns can lead to pronounced improvements in the ability of animals, including primates, to deal with complexity.

As mentioned earlier, enhancement could take the form of acceleration of cognitive activities, and thus allowing for more computations in the same time frame, or expansion of networks and potentially new types of operations. One route for testing the latter possibility would be to overtrain animals to the point at which optimal performance is fully established and then to determine if network facilitation through enhanced transmission allows the subject to go beyond normal limits. There is very little work of this kind for ampakines or any other putative enhancer but suggestive results have been described. The study noted above in which ampakines expanded the hippocampal response during learning (**Figure 6**) also found that overtrained rats significantly improved their learning scores under the influence of the drug. Remarkably, the animals then continued to perform at supra-normal levels in the absence of the ampakine. Detailed analyses showed that the animals shifted response strategies in a manner that reduced proactive interference between trials (Hampson et al., 1998a). In essence, the drugs opened the way to expanded networks and the development of higher order rules that cannot otherwise be acquired even with weeks of training. Another example of going well beyond normal limits has been described for monkeys performing a challenging delayed match-to-sample problem (Porrino et al., 2005). The animals were trained to asymptote to identify, as indicated by movement of a computer cursor, a previously seen real world cue from a group of similar objects. Performance on the task was increased dramatically with ampakine pretreatment. Brain imaging studies then uncovered a remarkable result: the ampakine intensified activity in frontal and temporal cortices but also led to the engagement of a superior parietal region, the precuneus, which was inactive during vehicle trials. The precuneus is thought to be critical for envisioning future actions by humans. In any case, these results in a primate provide an example in which expansion of cortical networks is associated with a lifting of limits on performance in a cognitively demanding problem.

These few studies using overtrained animals, exciting though the findings may be, are hardly sufficient to establish the general point that increases in network throughput result in beyond normal performance on challenging problems. Experiments of this type are not common because they involve major investments in time and technology. And it will be noted that they focus on problems that are sharply defined with regard to cues and appropriate responses. One can fairly ask if these conditions capture the essence of cognition as a free flowing processing of the enormous complexities generated by the exterior and interior worlds of humans. This point is picked up in the following section.

FUTURE NEUROBIOLOGICAL STUDIES ON COGNITIVE ENHANCEMENT

A question running through this review, and alluded to immediately above, concerns the extent to which we can consider problem solving by animals as a fair descriptor of cognition. One can hardly question the proposition that the analyses of different computations performed by distinct frontal subfields in rats (e.g., credit assignment to particular serial actions, set shifting, focusing of attention; Turner et al., 2004; Sugrue et al., 2005; Demeter and Sarter, 2013) will provide deep insights into how humans resolve real world issues. But here we encounter the problem of how to define cognition and whether or not it can be understood in simple computational terms. To be specific, what might be needed are studies testing whether putative enhancers improve the performance of sophisticated (highly experienced) subjects dealing with novel circumstances of great complexity and without the benefit of external supervision. If nothing else, this would bring experiments closer to the human condition and thereby help explain why animal studies on cognition and memory have such a poor record in predicting human outcomes.

Much of the present discussion centered on the proposition that enhancing network throughput will have positive effects on cognition (**Figures 7A,B**). It will be recognized that most of the material presented in support of this idea dealt with specific neuronal circuits or opportunistic discoveries of network expansion. A more systematic, agnostic description of how experimental compounds affect the vast number of forebrain circuits is badly needed. This could be obtained using activity-regulated immediate early gene expression to provide an index of the recent history of neuronal firing. Such analyses would provide a picture of the networks assembled to deal with complex circumstances, surely an initial step toward a mechanism based theory of cognitive operations, and add an information rich step for the screening of experimental compounds. There is also the possibility that network maps of drug effects

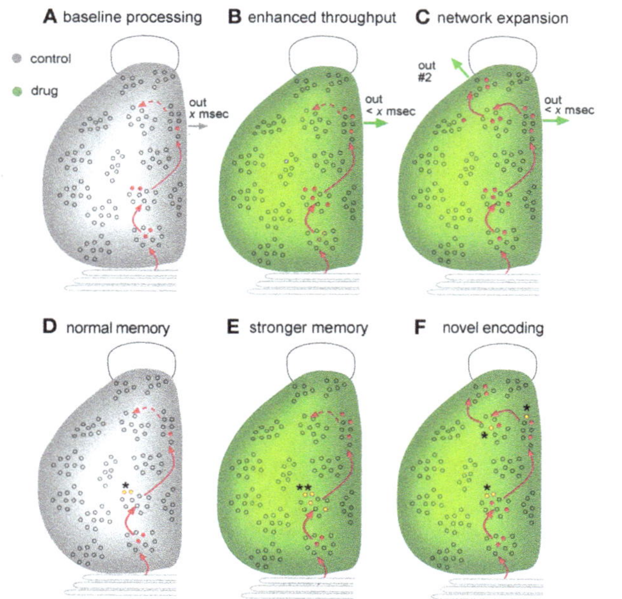

FIGURE 7 | Mapping as an endpoint measure for evaluating the effects of putative enhancers. Schematic illustration of a dorsal view of the left side of a rodent brain, with an open outline of the olfactory bulb at top and the cerebellum at bottom. Gray is for control subjects while green denotes results obtained in the presence of an experimental treatment. **(A–C)** Network Mapping. The figures describe the distribution of cells activated during learning of a novel environment, as could be determined from maps assembled from serial sections labeled for activation of Immediate-Early Genes (see text). Combining this information with neuroanatomy (red lines) would provide a picture of the extent to which known circuits were engaged during learning. **(A)** Interaction with the environment increases the number of cells firing (red dots) in three successive stages of a transcortical network, resulting in output from the third stage. A fourth region that that is weakly innervated by preceding network stages (dotted line) is not engaged. **(B)** A compound that facilitates excitatory synaptic transmission increases the number of neurons that respond to the input and thereby reduces circuit-throughput time (< *x* ms) and generates a more robust network output. **(C)** An additional possibility, supported by experimental work, is that improved transmission adds regions to the network, resulting in novel outputs ("out #2"). Potentially, the cortex in this instance would gain new capabilities for dealing with complex problems. **(D–F)** Mapping of encoding sites (engrams). Recent advances have made it possible to identify synapses that are modified by recent learning. Mapping studies for hippocampus strongly suggest that such effects are restricted to a small number of sites in a multiple stage network (see text). **(D)** Under control conditions, memory-related synaptic changes, such as LTP, are restricted to stage #2 (yellow dots, asterisk) of one network engaged during learning. **(E)** An enhancer could increase the number of neurons on which such synaptic changes occur in regions in which they are normally found (double asterisks). Such an effect is predicted to result in the formation of stronger memory (e.g., more resistant to extinction). **(F)** Improved transmission relating to an experimental treatment reduces the threshold for inducing memory-related synaptic alterations such as LTP. It follows from this that the manipulation could result in synaptic modifications in regions at which they do not normally occur (multiple asterisks). This is predicted to produce an elaborated, novel representation of the learned material.

would be predictive: measures of intensified activity within, or expansion of, behaviorally engaged circuits (**Figure 7C**) should lead to explicit hypotheses about the origins of psychological changes.

Another type of mapping may also prove useful in future searches for cognitive enhancers (**Figures 7D–F**). As noted, changes in the numbers of individual synapses associated with LTP-related actin regulatory proteins have been detected in hippocampus following learning. Notably, the labeled synapses were larger than their neighbors (Fedulov et al., 2007), an effect that was also seen with LTP (Chen et al., 2007). Continuing advances in the technology for identifying synapses engaged in plastic changes that underlie learning have made it possible to plot the distribution, across entire cross-sections of the hippocampus, of subfields that reliably contain many such contacts. A first study using the mapping method to plot synapses undergoing plasticity following learning of a new environment detected only three out of forty-two sampling zones within hippocampus that match this description; imposing a response contingency that interfered with free exploration eliminated the effect (Cox et al., 2014). These results cannot be taken as indicating that learning related synaptic adjustments only occur within these three sites; it is entirely possible that such effects are present in many regions but vary between subjects and/or are not numerically large enough to be detected with current procedures. But the results strongly suggest that encoding of one type of spatial information is not homogeneously distributed but instead occurs at high levels in a surprisingly small number of locations. In essence, they constitute a first, albeit crude memory map that covers one septo-temporal segment of the hippocampus.

Localizing memory has been a much discussed topic among brain scientists since the early days of the last century; subsequent attempts to map the distribution of encoding sites acquired an evocative title: "The search for the engram" (Thompson et al., 1976; Thompson and Krupa, 1994). Maps, or engrams, are of evident importance to the development of neurobiological theories of how memories are recalled but they are also of potential significance with regard to network events related to cognitive enhancement. The discussion to this point has stressed the effects of transiently facilitating network throughput but it is noteworthy that certain of the manipulations suggested for this purpose, such as increasing neurotrophic factor signaling, may also promote stable changes in connectivity. But would such changes simply increase the efficacy (e.g., throughput time) of extant circuits or would they allow for the emergence of new and persistent networks? This distinction returns to the earlier consideration of enhancement as reflecting faster processing or the introduction of new capabilities. The technology for mapping the location of learning-driven synaptic modifications may allow for neurobiological, as opposed to purely behavioral, tests of the question: does an experimental manipulation intensify the map (more synapses with LTP-related changes at normal sites) vs. creating additional regions with high numbers of modified connections (**Figures 7D–F**).

In all, a futuristic combination of network mapping with localization of synaptic changes could shift the evaluation of putative enhancers from exclusively behavioral endpoints to the presumed network substrates of cognitive operations. Such a step would likely lead to the many advantages in problem conceptualization historically associated with reductionism in science.

ACKNOWLEDGMENTS

Research described here was supported, in part, by grants NS045260 from NINDS, N0014-10-1-007 from ONR, and #1146708 from NSF, and an award to Gary Lynch from the UC Irvine Center for Autism Research and Translation. Conor D. Cox was supported by NSF fellowship DGE088392.

REFERENCES

Abraham, W. C. (2003). How long will long-term potentiation last? *Philos. Trans. R. Soc. Lond. B Biol. Sci.* 358, 735–744. doi: 10.1098/rstb.2002.1222

Abraham, W. C., and Williams, J. M. (2008). LTP maintenance and its protein synthesis-dependence. *Neurobiol. Learn. Mem.* 89, 260–268. doi: 10.1016/j.nlm.2007.10.001

Alarcon, J. M., Barco, A., and Kandel, E. R. (2006). Capture of the late phase of long-term potentiation within and across the apical and basilar dendritic compartments of CA1 pyramidal neurons: synaptic tagging is compartment restricted. *J. Neurosci.* 26, 256–264. doi: 10.1523/JNEUROSCI.3196-05.2006

Alkondon, M., and Albuquerque, E. X. (2001). Nicotinic acetylcholine receptor alpha7 and alpha4beta2 subtypes differentially control GABAergic input to CA1 neurons in rat hippocampus. *J. Neurophysiol.* 86, 3043–3055.

Andero, R., Daviu, N., Escorihuela, R. M., Nadal, R., and Armario, A. (2012). 7,8-dihydroxyflavone, a TrkB receptor agonist, blocks long-term spatial memory impairment caused by immobilization stress in rats. *Hippocampus.* 22, 399–408. doi: 10.1002/hipo.20906

Andero, R., Heldt, S. A., Ye, K., Liu, X., Armario, A., and Ressler, K. J. (2011). Effect of 7,8-dihydroxyflavone, a small-molecule TrkB agonist, on emotional learning. *Am. J. Psychiatry* 168, 163–172. doi: 10.1176/appi.ajp.2010.10030326

Arai, A., Black, J., and Lynch, G. (1994). Origins of the variations in long-term potentiation between synapses in the basal versus apical dendrites of hippocampal neurons. *Hippocampus* 4, 1–9. doi: 10.1002/hipo.450040103

Arai, A. C., Xia, Y. F., Rogers, G., Lynch, G., and Kessler, M. (2002). Benzamide-type AMPA receptor modulators form two subfamilies with distinct modes of action. *J. Pharmacol. Exp. Ther.* 303, 1075–1085. doi: 10.1124/jpet.102.040360

Arai, A., Kessler, M., Ambros-Ingerson, J., Quan, A., Yigiter, E., Rogers, G., et al. (1996). Effects of a centrally active benzoylpyrrolidine drug on AMPA receptor kinetics. *Neuroscience* 75, 573–585. doi: 10.1016/0306-4522(96)00263-1

Arai, A., and Lynch, G. (1998). The waveform of synaptic transmission at hippocampal synapses is not determined by AMPA receptor desensitization. *Brain Res.* 799, 230–234. doi: 10.1016/S0006-8993(98)00446-6

Araque, A., Parpura, V., Sanzgiri, R. P., and Haydon, P. G. (1999). Tripartite synapses: glia, the unacknowledged partner. *Trends Neurosci.* 22, 208–215. doi: 10.1016/S0166-2236(98)01349-6

Babayan, A. H., Kramar, E. A., Barrett, R. M., Jafari, M., Haettig, J., Chen, L. Y., et al. (2012). Integrin dynamics produce a delayed stage of long-term potentiation and memory consolidation. *J. Neurosci.* 32, 12854–12861. doi: 10.1523/JNEUROSCI.2024-12.2012

Balkowiec, A., and Katz, D. M. (2000). Activity-dependent release of endogenous brain-derived neurotrophic factor from primary sensory neurons detected by ELISA *in situ*. *J. Neurosci.* 20, 7417–7423.

Bari, A., Dalley, J. W., and Robbins, T. W. (2008). The application of the 5-choice serial reaction time task for the assessment of visual attentional processes and impulse control in rats. *Nat. Protoc.* 3, 759–767. doi: 10.1038/nprot.2008.41

Baudry, M., Kramar, E., Xu, X., Zadran, H., Moreno, S., Lynch, G., et al. (2012). Ampakines promote spine actin polymerization, long-term potentiation, and learning in a mouse model of Angelman syndrome. *Neurobiol. Dis.* 47, 210–215. doi: 10.1016/j.nbd.2012.04.002

Baumbarger, P. J., Muhlhauser, M., Zhai, J., Yang, R., and Nisenbaum, E. S. (2001). Positive modulation of alpha-amino-3-hydroxy-5-methyl-4-isoxazole propionic acid (AMPA) receptors in prefrontal cortical pyramidal neurons by a novel allosteric potentiator. *J. Pharmacol. Exp. Ther.* 298, 86–102.

Baxter, M. G., Lanthorn, T. H., Frick, K. M., Golski, S., Wan, R. Q., and Olton, D. S. (1994). C-cycloserine, a novel cognitive enhancer, improves spatial memory in aged rats. *Neurobiol. Aging.* 15, 207–213. doi: 10.1016/0197-4580(94)90114-7

Bernard, K., Danober, L., Thomas, J. Y., Lebrun, C., Munoz, C., Cordi, A., et al. (2010). Drug focus: S 18986: a positive allosteric modulator of AMPA-type glutamate receptors pharmacological profile of a novel cognitive enhancer. *CNS Neurosci. Ther.* 16, e193–212. doi: 10.1111/j.1755-5949.2009.00088.x

Bi, F., Broutman, G., Foy, M. R., Thompson, R. F., and Baudry, M. (2000). The tyrosine kinase and mitogen-activated protein kinase pathways mediate multiple effects of estrogen in hippocampus. *Proc. Natl. Acad. Sci. U.S.A.* 97, 3606–3607. doi: 10.1073/pnas.97.7.3602

Bliss, T. V., and Collingridge, G. L. (1993). A synaptic model of memory: long-term potentiation in the hippocampus. *Nature* 361, 31–39. doi: 10.1038/361031a0

Bliss, T. V. P., and Lomo, T. (1973). Long-lasting potentiation of synaptic transmission in the dentate area of the anesthetized rabbit following stimulation of the perforant path. *J. Physiol.* 232, 334–356.

Bollen, E., Vanmierlo, T., Akkerman, S., Wouters, C., Steinbusch, H. M., and Prickaerts, J. (2013). 7,8-dihydroxyflavone improves memory consolidation processes in rats and mice. *Behav. Brain Res.* 257, 8–12. doi: 10.1016/j.bbr.2013.09.029

Bouteiller, J. M., Allam, S. L., Hu, E. Y., Greget, R., Ambert, N., Keller, A. F., et al. (2011). Integrated multiscale modeling of the nervous system: predicting changes in hippocampal network activity by a positive AMPA receptor modulator. *IEEE Trans. Biomed. Eng.* 58, 3008–3011. doi: 10.1109/TBME.2011.2158605

Brennan, A. R., Dolinsky, B., Vu, M. A., Stanley, M., Yeckel, M. F., and Arnsten, A. F. (2008). Blockade of IP3-mediated SK channel signaling in the rat medial prefrontal cortex improves spatial working memory. *Learn. Mem.* 15, 93–96. doi: 10.1101/lm.767408

Brinton, R. D. (2009). Estrogen-induced plasticity from cells to circuits: predictions for cognitive function. *Trends Pharmacol. Sci.* 30, 212–222. doi: 10.1016/j.tips.2008.12.006

Buzsaki, G. (2005). Theta rhythm of navigation: link between path integration and landmark navigation, episodic and semantic memory. *Hippocampus* 15, 827–840. doi: 10.1002/hipo.20113

Cajal, S. R. (1894). La fine structure des centres nerveux. *Proc. R. Soc. Lond.* 55, 444–468. doi: 10.1098/rspl.1894.0063

Capocchi, G., Zampolini, M., and Larson, J. (1992). Theta burst stimulation is optimal for induction of LTP at both apical and basal dendritic synapses on hippocampal CA1 neurons. *Brain Res.* 591, 332–336. doi: 10.1016/0006-8993(92)91715-Q

Cepeda, N. J., Pashler, H., Vul, E., Wixted, J. T., and Rohrer, D. (2006). Distributed practice in verbal recall tasks: a review and quantitative synthesis. *Psychol. Bull.* 132, 354–380. doi: 10.1037/0033-2909.132.3.354

Chang, F.-L. F., and Greenough, W. T. (1984). Transient and enduring morphological correlates of synaptic activity and efficacy change in the rat hippocampal slice. *Brain Res.* 309, 35–46. doi: 10.1016/0006-8993(84)91008-4

Chen, L. Y., Rex, C. S., Casale, M. S., Gall, C. M., and Lynch, G. (2007). Changes in synaptic morphology accompany actin signaling during LTP. *J. Neurosci.* 27, 5363–5372. doi: 10.1523/JNEUROSCI.0164-07.2007

Chen, L. Y., Rex, C. S., Sanaiha, Y., Lynch, G., and Gall, C. M. (2010b). Learning induces neurotrophin signaling at hippocampal synapses. *Proc. Natl. Acad. Sci. U.S.A.* 107, 7030–7035. doi: 10.1073/pnas.0912973107

Chen, T. J., Gehler, S., Shaw, A. E., Bamburg, J. R., and Letourneau, P. C. (2006). Cdc42 participates in the regulation of ADF/cofilin and retinal growth cone filopodia by brain derived neurotrophic factor. *J. Neurobiol.* 66, 103–114. doi: 10.1002/neu.20204

Clarke, N. A., and Francis, P. T. (2005). Cholinergic and glutamatergic drugs in Alzheimer's disease therapy. *Expert Rev. Neurother.* 5, 671–682. doi: 10.1586/14737175.5.5.671

Commins, S., Cunningham, L., Harvey, D., and Walsh, D. (2003). Massed but not spaced training impairs spatial memory. *Behav. Brain Res.* 139, 215–223. doi: 10.1016/S0166-4328(02)00270-X

Cordoba Montoya, D. A., and Carrer, H. F. (1997). Estrogen facilitates induction of long term potentiation in the hippocampus of awake rats. *Brain Res.* 778, 430–438. doi: 10.1016/S0006-8993(97)01206-7

Cox, C. D., Rex, C. S., Palmer, L. C., Babayan, A. H., Pham, D. T., Corwin, S. D., et al. (2014). A map of LTP-related synaptic changes in dorsal hippocampus following unsupervised learning. *J. Neurosci.* 34, 3033–3041. doi: 10.1523/JNEUROSCI.4159-13.2014

Crystal, J. D., and Glanzman, D. L. (2013). A biological perspective on memory. *Curr. Biol.* 23, R728–731. doi: 10.1016/j.cub.2013.07.082

Dang, Y. H., Ma, X. C., Zhang, J. C., Ren, Q., Wu, J., Gao, C. G., et al. (2014). Targeting of NMDA receptors in the treatment of major depression. *Curr. Pharm. Des.* 19, 1–9. doi: 10.2174/1381612819666140110120435

Demeter, E., and Sarter, M. (2013). Leveraging the cortical cholinergic system to enhance attention. *Neuropharmacology* 64, 294–304. doi: 10.1016/j.neuropharm.2012.06.060

Demeter, E., Sarter, M., and Lustig, C. (2008). Rats and humans paying attention: cross-species task development for translational research. *Neuropsychology* 22, 787–799. doi: 10.1037/a0013712

Dickinson, J. A., Kew, J. N., and Wonnacott, S. (2008). Presynaptic alpha 7- and beta 2-containing nicotinic acetylcholine receptors modulate excitatory amino acid release from rat prefrontal cortex nerve terminals via distinct cellular mechanisms. *Mol. Pharmacol.* 74, 348–359. doi: 10.1124/mol.108.046623

Ding, Z. B., Wu, P., Luo, Y. X., Shi, H. S., Shen, H. W., Wang, S. J., et al. (2013). Region-specific role of Rac in nucleus accumbens core and basolateral amygdala in consolidation and reconsolidation of cocaine-associated cue memory in rats. *Psychopharmacology (Berl).* 228, 427–437. doi: 10.1007/s00213-013-3050-8

Dravid, S. M., Burger, P. B., Prakash, A., Gaballe, M. T., Yadav, R., Le, P., et al. (2010). Structural determinants of D-cycloserine efficacy at the NR1/NR2C NMDA receptors. *J. Neurosci.* 30, 2741–2754. doi: 10.1523/JNEUROSCI.5390-09.2010

Dunwiddie, T. V., and Haas, H. L. (1985). Adenosine increases synaptic facilitation in the *in vitro* rat hippocampus: evidence for a presynaptic site of action. *J. Physiol. (Lond).* 369, 365–377.

Eichenbaum, H., and Robitsek, R. J. (2009). Olfactory memory: a bridge between humans and animals in models of cognitive aging. *Ann. N.Y. Acad. Sci.* 1170, 658–663. doi: 10.1111/j.1749-6632.2009.04012.x

Fedulov, V., Rex, C. S., Simmons, D. A., Palmer, L., Gall, C. M., and Lynch, G. (2007). Evidence that long-term potentiation occurs within individual hippocampal synapses during learning. *J. Neurosci.* 27, 8031–8039. doi: 10.1523/JNEUROSCI.2003-07.2007

Flood, J. G., Morley, J. E., and Langhorn, T. H. (1992). Effect on memory processing by D-cycloserine, an agonist of the NMDA/glycine rceptor. *Eur. J. Pharmacol.* 221, 249–254. doi: 10.1016/0014-2999(92)90709-D

Foy, M. R., Xu, J., Xie, X., Brinton, R. D., Thompson, R. F., and Berger, T. W. (1999). 17beta-estradiol enhances NMDA receptor-mediated EPSPs and long-term potentiation. *J. Neurophysiol.* 81, 925–929.

Frey, U., and Morris, R. G. M. (1997). Synaptic tagging and long-term potentiation. *Nature* 385, 533–536. doi: 10.1038/385533a0

Frye, C. A., Duffy, C. K., and Walf, A. A. (2007). Estrogens and progestins enhance spatial learning of intact and ovariectomized rats in the object placement task. *Neurobiol. Learn. Mem.* 88, 208–216. doi: 10.1016/j.nlm.2007.04.003

Gall, C. M. (1992). Regulation of brain neurotrophin expression by physiological activity. *Trends Pharmacol. Sci.* 13, 401–403. doi: 10.1016/0165-6147(92)90123-N

Gioanni, Y., Rougeot, C., Clarke, P. B., Lepouse, C., Thierry, A. M., and Vidal, C. (1999). Nicotinic receptors in the rat prefrontal cortex: increase in glutamate release and facilitation of mediodorsal thalamo-cortical transmission. *Eur. J. Neurosci.* 11, 18–30. doi: 10.1046/j.1460-9568.1999.00403.x

Gold, P. E. (2008). Protein synthesis and memory. Introduction. *Neurobiol. Learn. Mem.* 89, 199–200. doi: 10.1016/j.nlm.2007.12.005

Gold, P. E., and Wrenn, S. M. (2012). Cycloheximide impairs and enhances memory depending on dose and footshock intensity. *Behav. Brain Res.* 233, 293–297. doi: 10.1016/j.bbr.2012.05.010

Granger, R., Deadwyler, S., Davis, M., Moskovitz, B., Kessler, M., Rogers, G., et al. (1996). Facilitation of glutamate receptors reverses an age-associated memory impairment in rats. *Synapse* 22, 332–337. doi: 10.1002/(SICI)1098-2396(199604)22:4%3C332::AID-SYN4%3E3.0.CO;2-C

Granger, R., Staubli, U., Davis, M., Perez, Y., Nilsson, L., Rogers, G. A., et al. (1993). A drug that facilitates glutamatergic transmission reduces exploratory activity and improves performance in a learning-dependent task. *Synapse* 15, 326–329. doi: 10.1002/syn.890150409

Grodstein, F. (2013). Hormone therapy in younger women and cognitive health. *JAMA Intern. Med.* 173, 1437–1438. doi: 10.1001/jamainternmed.2013.6827

Guzowski, J. F., Setlow, B., Wagner, E. K., and McGaugh, J. L. (2001). Experience-dependent gene expression in the rat hippocampus after spatial learning: a comparison of the immediate-early genes Arc, c-fos, and zif268. *J. Neurosci.* 21, 5089–5098.

Haditsch, U., Anderson, M. P., Freewoman, J., Cord, B., Babu, H., Brakebusch, C., et al. (2013). Neuronal Rac1 is required for learning-evoked neurogenesis. *J. Neurosci.* 33, 12229–12241. doi: 10.1523/JNEUROSCI.2939-12.2013

Hall, R. A., Kessler, M., Quan, A., Ambros-Ingerson, J., and Lynch, G. (1993). Cyclothiazide decreases [3H]AMPA binding to rat brain membranes: evidence that AMPA receptor desensitization increases agonist affinity. *Brain Res.* 628, 345–348. doi: 10.1016/0006-8993(93)90978-V

Hampson, R. E., Song, D., Opris, L., Santos, L. M., Shin, D. C., Gerhardt, G. A., et al. (2013). Facilitation of memory encoding in primate hippocampus by a neuroprosthesis that promotes task-specific neural firing. *J. Neural Eng.* 10, 066013. doi: 10.1088/1741-2560/10/6/066013

Hampson, R., Rogers, G., Lynch, G., and Deadwyler, S. (1998a). Facilitative effects of the ampakine CX516 on short-term memory in rats: enhancement of delayed-nonmatch-to-sample performance. *J. Neurosci.* 18, 2740–2747.

Hampson, R., Rogers, G., Lynch, G., and Deadwyler, S. (1998b). Facilitative effects of the ampakine CX516 on short-term memory in rats: correlations with hippocampal neuronal activity. *J. Neurosci.* 18, 2748–2763.

Hara, Y., Yuk, F., Puri, R., Janssen, W. G., Rapp, P. R., and Morrison, J. H. (2014). Presynaptic mitochondrial morphology in monkey prefrontal cortex correlates with working memory and is improved with estrogen treatment. *Proc. Natl. Acad. Sci. U.S.A.* 111, 486–491. doi: 10.1073/pnas.1311310110

Harvey, C. D., and Svoboda, K. (2007). Locally dynamic synaptic learning rules in pyramidal neuron dendrites. *Nature* 450, 1195–1200. doi: 10.1038/nature06416

Hasselmo, M. E. (2006). The role of acetylcholine in learning and memory. *Curr. Opin. Neurobiol.* 16, 710–715. doi: 10.1016/j.conb.2006.09.002

Hess, U. S., Whalen, S. P., Sandoval, L. M., Lynch, G., and Gall, C. M. (2003). Ampakines reduce methamphetamine-driven rotation and activate neocortex in a regionally selective fashion. *Neuroscience* 121, 509–521. doi: 10.1016/S0306-4522(03)00423-8

Hintzman, D. L. (1976). "Repetition and memory," in *The Psychology of Learning and Motivation,* ed G. H. Bower (New York, NY: Academic Press; Elsevier), 47–91.

Holmes, A. D., Copland, D. A., Silburn, P. A., and Chenery, H. J. (2011). Acute nicotine enhances strategy-based semantic processing in Parkinson's disease. *Int. J. Neuropsychopharmacol.* 14, 877–885. doi: 10.1017/S1461145710001665

Hosseini, R., Benton, D. C., Dunn, P. M., Jenkinson, D. H., and Moss, G. W. (2001). SK3 is an important component of K(+) channels mediating the after-hyperpolarization in cultured rat SCG neurones. *J. Physiol.* 535, 323–334. doi: 10.1111/j.1469-7793.2001.00323.x

Ikonen, S., and Riekkinen, P. Jr. (1999). Effects of apamin on memory processing of hippocampal-lesioned mice. *Eur. J. Pharmacol.* 382, 151–156. doi: 10.1016/S0014-2999(99)00616-0

Ingvar, M., Ambros-Ingerson, J., Davis, M., Granger, R., Kessler, M., Rogers, G. A., et al. (1997). Enhancement by an ampakine of memory encoding in humans. *Exp. Neurol.* 146, 553–559. doi: 10.1006/exnr.1997.6581

Isackson, P. J., Murray, K., Huntsman, M., and Gall, C. M. (1991). BDNF mRNA expression is increased in adult rat forebrain after limbic seizures: temporal patterns of induction distinct from NGF. *Neuron* 6, 937–948. doi: 10.1016/0896-6273(91)90234-Q

Jia, Y., Gall, C. M., and Lynch, G. (2010). Presynaptic BDNF promotes postsynaptic long-term potentiation in the dorsal striatum. *J. Neurosci.* 30, 14440–14445. doi: 10.1523/JNEUROSCI.3310-10.2010

Jiang, M., Peng, Q., Liu, X., Jin, J., Hou, Z., Zhang, J., et al. (2013). Small-molecule TrkB receptor agonists improve motor function and extend survival in a mouse model of Huntington's disease. *Hum. Mol. Genet.* 22, 2462–2470. doi: 10.1093/hmg/ddt098

Jin, R., Clark, S., Weeks, A. M., Dudman, J. T., Gouaux, E., and Partin, K. M. (2005). Mechanism of positive allosteric modulators acting on AMPA receptors. *J. Neurosci.* 25, 9027–9036. doi: 10.1523/JNEUROSCI.2567-05.2005

Jung, M. W., Larson, J., and Lynch, G. (1990). Long-term potentiation of monosynaptic EPSPs in rat piriform cortex *in vitro*. *Synapse* 6, 279–283. doi: 10.1002/syn.890060307

Katche, C., Bekinschtein, P., Slipczuk, L., Goldin, A., Izquierdo, I. A., Cammarota, M., et al. (2010). Delayed wave of c-Fos expression in the dorsal hippocampus involved specifically in persistence of long-term memory storage. *Proc. Natl. Acad. Sci. U.S.A.* 107, 349–354. doi: 10.1073/pnas.0912931107

Katche, C., Goldin, A., Gonzalez, C., Bekinschtein, P., and Medina, J. H. (2012). Maintenance of long-term memory storage is dependent on late posttraining Egr-1 expression. *Neurobiol. Learn. Mem.* 98, 220–227. doi: 10.1016/j.nlm.2012.08.001

Kessler, M., Baudry, M., and Lynch, G. (1989). Quinoxaline derivatives are high-affinity antagonists of the NMDA receptor-associated glycine sites. *Brain Res.* 489, 377–382. doi: 10.1016/0006-8993(89)90875-5

Klyuch, B. P., Dale, N., and Wall, M. J. (2012). Deletion of ecto-5′-nucleotidase (CD73) reveals direct action potential-dependent adenosine release. *J. Neurosci.* 32, 3842–3847. doi: 10.1523/JNEUROSCI.6052-11.2012

Kovalchuk, Y., Hanse, E., Kafitz, K. W., and Konnerth, A. (2002). Postsynaptic induction of BDNF-mediated long-term potentiation. *Science.* 295, 1729–1735. doi: 10.1126/science.1067766

Kowalczyk, T., Bocian, R., and Konopacki, J. (2013). The generation of theta rhythm in hippocampal formation maintained *in vitro*. *Eur. J. Neurosci.* 37, 679–699. doi: 10.1111/ejn.12091

Kramar, E. A., Babayan, A. H., Gavin, C. F., Cox, C. D., Jafari, M., Gall, C. M., et al. (2012b). Synaptic evidence for the efficacy of spaced learning. *Proc. Natl. Acad. Sci. U.S.A.* 109, 5121–5126. doi: 10.1073/pnas.1120700109

Kramar, E. A., Chen, L. Y., Brandon, N. J., Rex, C. S., Liu, F., Gall, C. M., et al. (2009). Cytoskeletal changes underlie estrogen's acute effects on synaptic transmission and plasticity. *J. Neurosci.* 29, 12982–12993. doi: 10.1523/JNEUROSCI.3059-09.2009

Kramar, E. A., Chen, L. Y., Lauterborn, J. C., Simmons, D. A., Gall, C. M., and Lynch, G. (2012a). BDNF upregulation rescues synaptic plasticity in middle-aged ovariectomized rats. *Neurobiol. Aging* 33, 708–719. doi: 10.1016/j.neurobiolaging.2010.06.008

Kramar, E. A., Lin, B., Lin, C. Y., Arai, A. C., Gall, C. M., and Lynch, G. (2004). A novel mechanism for the facilitation of theta-induced long-term potentiation by brain-derived neurotrophic factor. *J. Neurosci.* 24, 5151–5161. doi: 10.1523/JNEUROSCI.0800-04.2004

Kramar, E. A., Lin, B., Rex, C. S., Gall, C. M., and Lynch, G. (2006). Integrin-driven actin polymerization consolidates long-term potentiation. *Proc. Natl. Acad. Sci. U.S.A.* 103, 5579–5584. doi: 10.1073/pnas.0601354103

Kramar, E. A., and Lynch, G. (2003). Developmental and regional differences in the consolidation of long-term potentiation. *Neuroscience* 118, 387–398. doi: 10.1016/S0306-4522(02)00916-8

Labrie, V., and Roder, J. C. (2010). The involvement of the NMDA receptor d-serine/glycine site in the pathophysiology and treatment of schizophrenia. *Neurosci. Biobehav. Rev.* 34, 351–372. doi: 10.1016/j.neubiorev.2009.08.002

Larson, J., Wong, D., and Lynch, G. (1986). Patterned stimulation at the theta frequency is optimal for the induction of hippocampal long-term potentiation. *Brain Res.* 368, 347–350. doi: 10.1016/0006-8993(86)90579-2

Lauterborn, J. C., Lynch, G., Vanderklish, P., Arai, A., and Gall, C. M. (2000). Positive modulation of AMPA receptors increases neurotrophin expression by hippocampal and cortical neurons. *J. Neurosci.* 20, 8–21.

Lee, K., Oliver, M., Schottler, F., Creager, R., and Lynch, G. (1979). Ultrastructural effects of repetitive synaptic stimulation in the hippocampal slice preparation: a preliminary report. *Exp. Neurol.* 65, 478–480. doi: 10.1016/0014-4886(79)90114-6

Lee, K., Schottler, F., Oliver, M., and Lynch, G. (1980). Brief bursts of high-frequency stimulation produce two types of structural changes in rat hippocampus. *J. Neurophysiol.* 44, 247–258.

Lin, B., Kramar, E. A., Bi, X., Brucher, F. A., Gall, C. M., and Lynch, G. (2005). Theta stimulation polymerizes actin in dendritic spines of hippocampus. *J. Neurosci.* 25, 2062–2069. doi: 10.1523/JNEUROSCI.4283-04.2005

Liu, F., Day, M., Muniz, L. C., Bitran, D., Arias, R., Revilla-Sanchez, R., et al. (2008). Activation of estrogen receptor-beta regulates hippocampal synaptic plasticity and improves memory. *Nat. Neurosci.* 11, 334–343. doi: 10.1038/nn2057

Lynch, G. (1998). Memory and the brain: unexpected chemistries and a new pharmacology. *Neurobiol. Learn. Mem.* 70, 82–100. doi: 10.1006/nlme.1998.3840

Lynch, G. (2004a). AMPA receptor modulators as cognitive enhancers. *Curr. Opin. Pharmacol.* 4, 4–11. doi: 10.1016/j.coph.2003.09.009

Lynch, G., and Gall, C. M. (2013). Mechanism based approaches for rescuing and enhancing cognition. *Front. Neurosci.* 7:143. doi: 10.3389/fnins.2013.00143

Lynch, G., Kramar, E. A., Babayan, A. H., Rumbaugh, G., and Gall, C. M. (2013). Differences between synaptic plasticity thresholds result in new timing rules for maximizing long-term potentiation. *Neuropharmacology* 64, 27–36. doi: 10.1016/j.neuropharm.2012.07.006

Lynch, G., Palmer, L. C., and Gall, C. M. (2011). The likelihood of cognitive enhancement. *Pharmacol. Biochem. Behav.* 99, 116–129. doi: 10.1016/j.pbb.2010.12.024

Lynch, M. A. (2004b). Long-term potentiation and memory. *Physiol. Rev.* 84, 87–136. doi: 10.1152/physrev.00014.2003

Madau, P., Clark, A. G., Neale, S. A., Smith, L., Hamilton, N., Thompson, F., et al. and Lambert, J. J. (2009). "Program no. 613.2. Org 1, Org 2, and Org 3 potentiate NMDA-receptor mediated responses *in vitro*," in *Society for Neuroscience Annual Meeting Planner* (Chicago, IL: Society for Neuroscience).

Matsuzaki, M., Honkura, N., Ellis-Davies, G. C., and Kasai, H. (2004). Structural basis of long-term potentiation in single dendritic spines. *Nature.* 429, 761–766. doi: 10.1038/nature02617

McQuown, S. C., Barrett, R. M., Matheos, D. P., Post, R. J., Rogge, G. A., Alenghat, T., et al. (2011). HDAC3 is a critical negative regulator of long-term memory formation. *J. Neurosci.* 31, 764–774. doi: 10.1523/JNEUROSCI.5052-10.2011

Monaghan, D. T., Irvine, M. W., Costa, B. M., Fang, G., and Jane, D. E. (2012). Pharmacological modulation of NMDA receptor activity and the advent of negative and positive allosteric modulators. *Neurochem. Int.* 61, 581–592. doi: 10.1016/j.neuint.2012.01.004

Morris, R. G. (2003). Long-term potentiation and memory. *Philos. Trans. R. Soc. Lond. B Biol. Sci.* 358, 643–647. doi: 10.1098/rstb.2002.1230

Noetzli, M., and Eap, C. B. (2013). Pharmacodynamic, pharmacokinetic and pharmacogenetic aspects of drugs used in the treatment of Alzheimer's disease. *Clin. Pharmacokinet.* 52, 225–241. doi: 10.1007/s40262-013-0038-9

Normann, C., and Berger, M. (2008). Neuroenhancement: status quo and perspectives. *Eur. Arch. Psychiatry Clin. Neurosci.* 258(Suppl. 5), 110–114. doi: 10.1007/s00406-008-5022-2

Oliver, M. W., Kessler, M., Larson, J., Schottler, F., and Lynch, G. (1990). Glycine site associated with the NMDA receptor modulates long-term potentation. *Synapse* 5, 265–270. doi: 10.1002/syn.890050403

Olpe, H. R., Klebs, K., Kung, E., Campiche, P., Glatt, A., Ortmann, R., et al. (1987). Cholinomimetics induce theta rhythm and reduce hippocampal pyramidal cell excitability. *Eur. J. Pharmacol.* 142, 275–283. doi: 10.1016/0014-2999(87)90117-8

Ooishi, Y., Kawato, S., Hojo, Y., Hatanaka, Y., Higo, S., Murakami, G., et al. (2012). Modulation of synaptic plasticity in the hippocampus by hippocampus-derived estrogen and androgen. *J. Steroid Biochem. Mol. Biol.* 131, 37–51. doi: 10.1016/j.jsbmb.2011.10.004

Otto, T., Eichenbaum, H., Wiener, S. I., and Wible, C. G. (1991). Learning-related patterns of CA1 spike trains parallel stimulation parameters optimal for inducing hippocampal long-term potentiation. *Hippocampus* 1, 181–192. doi: 10.1002/hipo.450010206

Paul, S. M., Doherty, J. J., Robichaud, A. J., Belfort, G. M., Chow, B. Y., Hammond, R. S., et al. (2013). The major brain cholesterol metabolite 24(s)-hydroxycholesterol is a potent allosteric modulator of n-methyl-d-aspartate receptors. *J. Neurosci.* 33, 17290–17300. doi: 10.1523/JNEUROSCI.2619-13.2013

Perlmutter, L. S., Siman, R., Gall, C., Seubert, P., Baudry, M., and Lynch, G. (1988). The ultrastructural localization of calcium-activated protease 'calpain' in rat brain. *Synapse* 2, 79–88. doi: 10.1002/syn.890020111

Peters, J., and De Vries, T. J. (2013). D-cycloserine administration directly to infralimbic medial prefrontal cortex enhances extinction memory in sucrose-seeking animals. *Neuroscience* 230, 24–30. doi: 10.1016/j.neuroscience.2012.11.004

Plath, N., Ohana, O., Dammermann, B., Errington, M. L., Schmitz, D., Gross, C., et al. (2006). Arc/Arg3.1 is essential for the consolidation of synaptic plasticity and memories. *Neuron* 52, 437–444. doi: 10.1016/j.neuron.2006.08.024

Porrino, L., Daunais, J., Rogers, G., Hampson, R., and Deadwyler, S. (2005). Facilitation of task performance and removal of the effects of sleep deprivation by an ampakine (CX717) in nonhuman primates. *PLoS Biol.* 3:e299. doi: 10.1371/journal.pbio.0030299

Rex, C. S., Chen, L. Y., Sharma, A., Liu, J., Babayan, A. H., Gall, C. M., et al. (2009). Different Rho GTPase-dependent signaling pathways initiate sequential steps in the consolidation of long-term potentiation. *J. Cell Biol.* 186, 85–97. doi: 10.1083/jcb.200901084

Rex, C. S., Gavin, C. F., Rubio, M. D., Kramar, E. A., Chen, L. Y., Jia, Y., et al. (2010). Myosin IIb regulates actin dynamics during synaptic plasticity and memory formation. *Neuron.* 67, 603–617. doi: 10.1016/j.neuron.2010.07.016

Rex, C. S., Kramar, E. A., Colgin, L. L., Lin, B., Gall, C. M., and Lynch, G. (2005). Long-term potentiation is impaired in middle-aged rats: regional specificity and reversal by adenosine receptor antagonists. *J. Neurosci.* 25, 5956–5966. doi: 10.1523/JNEUROSCI.0880-05.2005

Rex, C. S., Lauterborn, J. C., Lin, C. Y., Kramar, E. A., Rogers, G. A., Gall, C. M., et al. (2006). Restoration of long-term potentiation in middle-aged hippocampus after induction of brain-derived neurotrophic factor. *J. Neurophysiol.* 96, 677–685. doi: 10.1152/jn.00336.2006

Rex, C. S., Lin, C. Y., Kramar, E. A., Chen, L. Y., Gall, C. M., and Lynch, G. (2007). Brain-derived neurotrophic factor promotes long-term potentiation-related cytoskeletal changes in adult hippocampus. *J. Neurosci.* 27, 3017–3029. doi: 10.1523/JNEUROSCI.4037-06.2007

Rioult-Pedotti, M. S., Friedman, D., and Donoghue, J. P. (2000). Learning-induced LTP in neocortex. *Science* 290, 533–536. doi: 10.1126/science.290.5491.533

Roman, F., Staubli, U., and Lynch, G. (1987). Evidence for synaptic potentiation in a cortical network during learning. *Brain Res.* 418, 221–226. doi: 10.1016/0006-8993(87)90089-8

Routtenberg, A. (2008). The substrate for long-lasting memory: if not protein synthesis, then what? *Neurobiol. Learn. Mem.* 89, 225–233. doi: 10.1016/j.nlm.2007.10.012

Sarter, M., Parikh, V., and Howe, W. M. (2009). nAChR agonist-induced cognition enhancement: integration of cognitive and neuronal mechanisms. *Biochem. Pharmacol.* 78, 658–667. doi: 10.1016/j.bcp.2009.04.019

Schmid, D. A., Yang, T., Ogier, M., Adams, I., Mirakhur, Y., Wang, Q., et al. (2012). A TrkB small molecule partial agonist rescues TrkB phosphorylation deficits and improves respiratory function in a mouse model of Rett syndrome. *J. Neurosci.* 32, 1803–1810. doi: 10.1523/JNEUROSCI.0865-11.2012

Schmitz, D., Mellor, J., Breustedt, J., and Nicoll, R. A. (2003). Presynaptic kainate receptors impart an associative property to hippocampal mossy fiber long-term potentiation. *Nat. Neurosci.* 6, 1058–1063. doi: 10.1038/nn1116

Seese, R. R., Babayan, A. H., Katz, A. M., Cox, C. D., Lauterborn, J. C., Lynch, G., et al. (2012). LTP induction translocates cortactin at distant synapses in wild-type but not Fmr1 knock-out mice. *J. Neurosci.* 32, 7403–7413. doi: 10.1523/JNEUROSCI.0968-12.2012

Seese, R. R., Chen, L. Y., Cox, C. D., Schulz, D., Babayan, A. H., Bunney, W. E., et al. (2013). Synaptic abnormalities in the infralimbic cortex of a model of congenital depression. *J. Neurosci.* 33, 13441–13448. doi: 10.1523/JNEUROSCI.2434-13.2013

Sheinin, A., Shavit, S., and Benveniste, M. (2001). Subunit specificity and mechanism of action of NMDA partial agonist D-cycloserine. *Neuropharmacology* 41, 151–158. doi: 10.1016/S0028-3908(01)00073-9

Shires, K. L., Da Silva, B. M., Hawthorne, J. P., Morris, R. G. M., and Martin, S. J. (2012). Synaptic tagging and capture in the living rat. *Nature Comm.* 3:1246. doi: 10.1038/ncomms2250

Shors, T. J., Servatius, R. J., Thompson, R. F., Rogers, G., and Lynch, G. (1995). Enhanced glutamatergic neurotransmission facilitates classical conditioning in the freely-moving rat. *Neurosci. Lett.* 186, 153–156. doi: 10.1016/0304-3940(95)11309-K

Simmons, D. A., Belichenko, N. P., Yang, T., Condon, C., Monbureau, M., Shamloo, M., et al. (2013). A small molecule TrkB ligand reduces motor impairment and neuropathology in R6/2 and BACHD mouse models of Huntington's disease. *J. Neurosci.* 33, 18712–18727. doi: 10.1523/JNEUROSCI.1310-13.2013

Simmons, D. A., Mehta, R. A., Lauterborn, J. C., Gall, C. M., and Lynch, G. (2011). Brief ampakine treatments slow the progression of Huntington's disease phenotypes in R6/2 mice. *Neurobiol. Dis.* 41, 436–444. doi: 10.1016/j.nbd.2010.10.015

Simmons, D. A., Rex, C. S., Palmer, L., Pandyarajan, V., Fedulov, V., Gall, C. M., et al. (2009). Up-regulating BDNF with an ampakine rescues synaptic plasticity and memory in Huntington's disease knockin mice. *Proc. Natl. Acad. Sci. U.S.A.* 106, 4906–4911. doi: 10.1073/pnas.0811228106

Sirvio, J., Larson, J., Quach, C. N., Rogers, G. A., and Lynch, G. (1996). Effects of pharmacologically facilitating glutamatergic transmission in the trisynaptic intrahippocampal circuit. *Neuroscience* 74, 1025–1035. doi: 10.1016/0306-4522(96)00170-4

Snider, J., Plank, M., Lynch, G., Halgren, E., and Poizner, H. (2013). Human cortical theta during free exploration encodes space and predicts subsequent memory. *J. Neurosci.* 33, 15056–15068. doi: 10.1523/JNEUROSCI.0268-13.2013

Staubli, U. (1992). A peculiar form of potentiation in mossy fiber synapses. *Epilepsy Res. Suppl.* 7, 151–157.

Staubli, U., and Lynch, G. (1987). Stable hippocampal long-term potentiation elicited by 'theta' pattern stimulation. *Brain Res.* 435, 227–234. doi: 10.1016/0006-8993(87)91605-2

Staubli, U., Rogers, G., and Lynch, G. (1994). Facilitation of glutamate receptors enhances memory. *Proc. Natl. Acad. Sci. U.S.A.* 91, 777–781. doi: 10.1073/pnas.91.2.777

Staubli, U., and Xu, F. B. (1995). Effects of 5-HT3 receptor antagonism on hippocampal theta rhythm, memory, and LTP induction in the freely moving rat. *J. Neurosci.* 15, 2445–2452.

Stefanko, D. P., Barrett, R. M., Ly, A. R., Reolon, G. K., and Wood, M. A. (2009). Modulation of long-term memory for object recognition via HDAC inhibition. *Proc. Natl. Acad. Sci. U.S.A.* 106, 9447–9452. doi: 10.1073/pnas.0903964106

Stephan, H., Frahm, H., and Baron, G. (1981). New and revised data on volumes of brain structures in insectivores and primates. *Folia Primatol.* 35, 1–29. doi: 10.1159/000155963

Sugrue, L. P., Corrado, G. S., and Newsome, W. T. (2005). Choosing the greater of two goods: neural currencies for valuation and decision making. *Nat. Rev. Neurosci.* 6, 363–375. doi: 10.1038/nrn1666

Sun, Y., Olson, R., Horning, M., Armstrong, N., Mayer, M., and Gouaux, E. (2002). Mechanism of glutamate receptor desensitization. *Nature* 417, 245–253. doi: 10.1038/417245a

Swanson, L. W. (1995). Mapping the human brain: past, present, and future. *Trends Neurosci.* 18, 471–474. doi: 10.1016/0166-2236(95)92766-J

Thompson, R. F., Berger, T. W., Cegavske, C. F., Patterson, M. M., Roemer, R. A., Teyler, T. J., et al. (1976). The search for the engram. *Am. Psychol.* 31, 209–226. doi: 10.1037/0003-066X.31.3.209

Thompson, R. F., and Krupa, D. J. (1994). Organization of memory traces in the mammalian brain. *Ann. Rev. Neurosci.* 17, 519–549. doi: 10.1146/annurev.ne.17.030194.002511

Tsai, G. E., Falk, W. E., Gunther, J., and Coyle, J. T. (1999). Improved cognition in Alzheimer's disease with sort-term D-cycloserine treatment. *Am. J. Psychiatry* 156, 467–469.

Tsunada, J., and Sawaguchi, T. (2012). Neuronal categorization and discrimination of social behaviors in primate prefrontal cortex. *PLoS ONE* 7:e52610. doi: 10.1371/journal.pone.0052610

Tully, T., Bourtchouladze, R., Scott, R., and Tallman, J. (2003). Targeting the CREB pathway for memory enhancers. *Nat. Rev. Drug Discov.* 2, 267–277. doi: 10.1038/nrd1061

Turner, D. C., Clark, L., Pomarol-Clotet, E., McKenna, P., Robbins, T. W., and Sahakian, B. J. (2004). Modafinil improves cognition and attentional set shifting in patients with chronic schizophrenia. *Neuropsychopharmacology* 29, 1363–1373. doi: 10.1038/sj.npp.1300457

Vertes, R. P. (2005). Hippocampal theta rhythm: a tag for short-term memory. *Hippocampus.* 15, 923–935. doi: 10.1002/hipo.20118

Vick, K. A. T., Guidi, M., and Stackman, R. W. Jr. (2010). *In vivo* pharmacological manipulation of small conductance Ca(2+)-activated K(+) channels influences motor behavior, object memory and fear conditioning. *Neuropharmacology* 58, 650–659. doi: 10.1016/j.neuropharm.2009.11.008

Vierk, R., Glassmeier, G., Zhou, L., Brandt, N., Fester, L., Dudzinski, D., et al. (2012). Aromatase inhibition abolishes LTP generation in female but not in male mice. *J. Neurosci.* 32, 8116–8126. doi: 10.1523/JNEUROSCI.5319-11.2012

Wall, M. J., and Dale, N. (2013). Neuronal transporter and astrocytic ATP exocytosis underlie activity-dependent adenosine release in the hippocampus. *J. Physiol.* 591, 3853–3871. doi: 10.1113/jphysiol.2013.253450

Whitlock, J. R., Heynen, A. J., Shuler, M. G., and Bear, M. F. (2006). Learning induces long-term potentiation in the hippocampus. *Science* 313, 1093–1097. doi: 10.1126/science.1128134

Wonnacott, S. (1997). Presynaptic nicotinic ACh receptors. *Trends Neurosci.* 20, 92–98. doi: 10.1016/S0166-2236(96)10073-4

Wu, F. S., Gibbs, T. T., and Farb, D. H. (1991). Pregnenolone sulfate: a positive allosteric modulator at the n-methyl-d-aspartate receptor. *Mol. Pharmacol.* 40, 333–336.

Zeeb, F. D., Robbins, T. W., and Winstanley, C. A. (2009). Serotonergic and dopaminergic modulation of gambling behavior as assessed using a novel rat gambling task. *Neuropsychopharmacology* 34, 2329–2343. doi: 10.1038/npp.2009.62

12

Understanding entangled cerebral networks: a prerequisite for restoring brain function with brain-computer interfaces

Emmanuel Mandonnet[1,2,3] and Hugues Duffau[4,5]*

[1] Department of Neurosurgery, Hôpital Lariboisière, Paris, France
[2] Department of Neurosurgery, Université Paris Diderot, Paris, France
[3] IMNC, UMR 8165, Orsay, France
[4] Department of Neurosurgery, Gui de Chauliac Hospital, Montpellier University Medical Center, Montpellier, France
[5] Team "Plasticity of Central Nervous System, Stem Cells and Glial Tumors," INSERM U1051, Institute for Neuroscience of Montpellier, Montpellier University Medical Center, Montpellier, France

Edited by:
Mikhail Lebedev, Duke University, USA

Reviewed by:
Yoshio Sakurai, Kyoto University, Japan
Philip Kennedy, Neural Signals Inc., USA

***Correspondence:**
Hugues Duffau, Department of Neurosurgery, Gui de Chauliac Hospital, Montpellier University Medical Center, 80 Av. Augustin Fliche, 34295 Montpellier, France
e-mail: h-duffau@chu-montpellier.fr

Historically, cerebral processing has been conceptualized as a framework based on statically localized functions. However, a growing amount of evidence supports a hodotopical (delocalized) and flexible organization. A number of studies have reported absence of a permanent neurological deficit after massive surgical resections of eloquent brain tissue. These results highlight the tremendous plastic potential of the brain. Understanding anatomo-functional correlates underlying this cerebral reorganization is a prerequisite to restore brain functions through brain-computer interfaces (BCIs) in patients with cerebral diseases, or even to potentiate brain functions in healthy individuals. Here, we review current knowledge of neural networks that could be utilized in the BCIs that enable movements and language. To this end, intraoperative electrical stimulation in awake patients provides valuable information on the cerebral functional maps, their connectomics and plasticity. Overall, these studies indicate that the complex cerebral circuitry that underpins interactions between action, cognition and behavior should be throughly investigated before progress in BCI approaches can be achieved.

Keywords: brain networks, movement, language, anatomo-functional connectivity, functional restoration, brain-computer interface

INTRODUCTION

Technological advances in electrodes design have opened a number of new possibilities for brain-computer interfaces (BCIs) that decode large-scale neuronal activity (Lebedev and Nicolelis, 2006). It is now feasible to simultaneously record single-unit activity of hundreds of brain neurons, or record local field potentials (LFPs) from several relatively small brain areas. However, these technological achievements are insufficient for a BCI that restores a specific function, unless the *network* of brain areas involved in that function is well understood.

Although localizationist theories of brain function have been influential in the past, it is becoming increasingly clear that they are, out of date and of little use for BCIs (Nicolelis and Lebedev, 2009). Instead of assigning a fixed function to each discrete brain area, the current hodotopical and plastic view on cerebral organization states that brain functions are subserved by multiple cortical areas. These densely areas, interconnected by white matter pathways, work together rather than representing isolated processing units, and constitute a functional network.

Many fundamental issues of such functional networks are under debate. For example, is it possible to subdivide a cognitive task into separate elementary subtasks (performed successively or simultaneously), each associated with a spatially distinct subnetwork? Such spatial separability is supported by the observation of dissociation and double dissociations in patients with focal lesions (Shadmehr and Krakauer, 2008). Direct electrical stimulation (DES) is a powerful methodology for the investigation of spatial separability. For this purpose, DES is applied in awake subjects to induce transient deficits in particular components of cognitive tasks. Here, we review DES studies of motor and language functions and we discuss the relevance of these results to BCIs.

NETWORKS FOR VOLUNTARY MOVEMENTS

Since the seminal work of Penfield (Penfield and Bolchey, 1937), it has been well known that, under local anesthesia, cortical stimulation of the precentral gyrus evokes movements on the

Abbreviations: EMG, electromyogram; BCI, brain computer interface; SMA, supplementary motor area; CMAr, rostral cingulate motor area; CMAv, ventral cingulate motor area; CMAd, dorsal cingulate motor area; PMd, premotor dorsal; PMv, premotor ventral; RCZa, anterior rostral cingulate zone; RCZp, posterior rostral cingulate zone; CCZ, caudal cingulate zone; NMA, negative motor area; IFG, inferior frontal gyrus; VAC, vertical anterior commissure; BMMP, bimanual modulatory motor pathway; DES, direct electrical stimulation; PPTT, pyramid palm tree test; GPi, internal globus pallidum; GPe, external globus pallidum; STN, subthalamic nucleus; SLF, superior longitudinal fasciculus; IFOF, inferior fronto-occipital fasciculus; BCBI, brain-computer-brain interface; BCIm, multiple brain computer interface; DBS, deep brain stimulation; vSMG, ventral supramarginal gyrus.

contra-lateral side of the body. This method reveals a cortical somatotopic map of the body, which is often called a "homunculus". A similar homunculus can be reconstructed from cortical lesion studies. Based on these results, many neurological textbooks have adopted a simplified model of brain function and connectivity, which maps each brain area to a body part and assigns it a fixed function. For example, motor functions are assigned to an area located in the precentral gyrus and called the primary motor cortex (M1). M1 is considered as the lowest level of cortical motor hierarchy because all cortical motor signals converge. M1 then utilizes its somatotopic map to issue commands to spinal motoneurons, to which it is connected through the corticospinal tract, as well as less direct projections relayed by subcortical nuclei.

This model of M1 function is often mimicked by BCIs (Lebedev and Nicolelis, 2006). For example, Hochberg and his colleagues employed a 96-channel microelectrode array implanted in M1 of tetraplegic patients to interface cortical activity and a robotic arm (Hochberg et al., 2012). This study provided an important proof-of-concept demonstration, but the patients were unable to achieve good accuracy in the control of the robotic arm. This observation suggested that recording from M1 only may not be sufficient to capture all details of voluntary movements. One way to improve the performance of such neural prosthesis would be to implant multiple brain areas with recording arrays (BCIm for multiple brain computer interface), coding for distinct subparts of intentional movement, instead of just M1 (Lebedev and Nicolelis, 2006; Nicolelis and Lebedev, 2009). The performance would improve because neuronal signals provided by multiple areas better capture a diversity of neuronal mechanisms involved in programming and execution of voluntary movements. Hence, there is a growing understanding that BCIs may benefit from the recordings of large-scale motor networks and the utilization of such networks' principles.

Important insights on the mechanisms of brain motor networks are provided by DES studies in humans. DES studies are conducted under three types of conditions: (i) pre-operative mapping with 50–60 Hz DES in pharmacoresistant epileptic patients; (ii) 60 Hz bipolar DES of gray and white matter during glioma surgery; and (iii) high-frequency deep brain stimulation (DBS) utilized for treatment of motor and psychiatric disorders. Motor responses can be evoked by DES of various cortical sites. Historically, Penfield and Bolchey (1937) reported that motor responses were not exclusively evoked from the precentral gyrus. For instance, they observed motor responses for about 25% of stimulated locations in the postcentral gyrus. Furthermore, they found that somatosensory responses were not localized to the postcentral gyrus either. They observed sensory responses in 25% of precentral recordings. Thus, these early experiments already questioned the segregation of sensory and motor functions in cortical areas traditionally believed to be purely motor or purely sensory. These results were somehow forgotten, but decisively rediscovered in 1996 (Nii et al., 1996). The functional significance of the mosaic pattern of sensory and motor representations within the primary motor and sensory areas remains to be elucidated.

Adding more sophistication to the function of somatosensory cortex, neurons in the primary motor and sensory areas exhibited responses to visual stimuli (Shokur et al., 2013). One influential theory explains such cross-modal responses in terms of a system of mirror neuron, first described in the premotor cortex of non-human primates and then in humans (Rizzolatti and Craighero, 2004). Mirror neurons respond to actions performed by a different person. Even in M1, neurons respond when a subject watches movement performed by somebody else (Vigneswaran et al., 2013). Despite these neurons having corticospinal projecting axons (pyramidal tract neurons), these M1 modulations do not evoke EMGs during observation only. This is possibly due to the fact that activation of M1 mirror neurons is accompanied by an inhibition of unwanted movement, for example unwanted imitation of the observed movements. Overall, these results indicate that M1 is not exclusively dedicated to motor execution. It has been suggested that M1 neurons that modulate their activity without producing overt movements can be utilized in BCIs (Schieber, 2011).

Apart from M1, motor responses can be evoked by DES applied to premotor areas. Premotor areas have direct connections to M1 *and* to the spinal cord (Dum and Strick, 1991). Premotor areas include four mesial (SMA proper, CMAr, CMAv, CMAd) and two lateral (PMd, PMv) areas (Dum and Strick, 2002). In humans, homologs of the mesial areas have been identified, and named SMA proper, RCZa, RCZp, and CCZ (Picard and Strick, 2001). DES of premotor areas induces movements, sometimes with complex pattern (Fried et al., 1991; Lim et al., 1996; Chassagnon et al., 2008; Basha et al., 2013).

The homologs of PMd and PMv are not clearly defined in humans, and stimulation of these areas often results in movement suppressions, called negative motor effects (Lüders et al., 1995; Mikuni et al., 2006). In negative motor areas (NMA), DES suppresses an ongoing movement on the contralateral side of the body. Such suppression can occur with or without associated speech arrest, and does not result in a loss of consciousness. As recently reviewed (Filevich et al., 2012), cortical NMA in humans have two epicenters: the pre-SMA (bilaterally) and the posterior part of the inferior frontal gyrus (right predominance). Additionally, several studies reported NMAs in PMd and PMv (Mikuni et al., 2006).

The physiological role of cortical NMAs is still debated. The classical interpretation is that 60 Hz stimulation may disturb neuronal networks responsible for sustained execution of movements. In this view, cortical NMAs would sustain the coding of (positive) motor programs that become jammed by DES. An alternative explanation is that these NMAs are physiologically involved in the inhibition of motor action; therefore their activation by DES inhibits movements. Note that pre-SMA and the IFG are not considered as premotor areas, meaning that this inhibition is probably not processed through direct projections to the spinal cord. We suggest that both interpretations are valid. In particular, the negative motor effect commonly elicited by the stimulation of the foot of the pre-central gyrus is likely due to a perturbation in the coding of the motor programs. This area is located just above the sylvian fissure, where Rizzolatti and Craighero reported the mirror neuron area of the ventral premotor cortex (vPMC; Rizzolatti and Craighero, 2004), as suggested in Mikuni et al. (2006). Because of the connections with parietal areas

(Matsumoto et al., 2012, 2007), this site is an ideal candidate for the storage of *state estimation* (see the model of optimal feedback control, Shadmehr and Krakauer (2008)). Hence, 60 Hz signals can be viewed as an increase of the noise in this system, causing motor action to stop (by some yet undiscovered mechanism). On the other hand, there is also evidence that pre-SMA and IFG stimulation effect could be mediated by a direct activation of an inhibiting area (Filevich et al., 2012). In support of such dual mechanism, resection of vPMC induces definitive articulatory deficits if the underlying connectivity is not preserved (van Geemen et al., 2014), while no permanent deficits are observed following a resection of pre-SMA and right IFG.

We next ask how is DES-induced inhibition enacted: is there a decrease in the firing of M1 neurons or is there an increase in the firing in some inhibitory circuits? These details have been recently clarified using white matter stimulation in awake patients undergoing glioma resection. Stimulation within the depth of the posterior SMA and posterior part of middle frontal gyrus (dorsal premotor areas)—more or less at the level of the VAC line in a sagittal plane—stopped an on-going movement (Schucht et al., 2013). It was proposed that the effect was mediated by a direct activation of corticospinal neurons that inhibit motoneurons at the level of a spinal circuitry. This mechanism should not come as a surprise because cortical control over fine movements requires both supra-spinal excitatory and inhibitory modulation of the spinal motoneurons (Filevich et al., 2012). The cortical origin of these fibers fits well with the depth of the pre-central sulcus.

A second pathway, distinct from the previous one, has been shown to generate a specific disruption of bimanual movements, performed either in phase or in anti-phase (Rech et al., 2014). The spatial distribution of the corresponding DES sites is very close to the one cited above for unilateral negative motor responses. They lie close to the VAC line in the sagittal plane and could take their origin in the caudal cingulate zone or in the depth of the pre-central sulcus, and running towards the head of caudate nucleus and the anterior arm of internal capsule (Rech et al., 2014). Based on these studies, the concept of bimanual modulatory motor pathway was introduced, and it was suggested that the stimulated fibers could belong to the subcallosal fasciculus (Kinoshita et al., 2012), also called frontal aslant tract (Catani et al., 2012). But again, it remains currently speculative whether this bilateral inhibitory effect should be interpreted as noise that perturbs the normal functioning of the BMMP or whether DES triggers the physiological inhibitory mechanism of the BMMP.

In addition to DES studies, similar questions have been regarding the action of DBS, stimulation approach widely used to treat movement disorders, such as Parkinson's disease. Here, computer modeling recently provided new insights. In these models, motor signs in parkinsonism are presumed to arise from the *bursting* activity of the GPi, which exerts an inhibitory effect onto the thalamus and compromises the fidelity of thalamocortical relay cells. This mechanism agrees with the recent suggestion that the thalamus is not simply a relay station but rather an active filter of the signals passing through cortico-thalamo-cortical loops, whose function is modulated by the basal ganglia output (Sherman and Guillery, 2011; Crosson, 2013). Computational simulations of the GPe-STN-GPi direct and indirect pathways showed that DBS can restore the thalamocortical transmission through *tonic* inhibition of the thalamocortical cells by GPi inputs, due to the prevention of the low-threshold calcium rebound bursts (Rubin and Terman, 2004; Guo et al., 2008; Rubin et al., 2012). Note that the pathological state is evoked by the *pattern* of activity within the network and not simply an average spiking neuronal rate in an area that correlates with the pathological state. Overall, computer simulation proved to be very helpful for better understanding of such networks.

In summary, we have a relatively good understanding of the motor system in non-human primates, but know very little about the organization and function of motor system in humans. Inferences from non-humans studies do not always hold true in humans. However, there is a growing understanding that motor systems in all primates function as distributed network of areas, each involved in multiple levels of motor control, rather than a collection of areas with specialized functions. Interestingly, DES studies in awake neurosurgical patients have provided important information on the organization of motor system in humans. Additional insights have been provided by computer modeling. We suggest that further research on the motor system in humans will be very beneficial for BCIs.

LANGUAGE NETWORKS

Unraveling the complex neural mechanisms of language is a real challenge. This challenge is even more difficult than the one for motor functions, because non-human primates cannot serve as a model. For many years, our knowledge came from the observations on speech deficits caused by brain lesions. These studies lead to the well-known model that describes a center of speech production (Broca's area), a center of speech comprehension (Wernicke's area), and a putative link between them made by the arcuate fasciculus. Following this model, the first BCI for language function utilized an array of microelectrodes implanted in the speech motor cortex (Kennedy et al., 2011).

Advances in non-invasive functional neuroimaging greatly enhanced our understanding of brain networks involved in language. It is now well recognized that distinct networks can be identified for different language aspects. In particular, a dual stream model of language has been proposed (Hickok and Poeppel, 2007). In this model, a left-lateralized dorsal stream is in charge of articulatory and phonological processes, whereas a bilateral ventral stream plays a central role in semantics. Observations of speech disturbances induced by axonal DES offer a unique tool to validate the model and to refine its axonal anatomical correlates. Indeed, errors induced by DES during a simple picture naming task, in awake patients operated for a glioma, allow to detect which subnetwork is transiently knocked out by the stimulation (Mandonnet et al., 2010). In these experiments, a speech therapist reports on-line the types of errors, e.g., dys- or anarthria, phonemic paraphasia, semantic paraphasia (Duffau et al., 2014). Dysarthria was observed when stimulating the opercular fronto-parietal loop that corresponds to the most lateral branch of superior longitudinal fasciculus (SLF III; Duffau et al., 2003). Phonemic paraphasia were elicited by stimulation of the arcuate branch of the SLF (Maldonado et al., 2011). Finally, semantic paraphasias were caused by stimulation of the inferior fronto-occipital fasiculus (IFOF; Duffau et al., 2005). On top of that, supramodal semantic abilities can also be tested by adding a semantic association test (PPTT) in the set of intraoperative tasks (Gatignol et al., 2004). Double dissociation patterns can be evidenced by alternating the picture naming test with the PPTT: during stimulation of deepest part of the IFOF, the patient can name the picture without being able to answer the PPTT, and conversely, during stimulation of a more superficial part of the IFOF, the patient has anomia while performing correctly the PPTT (Duffau et al., 2013; Moritz-Gasser et al., 2013). This disruption of semantic association can be viewed in the broader framework of an impairment of the noetic consciousness (Moritz-Gasser et al., 2013). Last but not least, the contextual rule linked to a given task is equally important. For example, the picture naming is not a *per-se* task: one could ask the patient to tell the color of the item, or to categorize items as animate/inanimate. The anatomical correlates of this contextual role and its interplay with the networks mentioned above still have to be discovered, although one can reasonably assume a major role of the deep gray nuclei (Gil Robles et al., 2005) and thalamus (Hebb and Ojemann, 2013).

Finally, studies in glioma patients provide important insights on the plasticity of language networks. Atlases of functional resectability provide a simple way to assign a quantitative value of plastic potential for each brain voxel (Mandonnet et al., 2007; Ius et al., 2011; De Witt Hamer et al., 2013) emphasizing the fundamental role of long-range connections for language processing, especially for the IFOF and SLF on the dominant side.

We suggest that future BCI applications for language function should take into consideration the new views on the neural mechanism of language function. In particular, it is important to consider that language processing is subserved by plastic, delocalized and synchronized networks that handle distinct language components. For example, in a locked-in patient with intact language networks, is it possible to decode words by interfacing a unique site or is it mandatory to use several recording devices, for example, in the phonological and semantic areas? At a first glance, it might seem advantageous to place the device in the speech motor cortex, which is the final encoding stage that generates speech output signal. However, the paradox is that this type of decoding may be way too complex. Indeed, since speech motor cortex encodes words at the level of muscles activity, this encoding includes information indirectly related to the targeted word (the speed, volume, timber at which the word is pronounced), which makes the decoding task very challenging. Hence, it might be much more efficient to interface areas that encode words at a higher level of abstraction, for instance its phonological (sequence of ordered phonemes) or semantic (either language modality dependant or even at the level of an amodal concept) representations. The problem when dealing with the higher level of coding is that the information is distributed over several interconnected areas, and one might not be able to retrieve the target word by recording a single area belonging to the network. One possibility would be to change the design of the electrodes so that we could record the area of convergence of the IFOF or arcuate fasciculus.

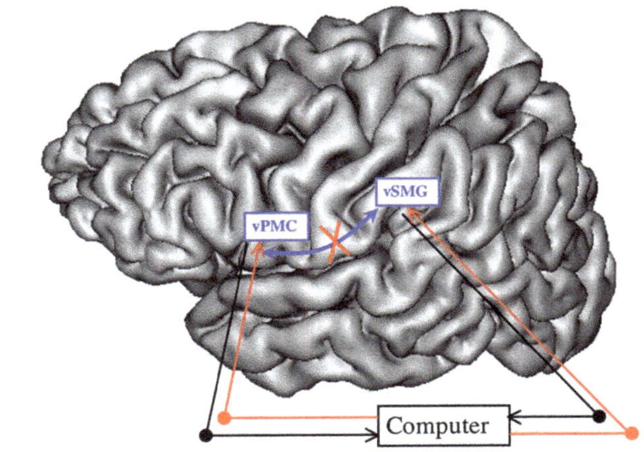

FIGURE 1 | Restoring the articulatory loop following white matter damage. This subnetwork is constituted by the ventral premotor cortex (vPMC) (BA 6) and the (antero-)ventral supramarginal gyrus (vSMG), linked through the third branch of the superior longitudinal fasciculus (SLF III). When this pathway is damaged, with cortical areas still intact, one has to recreate a bidirectional synchronized link: stimulation pattern over one area is computed from the recorded activity in the other area, introducing a time lag (see for example Jackson et al., 2006 for a short-range unidirectional version of such device).

Taking a different perspective, one can also envision BCI devices in aphasic patients following a stroke lesion, especially when one has to restore the long-range communication destroyed by the ischemia of the white matter. One possibility would be to build a brain-computer-brain interface (BCBI): two recording devices would be put in two distant disconnected areas still functional, and the activity of one area would shape the stimulation pattern over the other one, thus restoring a bidirectional synchronized link between both areas (see **Figure 1**).

CONCLUSION

DES studies greatly contributed to unravel the complex issue of separability of motor and language functions. Of note, neural networks subserving mentalizing and emotion can also be mapped with this method (Herbet et al., 2014). Combining this methodology with neuronal recordings (cortico-cortical evoked potentials (Matsumoto et al., 2004, 2007, 2012; Swann et al., 2012; Enatsu et al., 2013)) is currently the best way to characterize anatomically and electrophysiologically each subnetwork underlying an elementary subfunction. However, it is anticipated that computer modeling will play an essential role in the analysis of experimental data. In turn, better knowledge of the electrophysiological activity within a subnetwork will pave the way towards new BCI concepts, including mBCI and BCBI. In summary, the entangled circuits underpinning interactions between action, cognition and behavior should need to be better understood for BCIs to take a full advantage of brain modulations in a reliable and reasonable way for patients.

REFERENCES

Basha, M. M., Fernández-Baca Vaca, G., and Lüders, H. O. (2013). Mapping of cingulate motor function by cortical stimulation. *Epileptic Disord.* 15, 333–337. doi: 10.1684/epd.2013.0595

Catani, M., Dell'acqua, F., Vergani, F., Malik, F., Hodge, H., Roy, P., et al. (2012). Short frontal lobe connections of the human brain. *Cortex* 48, 273–291. doi: 10.1016/j.cortex.2011.12.001

Chassagnon, S., Minotti, L., Kremer, S., Hoffmann, D., and Kahane, P. (2008). Somatosensory, motor, and reaching/grasping responses to direct electrical stimulation of the human cingulate motor areas. *J. Neurosurg.* 109, 593–604. doi: 10.3171/JNS/2008/109/10/0593

Crosson, B. (2013). Thalamic mechanisms in language: a reconsideration based on recent findings and concepts. *Brain Lang.* 126, 73–88. doi: 10.1016/j.bandl.2012.06.011

De Witt Hamer, P. C., Hendriks, E. J., Mandonnet, E., Barkhof, F., Zwinderman, A. H., and Duffau, H. (2013). Resection probability maps for quality assessment of glioma surgery without brain location bias. *PLoS One* 8:e73353. doi: 10.1371/journal.pone.0073353

Duffau, H., Gatignol, P., Denvil, D., Lopes, M., and Capelle, L. (2003). The articulatory loop: study of the subcortical connectivity by electrostimulation. *Neuroreport* 14, 2005–2008. doi: 10.1097/00001756-200310270-00026

Duffau, H., Gatignol, P., Mandonnet, E., Peruzzi, P., Tzourio-Mazoyer, N., and Capelle, L. (2005). New insights into the anatomo-functional connectivity of the semantic system: a study using cortico-subcortical electrostimulations. *Brain* 128, 797–810. doi: 10.1093/brain/awh423

Duffau, H., Herbet, G., and Moritz-Gasser, S. (2013). Toward a pluri-component, multimodal and dynamic organization of the ventral semantic stream in humans: lessons from stimulation mapping in awake patients. *Front. Syst. Neurosci.* 7:44. doi: 10.3389/fnsys.2013.00044

Duffau, H., Moritz-Gasser, S., and Mandonnet, E. (2014). A re-examination of neural basis of language processing: proposal of a dynamic hodotopical model from data provided by brain stimulation mapping during picture naming. *Brain Lang.* 131, 1–10. doi: 10.1016/j.bandl.2013.05.011

Dum, R. P., and Strick, P. L. (1991). The origin of corticospinal projections from the premotor areas in the frontal lobe. *J. Neurosci.* 11, 667–689.

Dum, R. P., and Strick, P. L. (2002). Motor areas in the frontal lobe of the primate. *Physiol. Behav.* 77, 677–682. doi: 10.1016/s0031-9384(02)00929-0

Enatsu, R., Matsumoto, R., Piao, Z., O'Connor, T., Horning, K., Burgess, R. C., et al. (2013). Cortical negative motor network in comparison with sensorimotor network: a cortico-cortical evoked potential study. *Cortex* 49, 2080–2096. doi: 10.1016/j.cortex.2012.08.026

Filevich, E., Kühn, S., and Haggard, P. (2012). Negative motor phenomena in cortical stimulation: implications for inhibitory control of human action. *Cortex* 48, 1251–1261. doi: 10.1016/j.cortex.2012.04.014

Fried, I., Katz, A., McCarthy, G., Sass, K. J., Williamson, P., Spencer, S. S., et al. (1991). Functional organization of human supplementary motor cortex studied by electrical stimulation. *J. Neurosci.* 11, 3656–3666.

Gatignol, P., Capelle, L., Le Bihan, R., and Duffau, H. (2004). Double dissociation between picture naming and comprehension: an electrostimulation study. *Neuroreport* 15, 191–195. doi: 10.1097/00001756-200401190-00037

Gil Robles, S., Gatignol, P., Capelle, L., Mitchell, M.-C., and Duffau, H. (2005). The role of dominant striatum in language: a study using intraoperative electrical stimulations. *J. Neurol. Neurosurg. Psychiatry* 76, 940–946. doi: 10.1136/jnnp.2004.045948

Guo, Y., Rubin, J. E., McIntyre, C. C., Vitek, J. L., and Terman, D. (2008). Thalamocortical relay fidelity varies across subthalamic nucleus deep brain stimulation protocols in a data-driven computational model. *J. Neurophysiol.* 99, 1477–1492. doi: 10.1152/jn.01080.2007

Hebb, A. O., and Ojemann, G. A. (2013). The thalamus and language revisited. *Brain Lang.* 126, 99–108. doi: 10.1016/j.bandl.2012.06.010

Herbet, G., Lafargue, G., Bonnetblanc, F., Moritz-Gasser, S., Menjot de Champfleur, N., and Duffau, H. (2014). Inferring a dual-stream model of mentalizing from associative white matter fibers disconnection. *Brain* 137, 944–959. doi: 10.1093/brain/awt370

Hickok, G., and Poeppel, D. (2007). The cortical organization of speech processing. *Nat. Rev. Neurosci.* 8, 393–402. doi: 10.1038/nrn2113

Hochberg, L. R., Bacher, D., Jarosiewicz, B., Masse, N. Y., Simeral, J. D., Vogel, J., et al. (2012). Reach and grasp by people with tetraplegia using a neurally controlled robotic arm. *Nature* 485, 372–375. doi: 10.1038/nature11076

Ius, T., Angelini, E., Thiebaut de Schotten, M., Mandonnet, E., and Duffau, H. (2011). Evidence for potentials and limitations of brain plasticity using an atlas of functional resectability of WHO grade II gliomas: towards a "minimal common brain". *Neuroimage* 56, 992–1000. doi: 10.1016/j.neuroimage.2011.03.022

Jackson, A., Mavoori, J., and Fetz, E. E. (2006). Long-term motor cortex plasticity induced by an electronic neural implant. *Science* 444, 56–60. doi: 10.1038/nature05226

Kennedy, P., Andreasen, D., Bartels, J., Ehirim, P., Mao, H., Velliste, M., et al. (2011). Making the lifetime connection between brain and machine for restoring and enhancing function. *Prog. Brain Res.* 194, 1–25. doi: 10.1016/B978-0-444-53815-4.00020-0

Kinoshita, M., Shinohara, H., Hori, O., Ozaki, N., Ueda, F., Nakada, M., et al. (2012). Association fibers connecting the Broca center and the lateral superior frontal gyrus: a microsurgical and tractographic anatomy. *J. Neurosurg.* 116, 323–330. doi: 10.3171/2011.10.JNS11434

Lebedev, M. A., and Nicolelis, M. A. (2006). Brain-machine interfaces: past, present and future. *Trends Neurosci.* 29, 536–546. doi: 10.1016/j.tins.2006.07.004

Lim, S. H., Dinner, D. S., and Lüders, H. O. (1996). Cortical stimulation of the supplementary sensorimotor area. *Adv. Neurol.* 70, 187–197.

Lüders, H. O., Dinner, D. S., Morris, H. H., Wyllie, E., and Comair, Y. G. (1995). Cortical electrical stimulation in humans. The negative motor areas. *Adv. Neurol.* 67, 115–129.

Maldonado, I. L., Moritz-Gasser, S., de Champfleur, N. M., Bertram, L., Moulinié, G., and Duffau, H. (2011). Surgery for gliomas involving the left inferior parietal lobule: new insights into the functional anatomy provided by stimulation mapping in awake patients. *J. Neurosurg.* 115, 770–779. doi: 10.3171/2011.5.JNS112

Mandonnet, E., Jbabdi, S., Taillandier, L., Galanaud, D., Benali, H., Capelle, L., et al. (2007). Preoperative estimation of residual volume for WHO grade II glioma resected with intraoperative functional mapping. *Neuro Oncol.* 9, 63–69. doi: 10.1215/15228517-2006-015

Mandonnet, E., Winkler, P. A., and Duffau, H. (2010). Direct electrical stimulation as an input gate into brain functional networks: principles, advantages and limitations. *Acta Neurochir. (Wien)* 152, 185–193. doi: 10.1007/s00701-009-0469-0

Matsumoto, R., Nair, D. R., Ikeda, A., Fumuro, T., Lapresto, E., Mikuni, N., et al. (2012). Parieto-frontal network in humans studied by cortico-cortical evoked potential. *Hum. Brain Mapp.* 33, 2856–2872. doi: 10.1002/hbm.21407

Matsumoto, R., Nair, D. R., LaPresto, E., Bingaman, W., Shibasaki, H., and Lüders, H. O. (2007). Functional connectivity in human cortical motor system: a cortico-cortical evoked potential study. *Brain* 130, 181–197. doi: 10.1093/brain/awl257

Matsumoto, R., Nair, D. R., LaPresto, E., Najm, I., Bingaman, W., Shibasaki, H., et al. (2004). Functional connectivity in the human language system: a cortico-cortical evoked potential study. *Brain* 127, 2316–2330. doi: 10.1093/brain/awh246

Mikuni, N., Ohara, S., Ikeda, A., Hayashi, N., Nishida, N., Taki, J., et al. (2006). Evidence for a wide distribution of negative motor areas in the perirolandic cortex. *Clin. Neurophysiol.* 117, 33–40. doi: 10.1016/j.clinph.2005.08.021

Moritz-Gasser, S., Herbet, G., and Duffau, H. (2013). Mapping the connectivity underlying multimodal (verbal and non-verbal) semantic processing: a brain electrostimulation study. *Neuropsychologia* 51, 1814–1822. doi: 10.1016/j.neuropsychologia.2013.06.007

Nicolelis, M. A., and Lebedev, M. A. (2009). Principles of neural ensemble physiology underlying the operation of brain-machine interfaces. *Nat. Rev. Neurosci.* 10, 530–540. doi: 10.1038/nrn2653

Nii, Y., Uematsu, S., Lesser, R. P., and Gordon, B. (1996). Does the central sulcus divide motor and sensory functions? Cortical mapping of human hand areas as revealed by electrical stimulation through subdural grid electrodes. *Neurology* 46, 360–367. doi: 10.1212/wnl.46.2.360

Penfield, W., and Bolchey, E. (1937). Somatic motor and sensory representation in the cerebral cortex of man as studied by electrical stimulation. *Brain* 60, 389–443. doi: 10.1093/brain/60.4.389

Picard, N., and Strick, P. L. (2001). Imaging the premotor areas. *Curr. Opin. Neurobiol.* 11, 663–672. doi: 10.1016/s0959-4388(01)00266-5

Rech, F., Herbet, G., Moritz-Gasser, S., and Duffau, H. (2014). Disruption of bimanual movement by unilateral subcortical electrostimulation. *Hum. Brain Mapp.* doi: 10.1002/hbm.22413. [Epub ahead of print].

Rizzolatti, G., and Craighero, L. (2004). The mirror-neuron system. *Annu. Rev. Neurosci.* 27, 169–192. doi: 10.1146/annurev.neuro.27.070203.144230

Rubin, J. E., and Terman, D. (2004). High frequency stimulation of the subthalamic nucleus eliminates pathological thalamic rhythmicity in a computational model. *J. Comput. Neurosci.* 16, 211–235. doi: 10.1023/b:jcns.0000025686.47117.67

Rubin, J. E., McIntyre, C. C., Turner, R. S., and Wichmann, T. (2012). Basal ganglia activity patterns in parkinsonism and computational modeling of their downstream effects. *Eur. J. Neurosci.* 36, 2213–2228. doi: 10.1111/j.1460-9568.2012.08108.x

Schieber, M. H. (2011). Dissociating motor cortex from the motor. *J. Physiol.* 589, 5613–5624. doi: 10.1113/jphysiol.2011.215814

Schucht, P., Moritz-Gasser, S., Herbet, G., Raabe, A., and Duffau, H. (2013). Subcortical electrostimulation to identify network subserving motor control. *Hum. Brain Mapp.* 34, 3023–3030. doi: 10.1002/hbm.22122

Shadmehr, R., and Krakauer, J. W. (2008). A computational neuroanatomy for motor control. *Exp. Brain Res.* 185, 359–381. doi: 10.1007/s00221-008-1280-5

Sherman, S. M., and Guillery, R. W. (2011). Distinct functions for direct and transthalamic corticocortical connections. *J. Neurophysiol.* 106, 1068–1077. doi: 10.1152/jn.00429.2011

Shokur, S., O'Doherty, J. E., Winans, J. A., Bleuler, H., Lebedev, M. A., and Nicolelis, M. A. (2013). Expanding the primate body schema in sensorimotor cortex by virtual touches of an avatar. *Proc. Natl. Acad. Sci. U S A* 110, 15121–15126. doi: 10.1073/pnas 1308459110

Swann, N. C., Cai, W., Conner, C. R., Pieters, T. A., Claffey, M. P., George, J. S., et al. (2012). Roles for the pre-supplementary motor area and the right inferior frontal gyrus in stopping action: electrophysiological responses and functional and structural connectivity. *Neuroimage* 59, 2860–2870. doi: 10.1016/j.neuroimage.2011.09.049

van Geemen, K., Herbet, G., Moritz-Gasser, S., and Duffau, H. (2014). Limited plastic potential of the left ventral premotor cortex in speech articulation: evidence From intraoperative awake mapping in glioma patients. *Hum. Brain Mapp.* 35, 1587–1596. doi: 10.1002/hbm.22275

Vigneswaran, G., Philipp, R., Lemon, R. N., and Kraskov, A. (2013). M1 corticospinal mirror neurons and their role in movement suppression during action observation. *Curr. Biol.* 23, 236–243. doi: 10.1016/j.cub.2012.12.006

13

Robust sequential working memory recall in heterogeneous cognitive networks

Mikhail I. Rabinovich[1], Yury Sokolov[2]* and Robert Kozma[2]

[1] *BioCircuits Institute, University of California San Diego, La Jolla, CA, USA*
[2] *Department of Mathematical Sciences, University of Memphis, Memphis, TN, USA*

Edited by:
Mikhail Lebedev, Duke University, USA

Reviewed by:
Tara Thiagarajan, National Center for Biological Sciences, India
KongFatt Wong-Lin, University of Ulster, UK
Zachary P. Kilpatrick, University of Houston, USA

***Correspondence:**
Yury Sokolov, Department of Mathematical Sciences, University of Memphis, 373 Dunn Hall, Memphis, TN 38152, USA
e-mail: ysokolov@memphis.edu

Psychiatric disorders are often caused by partial heterogeneous disinhibition in cognitive networks, controlling sequential and spatial working memory (SWM). Such dynamic connectivity changes suggest that the normal relationship between the neuronal components within the network deteriorates. As a result, competitive network dynamics is qualitatively altered. This dynamics defines the robust recall of the sequential information from memory and, thus, the SWM capacity. To understand pathological and non-pathological bifurcations of the sequential memory dynamics, here we investigate the model of recurrent inhibitory-excitatory networks with heterogeneous inhibition. We consider the ensemble of units with all-to-all inhibitory connections, in which the connection strengths are monotonically distributed at some interval. Based on computer experiments and studying the Lyapunov exponents, we observed and analyzed the new phenomenon—clustered sequential dynamics. The results are interpreted in the context of the winnerless competition principle. Accordingly, clustered sequential dynamics is represented in the phase space of the model by two weakly interacting quasi-attractors. One of them is similar to the sequential heteroclinic chain—the regular image of SWM, while the other is a quasi-chaotic attractor. Coexistence of these quasi-attractors means that the recall of the normal information sequence is intermittently interrupted by episodes with chaotic dynamics. We indicate potential dynamic ways for augmenting damaged working memory and other cognitive functions.

Keywords: cognitive dynamics, memory disorders, inhibition, sequential intermittency, complex networks, heteroclinic chimeras

1. INTRODUCTION

The human brain is a complex net of functionally interconnected regions. Deeper understanding the dynamics of this network is very useful for describing how brain activities transform to task-dependent cognitive processes. This dynamical approach is providing new insights into abnormal brain organization in various psychiatric and neurological disorders. Advances in this area stimulate new discoveries on dynamical disorders related to network connectivity, such as obsessive-compulsive disorder, schizophrenia, dementia, and drug dependence (Chambers et al., 2009; Bystritsky et al., 2012; Hughes et al., 2013). Non-linear dynamical models studying psychopathology must focus on understanding how disturbances in the networks' architecture contribute to cognitive and affective dysfunctions. In particular, it is extremely important to separate emergent dynamics into pathological and non-pathological regimes concerning a specific cognitive task.

As well known, cognitive human resources are finite (Franconeri et al., 2013). When a person becomes sick or its cognitive problem worsens, the performance degrades. There are several possible mechanisms of cognitive resource limitations discuss in the literature; for a review, see Emrich et al. (2013). In this paper, we focus on sequential working memory (SWM) capacity and discuss the instability mechanism related to the length of the information items (chunks) sequence. SWM is a dynamical cognitive network that enables and sustains a set of sequentially ordered mental representations for further recall and processing. The capacity of SWM is quite limited, i.e., it is 5 ± 2 chunks of information at any time instant (Miller, 1956; Bick and Rabinovich, 2009; Rabinovich et al., 2014). The contents of SWM are generally thought to be conscious. The SWM cognitive network, as imaging experiments indicate, consists of several brain modules distributed in different areas of the frontal cortex, sensory cortical regions, hippocampus and some others. These modules interact through the attentional process (Postle, 2006), forming stimulus-dependent spatiotemporal informational modes.

In excitatory-inhibitory cognitive networks that perform SWM, these modes sequentially turn off/ turn on each other according to winnerless competition (WLC) principle. As a result, a stable time-ordered sequence of chunks is formed (Rabinovich et al., 2014). In experiments, the sequence of such switching looks like a chain of metastable states—each state corresponds to the specific mode lasting for a finite time (Stopfer et al., 2003; Jones et al., 2007; Bouchard et al., 2013). The mathematical image of the sequence of metastable states is a stable heteroclinic channel (SHC) in the phase space of the corresponding dynamical model (Afraimovich et al., 2004a; Rabinovich et al., 2012b).

If excitation is constant, cognitive inhibition plays a key role in SWM dynamics and it is the origin of WLC. Cognitive inhibition refers to the mind's ability to tune out stimuli that are irrelevant to the task/process at hand or to the mind's current state (Harnishfeger, 1995; MacLeod, 2007). Cognitive inhibition is caused by several different interacting biological factors. The first is the existence of inhibitory neurotransmitters, or chemicals emitted by brain cells to both communicate and inhibit communication between each other. GABA is an inhibitory transmitter that has been implicated in certain simple behavioral measures of inhibition and the control of behavior in normal and pathological cases; it has been identified in the cerebral cortex (Dempster and Corkill, 1999). Given the cerebral cortex's importance in many brain functions such as memory and thought, the presence of the inhibitory substance GABA supports the cognitive inhibition processes that go on in this area of the brain. Cognitive inhibition is playing a key role in schizophrenia (Westerhausen et al., 2011). The corresponding degradation of the sequence of information items stability is analyzed in this paper. In particular, we are interested in the dynamics of sequential switching in the case of heterogeneity of the SWM network as a result of decreasing cognitive inhibition.

For the description of the modes interaction in excitatory-inhibitory cognitive networks, we use here the traditional model of population dynamics and game theory—generalized Lotka-Volterra equation for N interacting agents (Hofbauer and Sigmund, 1998). In canonic form (see below) this model has N metastable states that are represented in the phase space by saddle fixed points on the axes corresponding to different agent-variables. We consider the case of all-to-all inhibitory connections between participants. Depending on the strengths of the anatomical connections of the subnetworks - motifs or clusters that are embedded in an original larger network can form. These are anatomical motifs. Here we show that in heterogeneous networks one can observe the emergence of dynamical clusters, or dynamical motifs in the phase space, which can be interpreted as temporal unification of different groups of agents.

Cognitive functions, including working memory and attention, involve interconnected networks of brain regions. Recent investigations indicated abnormalities in structural and functional networks in the case of schizophrenia and other disorders, such as depression, obsessive-compulsive disorder, and substance abuse. These conditions are associated with deficits of GABA-mediated synaptic transmission in the brain, when inhibitory connections become weaker in frontal-subcortical neuronal networks (Tekin and Cummings, 2002; Lewis et al., 2005; Murray et al., 2014a).

In contrast with GABA synaptic inhibition in neurophysiological networks, the inhibition in cognition is a concept that is based on behavioral and imaging experiments. In fact, it is a process that has been postulated and modeled by kinetic equations for the competitive cognitive modes (Rabinovich et al., 2012b). In the framework of such models, it is possible to explain changes and deteriorations in the cognitive performance in many domains of psychological and psychiatric research. There are many areas of psychology and cognitive science where the concept of inhibition in global brain networks has been used successfully (Aron, 1982; Constantinidis and Wang, 2004; Gorfein et al., 2007; Joorman et al., 2007; Engelhart et al., 2008; Baumeister et al., 2014; Deco et al., 2014).

Following previous studies, our results indicate potential dynamical ways for augmenting damaged working memory and other cognitive functions. Specifically, we hypothesize that psychiatric and cognitive conditions will express substantial changes in temporal dynamics during key cognitive functions. Furthermore, if these models are successful it would be of great interest to determine if manipulating the organization of the feedback between fMRI time series of working memory (WM) activity through repetitive transcranial stimulation targeting prefrontal cortex can modulate inhibitory WM network and thus provide some control of the chaotic dynamics.

This paper focuses on the analysis of two related cognitive processes, i.e., sequential working memory and attention sharing. The analysis of the dynamics of corresponding functional global networks with inhibitory heterogeneous connections between cognitive modes (information items) revealed a new type of network behavior, which is coined *clustering dynamics*. Clustering dynamics is a sequential activity that includes ordered switching between a few information items, interrupted by intervals with chaotic switching between some other ones. The mathematical image of such intermittent dynamics we named *heteroclinic chimera* as an analog to chimeras observed in networks of phase oscillators (see Omelchenko et al., 2013; Panaggio and Abram, 2014), inspired by neuroscience (Kozma, 1998; Henderson and Robinson, 2011). The observed phenomenon leads to decreasing capacity of the sequential working memory. Moreover, it causes serious impediments in the process of attention sharing among several objects.

2. RELATION TO OTHER MODELING STUDIES

In Loh et al. (2007), based on a statistical dynamical model of integrate-and-fire **neuronal** network, the stability of attractor states in prefrontal cortical networks has been analyzed. The authors showed that for the stability of network dynamics is important to have a balance between excitation (NMDA conductance) and inhibition (GABA conductance). In particular, decreasing inhibition reduced the basins of cognitive attractors and destabilized the cognitive task performance that models the schizophrenia symptoms. The concept of excitation-inhibition dynamical balance is supported also by other modeling (Murray et al., 2014b), and experimental studies. In their nice work Murray and coauthors have showed that with constant excitation disinhibition increases random drift and decreases memory precision.

It is important to note that dynamical modeling of sequential neural activities has a long history; for a review, see Rabinovich et al. (2006). In particular, about 30 years ago, two seminal papers have been published (Kleinfeld, 1986; Sompolinsky and Kanter, 1986), in which authors used the same idea, i.e., that sequential patterns were generated by neural networks with time-delayed connections. Recent work about robust sequential memory in networks with controllable steady-state period is related to this idea (Xia et al., 2009). Camperi and Wang (1998) analyzed visual working memory models using networks with cellular bistability. Szatmary and Izhikevich (2010) built a spike-timing network model of working memory using associative short-term synaptic plasticity (STDP). Buonomano (2000) has trained a biophysical network model of decoding temporal information using similar principles. In Seliger et al. (2003), the problem of recalling temporal sequence was solved in the framework of WLC networks. Concluding this obviously incomplete list, we notice that memory storage on short timescales can be maintained by neural activity that passed sequentially through a chain of network states (Goldman, 2009). This mechanism reminds the information propagation along heteroclinic channel in the phase space of WLC network (Rabinovich et al., 2012a).

3. MATERIALS AND METHODS

3.1. DYNAMICAL PRINCIPLES OF COGNITION: THE SIMPLEST CANONICAL MODEL

In order to build a non-linear dynamical model of sequential working memory, attention, and other cognitive functions in normal and pathological conditions, we use the following ideas based on brain imaging and behavioral experiments (see Rabinovich et al., 2012b): (i) the equations of the model have to be written for variables that represent the evolution of the temporal coherency of the brain components, and must have solution which correspond to metastable patterns (knowledge) in the brain; (ii) the model must be based on winnerless competitive (WLC) dynamics, a non-linear process of interaction of many informational items or spatiotemporal modes, which guarantees sequential switching between metastable states and potential robustness of transient creativity dynamics; (iii) the model is an open dissipative system where inhibition is balanced by excitation; and (iv) the dynamics of the model has to be sensitive to the changes in memory and environment information.

In our study, we consider a kinetic equation, which can be written as $\dot{x}_i = x_i F(x)$, where $F(x)$ is a vector function and $x = (x_1, \ldots, x_n)$. The Generalized Lotka Volterra (GLV) equation is a specific example of the kinetic equation. Thus, GLV is a non-linear population model with a simple quadratic nonlinearity. Moreover, it is known that a system of non-linear equations can be rewritten as system of GLV equations after some suitable transformations (Hernandez-Bermejo et al., 1998). Therefore, the "simple" Lotka Volterra equations can provide a powerful tool for the description of the dynamics of complex networks. Using this approach, one can write the model in the simplest canonical form of Generalized Lotka-Volterra equations (Rabinovich et al., 2006):

$$\tau_\ell \frac{dR_\ell}{dt} = R_\ell \left(\gamma_\ell - \sum_{k=1}^{N} a_{\ell,k} R_k \right), \quad (1)$$

where R_ℓ is the level of activity of ℓ-th mode , $\ell = 1, \ldots, N$. Information mode variable R_ℓ must be positive or equal to zero for all ℓ. N is the total number of modes describing the components that interact to perform a specific cognitive task. Time constants τ_ℓ are fixed for a given system ℓ, while parameters $a_{\ell,k}$ describe the inhibitory connections between mode ℓ and k, while $a_{\ell,\ell} = 1$ for any ℓ, and γ_ℓ is the strength of the stimulation of mode ℓ. It is important that, in general, the elements of this matrix are controlled by cognitive tasks.

The dynamics of the cognitive network is extremely sensitive to the diversity of inhibitory connections. In this work, we model cognitive diseases through heterogeneous decrease of inhibitory activity in the cortex.

It is very important to emphasize that the complexity of the corresponding model is determined by the numbers of variables (agents) and the task dependent functional hierarchical architecture of the cognitive networks (Rabinovich et al., 2014). The individual dynamics of the agents is of secondary importance and it can be selected based on a suitably simple model. While numerous models exist that explain various aspects of cortical behavior, even simple, parsimonious GLV models (Bick and Rabinovich, 2009; Rabinovich et al., 2010) can produce intermittent chaotic behavior by a change in inhibitory weights, which provide insights into dynamical behaviors that may mirror pathological conditions.

3.2. LOTKA-VOLTERRA NETWORKS. GALLERY OF THE PHENOMENA

GLV model is very important and popular model for the analysis of multi agent non-equilibrium dynamics in ecology, biochemistry, and neuroscience. There is a huge amount of publications about GLV dynamics. Here we recall the main phenomena that are described by this model, which have been observed over a wide range of the control parameters.

If the connection matrix is symmetric the GLV model is a gradient system and demonstrates monotonic dissipative dynamics (Hirsch and Smith, 2005). In particular, one can observe multistability like in associative memory neural networks (Hopfeld, 1982; Cohen and Grossberg, 1983; Yi et al., 2003). In the case of moderate inhibition, the typical regime is winner-share-all (Fukai and Tanaka, 1997). Phase portrait of such stable regime of the symmetric high-dimensional model Equation (1) is shown in **Figure 1A**.

If the connection matrix is non-symmetric, the GLV model dynamics is extremely rich. For $N > 3$ the dynamics of GLV system can be chaotic (Arneodo et al., 1982; Takeuchi, 1996; Varona et al., 2002; Rabinovich et al., 2012b). An example of chaotic behavior in the GLV model with 6-modes is shown in **Figure 1B**. Another example is the transient dynamics representing cognitive information processing such as attention switching or sequential working memory stability (Bick and Rabinovich, 2009; Rabinovich et al., 2014); stable heteroclinic transients are illustrated in **Figure 1C**.

The key issue for the present study is understanding the origin of the SHC instability in the framework of model Equation (1) with heterogeneous connections. The results are important for the description of sequential information processing; for a review, see Rabinovich et al. (2012a).

3.3. STABILITY OF THE INFORMATION SEQUENCE. SADDLE VALUES

Robust transient dynamics is organized in the phase space typically as a chain of sequentially switching of metastable states—saddle points. The mathematical image of such dynamics is a stable heteroclinic channel—the vicinity of the chain of saddles coupled sequentially by their unstable separatrices. The chain can be finite, i.e., ending at the simple attractor (stable fixed point), or it can be periodic, asymptotically reaching a heteroclinic cycle.

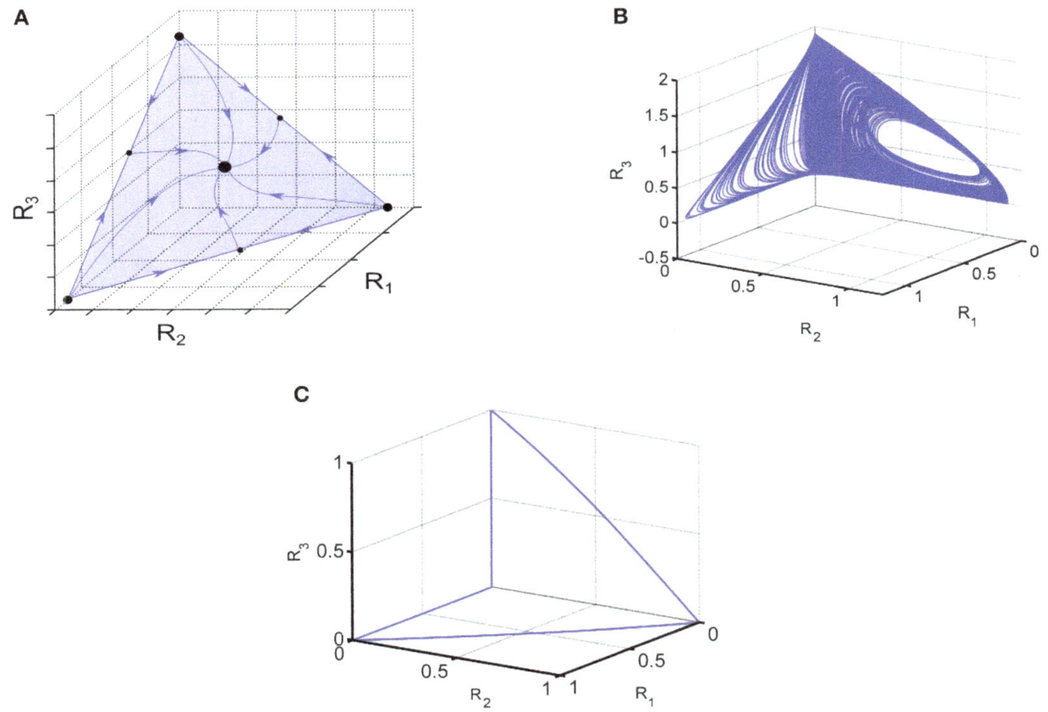

FIGURE 1 | Illustration of various dynamical regimes of the Lotka-Volterra system. (A) Example of a system when all trajectories converge to one stable fixed point, illustrating the coexistence of 3 modes. **(B)** Portrait of irregular switching in a 6-dimensional inhibitory LV network. 3D projection of the phase portrait of the observed strange attractor Equation (1). **(C)** Winnerless competitive dynamics of a network with random non-symmetric connections; 3D projection is shown; see Huerta and Rabinovich (2004).

Let $A_i = (0, \dots, 0, \gamma_i, 0, \dots, 0)$ be an equilibrium point of the system Equation (1), $i = 1, \dots, N$. If $\lambda_1^{(i)}, \dots, \lambda_N^{(i)}$ are eigenvalues of the matrix of the system linearized at A_i, that are ordered as follows $\lambda_1^{(i)} > \dots \geq \mathrm{Re}\lambda_{k_i}^{(i)} > 0 > \mathrm{Re}\lambda_{k_i+1}^{(i)} \geq \dots \geq \mathrm{Re}\lambda_N^{(i)}$ then A_i is a saddle with k_i-dimensional unstable manifold.

When the unstable manifolds of the saddles are one-dimensional, i.e., $k_i = 1$ for all i, the stability of a SHC depends on the ratios of the compression of the phase volume to the stretching of it in the vicinity of the channel. These ratios are called saddle values and they can be defined as $\nu_i = -\mathrm{Re}\lambda_2^{(i)}/\lambda_1^{(i)}$. Thus, if $\nu_i > 1$, the saddle is called dissipative and the trajectories get closer to the unstable manifold of the saddle after passing through its neighborhood. The mechanism of the SHC emergence in dissipative systems is the Winnerless Competition that can guarantee the sequential switching of agents activity in networks with non-symmetric inhibitory coupling (Rabinovich et al., 2006, 2012b; Bick and Rabinovich, 2010).

The conditions of the existence and stability of the heteroclinic contour with constant uniform stimulation strength $\gamma_i = 1$ for any i are given in Afraimovich et al. (2004a). The conditions of existence and stability of the heteroclinic sequence with different values of γ_i were obtained in Afraimovich et al. (2004b). To support the proposed interpretation of cognitive dynamics using heteroclinic chimera, we provide detailed mathematical analysis in the Appendix.

4. RESULTS

4.1. DEPENDENCE OF THE NETWORK DYNAMICS ON THE DISTRIBUTION OF INHIBITORY CONNECTIONS STRENGTHS

In this work, a system of 6 LV Equations (1) is studied. **Figure 2** illustrates the general structure of such system with all-to-all connections among 6 modes shown in 6 different colors; external inputs are marked by arrows pointing to each mode. We are able to select the parameters of the model to guarantee the regime of regular sequential working memory. In order to produce a system having robust heteroclinic contour, the inhibitory connections are chosen in two groups, i.e., with weights greater than one and smaller than one, respectively, while the self-inhibition weights are equal to one. Moreover, the weights in each of these subsets have a limited spread, i.e., they are concentrated around a particular value. Also, the strength of the inhibition is growing when the number of interacting modes increases; for details, see Bick and Rabinovich (2010). In the pathological case of weakened inhibition, on the other hand, we may expect that the strength of some inhibitory connections to approach zero.

4.2. DYNAMICAL CLUSTERING IN HETEROGENEOUS NETWORKS. INTERMITTENT SEQUENCES AND HETEROCLINIC CHIMERA

To analyze in detail the case of reduced/intermediate strength of coupling when quasi-periodic heteroclinic dynamics and chaos co-exist in a mutually coupled system, we performed extensive

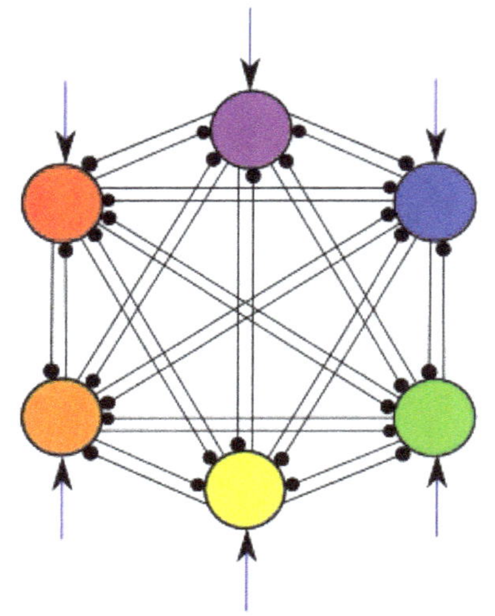

FIGURE 2 | All-to-all inhibitory interactions between 6 modes (information items) of the cognitive network; excitatory self connections are not shown. Black arrows represent incoming signals.

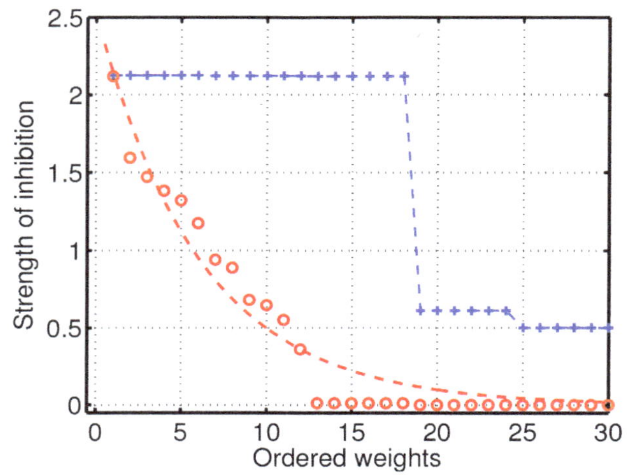

FIGURE 3 | Distribution of the strengths of the inhibitory connections in the GLV network with 6 participants. Blue: connectivity in a network producing normal SHC behavior; the large weights represent two triangle motifs with strong constant connectivity values, while there is a group of small weights describing weak connectivity between the motifs. Red: illustrates the pathological case with significantly reduced inhibitory connections with respect to normal SHC case, which are distributed over the parameter range; the dotted red line is a simple exponential fit shown for better visibility.

simulations with various sets of parameters. Examples of the distribution of the inhibitory weights in the GLV system with 6 modes are given in **Figure 3**. Blue color illustrates connectivity in a network producing normal SHC behavior, when the strong weights correspond to two triangle motifs, while there is a group of small weights describing weak connectivity between the motifs. The degraded (pathological) case is shown in red and it has significantly reduced inhibitory connection values with respect to the normal SHC case. The magnitudes of the weights are distributed over a range of parameters; the dotted red line illustrates a simple exponential fit for better visibility.

Takens' theorem (Takens, 1981) can be used to reconstruct high-dimensional attractors from the time series of a variable using time-delayed coordinate embedding. Note that time delay τ can be selected according to the given problem to produce a suitable display of the phase portrait. For example, $R_1(t)$ and its time-lagged copies $R_1(t-\tau)$ and $R_1(t-2\tau)$ are used in **Figure 4** to show the 3-dimensional phase portrait with time-lagged reconstruction. The case of $\tau = 150$ is used in this display; the direction of the trajectory is illustrated by arrows. **Figure 4A** shows the case of SHC corresponding to normal parameters. On the other hand, the attractor produced by reduced strength of coupling parameters given in **Figure 4** reflecting pathological conditions is shown in **Figure 4B**. Here a highly complex dynamics emerges resembling the Roessler strange attractor with two wings (Kennel et al., 1992). Specifically, the attractor in **Figure 4B** has a main wing and a secondary wing. The main wing is shown by overlapping red, orange, yellow, and green patches. There is a second wing, which is less pronounced and approaches but does not quite reach the blue and magenta dots. The secondary wing starts when the trajectories exit the main wing shown as *Exit* in **Figure 4B**, and later return to the main wing through the region shown as *Enter*. **Figure 4C** depicts a more detailed view of the two-wing attractor using more detailed computer simulations with about 10^5 time steps.

Quantitative evaluation of the Lyapunov exponents confirms the coexistence of heteroclinic cycles and chaos. Namely, we have two positive Lyapunov exponents, one small negative value close to zero, one small negative exponent, and two large negative exponents. The exact Lyapunov exponent values corresponding to parameters shown in **Figure 3** are as follows: $\lambda_1 = 0.0061 \pm 0.0005$, $\lambda_2 = 0.0008 \pm 0.0001$, $\lambda_3 = -0.0019 \pm 0.0015$, $\lambda_4 = -0.0127 \pm 0.0019$, $\lambda_5 = -0.6654 \pm 0.0004$, $\lambda_6 = -1.4409 \pm 0.0002$. We explored a variety of systems close and further away from the heteroclinic cycles. The above conclusions have been confirmed, i.e., we have two positive Lyapunov exponents, one close to zero, and the rest are negative. Our results show that two different dynamic regimes coexist in a single system of coupled agents with non-oscillatory intrinsic dynamics, similarly to the chimera states described recently in the literature (Abrams and Strogatz, 2004; Hagerstrom et al., 2012; Omelchenko et al., 2012). Earlier manifestations of chimera states have been in ensembles of phase oscillators. In our case of WLC, however, we observe amplitude clusterization.

Dynamical clustering means the separation of the phase flow into several qualitatively different components. In our example we have two components, one includes quasi-heteroclinic regular trajectories, while the other is a transient chaotic set. We named such complex image as **heteroclinic chimera**. We observe that the network's cooperative dynamics is dominated by the weak interaction between just a few (in our case two) dynamical sub-networks, although the monotonic heterogeneity of the connection strengths between agents would allow more distributed interaction dynamics.

We interpret this behavior as emergent granulation of the distributed dynamics into the interaction of just a few sub-networks.

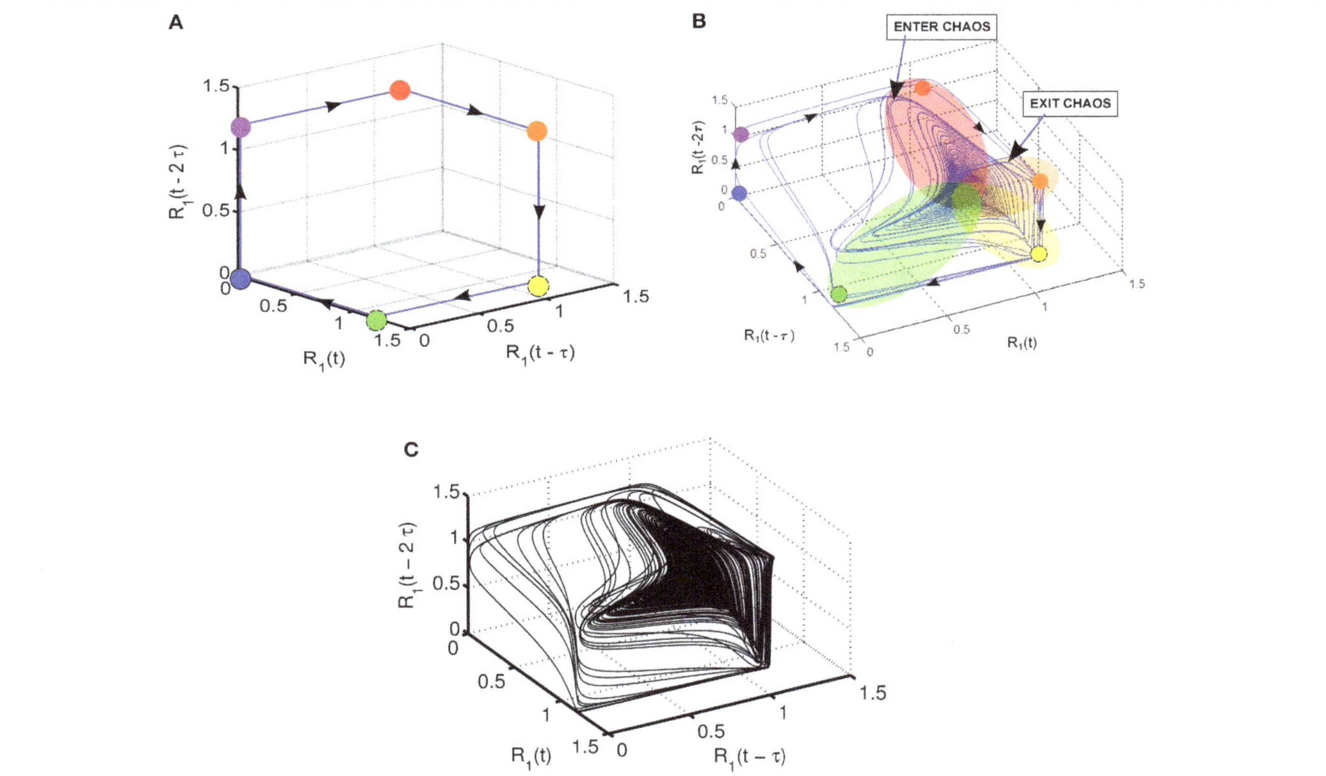

FIGURE 4 | Illustration of various dynamic regimes using 3-dimensional phase portrait with time-lagged reconstruction of R_1; (A) normal regime with stable heteroclinic channel (SHC); (B) abnormal regime: coexistence of SHC and quasi-chaotic attractor—heteroclinic chimera; (C) abnormal regime: coexisting SHC and quasi-chaotic attractor for longer time series with up to 10^5 points.

These sub-networks could be formed through the collaboration between agents R_i, $i = 1, \ldots, 6$ with the strongest mutual interaction between each others. We have tested this interpretation in the case of weak interaction between two strongly interconnected sub-networks, each with 3 modes (triangles). Our results indicate that in the case of coupled triangles we have topologically the same phase portrait of heteroclinic chimera as we observed in the original system with distributed parameters. We pointed out earlier, following Equation 1, that information mode variable R_i is either positive or zero, which determines the differences between the previously known phase chimera characterizing the dynamics of the network of phase oscillators, and the new heteroclinic chimera observed here in the case of the WLC processes. These results point to the importance of conducting a rigorous analysis in the case of weak inhibitory connections; details are given in the Appendix.

Figure 5 is the schematic image of a SHC modeling normal cognitive functions with sequential switching between various memory items. The consecutive patterns are symbolized by circles of different colors for simplicity. The appearance of the transient chaotic dynamics is illustrated in **Figure 6**, when the sequence of the patterns enters a *valley*, in which various colors are mixed in a chaotic fashion. This is the model of abnormal cognitive dynamics when the regular sequential memory dynamics breaks down. After some period of time, however, the trajectory leaves the chaotic *valley*, e.g., through the orange unit, and it resumes the regular sequential switching pattern.

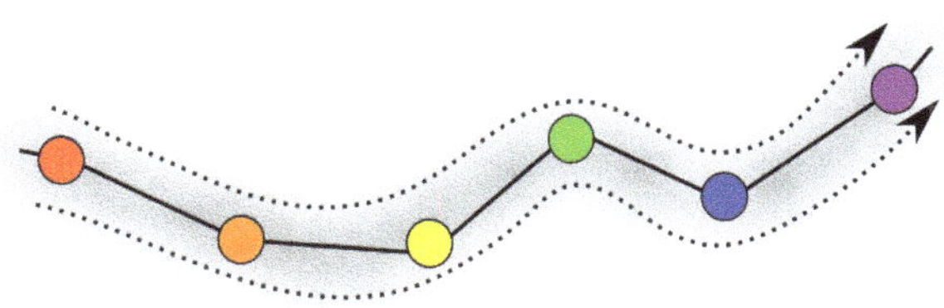

FIGURE 5 | Illustration of the trajectory in an SHC progressing through the sequence of saddle points; different memory patterns are shown in different colors, i.e., red, orange, yellow, green, blue, and violet.

Figure 7 illustrates heteroclinic chimera in a GLV network with degraded inhibitor weights. This GLV network has 6 units, from which two units are shown here, R_1 and R_2, respectively. **Figure 7A** depicts variable $R_1(t)$, which exhibits SHC regime with stable values over extended time periods. **Figure 7B** shows the temporal evolution of variable $R_2(t)$, which has frequent irregular oscillations. The determined positive Lyapunov exponent indicates the existence of chaos. The dynamics of all 6 variables R_i, $i = 1, \ldots, 6$ of the abnormal system is summarized in **Figure 8** using a raster plot. A given variable is shown in the plot

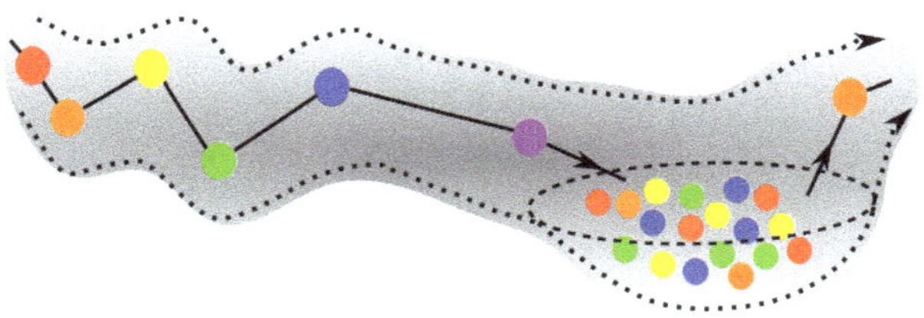

FIGURE 6 | Schematics of the trajectory of a pathological case of GLV equations, when the initial sequence enters a chaotic valley after the violet unit. The system stays in the valley for some time, but ultimately escapes it and resumes the regular SHC switching, see exit at the orange unit.

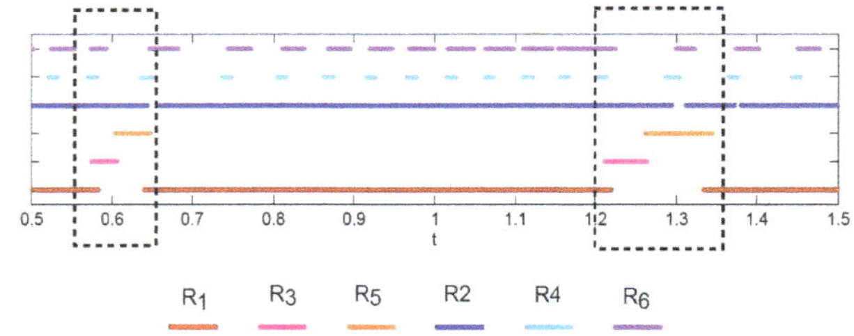

FIGURE 8 | Raster plot of intermittent sequences of the variables of the GLV system in the case of heteroclinic chimera dynamics; the 6 variables are shown as R_1, R_2, R_3, R_4, R_5, and R_6, respectively. A given variable is shown in the plot if its amplitude exceeds a threshold value; the threshold used here is 0.1. Note the preservation of sequential switching in the boxes marked by dashed lines.

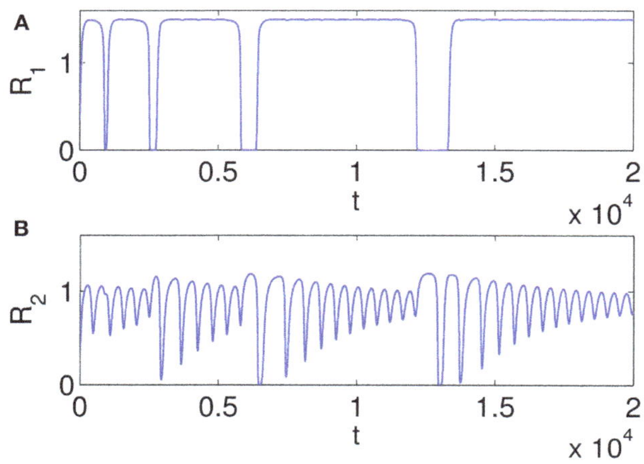

FIGURE 7 | Examples of time series illustrating heteroclinic chimera in a GLV network with degraded inhibitor weights; the GLV network has 6 units, and two units are shown here. (A) Variable $R_1(t)$ exhibits SHC regime with stable values over extended time periods; **(B)** Variable $R_2(t)$ has frequent irregular oscillations; the determined positive Lyapunov exponent indicates the existence of chaos.

if its amplitude exceeds a threshold value (of 0.1). Note the preservation of sequential switching in the boxes marked by dashed lines. While some of the variables apparently maintain stable heteroclinic trajectories, others exhibit intermittent oscillations and chaos, as a manifestation of heteroclinic chimera dynamics.

5. DISCUSSION

This paper analyzes the role of the heterogeneity of inhibitory connections in a cognitive network that models cognitive sequential information processing. The introduced model has been applied for the description and prediction of many cognitive processes like working memory, attention, and decision making. Here we suggested a plausible dynamical mechanism to study the deterioration of the working memory. Sequential order has been destroyed as the result of pathological heterogeneous decrease of some of the inhibitory connections. This mechanism is related to a new dynamical phenomenon: dynamical clustering of information items (cognitive modes) in networks with heterogeneous inhibitory connections.

The corresponding phenomenon is coined here "heteroclinic chimera." In the case of heteroclinic chimera, we observe the coexistence of chaotic and heteroclinic cycle behavior, thus the chimera property is expressed through sequential amplitude coordination. An important distinction between the previously described phase chimera and heteroclinic chimera is that phase chimera represents phase dynamics and it does not relate to the temporal sequence of items. The phenomenon of dynamical clustering described in this work in the case of heterogeneous inhibitory connections in model Equation 1 is robust. In Sokolov et al. (2014) the dynamics of the model is studied in the presence of multiplicative noise. It is shown that the noise does not change the qualitative picture of the dynamics.

Studies focusing on the analysis of sequential non-linear brain dynamics in the case of psychiatric disorders attract the interest of medical doctors. Results exist related to anxiety and depression (Bystritsky et al., 2014), and to obsessive-compulsive disorder (Bystritsky et al., 2012; Schiepek et al., 2013). Some psychiatrists anticipate that analysis of non-linear sequential dynamics will lead to changes in cognitive behavioral therapies (Kronemyer and Bystritsky, 2014).

There are several fMRI experiments that focused on the spatiotemporal analysis of the representation of informational items in short-time memory (Attout et al., 2014; D'Argembeau et al., 2014, and references therein). In addition, some experiments show the disruption of functional cortical networks in the case of psychiatric disorders including schizophrenia (Baker et al., 2014; Bittner et al., 2014). However, no comprehensive analysis have been completed yet concerning the spatiotemporal dynamics of functional cortical networks, in the case of patients with schizophrenia who do not recall ordered information from SWM. Together with our colleague Alan Simmons (UCSD Dept. of Psychiatry), we plan to conduct such analyses and compare the results with our predictions. In particular, we intend to measure the voxels in functional time series in pathological conditions, i.e., signal intensity vs. time activity in parietal and prefrontal cortexes, to characterize the performance of SWM recall. The modeling results are represented by the $R_i(t)$ time series. The mathematical image of the damaged SWM with heteroclinic chimera is in fact an intermittent chaotic dynamical regime. There are several successful methods for controlling chaotic dynamics; see, for example Sieber et al. (2014), which is a successful approach to modulate the irregular activities by feedback.

Observations in neuroimaging studies were used to describe the neural correlates of cognitive deficits in attention, working memory and executive functions in patients with Huntington's disease (Montoya et al., 2006). The chaotic behavior of clustered sequential dynamics can serve as a model of Huntington's Chorea.

A related important cognitive problem involves abnormalities in attention switching and focusing, which can be described by the proposed dynamical model; see also Rabinovich et al. (2013). Of the many clinical features of schizophrenia, disturbances in certain cognitive processes, such as impairments in attention, memory and executive functions (that is, the ability to plan, initiate, and regulate goal directed behavior), might represent the core features of the illness (Elvevag and Goldberg, 2000). There is increasing evidence indicating that such disorders are related to decreasing level of inhibition in cortical inhibitory circuits (Lewis et al., 2005). In recent studies, schizophrenia patients has been tested to answer the question: are they impaired relative to controls in sustaining attention, switching attention, or both (Smid et al., 2013). The results supported the hypothesis that schizophrenia is associated with attention switching, while the mechanisms of sustained attention remains largely intact. Our results give a dynamical interpretation to these observations.

If the GLV model suggested is successful in characterizing the differences in temporal dynamics in normal and pathological samples then it would be of great interest in determining if this could guide a potential intervention in these dynamics to either mimic or ameliorate the core symptomologies of these pathologies. We expect that it would be very promising to provide feedback based on functional sequential cortical activity during memory recall, i.e., the time series representing sequential switching between metastable states (Polyn et al., 2005; Norman et al., 2006), by repetitive transcranial brain stimulation. This feedback may involve either repetitive magnetic stimulation (Barr et al., 2013) or ultrasound stimulation (Hameroff et al., 2013; Mueller et al., 2014). Such feedback has to support the correct sequential switching between corresponding recalled information items from SWM.

SHC is the mathematical image of regular sequential switching of attention as it is postulated in Rabinovich et al. (2013). Regular sequential switching between attention modalities is maintained in our model at normal conditions. In the case of the pathological inhibitory strength distribution (selective decrease of inhibitory weights), the regular sequential switching of attention focus is impaired. As a result, the sequential switching is intermittently interrupted by periods of irregular/chaotic dynamics, and the attention switching process becomes uncontrolled. Our modeling results are also in agreement with recent works (Colzato et al., 2007; Tomasi et al., 2010) showing that chronic cocaine use is associated with disrupted inhibitory connections in the brain. In particular, findings in Tomasi et al. (2010) suggest that decreased functional dopaminergic inhibitory connectivity of the midbrain interferes with the activation and deactivation signals associated with sustained attention in cocaine addicts.

AUTHOR CONTRIBUTIONS

All co-authors have equal contribution to all steps of preparation of this article and they approved the version to be published.

ACKNOWLEDGMENTS

Thanks to Pablo Varona, Valentin Afraimovich and Karl Friston for useful discussions. Mikhail I. Rabinovich acknowledges support from ONR grant N00014310205. This material is based upon work supported by NSF to Robert Kozma in the CRCNS Program, grant number DMS-13-11165.

REFERENCES

Abrams, D., and Strogatz, S. (2004). Chimera states for coupled oscillators. *Phys. Rev. Lett.* 93, 174102. doi: 10.1103/PhysRevLett.93.174102

Afraimovich, V., Rabinovich, M., and Varona, P. (2004a). Heteroclinic contours in neural ensembles and the winnerless competition principle. *Int. J. Bifurcat. Chaos* 14, 1195. doi: 10.1142/S0218127404009806

Afraimovich, V. S., Zhigulin, V., and Rabinovich, M. I. (2004b). On the origin of reproducible sequential activity in neural circuts. *Chaos* 14, 1123–1129. doi: 10.1063/1.1819625

Arneodo, A., Coullet, P., Peyraud, J., and Tresser, C. (1982). Strange attractors in volterra equations for species in competition. *J. Math. Biol.* 14, 153–157. doi: 10.1007/BF01832841

Aron, A. (1982). The neural basis of inhibition in cognitive control. *Neuroscientist* 13, 153–157.

Attout, L., Fias, W., Salmon, E., and Majerus, S. (2014). Common neural substrates for ordinal representation in short-term memory, numerical and alphabetical cognition. *PLoS ONE* 9:e9204. doi: 10.1371/journal.pone.009204

Baker, J., Holmes, A., Maste, G., Yeo, B., Krienen, F., Buckner, R., et al. (2014). Disruption of cortical association networks in schizophrenia and psychotic bipolar disorder. *AMA Psychiatry* 71, 109–118. doi: 10.1001/jamapsychiatry.2013.3469

Barr, M., Farzan, F., Rajji, T., Voineskos, A., Blumberger, D., Arenovich, T., et al. (2013). Can repetitive magnetic stimulation improve cognition in schizophrenia? pilot data from a randomized controlled trial. *Biol. Psychiatry* 73, 510–517. doi: 10.1016/j.biopsych.2012.08.020

Baumeister, S., Hohmann, S., Wolf, I., Plichta, M., Rechtsteiner, S., Zangl, M., et al. (2014). Sequential inhibitory control processes assessed through simultaneous eeg-fmri. *Neuroimage* 94, 349–359. doi: 10.1016/j.neuroimage.2014.01.023

Bick, C., and Rabinovich, M. I. (2009). Dynamical origin of the effective storage capacity in the brain's working memory. *Phys. Rev. Lett.* 103:218101. doi: 10.1103/PhysRevLett.103.218101

Bick, C., and Rabinovich, M. I. (2010). On the occurrence o stable heteroclinic channels in lotka-volterra models. *Dyn. Syst.* 25, 1–14. doi: 10.1080/14689360903322227

Bittner, R., Linden, D., Roebroeck, A., Hartling, F., Rotarska-Jagiela, A., Maurer, K., et al. (2014). The when and where of working memory dysfunction in early-onset schizophrenia—a functional magnetic resonance imaging study. *Cereb. Cortex.* doi: 10.1093/cercor/bhu050. [Epub ahead of print].

Bouchard, K. E., Mesgarani, N., Johnson, K., and Chang, E. F. (2013). Functional organization of human sensorimotor cortex for speech articulation. *Nature* 495, 327–332. doi: 10.1038/nature11911

Buonomano, D. V. (2000). Decoding temporal information: a model based on short-term synaptic plasticity. *J. Neurosci.* 20, 1129–1141.

Bystritsky, A., Danial, J., and Kronemeyer, D. (2014). Interactions between diabetes and anxiety and depression: implications for treatment. *Endocrinol. Metab. Clin. N Am.* 43, 269–283. doi: 10.1016/j.ecl.2013.10.001

Bystritsky, A., Nierenberg, A. A., Feusner, J. D., and Rabinovich, M. (2012). Computational non-linear dynamical psychiatry: a new methodological paradigm for diagnosis and course of illness. *J. Psychiatry Res.* 46, 428–435. doi: 10.1016/j.jpsychires.2011.10.013

Camperi, M., and Wang, X. (1998). A model of visuospatial working memory in prefrontal cortex: recurrent network and cellular bistability. *J. Comput. Neurosci.* 5, 383–405. doi: 10.1023/A:1008837311948

Chambers, C., Garavan, H., and Bellgrove, M. (2009). Insights into the neural basis of response inhibition from cognitive and clinical neuroscience. *Neurosci. Biobehav. Rev.* 33, 631–646. doi: 10.1016/j.neubiorev.2008.08.016

Cohen, M., and Grossberg, S. (1983). Absolute stability of global pattern formation and parallel memory storage by competitive neural networks. *IEEE Trans. Syst. Man Cybernet.* 13, 288–307.

Colzato, L., van den Wildenberg, W., and Hommel, B. (2007). Impaired inhibitory control in recreational cocaine users. *PLoS ONE* 2:e1143. doi: 10.1371/journal.pone.0001143

Constantinidis, C., and Wang, X. (2004). A neural circuit basis for spatial working memory. *Neuroscientist* 10, 553–565. doi: 10.1177/1073858404268742

D'Argembeau, A., Jeunehomme, O., Majerus, S., Bastin, C., and Salmon, E. (2014). The neural basis of temporal order processing in past and future thought. *J. Cogn. Neurosci.* doi: 10.1162/jocn_a_00680. [Epub ahead of print].

Deco, G., Ponce-Alvarez, A., Hagmann, P., Romani, G., Mantini, D., and Corbetta, M. (2014). How local excitation-inhibition ratio impacts the whole brain. *Dynam. J. Neurosci.* 34, 7886–7898. doi: 10.1523/JNEUROSCI.5068-13.2014

Dempster, F., and Corkill, A. (1999). "The development of intelligence. Studies in developmental psychology," in *Chapter Neo-Interference Research and The Development of Intelligence*, ed M. Anderson (East Sussex: Psychology Press Limited), 215–243.

Elvevag, B., and Goldberg, T. E. (2000). Cognitive impairment in schizophrenia is the core of the disorder. *Crit. Rev. Neurobiol.* 14, 1–21. doi: 10.1615/CritRevNeurobiol.v14.i1.10

Emrich, S., Riggall, A., LaRocque, J., and Postle, B. (2013). Distributed patterns of activity in sensory cortex reflect the precision of multiple items maintained in visual short-term memory. *J. Neurosci.* 33, 6516–6523. doi: 10.1523/JNEUROSCI.5732-12.2013

Engelhart, P., Nigg, J., Carr, L., and Ferreia, F. (2008). Cognitive inhibition and working memory in attention-deficient/hyperactivity disorder. *J. Abnorm. Psychol.* 117, 591–605. doi: 10.1037/a0012593

Franconeri, S., Alvarez, G., and Cavanagh, P. (2013). Flexible cognitive resources: competitive content maps for attention and memory. *Trends Cogn. Sci.* 17, 134–141. doi: 10.1016/j.tics.2013.01.010

Fukai, T., and Tanaka, S. (1997). A simple neural network exhibiting selective activation of neuronal ensemblies: from winner-take-all to winners-share all. *Neural Comput.* 9, 77–97. doi: 10.1162/neco.1997.9.1.77

Goldman, M. (2009). Memory without feedback in a neural network. *Neuron* 61, 621–634. doi: 10.1016/j.neuron.2008.12.012

Gorfein, D. S., MacLeod, C. M., and Colin, M. (2007). *Inhibition in Cognition*. Washington, DC: American Psychological Association. doi: 10.1037/11587-000

Hagerstrom, A. M., Murphy, T. E., Roy, R., Hövel, P., Omelchenko, I., and Schöll, E. (2012). Experimental observation of chimeras in coupled map lattices. *Nat. Phys.* 8, 658. doi: 10.1038/nphys2372

Hameroff, S., Trakas, M., Duffield, C., Annabi, E., Gerace, M. B., Boyle, P., et al. (2013). Transcranial ultrasound (tus) effects on mental states: a pilot study. *Brain Stimul.* 6, 409–415. doi: 10.1016/j.brs.2012.05.002

Harnishfeger, K. (1995). *The Development of Cognitive Inhibition*. San Diego, CA: Academic Press, Inc.

Henderson, J. A., and Robinson, P. A. (2011). Geometric effects on complex network structure in the cortex. *Phys. Rev. Lett.* 107, 018102. doi: 10.1103/PhysRevLett.107.018102

Hernandez-Bermejo, B., Fairen, V., and Leon, B. (1998). Algebraic recasting of nonlinear systems of odes into universal formats. *J. Phys. A Math. Gen.* 31, 2415. doi: 10.1088/0305-4470/31/10/016

Hirsch, M. W., and Smith, H. (2005). *Handbook of Differential Equations: Ordinary Differential Equations*. Amsterdam: Elsevier.

Hofbauer, J., and Sigmund, K. (1998). *Evolutionary Games and Population Dynamics*. Cambridge, UK: Cambridge University Press. doi: 10.1017/CBO9781139173179

Hopfeld, J. (1982). Neural networks and physical systems with emergent collective computational abilities. *Proc. Natl. Acad. Sci. U.S.A.* 79, 2554–2558. doi: 10.1073/pnas.79.8.2554

Huerta, R., and Rabinovich, M. (2004). Reproducible sequence generation in random neural ensembles. *Phys. Rev. Lett.* 93:238104. doi: 10.1103/PhysRevLett.93.238104

Hughes, L., Ghosh, B., and Rowe, J. (2013). Reorganization of brain networks in frontotemporal dementia and progressive supranuclear palsy. *Neuroimage Clin.* 2, 459–468. doi: 10.1016/j.nicl.2013.03.009

Jones, L. M., Fontanini, A., Sadacca, B. F., Miller, P., and Katz, D. B. (2007). Natural stimuli evoke dynamic sequences of states in sensory cortical ensembles. *Proc. Natl. Acad. Sci. U.S.A.* 104, 18772–18777. doi: 10.1073/pnas.0705546104

Joorman, J., Yoon, K., and Zetsche, U. (2007). Cognitive inhibition in depression. *Appl. Prevent. Psychol.* 12, 128–139. doi: 10.1016/j.appsy.2007.09.002

Kennel, M. B., Brown, R., and Abarbanel, H. D. (1992). Determining embedding dimension for phase-space reconstruction using a geometrical construction. *Phys. Rev. A* 45, 3403. doi: 10.1103/PhysRevA.45.3403

Kleinfeld, D. (1986). Sequential state generation by model neural networks. *Proc. Nati. Acad. Sci. USA* 83, 9469–9473. doi: 10.1073/pnas.83.24.9469

Kozma, R. (1998). Intermediate-range coupling generates low-dimensional attractors deeply in the chaotic region of one-dimensional lattices. *Phys. Lett. A* 244, 85–91. doi: 10.1016/S0375-9601(98)00275-8

Kronemyer, D., and Bystritsky, A. (2014). A non-linear dynamical approach to belief revision in cognitive behavioral therapy. *Front. Comput. Neurosci.* 8:55. doi: 10.3389/fncom.2014.00055

Lewis, D., Hashimoto, T., and Volk, D. (2005). Cortical inhibitory neurons and schizophrenia. *Nat. Rev. Neurosci.* 6, 312–324. doi: 10.1038/nrn1648

Loh, M., Rolls, E., and Deco, G. (2007). A dynamical systems hypothesis of schizophrenia. *PLoS Comput. Biol.* 3:e228. doi: 10.1371/journal.pcbi.0030228

MacLeod, C. (2007). "Inhibition in cognition," in *Chapter The Concept of Inhibition in Cognition*, eds D. S. Gorfein and C. M. MacLeod (Washington, DC: American Psychological Association), 3–23.

Miller, G. A. (1956). The magical number seven, plus or minus two: some limits on our capacity for processing information. *Psychol. Rev.* 63, 81–97. doi: 10.1037/h0043158

Montoya, A., Price, B., Menear, M., and Lepage, M. (2006). Brain imaging and cognitive dysfunctions in huntington's disease. *J. Psychiatry Neurosci.* 31, 21–29.

Mueller, J., Legon, W., Opitz, A., Sato, T., and Tyler, W. J. (2014). Transcranial focused ultrasound modulates intrinsic and evoked eeg dynamics. *Brain Stimul.* doi: 10.1016/j.brs.2014.08.008. [Epub ahead of print].

Murray, J., Anticevic, A., Gancsos, M., and Ichinose, M. (2014a). Linking microcircuit dysfunction to cognitive impairment: effects of disinhibition associated with schizophrenia in a cortical working memory model. *Cereb. Cortex* 24, 859–872. doi: 10.1093/cercor/bhs370

Murray, J., Anticevic, A., Gancsos, M., Ichinose, M., Corlett, P., Krystal, J., et al. (2014b). Linking microcircuit dysfunction to cognitive impairment: effects of disinhibition associated with schizophrenia in a cortical working memory model. *Cereb. Cortex* 24, 859–872. doi: 10.1093/cercor/bhs370

Norman, K. A., Polyn, S. M., Detre, G. J., and Haxby, J. V. (2006). Beyond mind-reading: multi-voxel pattern analysis of fmri data. *Trends Cogn. Sci.* 10, 424–430. doi: 10.1016/j.tics.2006.07.005

Omelchenko, I., Omelchenko, O., Hövel, P., and Schöll, E. (2013). When nonlocal coupling between oscillators becomes stronger: patched synchrony or multichimera states. *Phys. Rev. Lett.* 110:224101. doi: 10.1103/PhysRevLett.110.224101

Omelchenko, I., Riemenschneider, B., Hövel, P., Maistrenko, Y., and Schöll, E. (2012). Transition from spatial coherence to incoherence in coupled chaotic systems. *Phys. Rev. E* 85, 026212. doi: 10.1103/PhysRevE.85.026212

Panaggio, M., and Abram, D. (2014). Chimera states: coexistence of coherence and incoherence in networks of coupled oscillators. arXiv:1403.6204v2

Polyn, S. M., Natu, V. S., Cohen, J. D., and Norman, K. A. (2005). Category-specic cortical activity precedes retrieval during memory search. *Science* 310, 1963–1966. doi: 10.1126/science.1117645

Postle, B. (2006). Working memory as an emergent property of the mind and brain. *Neuroscience* 139, 23–38. doi: 10.1016/j.neuroscience.2005.06.005

Rabinovich, M. I., Afraimovich, V. S., Bick, C., and Varona, P. (2012a). Information flow dynamics in the brain. *Phys. Life Rev.* 9, 51–73. doi: 10.1016/j.plrev.2011.11.002

Rabinovich, M. I., Friston, K., and Varona, P. (2012b). *Principles of Brain Dynamics: Global State Interactions*. Cambridge, MA: MIT Press.

Rabinovich, M. I., Muezzinoglu, M. K., Strigo, I., and Bystritsky, A. (2010). Dynamical principles of emotion-cognition interaction: mathematical images of mental disorders. *PLoS ONE* 5:e12547. doi: 10.1371/journal.pone.0012547

Rabinovich, M. I., Tristan, I., and Varona, P. (2013). Neural dynamics of attentional cross-modality control. *PLoS ONE* 8:e64406. doi: 10.1371/journal.pone.0064406

Rabinovich, M. I., Varona, P., Tristan, I., and Afraimovich, V. S. (2014). Chunking dynamics: heteroclinics in mind. *Front. Comput. Neurosci.* 8:22. doi: 10.3389/fncom.2014.00022

Rabinovich, M. I., Varona, P., Selverston, A., and Abarbanel, H. (2006). Dynamical principles in neuroscience. *Rev. Mod. Phys.* 78, 1213–1265. doi: 10.1103/RevModPhys.78.1213

Schiepek, G., Tominschek, I., Heinzel, S., Aigner, M., and Dold, M., (2013). Discontinuous patterns of brain activation in the psychotherapy process of obsessive-compulsive disorder: converging results from repeated fmri and daily self-reports. *PLoS ONE* 8:e71863. doi: 10.1371/journal.pone.0071863

Seliger, P., Tsimring, L., and Rabinovich, M. (2003). Dynamics-based sequential memory: winnerless competition of patterns. *Phys. Rev. E* 67, 1–4. doi: 10.1103/PhysRevE.67.011905

Sieber, J., Omel'chenko, O. E., and Wolfrum, M. (2014). Controlling unstable chaos: stabilizing chimera states by feedback. *Phys. Rev. Lett.* 112:054102. doi: 10.1103/PhysRevLett.112 054102

Smid, H., Martens, S., de Witte, M., and Bruggeman, R. (2013). Inflexible minds: impaired attention switching in recent-onset schizophrenia. *PLoS ONE* 8:e78062. doi: 10.1371/journal.pone.0078062

Sokolov, Y., Kozma, R., and Rabinovich, M. (2014). "Noise effects in a dynamical model of attentional switching," in *Biomedical Science and Engineering Center Conference (BSEC), 2014 Annual Oak Ridge National Laboratory* (Oak Ridge, TN).

Sompolinsky, H., and Kanter, I. I. (1986). Temporal association in asymmetric neural networks. *Phys. Rev. Lett.* 57, 2861–2864. doi: 10.1103/PhysRevLett.57.2861

Stopfer, M., Jayaraman, V., and Laurent, G. (2003). Intensity versus identity coding in an olfactory system. *Neuron* 39, 991–1004. doi: 10.1016/j.neuron.2003.08.011

Szatmary, B., and Izhikevich, E. (2010). Spike-timing theory of working memory. *PLoS Comput. Biol.* 6:e1000879. doi: 10.1371/journal.pcbi.1000879

Takens, F. (1981). *Dynamical Systems and Turbulence.* New York, NY: Springer-Verlag.

Takeuchi, Y. (1996). *Global Dynamical Properties of Lotka-Volterra Systems.* Singapore: World Scientific.

Tekin, S., and Cummings, J. (2002). Frontal-subcortical neuronal circuits and clinical neuropsychiatry: an update. *J. Psychosom. Res.* 53, 647–654. doi: 10.1016/S0022-3999(02)00428-2

Tomasi, D., Volkow, N., Wang, R., Carrillo, J., Maloney, T., Alia-Klein, N., et al. (2010). Disrupted functional connectivity with dopaminergic midbrain in cocaine abusers. *PLoS ONE* 5:e10815. doi: 10.1371/journal.pone.0010815

Varona, P., Rabinovich, M., Selverston, A., and Arshavsky, Y. (2002). Winnerless competition between sensory neurons generates chaos: a possible mechanism for molluscan hunting behavior. *Chaos* 12, 672–677. doi: 10.1063/1.1498155

Westerhausen, R., Kompus, K., and Hugdahl, K. (2011).) impaired cognitive inhibition in schizophrenia: a meta-analysis of the stroop interference effect. *Schizophr. Res.* 133, 172–181. doi: 10.1016/j.schres.2011.08.025

Xia, M., Fang, J., Pan, F., and Bai, E. (2009). Robust sequence memory in sparsely-connected networks with controllable steady-state period. *Neurocomputing* 72, 1213–1265. doi: 10.1016/j.neucom.2009.03.004

Yi, Z., Tan, K., and Lee, T. (2003). Multistability analysis for recurrent neural networks with unsaturating piecewise linear transfer functions. *Neural Comput.* 15, 639–662. doi: 10.1162/089976603321192112

APPENDIX

Here the case of GLV with weak inhibitory connections are studied. For convenience, let us introduce the notation for foregoing sub-networks S_1 and S_2, respectively. Both subsystems have 3 modes, S_1 contains modes R_1, R_3, and R_5, while S_2 includes R_2, R_4, and R_6. We consider the case of weak, uniform connections between the two subsystems. Accordingly, κ_1 and κ_2 denote the connection strength from S_1 to S_2 and from S_2 to S_1, respectively. For the sake of simplicity, here we assume $\kappa_2 = 0$ and we study bifurcation only with respect to one parameter $\kappa = \kappa_1$. Note that the results of this section are readily extendable to the case $\kappa_2 \neq 0$.

Based on the definition of subsystems S_1 and S_2, clearly two independent stable heteroclinic cycles exist for $\kappa_1 = 0$. Further, it is expected that the two heteroclinic cycles are maintained for very weak coupling $0 < \kappa << 1$. Increasing κ in the small to intermediate coupling levels, complex dynamics may emerge, such as simultaneous presence of chaos and heteroclinic cycles. The upper bound of this region is marked as κ^*. Finally, the cycles must collapse if coupling exceeds a high threshold value ($\kappa >> 1$).

We start with the definition of several quantities, which allow us to separate the whole domain of coupling parameter κ into regions with different types of behavior. The threshold values are expressed as follows: $\kappa^* = max_i\{\gamma_{i+1}/\gamma_i\},\ i = 1, \ldots, 6$, where γ_i is the strength of stimulation of mode i (see Equation 1). Further, let us characterize each equilibria. In the following considerations, all indices are written with respect to $(mod\ 6)$ and we use of the following convention $\{i \in \{0, \ldots, n\} | i = n \pmod{n}\} = n$. Let us define for each $i = 1, \ldots, 6$ the corresponding set of two numbers $\bar{i} = \{(i \pm 2)\ mod\ 6\}$.

Further notations are: $k^*_{odd} = \max\{k_1, k_3, k_5\}$ and $k^*_{even} = \max\{k_2, k_4, k_6\}$, and indexes defined as $i^*_{odd} = \arg\max\{k^*_{odd}\}$ and $i^*_{even} = \arg\max\{k^*_{even}\}$, where k_i is defined by

$$k_i = \frac{\gamma_{(i+1)}(-\sum_{k\in\bar{i}} \gamma_k a_{ki} + \gamma_i \prod_{k\in\bar{i}} a_{ki})}{\prod_{k\in\bar{i}} (\gamma_k - \gamma_i a_{ki})} \tag{2}$$

In the following considerations, we use quantities $k' = \max\{k_{i^*_{odd}-2}, k_{i^*_{odd}+2}\}$ and $k" = \max\{k_{i^*_{even}-2}, k_{i^*_{even}+2}\}$. It is easy to see that k' and $k"$ are larger than the other thresholds. In the following description, we assume that $k' < k"$ unless it is specified otherwise.

There exists a value of coupling parameter $0 < k^0 << 1$ such that for $\kappa \in (0, k^0)$ the coupled system exhibits two heteroclinic cycles. For $\kappa \in (k^o, \kappa^*)$ various complex behaviors emerge, with the possibility of co-existing chaotic attractor and heteroclinic cycle. In the case of $\kappa \in (\kappa^*, k')$ the system converges to a fixed point. For $\kappa \in (k', k")$, a heteroclinic cycle in one system coexists with zero fixed points in the other system. Finally, for $\kappa > k"$ the coupled system collapses. Thus, we have the following regions

$$0 < k^o < \kappa^* < k' \leq k" < \infty. \tag{3}$$

If $k' = k"$ then the conclusion still holds with the difference that the behavior corresponding to values between k' and $k"$ does not occur. The present results were derived based on the dissipative property of the saddle point. In other words, the equilibrium point attracts trajectories in its neighborhood if it is dissipative point. However, if the dissipative property of the saddle point changes, i.e., the saddle value is no more greater than one due to the increase of κ, we may observe that the orbits move in directions away from equilibria. For this reason, when the coupling parameter is large ($\kappa > k'$), the origin will attract the trajectories of one of the subsystems. Under this scenario, we have one subsystem (i.e., $S1$ or $S2$) embedded in 6 dimension, and this subsystem behaves as in the case $\kappa = 0$. In other words, considering the phase space $\mathbb{R}^6 = \mathbb{R}^3 \oplus \mathbb{R}^3$, if one subsystem vanishes we deal with the subspace where all coordinates of this subsystem are zero, so the other subsystem behaves like in the case $\kappa = 0$.

In the case of $\kappa \in (\kappa^*, k')$, the central eigenspace of each equilibria stays the same. However, the number of stable non-leading eigenvalues is increased to the maximum possible value, thus fixed points appear. In the most challenging case when $\kappa \in (k^0, \kappa^*)$, the equilibria which form the heteroclinic cycles have different number of stable and unstable non-leading eigenvalues. This case is possible due to the non-symmetry of the equations, which describe the coupled system with mutual inhibition between its subsystems. To put it simply, there is no symmetry group between its subsystems coupling.

14

Classification of single-trial auditory events using dry-wireless EEG during real and motion simulated flight

Daniel E. Callan[1,2]*, Gautier Durantin[3] and Cengiz Terzibas[2]

[1] Center for Information and Neural Networks (CiNet), National Institute of Information and Communications Technology (NICT), Osaka University, Osaka, Japan
[2] Multisensory Cognition and Computation Laboratory Universal Communication Research Institute, National Institute of Information and Communications Technology, Kyoto, Japan
[3] Centre Aéronautique et Spatial, Institut Supérieur de l'Aéronautique et de l'Espace, Université de Toulouse, Toulouse, France

Edited by:
Mikhail Lebedev, Duke University, USA

Reviewed by:
Alistair McEwan, The University of Sydney, Australia
Raja Parasuraman, George Mason University, USA

***Correspondence:**
Daniel E. Callan, Center for Information and Neural Networks (CiNet), National Institute of Information and Communications Technology (NICT), Osaka University, 1-4 Yamadaoka, Suita City, Osaka 565-0871, Japan
e-mail: dcallan@nict.go.jp

Application of neuro-augmentation technology based on dry-wireless EEG may be considerably beneficial for aviation and space operations because of the inherent dangers involved. In this study we evaluate classification performance of perceptual events using a dry-wireless EEG system during motion platform based flight simulation and actual flight in an open cockpit biplane to determine if the system can be used in the presence of considerable environmental and physiological artifacts. A passive task involving 200 random auditory presentations of a chirp sound was used for evaluation. The advantage of this auditory task is that it does not interfere with the perceptual motor processes involved with piloting the plane. Classification was based on identifying the presentation of a chirp sound vs. silent periods. Evaluation of Independent component analysis (ICA) and Kalman filtering to enhance classification performance by extracting brain activity related to the auditory event from other non-task related brain activity and artifacts was assessed. The results of permutation testing revealed that single trial classification of presence or absence of an auditory event was significantly above chance for all conditions on a novel test set. The best performance could be achieved with both ICA and Kalman filtering relative to no processing: Platform Off (83.4% vs. 78.3%), Platform On (73.1% vs. 71.6%), Biplane Engine Off (81.1% vs. 77.4%), and Biplane Engine On (79.2% vs. 66.1%). This experiment demonstrates that dry-wireless EEG can be used in environments with considerable vibration, wind, acoustic noise, and physiological artifacts and achieve good single trial classification performance that is necessary for future successful application of neuro-augmentation technology based on brain-machine interfaces.

Keywords: EEG, dry EEG, brain machine interface, independent component analysis, Kalman filter, auditory evoked response, single trial, classification

INTRODUCTION

Technology capable of augmenting human performance by means of feedback of decoded neural states has potential for many types of neuroergonimic applications. Neuroergonomics is the study of the human brain in relation to performance at work, at home, in transportation, and in everyday settings with the goal of using this knowledge to design technologies and work environments to augment human behavior to enhance safety, usability, efficiency and enjoyment (Parasuraman, 2003; Parasuraman and Rizzo, 2008). Because of the inherent dangers in aviation and space operations these fields may be particularly well suited for neuroergonomic applications to increase performance and safety. There are many challenges for effective implementation of neuroergonomic technology in real-world situations. Unlike the laboratory where brain recordings can be made under controlled conditions, in real world situations there is considerable additional physiological and environmental noise that must be dealt with. In addition it is likely the case that brain dynamics differ in real-world environments compared to those of the laboratory (McDowell et al., 2013; Lin et al., 2014).

Pilots' often face periods of excessive workload, stress, fatigue, attentional deficits, etc... during flight operations that may affect performance. The ability to decode the mental state of the pilot and augment these states by neuro- adaptive feedback and/or automation has great potential in improving training, performance, and safety. In this article we are particularly interested in investigating brain potentials that occur as a result of passive presentation of an auditory stimulus during flight. This research has relevance to the phenomenon of inattentional deafness in which pilots' sometimes miss audio alarms. Missed audio alarms are responsible for a significant number of aviation accidents (Bliss, 2003; Scannella et al., 2013; Dehais et al., 2014).

There have been a number of studies in which brain activity has been measured with electroencephalography EEG during aviation (Sem-Jacobsen et al., 1959; Blanc et al., 1966; Caldwell and Lewis, 1995) and space operations (Maulsby, 1966; Cheron et al., 2009). EEG has been successfully collected in flight since the late 1950's (Sem-Jacobsen et al., 1959). These studies showed that although the in flight environment is subject to noise caused by vibration and greater physical movement of the pilot that are not present during laboratory based experiments, the EEG signals recorded are able to show changes in various frequency bands and additional specific features that are associated with flight performance (Sterman et al., 1987) as well as workload (Howitt et al., 1978; Hankins and Wilson, 1998; Dussault et al., 2005) and fatigue (Howitt et al., 1978; Sauvet et al., 2014). Experiments conducted aboard the International Space Station have shown changes in the rhythmic brain activity of astronauts as a result of microgravity (Cheron et al., 2009). In an experiment conducted during parabolic flight it was found that a mental imagery (Thinking of moving arm vs. thinking of words) based brain machine interface (BMI) task could achieve between 72%–79% single trial classification performance across the various g-force conditions ranging from 0 to 2 g (Millàn Jdel et al., 2009).

A BMI is a device that provides for the ability to transfer and use information from distinct brain states for communicating with a machine (Blankertz et al., 2010). BMI based on electroencephalography EEG have been used in many applications including, but not limited to, modulating brain rhythms to control movement of a cursor on a screen (Wolpaw et al., 2002) as well as a quadrocopter in the real world (LaFleur et al., 2013), decoding brain states such as attention, performance capability, workload, etc... (Dornhege et al., 2007; Müller et al., 2008; Blankertz et al., 2010), decoding various perceptual events (Birbaumer et al., 1999; Wang et al., 2006; Bin et al., 2009). A primary goal of BMI research is to augment human behavior to allow for enhanced performance. Notably, there are considerable improvements in performance for some medical applications of BMI when the user's motor system is severely incapacitated. For example patients with locked-in syndrome who are not able to communicate through standard pathways or assistive technology can learn to spell and initiate dialogs using P300 based BMI (Sellers et al., 2014). Non-medical application of the BMI P300 speller in normal healthy individuals is not practical since normal channels of communication are considerably better.

There are several limitations for the practical neuroergonomic application of many of these BMIs in real-world situations (Blankertz et al., 2010). Many of these BMIs take a considerable amount of time for operator training, on the order of months. This is true especially for implementations when the user needs to learn how to modulate various brain rhythms (Wolpaw et al., 2002; LaFleur et al., 2013). For practical application there should be very little if any operator training in control of the BMI. Many BMIs require considerable mental workload to operate, such as those requiring mental imagery and those utilizing focused attention away from the primary task environment. The amount of cognitive resources required to operate such BMI can be so high, that the operator's usual channels of perceptual, motor, and cognitive processing are greatly impaired. For example, it is obvious that if one is actively involved with mentally imaging movement of their left hand to move a vehicle left, mentally imaging movement of both arms to move a vehicle right, mentally imaging walking to move forward, and mental word association to move back, that this will drastically compromise the operators ability to speak, walk, and move their hands while engaged in operating the BMI. However, if one uses a joystick to move a vehicle the operator will still be able to speak, walk, and move their hands around without drastically compromising performance depending on the difficulty of the task at hand. While P300 based BMI have advantages in that they do not require extensive subject training, they often require directed attention away from the environment in which they are suppose to operate in. For example subjects using a P300 based BMI to control various items in a virtual apartment reported a far lower sense of presence, which they attributed to increased workload, in interacting in the environment than did control subjects not using BMI (Groenegress et al., 2010). In order for a BMI to be effective it is necessary to utilize naturally occurring brain states for control. Another limitation of many of these BMI implementations is that they utilize rather bulky EEG systems that are not portable and use gel that takes a considerable amount of time and assistance to apply.

Practical application of EEG in real-world situations requires the use of technology that is easy to wear without the use of gel and one that is wireless to transmit data to a computer for real-time processing. There are many dry-wireless EEG systems available that have been used for many different applications including drowsiness detection (Park et al., 2011), gaming (Liao et al., 2012; Zao et al., 2014), and detection of perceptual events (Lin et al., 2014). Of particular interest in relation to real-world application of BMI is the study conducted by Lin et al. (2014) investigating the impact of walking locomotion on the ability to detect steady state visual evoked potentials (SSVEP) using a dry-wireless EEG system. The SSVEP is a frequency coded neural response that is modulated by the presentation frequency of the visual stimuli (Lin et al., 2014). The classification performance was good but decreased as a result of walking speed from 84.87% for standing to 83.03% for 1 MPH walking, 79.47% for 2 MPH walking, and 75.26% for 3 MPH walking (Lin et al., 2014). The decrease in performance as a function of walking speed may result from increasingly larger artifacts in the EEG as well as to greater difficulty in fixated attention to the visual stimuli as one moves more. Dry electrodes are more susceptible to movement related artifacts than gel based EEG recording (Guger et al., 2012; Lin et al., 2014). One limitation for utilization of the SSVEP for many BMI applications is that the task requires the subject to attend to the visual stimuli presented on the computer screen. This requirement is not practical in many real-world situations where perceptual motor control requires the use of the visual system such as in aviation and space operations.

The goal of this study is to determine the extent to which perceptually evoked brain related EEG signals, recorded with a dry-wireless system in noisy real-world environments can be decoded for potential use in BMIs to augment human performance. With a focus on aviation related applications we conducted our experiment in two environmental conditions.

One environmental condition was the use of a motion platform based flight simulator the other was an open cockpit biplane. In order to avoid practical problems in controlling the airplane by using a visual based perceptual presentation task, an auditory stimulus presentation task was used to assess single trial classification performance. The advantage of using an audio stimulus presentation task (100 ms chirp sound) is that it can be played passively in the background while the pilot attends to flying the plane. The goal for the classifier was to determine from the EEG data the presentation of the audio stimulus (chirp) from periods of no audio stimulus (silence) presentation.

A control condition was used for both environmental conditions. In the motion platform condition the experiment was conducted with the platform and flight simulator off (a relatively noise free condition) and with the motion platform on while flying aerobatic maneuvers in the flight simulator (Platform Off and Platform On conditions). In the platform on condition there is considerable movement of the individuals arms, legs, eyes, neck, and entire body as well as potential electrical noise from the motion platform motors. In the biplane condition the experiment was conducted with the engine and avionics off while sitting on the tarmac (a relatively noise free condition) and with the engine and avionics on while piloting the plane in cruise flight. The open cockpit biplane may constitute one of the most challenging environments for EEG recording in which there is an incredible amount of vibration, wind, acoustic noise, as well as considerable movement of the individual's arms, legs, eyes, neck, and entire body.

There are considerable sources of noise that make recording of EEG in real-world environments challenging including non-neurological electrophysiological signals (e.g., muscle activity), electronic noise, and mechanical vibrations. In order to be able to clean the data of the artifacts and extract brain activity related to the auditory evoked responses several procedures within EEGLAB (Swartz Center for Computational Neuroscience, Delorme and Makeig, 2004) are used including independent component analysis (ICA). In addition to these artifact-cleaning procedures a Kalman (1960) filter implementing a dynamical model of the single-trial auditory evoked responses was also used to help extract brain activity related to presentation of the audio stimuli. Based on the results of Lin et al. (2014) using a similar dry-wireless EEG system it is predicted that above chance classification performance in detecting single trial audio stimulus presentation will be achieved in all conditions. Furthermore, it is predicted that both ICA and Kalman filtering will improve classification performance across all conditions.

METHODS

SUBJECTS

The same subject was used for all studies. The subject was male, right handed, 45 years old, with normal hearing. One of the authors served as the subject in this experiment. He has 5 years of flying experience with more than 250 h total time and 200 h in biplanes of the same make and model. The subject gave informed consent for experimental procedures approved by the ethics committee of the National Institute of Information and Communications Technology in accordance with the principles expressed in the Declaration of Helsinki.

Motion Platform Flight Simulator

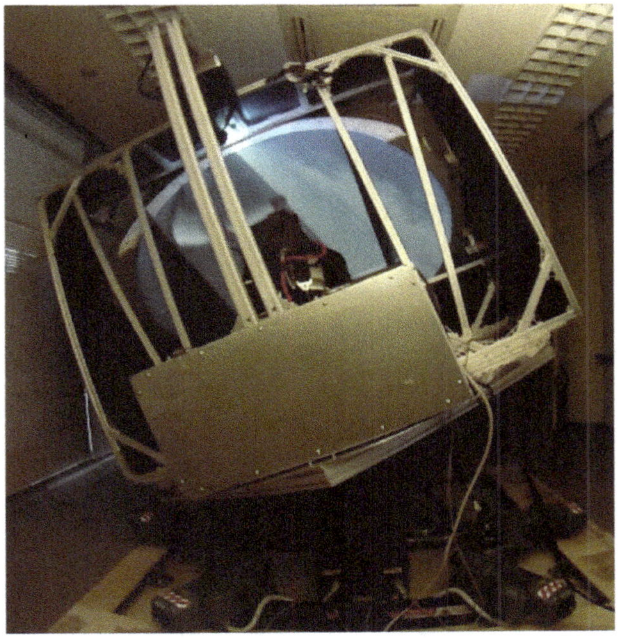

FIGURE 1 | Motion Platform Flight Simulator composed of the CKAS V7 6 degree of freedom Motion System (CKAS Mechatronics, Melborn, Australia) with a custom built cockpit utilizing dome projection for video. The flight controls consist of 1. A control stick to manipulate the elevator (pitch) and ailerons (roll), 2. Rudder pedals to manipulate the rudder (yaw), and 3. A Throttle to manipulate thrust. Single-trial auditory events using dry-wireless EEG were evaluated while the subject was flying through a simulated Redbull Air Race course.

PROCEDURE

The experimental task consisted of passively listening to a chirp sound (0.1 s duration) in different environmental settings while recording brain activity using the Cognionics 64 channel dry wireless EEG system. The chirp sound was presented 200 times spaced randomly by at least 0.6–2.5 s of silence. Within these periods of silence 200 independent 0.5 s segments were randomly extracted. The different environmental settings and conditions are as follows: Electric Motion Platform (Platform Off, Platform On) and open cockpit Biplane (Engine Off, Engine On).

The CKAS V7 6 degree of freedom Motion System (CKAS Mechatronics, Melborn, Australia) with a custom built cockpit utilizing dome projection for video was used (see **Figure 1**). In the motors off condition the subject was sitting still in the chair mounted on the platform. In the motors on condition the subject was engaging in aerobatic flight simulation (X-Plane Laminar Research) through the same Redbull Air Race course as used in a previous fMRI study (Callan et al., 2012). See Callan et al. (2012, 2013) for details on the implementation of the flight simulator system for brain imaging experiments. Just as in a

Open Cockpit Biplane used in Experiment

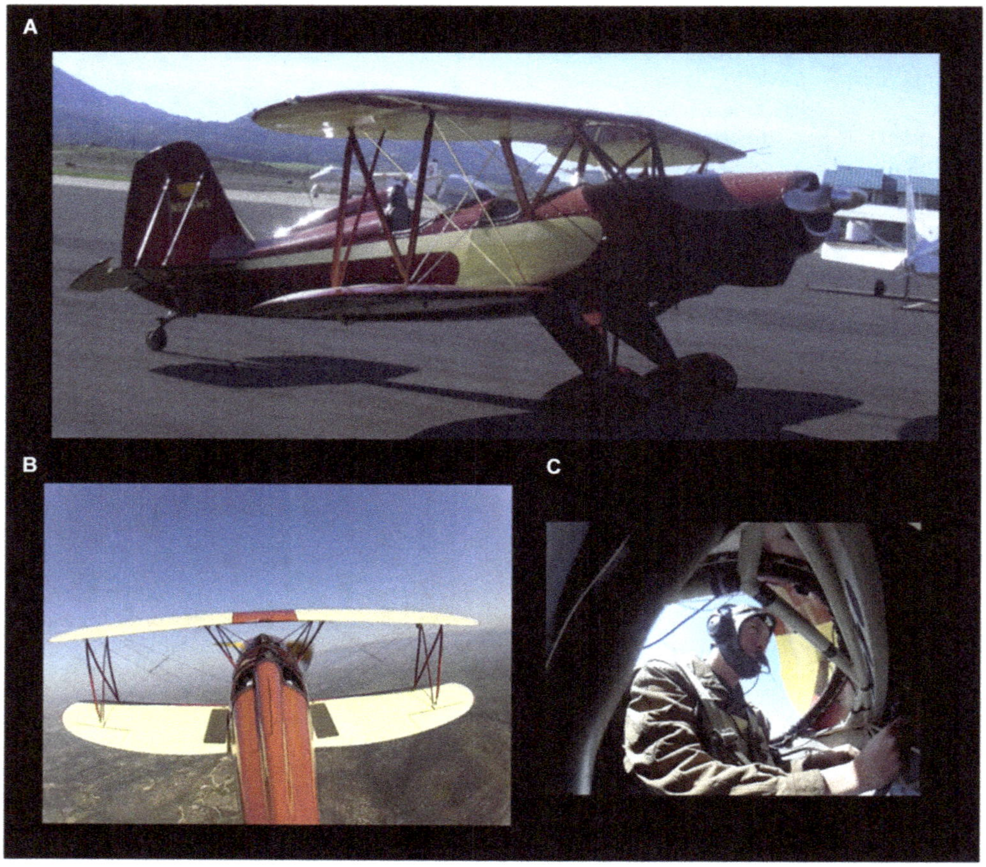

FIGURE 2 | Open Cockpit Starduster SA300 Biplane used for in flight and ground testing of single-trial auditory events using dry-wireless EEG. **(A)** View off the biplane on the ground. **(B)** View of the biplane in the air. **(C)** Picture of the subject wearing the Cognionics 64 channel dry-wireless EEG under the leather flight helmet. This is the same EEG system pictured in **Figure 3**.

real airplane, the subject controlled the ailerons and elevator by stick with the right hand, the throttle lever with the left hand, and the rudders with foot pedals. The motors of the motion platform moved in relation to the accelerations of the aircraft in the flight simulator. No sound was presented from the flight simulator. In both the platform off and platform on conditions the audio stimuli were presented using the Clarity Aloft Pro aviation headset using the same sound level. The experiment took approximately 10 min for each condition. The platform on condition was conducted first followed by the platform off condition.

The biplane used in the experiment was an open cockpit two passenger Starduster SA300 (see **Figure 2**). In the engine off condition the subject was sitting in the front seat of the biplane on the tarmac with avionics off. In the engine on condition the subject was piloting the plane during cruise flight from the front seat with avionics on. In the engine on condition there was extreme vibration, acoustic noise, and wind. In both the engine off and engine on conditions the Cognionics EEG system was worn underneath a leather flight cap. The audio stimuli were presented using the Bose A20 active noise canceling aviation headset using the same sound level. The experiment took approximately 10 min for each condition. The engine off condition was conducted first followed by the engine on condition.

EEG RECORDING AND ANALYSIS

EEG was recorded using the Cognionics HD-72 dry wireless EEG headset (Cognionics, Inc., San Diego[1]). The same 64-channel EEG system was used by Mullen et al. (2013) and shares the same underlying technology as the 32-channel system reported in Chi et al. (2013) and Lin et al. (2014).

The EEG headset consists of a mechanically flexible spine to provide structure and ease of handling. Each segment of the spine contains a row of electrodes. The 64 electrodes provide full scalp coverage. An internal active shield, covering all sensor positions, spans the entire headset to minimize external noise pickup and

[1] http://www.cognionics.com/

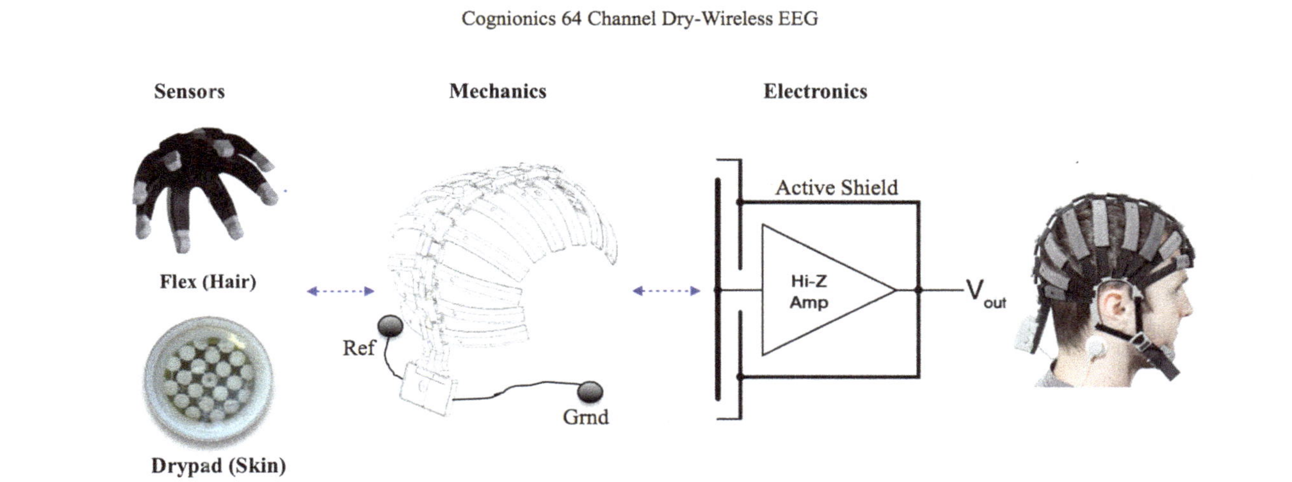

FIGURE 3 | Cognionics 64 Channel Dry-Wireless EEG Headset. Two types of dry sensors are used: The flex sensors are placed over hair and the Drypad sensors are placed over bearskin, such as the forehead. In our setup, we utilized 7 Drypad sensors on the forehead (first band) and 54 flex sensors across the rest of the array. Each band of the headset is user adjustable to enable proper fit and sensor pressure over different head sizes and shapes. An internal flexible conductive layer forms an active shield, which spans the entire headset, to minimize external noise pickup even with high-impedance dry electrodes. Ground (Grnd) and reference (Ref) electrodes are placed under the ear as shown in the figure. The same cap pictured here is in **Figure 2** underneath the leather flight helmet. See the text in the Methods section for further details.

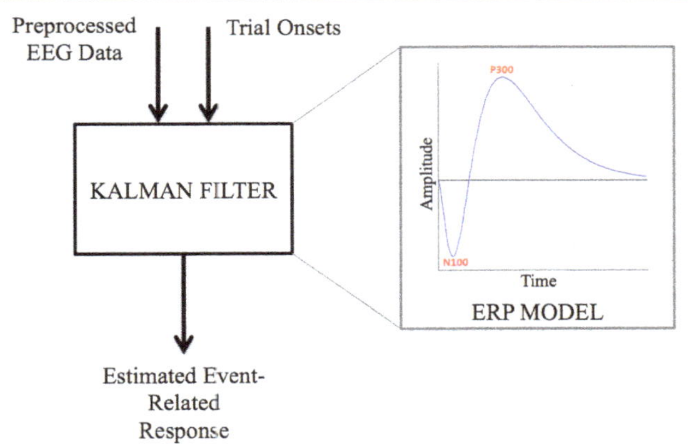

FIGURE 4 | Kalman filter functional model. Kalman filter is designed from an Event Related Potential (ERP) dynamical model (on the right), and uses both preprocessed EEG data and trial onsets to estimate the instantaneous event-related response.

artifacts. Reference and ground are placed on the mastoids with by two standard ECG adhesive electrodes (see **Figure 3**).

Two sensor options are compatible with the headset and connect via a miniature snap receptacle. In the setup, seven Drypad sensors were placed on the forehead (**Figure 3**). The Drypad electrode is a cushioned membrane that is optimized for bare skin contact. For the remaining 57 positions, we used the Flex sensors designed for thru-hair measurements. The Flex sensor is specifically designed to brush aside hair and make direct scalp contact with legs that gently bend and deform under modest pressure. Compared to previous metal pin sensors (e.g., Liao et al., 2011), the Flex sensors offer improved comfort and safety since the sensors can completely flatten under hard impacts. Contact impedances with both sensors typically range from 100 k to 1 MOhm (Mullen et al., 2013) on unprepared skin.

To adequately acquire EEG signals with high electrode impedances, the Cognionics system utilizes a combination of active shielding, high input impedance amplifiers and active grounding to cancel and minimize environmental noise. Data is sampled at 300 Hz (DC-80 Hz bandwidth) with 24-bit ADCs to maximize dynamic range and quickly recover from overload artifacts. Total noise within the EEG band (1–50 Hz) is 0.7 microVolts RMS. The signal quality of the sensors, electrodes, and the data acquisition circuitry has been shown to be comparable to wet electrode based EEG systems with a correlation between simultaneously recorded evoked potentials of $r > 0.9$ (Chi et al., 2013; Mullen et al., 2013).

All electronics are housed in a miniature box at the base of the headset, which weighs a total of only 350 g making the entire system lightweight, portable and wearable. Data transmission is accomplished by a custom 5 GHz WiFi module. The headset radio communicates directly to an embedded WiFi host, in a point-to-point network, running on a USB dongle to minimize the overhead associated with a typical access point and PC-based software protocol stack, thereby minimizing latency and jitter. The receiving computer was a Panasonic CF-AX2 running Ubuntu Linux operating system. The average delay in receiving the signal was less than 1 ms. Audio stimuli were presented from the same computer as used to record the EEG by means of the auxiliary input to the aviation headset. The presentation of the audio signals was given time stamps in correspondence with the time stamps given for each of the recorded EEG samples. The high temporal precision of the wireless link and the presentation software allows for accurate time registration between stimulus and EEG without the use of wire-line markers.

The EEG data was preprocessed using artifact-cleaning procedures available in EEGLAB (Delorme and Makeig, 2004). The data was first filtered using a FIR band pass filter between 2 and 30 Hz with a filter order of 496. The data was separated into a training set of 75% of the stimuli (150 chirp stimuli and 150 silent stimuli) and a testing set of 25% of the stimuli (50 chirp stimuli and 50 silent stimuli) for the platform off and on conditions and the biplane engine off and on conditions. The rational for choosing 75% of the trials for training and 25% for testing is that we believed this division would provide enough training data to generalize to a novel testing set while maintaining enough trials in the testing set to be a reasonable representation of the population. Although we did not attempt to train and test on a 50% split of the data we believed that the amount of training data may not have been sufficient for generalization to the novel test set. The artifact cleaning procedures were applied only to the training sets. The results of which were then applied to the corresponding test sets. The exact same cleaning procedures were then applied to the corresponding testing sets, with the same parameters.

Channels were considered to be bad and were removed from the training data based on the following: Maximum amplitude in the channel is greater than 100 microvolts; Channel flatline duration is greater than 5 s; Channel is correlated at less than 0.8 to its robust estimate based on other channels; Channel has more line noise relative to its signal than 4 standard deviations from the channel population mean. These same channels were then removed from the corresponding test sets.

The next step was to clean the multi-channel training data with the artifact subspace reconstruction (ASR) method using the defaults given in the clean_artifacts software within EEGLAB. ASR allows for the removal of non-stationary high-variance signals from EEG and reconstructs missing data using a spatial mixing matrix (See EEGLAB software by Christian Kothe and the following for details[2]). Calibration data from clean segments of the training data were used to determine the ASR filters separately for each of the four conditions. The ASR filter was then applied to the corresponding test data.

Following cleaning of the data by ASR, ICA using the extended infomax algorithm (Bell and Sejnowski, 1995) in EEGLAB was applied in order to separate brain activity related to the auditory evoked potentials from other brain and artifact related components. The weights of the ICA were determined only from the training data separately for each of the four conditions (platform off, platform on, engine off, engine on). These weights were then applied to the corresponding test data to determine the ICA activation waveforms. See **Figure 5** for an example of the continuous data before ASR, after ASR, and after ICA.

Kalman filtering (Kalman, 1960) was applied to the ASR filtered data both before and after ICA, to produce an estimate of the single-trial auditory evoked response. Kalman filtering is a linear quadratic estimation method, which relies on both the measurements and a modelization of the Event-Related Potential (ERP) dynamics to product an estimate in real-time. This method has been successfully applied to single-trial event related potentials estimation (Georgiadis et al., 2005). In our case, the parameters used as a model for the Kalman filter design were the N100 and P300 waves, generic features of the auditory evoked potential (see **Figure 4**). Both waves were modeled by a third-order impulse response with peaks respectively at 100 ms and 300 ms. The state noise was considered as white noise (Georgiadis et al., 2005), and the measurement noise covariance to state noise covariance ratio was fixed to 0.001, so that the Kalman estimate would put confidence in the measurements (Grewal and Andrews, 2008).

TRAINING AND TESTING THE CLASSIFIER

The Matlab Least Squares Probabilistic Classification (LSPC) toolbox (Sugiyama, 2010) was used to determine how well single trial audio presented stimuli could be identified in the EEG signal from periods of audio silence. LSPC uses a linear combination of kernel function to model the class-posterior probability. Regularized least-squares fitting of the true class-posterior probability is used to learn its parameters (Sugiyama, 2010). The use of least-squares fitting to determine a linear model allows for a global solution to be made analytically providing a considerable speedup in computational time. The default parameters were used in training of the LSPC models (see Matlab code: Sugiyama, 2010).

The features used to train the classifier consisted of the samples from onset to 500 ms after stimulus onset (150 samples) for both chirp and silent stimuli. In the case of ICA data the components selected to be included in the LSPC model were determined by visual inspection of the mean of the activation waveform of the chirp training data stimuli that showed a characteristic auditory evoked potential. For the pre-ICA data all of the channels were included in the LSPC model. The large number of features relative to the number of trials used to train the classifiers has the potential for over-fitting, resulting in poor generalization to the novel test data. We utilized inner cross-validation procedures for model selection in part to assess and protect against potential over-fitting.

The following inner cross-validation procedures were used for model selection and testing: Randomized ten fold cross-validation was used on the training data and the trained model with the best performance was selected for evaluating performance on the test data. One fold of the training data consisted of 135 chirp and 135 silent stimuli and one fold upon which the model was evaluated for selection consisted of 15 chirp and 15 silent stimuli. The final test data consisted of 50 chirp and 50 silent stimuli. This procedure was conducted 100 times to determine the distribution of performance of the model given random aspects of training (e.g., the trials selected for training and their order into the model).

Several conditions were evaluated to assess the efficacy of ICA and Kalman filtering in improving classification performance on the data. These conditions included the four environmental

[2]http://sccn.ucsd.edu/eeglab/plugins/ASR.pdf

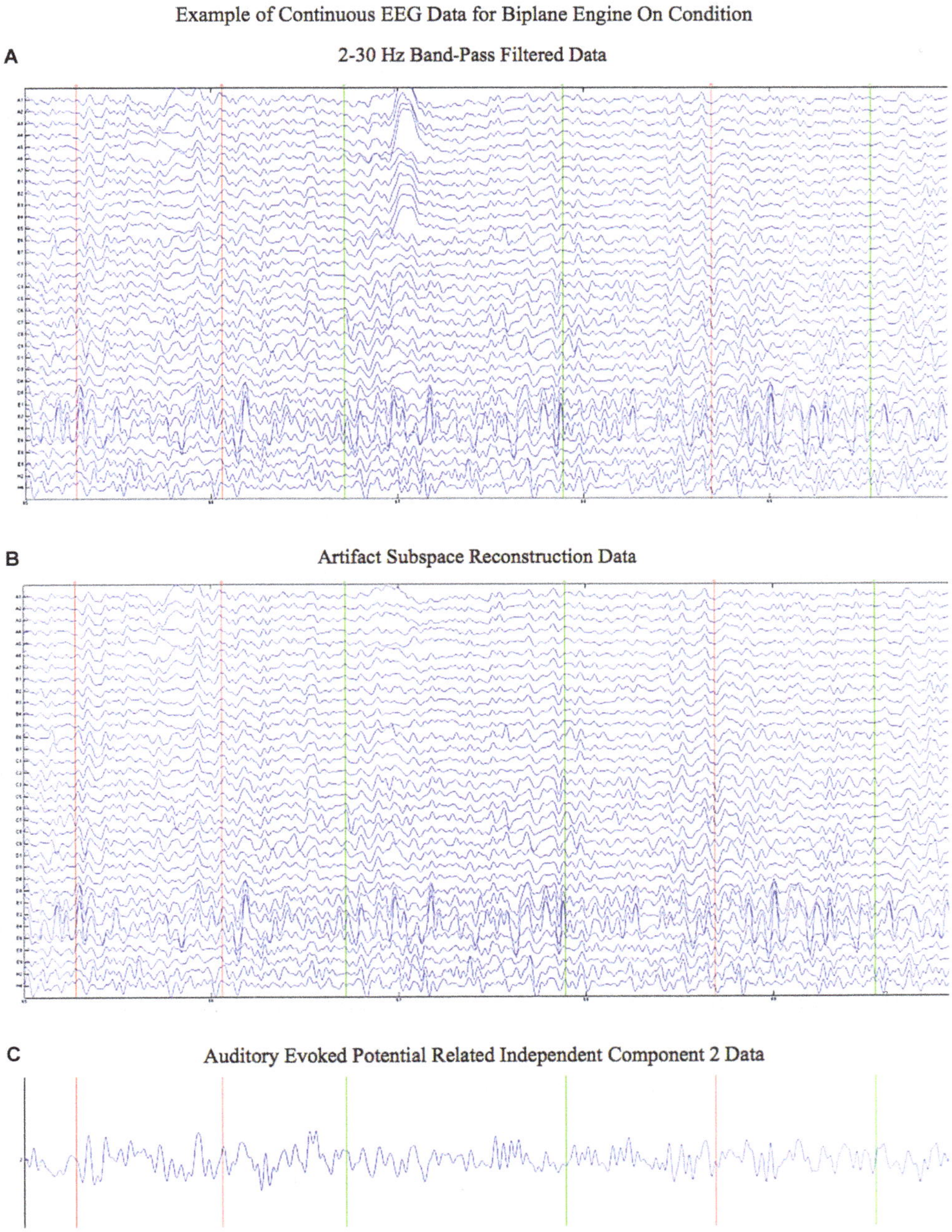

FIGURE 5 | Example of Continuous EEG Data for the Biplane Engine On Condition. **(A)** Five seconds of continuous data from the test set that has been band pass filtered from 2–30 Hz for the 34 electrodes included. **(B)** Five seconds of continuous data from the test set that has undergone artifact subspace reconstruction as well as band pass filtered from 2–30 Hz for the 34 electrodes included. Notice how ASR has cleaned up the artifact present in many of the channels (compare with **(A)** above). **(C)** Five seconds of continuous data from the test set for auditory evoked potential related independent component number 2. The ICA was carried out over the data in **(B)**. Green lines denote the onset of audio stimuli and Red lines denote the onset of silent trials.

conditions (Platform Off, Platform On, biplane Engine Off, biplane Engine On) and four preprocessing conditions (pre-ICA constituting the baseline no processing condition, ICA, pre-ICA Kalman filtered, ICA Kalman filtered) for a total of 16 analyses.

The statistical significance between the various conditions was determined by repeating the nested cross-validation process ten times for each condition. The nested cross-validation procedure is commonly used to estimate the stability of the model across conditions (Shenoy et al., 2008). At each step, we computed the

Table 1 | Classification performance for the platform condition on the test data.

	Platform off				Platform on			
	Accuracy (%)	False positive rate (%)	False negative rate (%)	d'	Accuracy (%)	False positive rate (%)	False negative rate (%)	d'
Pre-ICA	78.3 (0.33)	19.8 (0.20)	23.6 (0.65)	1.69 (0.01)	71.6 (0.56)	35.4 (1.52)	21.4 (0.60)	0.75 (0.08)
ICA	81.0 (0.49)	21.4 (0.99)	16.6 (0.73)	1.59 (0.07)	73.7 (0.52)	26.8 (1.91)	25.8 (1.75)	1.26 (0.12)
Pre-ICA + Kalman Filter	77.8 (0.55)	20.2 (1.05)	24.2 (1.94)	1.68 (0.07)	72.8 (0.53)	36.6 (1.58)	17.8 (1.94)	0.69 (0.08)
ICA + Kalman Filter	83.4 (0.27)	17.2 (0.53)	16.0 (0.60)	1.90 (0.04)	73.1 (0.8)	28.4 (2.61)	25.4 (1.79)	1.18 (0.16)

The standard error is given in parentheses below each mean value of the 10 nested cross-validation iterations.

Table 2 | Classification performance for the biplane condition on the test data.

	Biplane engine off				Biplane engine on			
	Accuracy	False positive rate	False negative rate	d'	Accuracy	False positive rate	False negative rate	d'
Pre-ICA	77.4 (1.01)	20.2 (2.72)	25.0 (2.20)	1.75 (0.21)	66.1 (0.75)	38.0 (1.23)	29.8 (1.31)	0.61 (0.06)
ICA	78.5 (0.72)	20.0 (1.58)	23.0 (0.68)	1.71 (0.11)	77.3 (0.45)	23.6 (1.26)	21.8 (0.81)	1.45 (0.08)
Pre-ICA + Kalman Filter	77.0 (0.97)	14.6 (1.16)	31.4 (2.53)	2.13 (0.1)	65.3 (0.96)	35.4 (2.78)	34.0 (2.40)	0.78 (0.17)
ICA + Kalman Filter	81.1 (0.35)	10.0 (1.19)	27.8 (1.35)	2.65 (0.18)	79.2 (0.39)	22.6 (1.12)	19.0 (1.16)	1.51 (0.07)

The standard error is given in parentheses below each mean value of the 10 nested cross-validation iterations.

classification accuracy, false positive rate and false negative rate. The differences between the classification results obtained from each of the preprocessing conditions were then compared using Wilcoxon sign-rank test.

RESULTS

The number of channels not rejected out of the 64 by the preprocessing steps for the various conditions are as follows: Platform Off (46), Platform On (20), Biplane Engine Off (30), Biplane Engine On (34). The independent components showing auditory evoked potentials used to train the LSPC models were the following for the various conditions: Platform Off (2, 3), Platform On (1, 3), Biplane Engine Off (2, 3), Biplane Engine On (2, 16). The components are sorted in descending order of mean projected variance. Therefore, the lower the component number the larger is the projected variance. Parentheses.

The results of the single trial classification performance for audio chirp verses silent stimuli for all environmental and analysis method conditions were significantly above chance ($p < 0.05$) based on permutation testing of 100 random shuffling of the labels compared to the mean performance of the respective models trained with correct labels. The accuracy, false positive rate, false negative rate, and d' (sensitivity) along with the standard errors in parentheses for the platform off and platform on conditions for the four analysis conditions (Pre-ICA, ICA Pre-ICA + Kalman Filter, and ICA + Kalman Filter) are given in **Table 1**. The corresponding results for the biplane Engine Off and Engine On conditions are given in **Table 2**. The statistical significance of model stability for accuracy on the contrasts of pre-ICA vs. ICA, Off vs. On, and No Kalman filter vs. Kalman filter are given in **Tables 3A–C**. Testing for significance based on the 100 trials of the test set across the various contrasts using the Wilcoxon sign-rank test is given in **Tables 4A–D**.

DISCUSSION

The primary objective of this experiment was to show as a proof of concept that a dry-wireless EEG system could be used in extremely noisy real-world environments while the operator is carrying out complex perceptual motor tasks and still show good classification performance of a perceptual event. Both the motion platform based flight simulation and the open cockpit biplane environments produced considerable artifacts challenging the ability for accurate classification of a perceptual event from EEG data. In the platform on condition the subject was flying through a Redbull Air Race course making abrupt banks to go through the cones in the correct orientation (Callan et al., 2013). The movement of the platform and the head and body to these banks produces large artifacts in the EEG trace. In the open cockpit biplane there is considerable vibration, wind, acoustic noise, and physiological noise resulting from control of the plane and movement of the body that produces large artifacts in the EEG trace.

Despite these challenging environments our study showed that far above chance classification performance can be achieved for all environmental conditions (Platform Off, Platform On, Biplane Engine Off, Biplane Engine On) and for all analysis conditions (Pre-ICA, Pre-ICA Kalman filtered, ICA, and ICA Kalman filtered) (See **Tables 1–4**). The classification performance was the best when applying both ICA and Kalman filtering to the data. This was especially true in the Biplane Engine On condition in which classification performance improved from 66.1% in the baseline pre-ICA no processing condition to 79.2% in the ICA Kalman filtering condition (See **Tables 2–4**). This

Table 3 | Statistical significance of the various contrasts using nested cross-validation to evaluate model stability.

A. ICA vs. Baseline Pre-ICA

Overall	Platoff	Platon	Engoff	Engon	Platoff + Kalman	Platon + Kalman	Engoff + Kalman	Engon + Kalman
***		**		**		**		**

B. Off vs. On

Overall	Platform Pre-ICA	Engine Pre-ICA	Platform Pre-ICA + Kalman	Engine Pre-ICA + Kalman	Platform ICA	Engine ICA	Platform ICA + Kalman	Engine ICA + Kalman
***	**	**	**	**	**		**	*

C. Kalman Filter vs. no Kalman Filter

Overall	Platform Off Pre-ICA	Platform On Pre-ICA	Engine Off Pre-ICA	Engine On On Pre-ICA	Platform Off ICA	Platform On ICA	Engine Off ICA	Engine On ICA
*					**		*	**

*Significance (one-tailed) is determined using the Wilcoxon sign-rank test. * = p < 0.05; ** = p < 0.01; *** = p < 0.001.*

Table 4 | Statistical significance evaluated across trials of the test set for the various contrasts.

A. ICA vs. Baseline Pre-ICA

Overall	Platform	Biplane	Platoff	Platon	Engoff	Engon
**		**				**

B. ICA + Kalman vs. Baseline Pre-ICA

Overall	Platform	Biplane	Platoff	Platon	Engoff	Engon
**		**			*	**

C. Off vs. On

Overall	Platform	Biplane
***	**	*

D. ICA + Kalman vs. ICA

Overall	Platform	Biplane	Platoff	Platon	Engoff	Engon
		*			*	

*Significance (one-tailed) is determined using the Wilcoxon sign-rank test. * = p < 0.05; ** = p < 0.01; *** = p < 0.001.*

classification performance was comparable to that of the Engine Off condition (81.1%) in which the biplane was sitting on the tarmac. It is unclear why the Platform On condition did not show the same beneficial effects of ICA Kalman filtering vs. the baseline no processing condition (73.1% vs. 71.6% respectively), as did the Biplane Engine On condition (See **Tables 1–4**). One possibility is that the abrupt movement of the body and head during the flight task produced non-stationary artifacts that could not be separated by the EEGLAB artifact cleaning methods or by ICA and Kalman filtering. In the future utilizing data from an accelerometer mounted on the head as a regressor of non-interest may be able to extract possible movement related artifacts and improve classification performance. The significantly greater accuracy for the Off over the On conditions is to be expected (See **Tables 1–4**) not only because of the much greater artifacts present in the On conditions but also because auditory responses are decreased depending on attention (Paul et al., 2014). It is likely that the attention needed for piloting in the On conditions reduced attention to the auditory stimuli.

The use of Kalman filtering was most effective when conducted on ICA processed data. Kalman filtering on pre-ICA data did not show improvement in performance compared to that of ICA processed data (See **Tables 1–4**). One possible explanation for these results is that ICA is able to separate the brain activity related to the auditory event from other brain activity and artifacts allowing for better estimation by the Kalman filter that utilizes generic information about the auditory evoked response as a dynamical model. In the pre-ICA data the brain activity for various processes as well as artifacts are mixed within all the channels and estimation of the auditory events by the Kalman filter model may be more difficult for these signals.

Because the results are only of a single subject it is not clear how well they generalize to other individuals. It is likely that different individuals with different levels of flight experience may show more/or less movement and physiological artifacts that may decrease/increase classification performance. The Cognionics dry wireless EEG system has already been shown to give good classification performance on a SSVEP test across a number of subjects (Lin et al., 2014). The Lin et al. (2014) study demonstrates that the Cognionics EEG system is able to extract from a group of individuals and is not just limited to a few special individuals. ICA has additionally been shown to be very good at extracting artifacts and task related components from EEG data (Delorme et al., 2007). This was also demonstrated for the data collected in this study and it is unlikely that it is only applicable to the single subject that participated. Despite these limitations the results do stand as a demonstration that it is possible to collect data in real-world environments that have considerable noise, both environmental and physiological, using dry-wireless EEG and obtain classification performance sufficient for some BMI augmentive neuroscience based applications. The research presented here lays a foundation for future aviation based studies where subject variability in EEG responses can be evaluated.

For effective use in implementing BMI in real-world applications it is necessary that the processes used for classification be fast enough for online control either in terms of manipulating robotic devices, giving feedback to the operator, and/or utilizing adaptive automation to augment human performance (Byrne and Parasuraman, 1996; Wilson and Russell, 2007). One of the key elements of this study was that the training set came from the first 75% of the data and the novel test set came from the last 25% of the data. All of the artifact-cleaning methods were applied to the training set and the same criteria and weights were then applied to the testing set. ASR, ICA, and LSPC classifier model selection by cross-validation requires some processing time depending on computer speed. In our case running the programs in Matlab on a MacBook Pro took around 10 min. The largest portion of time was spent computing the ICA. Therefore, implementation of a BMI would require a delay of approximately 10 min after the training data is collected before it could be applied if ICA is used. Just a couple minutes for model selection and training are required if ICA is not used. The extraction of channels, the ASR model, and the ICA weights from the training data as well as the Kalman filter can be applied without delay (the delay is the same as the sampling rate) to the test set. In this case the features used in the classification model were samples for 500 ms after stimulus onset. Therefore, depending on the type of initial band-pass filtering, the processing delay to control the BMI could be around 515 ms. Although the initial band-pass filter order for processing this data set was 496 samples, which would create a considerable delay it is possible to implement different types of filters with a lower order to decrease the processing delay. A delay of less than a second could certainly be used in a BMI to give a warning signal to the pilot or engage adaptive automation (Byrne and Parasuraman, 1996; Wilson and Russell, 2007), however, it is not sufficient for closed-loop control.

Given the significant number of aviation accidents that result from missed auditory alarms (Bliss, 2003; Scannella et al., 2013; Dehais et al., 2014), a BMI based on detection of auditory events could be quite important in giving alternate forms of feedback to warn the pilot when necessary. It is well known that high workload decreases the ability to perceive task-irrelevant and/or unattended visual and auditory information (Lavie, 1995, 2005, 2010). This phenomenon is called inattentional blindness with respect to vision (Mack and Rock, 1998) and inattentional deafness with respect to audition (Wood and Cowan, 1995; Macdonald and Lavie, 2011; Dehais et al., 2014). Inattentional deafness is known to be a critical factor in missing of auditory alarms in aeronautics (Dehais et al., 2014). It is interesting that although task irrelevant auditory stimuli can be presented in the background without any decrement in task related performance, the evoked brain potentials to these auditory events is modulated by workload on the primary task (Krammer et al., 1995). As such, it may be possible to assess the workload of the pilot and likely occurrences of inattentional deafness by investigating brain response to auditory events. An EEG based BMI system could potentially be used to decode the mental state of the pilot for occurrence of inattantional deafness and augment their mental state by feedback through a different modality or engage adaptive automation. Considerably more research needs to be conducted to determine on a single event basis whether an incidence of inattentional deafness is present or not before such a system can be implemented.

When one considers that brain dynamics are different while undergoing complex tasks in natural environments from that of the laboratory (McDowell et al., 2013; Lin et al., 2014) and that dry EEG systems are susceptible to movement-based artifacts (Guger et al., 2012; Lin et al., 2014) the single-trial classification performance of auditory perceptual events by a dry-wireless EEG system in the robust flight conditions of our study are quite impressive. This research demonstrates the feasibility of new avenues for investigating brain processes in real-world situations that cannot be conducted in the laboratory. In addition the research presented here also demonstrates that plausible BMI using dry-wireless EEG can be implemented in real-world settings to augment human performance.

ACKNOWLEDGMENTS

I would like to thank Makoto Miyakoshi and John Iversen for assistance with pre-processing techniques in EEGLAB and Mike Chi for assistance with the Cognionics EEG system. I would also like to thank James Zapata for piloting assistance in carrying out the experiment in the biplane. In addition I would like to give special thanks to Wayne Spani and sons for all their great work on the Starduster.

REFERENCES

Bell, A. J., and Sejnowski, T. J. (1995). An information-maximization approach to blind separation and blind deconvolution. *Neural Comput.* 7, 1129–1159. doi: 10.1162/neco.1995.7.6.1129

Bin, G., Gao, X., Yan, Z., Hong, B., and Gao, S. (2009). An online multichannel SSVEP-based brain-computer interface using a canonical correlation analysis method. *J. Neural Eng.* 6:046002. doi: 10.1088/1741-2560/6/4/046002

Birbaumer, N., Ghanayim, N., Hinterberger, T., Iversen, I., Kotchoubey, B., Kübler, A., et al. (1999). A spelling device for the paralysed. *Nature* 398, 297–298. doi: 10.1038/18581

Blanc, C., Lafontain, E., and Medvadeff, M. (1966). Radiotelemetric recordings of the electroencephalograms of civil aviation pilots during flight. *Aerosp. Med.* 37, 1060–1065.

Blankertz, B., Tangermann, M., Vidaurre, C., Fazli, S., Sannelli, C., Haufe, S., et al. (2010). The Berlin brain-computer interface: non-medical uses of BCI technology. *Front. Neurosci.* 4:198. doi: 10.3389/fnins.2010.00198

Bliss, J. P. (2003). Investigation of alarm-related accidents and incidents in aviation. *Int. J. Aviat. Psychol.* 13, 249–268. doi: 10.1207/s15327108ijap1303_04

Byrne, E. A., and Parasuraman, R. (1996). Psychophysiology and adaptive automation. *Biol. Psychol.* 42, 249–268. doi: 10.1016/0301-0511(95)05161-9

Caldwell, J. A., and Lewis, J. A. (1995). The feasibility of collecting in-flight EEG data from helicopter pilots. *Aviat. Space Environ. Med.* 66, 883–889.

Callan, D. E., Gamez, M., Cassel, D. B., Terzibas, C., Callan, A., Kawato, M., et al. (2012). Dynamic visuomotor transformation involved with remote flying of a plane utilizes the 'Mirror neuron' system. *PLoS One* 7:e33873. doi: 10.1371/journal.pone.0033873

Callan, D. E., Terzibas, C., Cassel, D. B., Callan, A., Kawato, M., and Sato, M. A. (2013). Differential activation of brain regions involved with error-feedback and imitation based motor simulation when observing self and an expert's actions in pilots and non-pilots on a complex glider landing task. *Neuroimage* 72, 55–68. doi: 10.1016/j.neuroimage.2013.01.028

Cheron, G., Cebolla, A. M., Petieau, M., Bengoetxea, A., Palmero-Soler, E., Leroy, A., et al. (2009). Chapter 13 adaptive changes of rhythmic EEG oscillations in space: implications for brain-machine interface applications. *Int. Rev. Neurobiol.* 86, 171–187. doi: 10.1016/s0074-7742(09)86013-3

Chi, Y. M., Wang, Y., Wang, Y.-T., Jung, T.-P., Kerth, T., and Cao, Y. (2013). "A practical mobile dry EEG system for human computer interfaces," in *Foundations of Augmented Cognition*, eds D. Schmorrow and C. Fidopiastis (Berlin, Heidelberg: Springer), 649–655.

Dehais, F., Causse, M., Vachon, F., Régis, N., Menant, E., and Tremblay, S. (2014). Failure to detect critical auditory alerts in the cockpit: evidence for inattentional deafness. *Hum. Factors* 56, 631–644. doi: 10.1177/0018720813510735

Delorme, A., and Makeig, S. (2004). EEGLAB: an open source toolbox for analysis of single-trial EEG dynamics including independent component analysis. *J. Neurosci. Methods* 134, 9–21. doi: 10.1016/j.jneumeth.2003.10.009

Delorme, A., Sejnowski, T., and Makeig, S. (2007). Improved rejection of artifacts from EEG data using high-order statistics and independent component analysis. *Neuroimage* 34, 1443–1449. doi: 10.1016/j.neuroimage.2006.11.004

Dornhege, G., del, R., Millan, J., Hinterberger, T., McFarland, D. J., and Muller, K. (eds) (2007). *Toward Brain-Computer Interfacing.* Cambridge, MA: MIT Press.

Dussault, C., Jouanin, J. C., and Guezennec, C. Y. (2005). EEG and ECG changes during selected flight sequences. *Aviat. Space Environ. Med.* 75, 889–897.

Georgiadis, S. D., Ranta-aho, P. O., Tarvainen, M. P., and Karjalainen, P. A. (2005). Single-trial dynamical estimation of event-related potentials: a Kalman filter-based approach. *IEEE Trans. Biomed. Eng.* 52, 1397–1406. doi: 10.1109/tbme.2005.851506

Grewal, M. S., and Andrews, A. P. (2008). *Kalman Filtering: Theory and Practice using MATLAB.* Hoboken, NJ: John Wiley and Sons.

Groenegress, C., Holzner, C., Guger, C., and Slater, M. (2010). Effects of P300-based BCI use on reported presence in a virtual environment. *Presence* 19, 1–11. doi: 10.1162/pres.19.1.1

Guger, C., Ktausz, G., Allison, B. Z., and Edlinger, G. (2012). Comparison of dry and gel based electrodes for p300 brain-computer interfaces. *Front. Neurosci.* 6:60. doi: 10.3389/fnins.2012.00060

Hankins, T. C., and Wilson, G. F. (1998). A comparison of heart rate, eye activity, EEG and subjective measures of pilot mental workload during flight. *Aviat. Space Environ. Med.* 69, 360–367.

Howitt, J. S., Hay, A. E., Shergold, G. R., and Ferres, H. M. (1978). Workload and fatigue–in-flight EEG changes. *Aviat. Space Environ. Med.* 49, 1197–1202.

Kalman, R. E. (1960). A new approach to linear filtering and prediction problems. *J. Fluids Eng.* 82, 35–45. doi: 10.1115/1.3662552

Krammer, A. F., Trejo, L. J., and Humphrey, D. (1995). Assessment of mental workload with task-irrelevant auditory probes. *Biol. Psychol.* 40, 83–100. doi: 10.1016/0301-0511(95)05108-2

LaFleur, K., Cassady, K., Doud, A., Shades, K., Rogin, E., and He, B. (2013). Quadcopter control in three-dimensional space using a noninvasive motor imagery-based brain-computer interface. *J. Neural Eng.* 10:046003. doi: 10.1088/1741-2560/10/4/046003

Lavie, N. (1995). Perceptual load as a necessary condition for selective attention. *J. Exp. Psychol. Hum. Percept. Perform.* 21, 451–468. doi: 10.1037//0096-1523.21.3.451

Lavie, N. (2005). Distracted and confused?: selective attention under load. *Trends Cogn. Sci.* 9, 75–82. doi: 10.1016/j.tics.2004.12.004

Lavie, N. (2010). Attention, distraction and cognitive control under load. *Curr. Dir. Psychol. Sci.* 19, 143–148. doi: 10.1177/0963721410370295

Liao, L. D., Chen, C. Y., Wang, I. J., Chen, S. F., Li, S. Y., Chen, B. W., et al. (2012). Gaming control using a wearable and wireless EEG-based brain-computer interface device with novel dry foam-based sensors. *J. Neuroeng. Rehabil.* 9:5. doi: 10.1186/1743-0003-9-5

Liao, L. D., Wang, I. J., Chen, S. F., Chang, J. Y., and Lin, C. T. (2011). Design, fabrication and experimental validation of a novel dry-contact sensor for measuring electroencephalography signals without skin preparation. *Sensors* 11, 5819–5834. doi: 10.3390/s110605819

Lin, Y. P., Wang, Y., Wei, C. S., and Jung, T. P. (2014). Assessing the quality of steady-state visual-evoked potentials for moving humans using a mobile electroencephalogram headset. *Front. Hum. Neurosci.* 8:182. doi: 10.3389/fnhum.2014.00182

Macdonald, J. S., and Lavie, N. (2011). Visual perceptual load induces inattentional deafness. *Atten. Percept. Psychophys.* 73, 1780–1789. doi: 10.3758/s13414-011-0144-4

Mack, A., and Rock, I. (1998). *Inattentional Blindness.* Cambridge: MIT Press.

Maulsby, R. (1966). Electroencephalogram during orbital flight. *Aerosp. Med.* 37, 1022–1026.

McDowell, K., Chin-Teng, L., Oie, K. S., Jung, T. P., Gordon, S., Whitaker, K., et al. (2013). Real-world neuroimaging technologies. *IEEE Access* 1, 131–149. doi: 10.1109/access.2013.2260791

Millàn Jdel, R., Ferrez, P. W., and Seidl, T. (2009). Chapter 14 validation of brain-machine interfaces during parabolic flight. *Int. Rev. Neurobiol.* 86, 189–197. doi: 10.1016/s0074-7742(09)86014-5

Mullen, T., Kothe, C., Chi, Y. M., Ojeda, A., Kerth, T., Makeig, S., et al. (2013). "Real-time modeling and 3D visualization of source dynamics and connectivity using wearable EEG," in *EMBC, 25th Annual International Conference of the IEEE* (Osaka: IEEE), 2184–2187.

Müller, K., Tangermann, M., Dornhege, G., Krauledat, M., Curio, G., and Blankertz, B. (2008). Machine learning for real-time single-trial EEG-analysis: from brain-computer interfacing to mental state monitoring. *J. Neurosci. Methods* 167, 82–90. doi: 10.1016/j.jneumeth.2007.09.022

Parasuraman, R. (2003). Neuroergonomics; research and practice. *Theor. Issues Ergon. Sci.* 4, 5–20. doi: 10.1080/14639220210199753

Parasuraman, R., and Rizzo, M. (2008). *Neuroergonomics: The Brain at Work.* New York, NY: Oxford University Press.

Park, J., Xu, L., Sridhar, V., Chi, M., and Cauwenberghs, G. (2011). "Wireless dry EEG for drowsiness detection," in *33rd Annual International Conference of the IEEE EMBS* (Boston, Massachusetts USA: IEEE).

Paul, B. T., Bruce, I. C., Bosnyak, D. J., Thompson, D. C., and Roberts, L. E. (2014). Modulation of electrocortical brain activity by attention in individuals with and without Tinnitus. *Neural Plast.* 2014:127824. doi: 10.1155/2014/127824

Sauvet, F., Baugard, C., Coroenne, M., Lely, L., Van Beers, P., Elbaz, M., et al. (2014). In-flight automatic detection of vigilance states using a single EEG channel. *IEEE Trans. Biomed. Eng.* 61, 2840–2847. doi: 10.1109/TBME.2014.2331189

Scannella, S., Causse, M., Chauveau, N., Pastor, J., and Dehais, F. (2013). Effects of the audiovisual conflict on auditory early processes. *Int. J. Psychophysiol.* 89, 115–122. doi: 10.1016/j.ijpsycho.2013.06.009

Sellers, E. W., Ryan, D. B., and Hauser, C. K. (2014). Noninvasive brain-computer interface enables communication after brainstem stroke. *Sci. Transl. Med.* 6:257re7. doi: 10.1126/scitranslmed.3007801

Sem-Jacobsen, C. W., Nilseng, O., Patten, C., and Eriksen, O. (1959). Electroencephalographic recording in simulated combat flight in a jet fighter plane. *Electroencephalogr. Clin. Neurophysiol.* 11, 154–155. doi: 10.1016/0013-4694(59)90018-5

Shenoy, P., Miller, K. J., Ojemann, J. G., and Rao, R. P. (2008). Generalized features for electrocorticographic BCIs. *IEEE Trans. Biomed. Eng.* 55, 273–280. doi: 10.1109/tbme.2007.903528

Sterman, M., Schummer, G., Dushenko, T., and Smith, J. (1987). "Electroencephalographic correlates of pilot performance: simulation and in-flight studies," in *Electrical and Magnetic Activity of the Central Nervous System: Research and Clinical Applications in Aerospace Medicine* (Neuilly Sur Seine, France: Nato. AGARD CP No. 432), 1–16.

Sugiyama, M. (2010). Superfast-trainable multi-class probabilistic classifier by least-squares posterior fitting. *IEICE Trans. Inf. Syst.* 93-D, 2690–2701.

Wang, Y., Wang, R., Gao, X., Hong, B., and Gao, S. (2006). A practical VEP-based brain-computer interface. *IEEE Trans. Neural Syst. Rehabil. Eng.* 14, 234–239. doi: 10.1109/tnsre.2006.875576

Wilson, G. F., and Russell, C. A. (2007). Performance enhancement in an uninhabited air vehicle task using psychophysiologically determined adaptive aiding. *Hum. Factors* 49, 1005–1018. doi: 10.1518/001872007x249875

Wolpaw, J. R., McFarland, D. J., and Vaughan, T. M. (2002). Brain computer interface research at the Wadsworth center. *IEEE Trans. Rehabil. Eng.* 8, 222–226. doi: 10.1109/86.847823

Wood, N. L., and Cowan, N. (1995). The cocktail party phenomenon revisited: attention and memory in the classic selective listening procedure of Cherry (1953). *J. Exp. Psychol. Gen.* 124, 243–262. doi: 10.1037/0096-3445.124.3.243

Zao, J. K., Gan, T. T., You, C. K., Chung, C. E., Wang, Y. T., Rodríguez Méndez, S. J., et al. (2014). Pervasive brain monitoring and data sharing based on multi-tier distributed computing and linked data technology. *Front. Hum. Neurosci.* 8:370. doi: 10.3389/fnhum.2014.00370

15

Attitudes toward pharmacological cognitive enhancement

Kimberly J. Schelle[1], Nadira Faulmüller[2,3]*, Lucius Caviola[2] and Miles Hewstone[2]

[1] Department of Industrial Design, Eindhoven University of Technology, Eindhoven, Netherlands
[2] Department of Experimental Psychology, University of Oxford, Oxford, UK
[3] Department of Values, Technology and Innovation, Delft University of Technology, Delft, Netherlands

Edited by:
Mikhail Lebedev, Duke University, USA

Reviewed by:
Veljko Dubljevic, McGill University, Canada
Wayne Denis Hall, University of Queensland, Australia

***Correspondence:**
Nadira Faulmüller, Department of Experimental Psychology, University of Oxford, 9 South Parks Road, Oxford, OX1 3UD, UK
e-mail: nadira.faulmueller@psy.ox.ac.uk

A primary means for the augmentation of cognitive brain functions is "pharmacological cognitive enhancement" (PCE). The term usually refers to the off-label use of medical substances to improve mental performance in healthy individuals. With the final aim to advance the normative debate taking place on that topic, several empirical studies have been conducted to assess the attitudes toward PCE in the public, i.e., in groups outside of the academic debate. In this review, we provide an overview of the 40 empirical studies published so far, reporting both their methodology and results. Overall, we find that several concerns about the use of PCE are prevalent in the public. These concerns largely match those discussed in the normative academic debate. We present our findings structured around the three most common concerns: medical safety, coercion, and fairness. Fairness is divided into three subthemes: equality of opportunity, honesty, and authenticity. Attitudes regarding some concerns are coherent across studies (e.g., coercion), whereas for others we find mixed results (e.g., authenticity). Moreover, we find differences in how specific groups—such as users, nonusers, students, parents, and health care providers—perceive PCE: a coherent finding is that nonusers display more concerns regarding medical safety and fairness than users. We discuss potential psychological explanations for these differences.

Keywords: cognitive enhancement, neuroenhancement, brain function augmentation, medical safety, coercion, fairness, authenticity, smart drugs

INTRODUCTION

Brain enhancement is a topic of huge interest in the media and the academic literature. An often discussed form of brain enhancement is *pharmacological cognitive enhancement* (PCE) which usually refers to the use of certain prescription substances. Schermer et al. (2009) define these sorts of enhancements as "pharmacological interventions that are intended to improve certain mental functions and that go beyond currently accepted medical indications" (p. 77). PCE is not only a topic that is debated in academia—mainly in neuroscience, law, and ethics—but also a reality: several surveys show that students, but also other groups such as academics and surgeons, use substances to enhance their cognitive performance (e.g., Maher, 2008; Smith and Farah, 2011; Franke et al., 2013). Examples of seemingly common pharmacological enhancers are methylphenidate (e.g., Ritalin®), mixed amphetamine salts (e.g., Aderall®), and modafinil (e.g., Provigil®). Originally, the first two were developed as treatment for Attention Deficit Hyperactivity Disorder and the latter as treatment for Narcolepsy, but now they are being used to enhance performance in healthy individuals.

Although there are considerable intra- and interpersonal differences in the effects of these substances (e.g., Husain and Mehta, 2011; Van Der Schaaf et al., 2013), average effects have been reported. In their overview of findings and meta-analysis of the effects of methylphenidate and modafinil in healthy individuals, Repantis et al. (2010) assessed mood, motivation and four categories of cognitive processes: wakefulness, attention and vigilance, memory and learning, and executive functions and information processing. The available data about methylphenidate did not provide enough information to draw a firm conclusion about the effects of methylphenidate on enhancing or maintaining performance, although evidence for a positive effect on memory was found. An enhancing effect on attention was not verified, conflicting with the goal of increasing concentration and alertness that users of enhancement substances often have (Teter et al., 2005). The aggregated findings of potential enhancing effects of modafinil indicate that it improves attention for well-rested individuals. Furthermore, it helps in maintaining a higher degree of wakefulness, memory and executive functions over a period of sleep deprivation (Repantis et al., 2010). The authors suggest that these effects led to a growing popularity of modafinil, and strongly recommend a public debate on the ethics of the use of PCE which takes this into account. However, other reviews did not find any effect or even suggested that the non-cognitive effects of the substances, e.g., on confidence and motivation, might be responsible for enhanced performance (Farah et al., 2014).

In the normative debate about whether or not PCE is to be endorsed, certain concerns about its use are often raised and have been discussed by several authors (e.g., Farah et al., 2004; Bostrom and Sandberg, 2009; Schermer et al., 2009; Hyman, 2011). In this review, we focus on three concerns that are most often emphasized by the public, but are also discussed in the normative debate.

First, the *medical safety* of the aforementioned substances has been discussed, in particular in terms of short- or long-term side effects. A second topic of discussion is *coercion*, relating to concerns about the explicit and implicit pressures that can arise from the availability of PCE, forcing people to use these substances to be able to compete, for example at the workplace or in school. The third concern relates to the *fairness* of the use of PCE. This concern includes several subtopics such as a possible unequal distribution of access to such enhancers, their use in competitive environments being seen as cheating, and also to what degree performance brought about under PCE can be seen as authentic.

There are good reasons to examine the *attitudes of the public* toward PCE in addition to this normative debate. In their plea for the inclusion of public views on developments in biomedicine and technology, Schicktanz et al. (2012) underline a view already suggested a few years ago by Sarewitz (2010) in a column in *Nature*. They propose three general arguments for the inclusion of the public in ethical reasoning. First, views and attitudes of the public can point to remote or emerging moral problems. Second, empirical research can be used to examine premises about human behavior and social consequences of actions that underlie several applied ethical arguments. Third, research on public opinions can increase the context-sensitivity of ethical reasoning by pointing out consequences of concrete decisions in social policy. They argue that any bioethical discussion that avoids a confrontation with public opinions "not only runs the risk of missing important aspects, ideas, and arguments. It also arouses strong suspicion of being indeed one-sided, biased or ideological—thus illegitimate." (Schicktanz et al., 2012, p. 136). Apart from the aforementioned general arguments to include the public's attitude in certain bioethical discussions, specific arguments for the case of PCE are also made. Faulmüller et al. (2013) describe how PCE, as long as it is perceived negatively by the public, might give rise to indirect psychological costs for users: they might be treated in ways that damage their psychological well-being, for example by a misattribution of their success to the enhancer rather than themselves, or by dehumanization or ostracism. More insight into the public's view can lead to more insight into these potential indirect psychological costs. In addition, Banjo et al. (2010) argue that physicians are and will be "gatekeepers" in dispensing at least a portion of PCE substances. Although there is discussion on if and how their views might affect social policy or legal regulation on PCE (Delaney and Martin, 2011), PCE is part of their clinical reality. Therefore their views can provide specific insights that are of importance to the general debate (Ott et al., 2012).

The current article is based on an extensive literature search. We used two databases, Web of Science and Scopus, and included all articles published in English between 1990 and 2014. The search terms we used were [("cognitive enhancer" OR "cognitive enhancement" OR "pharmacological enhancement" OR "prescription drug" OR "performance enhancing drug" OR neuroenhancement OR "human enhancement") AND (view OR perspective OR opinion OR attitude OR judgment OR motive OR justification)] as part of the title, abstract or keyword of the text. This search resulted in 447 articles in Web of Science and 4162 articles in Scopus. Based on a careful check of titles and abstracts, we selected all articles that reported empirical studies on the opinions of groups outside the normative academic debate (such as students or physicians) on the use of PCE. We also cross-checked the reference lists of the studies found this way to identify additional relevant literature matching our inclusion criteria. Moreover, we checked Google Scholar and asked colleagues publishing in this area to direct us to relevant publications. Overall, this search resulted in 40 publications reporting qualitative or quantitative examinations of attitudes, opinions, and views of the general public and more often specific sub-populations toward PCE, which we included in this review. These 40 publications are marked with an asterisk in the reference list.

Our overarching finding is that in the public several concerns about the use of PCE substances are prevalent: they agree on several concerns when being asked specifically and raise concerns themselves when being asked for their opinion. These concerns widely match the normative debate. Hence, this review is structured around the common concerns reflected in the academic and public debate: (1) medical safety, (2) coercion, and (3) fairness. Each section in this review will be introduced with a short description of the academic debate on the respective concern. Then, the relevant empirical studies are reported. We also try to pinpoint some shortcomings in the current literature and suggest potential paths for future research. **Table 1** provides an overview of key methodological aspects of all studies reviewed, containing information about the concerns investigated, the research method by which the data were obtained, the country where the study took place, and the sample (occupation of participants, sample size, sampling method, and response rate).

MEDICAL SAFETY

The normative debate about the safety of PCE usually focuses on potential trade-offs between benefits and risks. As with all medical procedures, there might be side effects and yet-unknown long-term health risks with substances such as methylphenidate or modafinil (King et al., 2006). Schermer et al. (2009) point out that the harm-benefit ratio of PCE deserves special consideration, as the life-improving benefits might not outweigh the potential risks for consumers who use them for enhancement purposes, instead of the therapeutic purposes for which the substances were originally developed. However, Dubljevic (2013) emphasizes the importance of analyzing different substances in a case-by-case approach, as some entail greater health and addiction risks than others (Kociancic et al., 2004). Several studies have examined people's health concerns about such cognitive enhancers. Interestingly both users and nonusers systematically overestimate the cognitive-enhancing effects of PCE (Finger et al., 2013; Ilieva et al., 2013), but a sharp discrepancy between their risk estimations is revealed. While nonusers generally have strong concerns regarding the safety of PCE, users show less concern.

Nonusers tend to believe that such substances are addictive, might induce sleep disorders and may even lead to mental health problems, which was shown in an interview study with 19 Australian students (Partridge et al., 2013). In two surveys conducted on a UK university campus with a total of 357 students, Scheske and Schnall (2012) observed that moral reservations against PCE stem mostly from these safety concerns: the riskier the substances, the more student respondents morally object to

Table 1 | Overview of the empirical studies discussed in this review.

Authors	Country	Occupation of participants	Sampling method	Research method	Response rate	Sample size	Concerns
Aikins, 2011	USA	University students	Purposive sampling	Semi-structured interview	n/a	12	Safety, fairness
Asscher and Schermer, 2013	The Netherlands	General public	Purposive sampling	Focus groups	n/a	37	Safety
Ball and Wolbring, 2014	Canada	Parents	Purposive sampling	Semi-structured interview	n/a	12	Safety
Banjo et al., 2010	USA and Canada	Physicians	Convenience sampling	Web-based survey	n/a	212	Safety, coercion, Fairness
Bell et al., 2013	Australia	University students	Convenience sampling	Interview	n/a	19	Safety, coercion
Bergström and Lynöe, 2008	Sweden	General public	Random sampling	Paper and pencil questionnaire	52%	517	Safety
		Physicians			39%	108	
Bossaer et al., 2013	USA	University students	All students at one university invited	Web-based survey	59.9%	372	Safety, fairness
Desantis and Hane, 2010	USA	University students	Convenience sampling	Interview	n/a	175	Safety
Dodge et al., 2012	USA	University students	All students at one university invited	Web-based survey	37%	±1200	Fairness
Dubljević et al., 2013*	Germany	University students	Three stage cluster sampling (universities, disciplines, students)	Web-based survey	First wave 53.5%	5882	Fairness
					Second wave 69.1%	3486	
Eickenhorst et al., 2012	Germany	University students	Convenience sampling	Web-based survey	n/a	1218	Safety
		University graduates				106	
European Citizens Panel, 2006	Belgium, Denmark, France, Germany, Greece, Hungary, Italy, the Netherlands, UK	General public	Stratified random sampling (age, profession, gender)	Citizen's deliberation	n/a	126	Coercion
Fitz et al., 2013	USA and Canada	General public	Convenience sampling, Amazon's Mechanical Turk recruitment	Web-based survey	n/a	4011	Safety, coercion, fairness

(Continued)

Table 1 | Continued

Authors	Country	Occupation of participants	Sampling method	Research method	Response rate	Sample size	Concerns
Forlini and Racine, 2009	Canada	University students	Purposive sampling	Focus groups	n/a	29	Coercion
		Parents				21	
		Health care providers				15	
Forlini and Racine, 2012a	Canada	University students	Purposive sampling	Focus groups	n/a	29	Safety, coercion, fairness
		Parents				21	
		Health care providers				15	
Forlini and Racine, 2012b	Canada	University students	Purposive sampling	Focus groups	n/a	29	Safety, fairness
		Parents				21	
		Health care providers				15	
Franke et al., 2012a*	Germany	High school students	All students at 12 public grammar and vocational schools, and students of three departments of one university invited	Paper and pencil questionnaire	83%	1035	Safety, coercion, fairness
		University students				512	
Franke et al., 2012b	Germany	University students	Convenience sampling	Interview	n/a	22	Safety, coercion, fairness
Franke et al., 2014	Germany	Physicians	All primary care physicians in one state invited	Paper and pencil questionnaire	30.2%	832	Safety
Hotze et al., 2011	USA	Physicians	Random sampling	Paper and pencil questionnaire	46.6%	633	Fairness
Judson and Langdon, 2009	USA	University students	All students at two colleges invited	Paper and pencil questionnaire	10%	333	Safety
Kudlow et al., 2013	Canada	University students	All medical students at one medical school invited	Web-based survey	50%	326	Safety
Maier et al., 2013	Switzerland	University students	All students at three educational institutions invited	Web-based survey	22.3%	6275	Coercion
Maslen et al., in press	Germany	University students	Convenience sampling	Paper and pencil questionnaire	n/a	80	Coercion
Mazanov et al., 2013	Australian	University students	Convenience sampling	Web-based survey	n/a	1729	General, fairness
Ott and Biller-Andorno, 2013	Switzerland	University students	Convenience sampling	Web-based survey and separate paper and pencil questionnaire	n/a	1765	Safety, fairness

(Continued)

Table 1 | Continued

Authors	Country	Occupation of participants	Sampling method	Research method	Response rate	Sample size	Concerns
Ott et al., 2012	Switzerland	Physicians	Stratified random sampling (profession, gender, years of training, language)	Paper and pencil questionnaire	23.9%	379	Safety
Partridge et al., 2012	Australia	General public	Random sampling	Telephone interview	31.9%	1265	General
Partridge et al., 2013	Australia	University students	Convenience sampling	Interview	n/a	19	Safety
Riis et al., 2008	USA	University students	*No information provided*	Web-based survey	n/a	357	Fairness
Sabini and Monterosso, 2005	USA	University students	Convenience sampling	Paper and pencil questionnaire	n/a	185	Fairness
Santoni de Sio et al., in press	United Kingdom	University students	Convenience sampling	Paper and pencil questionnaire	n/a	102	Safety, fairness
Sattler et al., 2013a*	Germany	University students	Three stage cluster sampling (universities, disciplines, students)	Web-based survey	87.1%	1852	Safety, fairness
(Sattler et al., 2013b)*	Germany	University teachers	Three stage cluster sampling (universities, disciplines, students/teachers)	Web-based survey	33.5%	1402	Safety
		University students			69.1%	3486	
Sattler et al., 2014*	Germany	University students	Three stage cluster sampling (universities, disciplines, students); only second time wave	Web-based survey	69.1%	3486	Safety, coercion, fairness
Sattler and Wiegel, 2013*	Germany	University students	Three stage cluster sampling (universities, disciplines, students); only second time wave	Web-based survey	First wave 53.5%	5882	Safety
					Second wave 69.1%	3486	
Scheske and Schnall, 2012	UK	University students	Convenience sampling, two studies - two samples	Paper and pencil questionnaire	n/a	50	Safety, fairness
						306	
Schildmann et al., 2013	Germany	University students	*No information provided*	Survey	n/a	1026	Coercion, fairness

(Continued)

Table 1 | Continued

Authors	Country	Occupation of participants	Sampling method	Research method	Response rate	Sample size	Concerns
Schuijff and Brom, 2013	The Netherlands	All	Purposive sampling	Focus groups	n/a	38	Safety, coercion, fairness
Sweeney, 2010	USA	University students	Convenience sampling	Paper and pencil questionnaire	n/a	100	Safety, fairness

Convenience sampling and purposive sampling require no random selection of participants, whereas random sampling, stratified random sampling and cluster sampling do. Purposive sampling requires obtaining a sample of people who meet a predetermined criterion, whereas convenience sampling does not. For stratified random sampling, a population is divided in strata (subgroups) from which participants are randomly selected to make sure all strata are represented in the sample in proportion to their prevalence in the population. Cluster sampling requires a list of clusters, e.g., disciplines in a university, from which a few clusters are randomly chosen. Instead of randomly selecting participants from a list of potential participants, e.g., all students of the university, every member of the selected cluster is invited to participate (Cozby, 2009).

**The authors explicitly state that N is not equal for each analysis due to missing data or specific criteria employed.*

their non-medical use. Similarly, in a survey involving 102 UK Science students, Santoni de Sio et al. (in press) found that the concern against enhancement use that was raised most often by respondents related to potential unintended side-effects.

A plausible consequence is that students are less willing to engage in PCE the higher the severity and risk of the resulting health issues are perceived to be. This was shown in two German factorial design online surveys based on a large pool of vignettes with a sample of 1852 students in the first study (Sattler et al., 2013a) and 3486 students and 1402 university teachers in the second study (Sattler et al., 2013b; these are results of the second wave of a biannual project; also see Sattler and Wiegel, 2013 and Dubljević et al., 2013 for findings on the first and second wave, and (Sattler et al., 2014) for other results on the second wave). Moreover, Franke et al. (2012a) showed in an extensive paper-and-pencil questionnaire study with a sample of 1547 German students that the majority would consider taking PCE substances only if their safety could be assured.

The relation between willingness to use PCE and the perceived risk of PCE might also be an explanation for the results from a focus group study on several human enhancement technologies conducted with 38 Dutch participants divided into five groups (Schuijff and Brom, 2013). (A focus group study is a qualitative research technique in which a group of participants discuss their opinions on a given topic.) After more information on the effects and risks of using methylphenidate as an enhancer was provided, fewer participants stated they would consider using the substance for enhancement purposes than before receiving the information. Participants in this study were not familiar with the concept of human enhancement, in contrast to participants in most of the other studies, and therefore might have underestimated the risks accompanying the use of PCE. In another Dutch focus group study with 37 participants divided into five groups, several examples of the use of medical means to fulfill non-medical wishes were investigated. An example related to PCE, taking β-blockers during a driving test, raised several concerns about medical risks (Asscher and Schermer, 2013). In a semi-structured interview study with twelve Canadian parents of either cognitively disabled or non-disabled children, Ball and Wolbring (2014) observed that all parents unanimously agreed that medical safety has to be insured in order to administer PCE to their children.

Sattler and Wiegel (2013) provided the first evidence on the influence of the perceived severity of side effects and risk attitudes on actual PCE use. In a large- scale online survey with 5882, in a first wave, and 3486 respondents, in a second wave, a lower proneness to risk and an expectation of more severe drug-related side effects were associated with more PCE use at the first time point and increased use of PCE over a 6-months period. However, other results in the second wave of the same project did not show the relation between the expected severity of side effects or risk attitudes and willingness to use PCE (Sattler et al., 2014). The authors did, though, find in the second wave that a higher expected likelihood of side effects decreased the willingness to use PCE.

Other findings suggest that natural remedies are perceived as less harmful than PCE substances, as shown in a questionnaire study involving the Swedish general public and physicians with a sample size of 625 in total (Bergström and Lynöe, 2008). Furthermore, people morally object more to the application of PCE substances if they are artificial rather than natural, and if they are taken in the form of injections rather than pills (Scheske and Schnall, 2012). Focus group participants in the Netherlands referred to natural remedies, placebo, and psychological treatment as alternatives to a specific example of PCE (taking β-blockers during a driving test; Asscher and Schermer, 2013). However, these results may depend on the familiarity of the sample with medical substances. An online survey among 326 Canadian medical students showed that there were no significant differences between attitudes toward pharmacological or natural supplements for cognitive enhancement (Kudlow et al., 2013).

Furthermore, 212 US American and Canadian physicians, reported in an online survey, being less comfortable prescribing PCE substances for non-medical use to young adults, compared to older patients (Banjo et al., 2010). Franke et al. (2014) confirmed these findings in a paper and pencil questionnaire study among 832 German physicians. In both studies, physicians worried about misuse and deemed PCE for young people to be unnecessary. Yet, this applied less to the treatment (i.e., medical use) of older patients. Consistent with these findings, an experimental vignette study conducted online with 4011 respondents found that the US American and Canadian public is more tolerant of side effects when they can be seen as the result of necessary therapy instead of enhancement (Fitz et al., 2013). This touches upon a big debate in medical ethics about the distinction between treatment and enhancement, since this is not a distinction based on biological facts, but, rather, reflecting subjective valuation (Parens, 1998; Daniels, 2000; Hyman, 2011). This is also reflected in a survey by Ott et al. (2012), who concluded that subjective suffering is taken into account as a criterion for disease. From the respondents, 379 Swiss general practitioners and psychiatrists, 88% reported being influenced by the degree of subjective suffering in prescribing an enhancer in four different scenarios. When asked if they would prescribe a PCE substance if a student requested a prescription to stay awake to study more, only 15% confirmed without any doubt, although 54% would prescribe if there were no therapeutic alternative. Around half of the respondents reported being confronted in their practice with such requests for prescriptions.

In contrast to these consistent findings on nonusers, *users* of PCE differ in their estimation of the safety of PCE substances. In an online survey with 1324 German students, users tended to rate the health consequences of PCE as less dangerous than nonusers did (Eickenhorst et al., 2012). This could be explained by users' higher ratings of willingness to take risks, found in a large-scale online survey involving 1765 Swiss students (Ott and Biller-Andorno, 2013). Moreover, fewer individuals (63.9%) from this latter survey's "user group" of 108 students reported worrying about side effects than individuals from the "nonuser group" of 1689 students (81.9%). Similarly, in a semi-structured interview study with 12 US American students who were illicitly or licitly using PCE, most participants believed that the benefits of PCE outweighed the potential negative side effects (Aikins, 2011). Another study with 333 US American students revealed that students who were illicitly using PCE had even more positive attitudes to the use of PCE with regard to medical safety issues compared to licit users (Judson and Langdon, 2009). In another interview study with 22 German students who used both caffeine and PCE, participants saw differences between the two forms of enhancement: in particular they estimated both the desired effects and the negative side effects as more pronounced in the case of PCE (Franke et al., 2012b). Also, Sweeney (2010) presents in her thesis results of a campus survey with a sample of 100 US American students, which demonstrate that students who are illicitly using cognitive enhancers seem to be more likely than nonusers to believe that the substances are harmless.

The aforementioned findings concerning differences between users and nonusers in their estimation of risks and harmfulness might also explain the large difference between the attitudes of users and nonusers found in other studies. A study on attitudes toward the acceptableness of PCE amongst 1265 members of the general public in Australia found that respondents who were familiar with PCE—either by using it themselves or by knowing somebody who used PCE—were twice as likely to find PCE acceptable than respondents who were not familiar with it (Partridge et al., 2012). Also users of PCE among a group of Canadian medical students tended to have more favorable attitudes toward PCE than nonusers (Kudlow et al., 2013). Lastly, a survey of 1729 students from Australian universities revealed differences in attitudes between users and nonusers of PCE, with users more often finding the use of study drugs "moral" than nonusers (Mazanov et al., 2013). The latter three studies did not specifically present the reason why respondents had a certain attitude toward PCE, and thus their opinions might not be related to medical safety. Still, these results are in line with a common finding in drug epidemiology, revealing that positive attitudes toward a drug, in particular low perceived risk, correlate with its use (e.g., Bachman et al., 1998; Bavarian et al., 2013; Cabriales et al., 2013).

In addition, users justify their practice and underestimate potential health risks for themselves and for others as shown in an interview-based survey with 175 US American students (Desantis and Hane, 2010). Conversely, Franke et al. (2012a) found that users and nonusers estimate addictive risks similarly, perhaps because there is a greater likelihood of substance dependency for users (Kroutil et al., 2006). However, Franke et al. (2012a) did not specifically test for PCE dependency in their study. In the abovementioned study by Desantis and Hane (2010), it was revealed that users argue for the substances' safety and downplay potential health risks by contrasting PCE to street-drugs (e.g., cocaine, heroin, etc.) and by pointing toward their acceptance within the medical establishment. This relates to the observation that students who believe that they know enough in order to safely use PCE are more likely to state that PCE is harmless (Sweeney, 2010). The fact that users tend to estimate PCE usage as harmless might explain why they find its application to be morally and socially acceptable (Desantis and Hane, 2010).

Hence, there is a general discrepancy between the views of users and nonusers with regard to the associated health risks of PCE and its moral acceptance, with users being less concerned than nonusers.

COERCION

The question of coercion relates to autonomy, i.e. the freedom to decide about one's personal life, and is a central issue in the normative debate on PCE. A main concern is that people are being pressured or even coerced into enhancing themselves. This might happen either indirectly in the form of peer pressure (Warren et al., 2009), or potentially directly in certain workplaces with long working hours and high demands on cognitive functioning, such as in the military or in surgery (Schoomaker, 2007; Maslen et al., in press). While opponents of enhancement consider it a "threat to the responsibility one bears for one's own life" (Habermas, 2003, p. 61), proponents instead focus on its advantages. They point out that PCE in particular entails the possibility of enhancing autonomy itself by increasing the reasoning abilities required to engage in such autonomous decisions (Schaefer et al., 2013).

The participants in Schuijff and Brom's (2013) focus group study indicated implicit peer pressure and explicit demand by employers to use human enhancement technologies to be a major concern for them. Maslen et al. (in press) found in a survey of 80 UK students clear and strong objection against the idea that people in professions with high responsibility, such as pilots and physicians, might even have a moral obligation to enhance their performance, with only one respondent agreeing to such an obligation and 44% completely disagreeing. Two other surveys among German students found that the majority of students did not approve of PCE in jobs with high responsibilities: in one survey only 26% of the 1026 respondents approved of the use of PCE in highly responsible jobs (Schildmann et al., 2013), the second found that approximate 20% of their 1547 respondents approved the use of PCE for individuals with high responsibility (Franke et al., 2012a).

Forlini and Racine (2009) conducted one of the (very few) studies investigating people's attitudes on autonomy and coercion specifically with regards to PCE, again with the use of focus groups. Their participants, 65 Canadians assigned to one of nine groups consisting of either students, parents, or healthcare providers, agreed that PCE should be a matter of personal choice. This seems in line with one of the recommendations of a "European citizens' panel" held in 2005 and 2006, a citizens' deliberation on brain science involving 126 individuals from nine European countries. (A citizen's deliberation is a form of public participation in consultation about science, but can be less structured than a focus group study because groups can change during the deliberation.) One of the topics touched upon briefly was human enhancement. The participants' highest ranked recommendation was that people should be given the right to take "whatever drug they want," but enough information about the effects and dangers should be available; however, they did not support use of PCE in situations in which people have to pass exams (European Citizens Panel, 2006).

Participants in Forlini and Racine's (2009) study held the descriptive view that users are generally deciding to take such substances as a result of a voluntary decision. At the same time, however, they believed that this decision can be influenced by perceived social pressure or by competitive environments, such as academia or the job market, where people are striving for success and feel they have to perform better than average. Health care providers amongst the participants admitted that students who don't take enhancers may be disadvantaged because demands are getting higher and PCE is becoming more prevalent. They regarded peer pressure as an important contributing factor to the perceived need to take cognitive enhancers. Parents, in contrast, were aware of the pressure being put on students and consequently felt worry and sadness. They feared that the use of PCE may become a new standard.

However, peer pressure seems to be a more complex phenomenon than one might assume. Sattler et al. (2014) show that willingness to take PCE drugs does not increase when others encourage it, but it decreases when disapproval of the use of PCE by others rises. Furthermore, on the one hand, Forlini and Racine (2009) observe the desire of students not to be at a disadvantage, while on the other hand, less than 10% of 1547 German students stated in a survey by Franke et al. (2012a) that they would use PCE if others did so. In an online study amongst 6275 Swiss students less than 3% agreed that other people's use of substances would justify the use of PCE, compared to over 66% who agreed that increased learning would justify the use (Maier et al., 2013). One methodological reason for these diverging findings might be that even though a qualitative approach as used by Forlini and Racine (2009) can reveal aspects that might stay undiscovered in quantitative approaches like surveys, the small sample size might limit the generalizability of the findings. Going beyond methodology, we might speculate that it is not other people using PCE *per se*, but other people performing better, that puts pressure on students and leads them to consider taking such substances. In general, student participants in Forlini and Racine's (2009) focus groups viewed PCE as a personal lifestyle choice and emphasized the importance of personal integrity, i.e., they accepted the use of PCE conditional on the fact that one remains faithful to one's personal values. At the same time, they recognized the difficulty of that endeavor when social pressure is high and when abstinence could lead to personal disadvantage. Parents of university students, on the other hand, maintained a paternalistic view: students should be informed about cognitive enhancement, and, as a consequence, they should be held responsible and accountable for the decision to engage in PCE.

Thus, people consider the role of peer pressure as problematic and agree on the importance of deciding autonomously whether to engage in PCE. However, since the few studies reported here reveal mixed results, more research is needed to investigate the topic in greater depth.

FAIRNESS

The normative debate around the fairness of PCE is perhaps the least clearly defined. The term "fairness" seems to raise different distinct concepts in the lay mind, and thus creates a difficulty in comparing different studies that ask for opinions on the fairness of PCE use without defining what is meant by "fair." Overall, fairness related concerns seem to play an important role in the public, since they have been the second most common argument, after unintended side effects, against the use of enhancement raised by participants in Santoni de Sio et al.'s (in press) survey. Forlini and Racine's (2012a also c.f. Forlini and Racine, 2009) focus-group study explored lay statements about fairness of PCE in greater detail. They developed a model to describe three different subthemes: they suggest that judgments of fairness can (apart from external factors like legislation) be defined by a relationship between *equality of opportunity*, *honesty*, and *authenticity*. Participants who valued the equality of opportunity described the importance of an equal distribution of opportunities to obtain PCE substances and opportunities deriving from their use. Honesty and authenticity are both related to effort that has to be invested to achieve a certain task. The underlying assumption is that when high performance is achieved with less effort—as might be the case when PCE substances are taken—this might be less fair compared to performance that is achieved with substantial effort. Honesty relates to the social aspect of this assumption and reflects the effect of PCE use on other individuals, for example in a competitive environment where PCE use might be seen as cheating. Authenticity relates to the individual PCE user and questions whether his/her performance under PCE, often seen as a situation in which effort is discounted, is an authentic performance. It is based on the underlying belief that putting in effort shapes the experience of an individual and thus affects a "future" individual that does not gain the same experience while using PCE. Although the above separation of concepts is too coarse to fully reflect the depth of the academic normative debate, the concerns of the public can be grouped around these subthemes of fairness.

EQUALITY OF OPPORTUNITY

First, we discuss equality of opportunity, the fear that inequality in access to enhancement substances might increase inequalities in society. Farah et al. (2004) describe how certain groups might experience cost barriers and social barriers to access PCE. (In this section, we do not consider concerns about restrictions of freedom to follow personal preferences, as these are discussed in the previous section about coercion). Equality of opportunity is also referred to as *distributive fairness* (e.g., Scheske and Schnall, 2012), *distributive justice* (Farah et al., 2004), or the *concern of inequality* (e.g., Bostrom and Sandberg, 2009). Note that the notion of equality of opportunity relates to a certain underlying theory of justice (cf. Rawls, 1971), which can be contrasted, for example, to the notion of equality of outcome. However, these underlying theories are not distinguished yet in empirical research on the public's opinions about PCE.

Although healthcare providers, students and parents who participated in the focus group study by Forlini and Racine (2012a) believed that, currently, everybody who wanted could find PCE substances one way or another, they did emphasize the importance of the value of equality of opportunity as part of their judgment on the fairness of the use of PCE. Correspondingly, in survey research by Sattler et al. (2013a) amongst 1852 respondents, a lower score on both willingness-to-use a PCE and moral acceptability of PCE substances was reported when judging an imaginary situation where no other students take this PCE substance, compared to situations in which half of the other students or all fellow students were taking the PCE substance. Possibly, they read the "no other student" situation as one where there is inequality in opportunity with them having, and other students not having, access and found this to be morally unacceptable. However, Sattler et al.'s (2013a) finding could also point to the experience of a "social norm," following from the prevalence of use that influences the judgment of moral acceptability.

In a survey, Hotze et al. (2011) presented 633 US American general practitioners with two statements related to this topic: a slight majority agreed that society should prevent economic advantages turning into biological advantages (57%), and that everyone should have equal access to medical enhancers (55%). Scheske and Schnall (2012) showed that the use of PCE substances is perceived as more wrong if not everybody can afford them, compared to situations in which everybody can. Fitz et al. (2013) investigated fairness by using the contrastive vignette technique online. Their 4011 respondents, recruited via Amazon's Mechanical Turk, were randomly assigned to one of 22 different vignettes that described the use of PCE diverging in terms of alleged safety, societal and peer pressure, fairness and authenticity. Respondents saw it as less fair if a student obtained an enhancer with the help of money given by his parents rather than with money earned by own work. The 185 US American respondents in Sabini and Monterosso's (2005) study endorsed the so-called "interaction view" (p. 91): their judgments of fairness depended on the group that was affected by the drug. Although their fairness ratings of PCE use were always close to or lower than the midpoint of the scale—thus generally regarding it as rather unfair—respondents believed the use by the worst performing 10% of students to be fairer than the use by everybody or the top 10%. The "interaction view" corresponds to what John Rawls (1971, 1985) calls the "difference principle": inequality is acceptable only if the current situation for those least advantaged is improved.

A survey amongst 1026 German students demonstrated that 27% of the respondents approved the use of PCE by worse performing classmates, while 57% approved the use for elderly with declining cognitive performance (Schildmann et al., 2013). Correspondingly, over a quarter of the respondents of another study among German students reported that classmates with low academic performance should be allowed to use PCE, while 50% indicated that the use of PCE by cognitively impaired elderly should be allowed (Franke et al., 2012a). The percentage of respondents who endorsed the use of PCE by classmates with low academic performance was higher among PCE users than nonusers. It is clear that although the interaction view is endorsed, previous performance is of less influence on judgments of fairness of the use of PCE than age. However, this is perhaps because the samples are both young students who are in competition with other young students, so that age and performance variables could be said to be confounded in the sample. Future studies need to investigate the attitudes of young students in competition with elderly students, and compare elderly students with elderly non-students, so that attitudes toward these factors could be separated. Sabini and Monterosso (2005) explain the interaction view by arguing that a substance that would affect the worst performing 10% only can better be seen as a normalizer instead of an enhancer, suggesting that in this case it might be closer to a treatment than to an enhancement. If this explanation is correct, it would seem that both the acceptance of side effects as well as the acceptance of a certain unequal distribution is greater in the case of a treatment compared to enhancement.

In general, healthcare providers, students, and parents seem to agree that an unequal distribution of PCE is unfair, if the unequal distribution is related to factors that are changeable, such as wealth. If the unequal distribution exists due to biological dispositions, such as having a low attention span, an unequal distribution is seen as less relevant to moral judgments. This is related to the distinction between treatment and enhancement, in which the former is generally believed to be seen as more acceptable (Parens, 1998; Daniels, 2000; Hyman, 2011). Users find it more acceptable than nonusers that fellow students with low academic performance use PCE, but research investigating the reasons for these diverging views of users and nonusers is still lacking.

HONESTY

Honesty relates to the question of whether the use of PCE might give a user an unfair advantage over people who do not use PCE, and thus might need to exert more effort to achieve the same result. Scheske and Schnall (2012) refer to honesty as *competitive fairness* and Bostrom and Sandberg (2009) discuss it in relation to *cheating*. Using an example and taking a normative stance, Bostrom and Sandberg (2009) describe how goals and rules define whether an act qualifies as cheating: if the primary goal of schooling is acquiring knowledge, PCE might be legitimate. In the case of a competition for grades or admission, however, PCE could be seen as cheating if it were against the rules or if access were unequally distributed.

Quantitative accounts of the public's opinion on honesty related to PCE use can be found in several studies. Students of a highly competitive UK university deemed the competitive advantage PCE can give as one of the most important concerns regarding its use: an advantage due to PCE use was found most morally wrong when no other competitors were taking the substance, relating competitive to distributive fairness and peer pressure (Scheske and Schnall, 2012). Moreover, an online survey by Bossaer et al. (2013) demonstrated that 60% of the 372 student respondents agreed that PCE provides users with an unfair advantage over other students. An almost identical amount of just over half of the respondents (56%) believed that PCE use for study purposes could be seen as academic dishonesty. In a large-scale online survey, with respectively 5882 and 3486 participants in the first and second wave, (Dubljević et al., 2013) found that German students deem the use of PCE with the intention to increase study performance to be morally less acceptable than traditional forms of academic misconduct, such as cheating in exams, fabrication, or plagiarism. Schildmann et al. (2013) reported that half of the respondents of their questionnaire study thought the use of PCE by others was unfair, another quarter was unsure of their thoughts about the statement, and only a quarter "rather" or "absolutely" agreed that the use of PCE by others was fair. Over half of the respondents in Franke et al. (2012a) indicated in a questionnaire that they found PCE fair "under no circumstances" or "probably not." This percentage was higher among females and among nonusers. Although exact percentages are not provided, Sweeney (2010) also discusses a survey amongst 100 students in which nonusers felt more troubled than users by academic advantages obtained by PCE. This difference between users and nonusers was also found in the online survey by Ott and Biller-Andorno (2013). They show that a little over 40% of nonusers agree that with using PCE, one would be betraying others who do not use PCE, while less than 20% of users agree to this statement. An online study with 1200 male US American student participants revealed that the misuse of performance enhancement substances in the sporting domain received a higher rating on a scale that measured the degree of cheating than the use of PCE in academia (Dodge et al., 2012).

As described above, Fitz et al. (2013) showed that when obtaining PCE takes less effort, it is seen as more unfair. This was reflected in reduced fairness ratings in a scenario in which one individual could use PCE and another could not. The effort needed to obtain PCE was manipulated, as well as a second variable, that of the effect of the PCE as either reducing the effort needed to study or increasing the number of hours that one could study for. The combination of diminished effort in obtainment and reduced study effort produced the lowest ratings of fairness. Thus, any variation of the description that would result in a reduction of effort for the user of PCE in comparison to a nonuser resulted in respondents judging PCE as less fair.

Qualitative studies provide a more elaborate but also more ambiguous perspective on honesty in relation to PCE. In an interview study amongst 19 Australian students by Bell et al. (2013 also c.f. Partridge et al., 2013) fairness appeared at the top of the list of concerns mentioned. More than half of the participants described PCE as a form of cheating, while most of the others explicitly reported that they did not find it unfair in comparison to other available methods for performance improvement (e.g., coffee). In contrast to coffee, focus group participants saw PCE as a form of cheating similar to the use of steroids (Forlini and Racine, 2012b). Also, participants showed dissent and indecision about whether PCE use should be seen as cheating or not (Forlini and Racine, 2012a). Each subgroup of students, parents, and health care providers included some individuals who saw PCE as an unfair shortcut, putting others at a disadvantage, but also individuals who considered PCE a study tool like any other.

To summarize, a little over half of the public believes that the use of PCE provides an unfair advantage to users, a situation that is seen as cheating, especially in highly competitive environments. Nonusers provide lower ratings of honesty than users in quantitative studies. In general there seems to be dissent on whether PCE qualifies as cheating or not. Qualitative studies give more insight into the different perspectives on this question.

AUTHENTICITY

In the normative debate, critics of PCE argue that users, compared with nonusers, of enhancement substances experience the value of exerting effort on a task less. This makes activities less meaningful and facilitates fewer experiences of self-development (see Schermer, 2008, for an analysis of this argument). Part of the debate therefore relates to authentic performance, for which effort is seen as a necessary condition (e.g., President's Council on Bioethics, 2003). Goodman (2010) specifies that this is true for what he calls process goods, for which the activity itself is seen as central. For so-called outcome goods, however, for which the result of an activity counts, effort is less relevant.

We can apply the distinction between process goods and outcome goods to the list of 19 traits rated by 357 respondents in an online study by Riis et al. (2008). For each trait they had to rate their willingness to enhance it using pharmacological means, if they could. Outcome related traits, such as memory, received higher scores on willingness-to-enhance than more process related traits, such as mood and social comfort. These higher ratings for what we deem outcome related traits might be explained by respondents valuing the notion of effort. Furthermore, respondents were less willing to enhance traits that were rated as more fundamental to the self, such as kindness and empathy.

Participants in the focus group study by Forlini and Racine (2012a) explicitly related effort to judgments of the fairness of PCE. Students, parents, and healthcare providers commented on effort and authenticity. They displayed both positive (nonproblematizing) and negative (problematizing) views toward PCE in relation to effort and authenticity in equal proportions, as can be seen in the following examples. Participants of each target group (students, parents, and healthcare providers) noted that even with the use of FCE, effort still had to be put in to complete certain tasks. However, participants also discussed how enhancement may compromise certain social and personal values that shape an individual's behavior. Also some of the student participants in the interview study by Bell et al. (2013) described PCE as a quick fix rather than a true reflection of an individual's abilities, while other participants neither reported effort nor authenticity as being corrupted by the use of PCE. Two thirds of the student respondents in the survey by Schildmann et al. (2013) agreed that performances done with PCE were "less commendable than comparable performances that are done without these substances" (p. 25). In addition, 63% of the 644 physicians who completed the survey by Hotze et al. (2011) viewed PCE as a threat to the value of human achievement. Moreover, an online survey by Banjo et al. (2010) showed that the respondents, 212 physicians, ranked "PCE undermines the values of personal effort" as the fourth most important reason (of 13 presented) to feel uncomfortable about prescribing PCE to non-elderly people. However, an online survey among 1729 Australian students showed that users of prescription amphetamines had fewer concerns regarding the integrity of authentic and moral actions than did nonusers (Mazanov et al., 2013).

Finally, in their experimental vignette study Fitz et al. (2013) found that respondents rated an individual's performance as significantly less authentic when PCE was used, compared to when it was not used. However, this opinion did not completely transfer to judgments of worthiness for a promotion when the character would be assigned a new project in his job. Respondents judged a PCE user as significantly more worthy when successful without enhancement compared to with enhancement, but they also indicated that people who succeeded with the help of PCE were more worthy of promotion than people who did not use PCE and failed.

To summarize, in general people are more likely to enhance outcome related traits than process related traits. However, in direct discussions about effort and authenticity in relation to fairness, individuals display divergent opinions on the importance of these topics. The proportion of people who believe effort is discounted and authenticity violated when using PCE is a little over half of the respondents in most studies. This implies that little less than half of the public is not that concerned about effort and authenticity in relation to PCE. One reason that is given is that effort still has to be invested to achieve certain goals, even when PCE is used.

CONCLUSION

This review provides an overview of 40 studies on the public's opinion about PCE. Our main finding is that in groups outside the normative academic debate several concerns about the use of pharmacological substances for performance enhancement are either raised or endorsed. These concerns that are discussed in the current review of research on opinions about PCE widely match the normative debate. These similarities between the public's opinion and the normative debate are also found in studies on other ethical issues, for example the sex selection of embryos (Banks et al., 2006) and life extension technologies (Partridge et al., 2009). The findings we present are divided between three concerns regarding PCE use which are common in both the ethical and lay debate: medical safety, coercion, and fairness.

Several studies have shown that *medical safety* is regarded as central by nonusers of PCE, and insecurity about it provides a reason for them to refuse the use of PCE. Related to this concern are findings that point toward a preference for natural over artificial enhancers. A similar preference can be seen for interventions that might be closer to treatment than to enhancement. Users, on the other hand, do not display these preferences and indicate conflicting results on judgments of (subjective) health risks associated with PCE. They are concerned about addiction, but do not worry about other health risks, and deem PCE more often harmless than nonusers do. A more convergent view can be found on the theme of *coercion*. Different subgroups agree that PCE should be a matter of personal choice. They believe that decisions concerning use are, in general, made voluntarily, although they can be influenced by perceived social pressure or by competitive environments. It is shown that peer pressure is a complex phenomenon, as students might not always be influenced by other people's PCE use itself, but only when these others achieve a higher performance compared to their own. However, only a few studies have investigated coercion to date and we call for future research to fill this gap. Finally, we discussed *fairness*, divided into three subthemes: equality of opportunity, honesty, and authenticity. An unequal distribution of PCE substances that might develop due to changeable factors—such as wealth—is seen as unfair, while an unequal distribution due to biological dispositions—such as a low attention span—is seen as less relevant to judgments of fairness. This might relate to a general finding that treatments are seen as more acceptable than enhancements. The public's opinion on the subthemes of honesty and authenticity shows a more complex pattern. Nonusers believe more often than users that the use of PCE provides an unfair advantage, although in general only half of the public raises concerns about this topic of honesty and cheating. Several studies show that around the theme of authenticity both problematizing and non-problematizing views on PCE arise in equal proportions. While some respondents indicate that "the work has still to be done" even when PCE is used, others believe that PCE is a quick fix and undermines an authentic performance.

One important distinction within the public can be found between users and nonusers, who tend to differ in their perspectives on the medical safety and subthemes of the fairness of PCE: while users generally deem PCE to be safe and fair, nonusers do not. These results imply that users are either more willing to engage in PCE because of their positive attitude toward it, or that they adopted their positive attitude as a result of personal usage. In either case, the differences in users' and nonusers' attitudes toward PCE might be driven by cognitive biases. It is possible, for example, that nonusers display a more negative view toward PCE because they experience the so-called status quo bias, which describes the irrational preference for an option only because it preserves the current state of affairs (Kahneman and Tversky, 2000). As currently PCE use is not seen as a common way to improve cognitive performance, this bias might result in the preference to not use PCE. This tendency, to use the status quo as a reference point, might explain why people prefer interventions when they are seen as treatments as opposed to enhancements (Bostrom and Ord, 2006). It is also possible, however, that users adopt a more positive view toward PCE in order to reduce their cognitive dissonance, the discomfort experienced when one's actions don't reflect one's beliefs (Festinger, 1957). This would reflect a situation in which users adapt their attitudes toward their PCE use, that is, their behavior. Future research is called to examine in greater depth which biases might influence people's attitudes toward PCE and the causal direction explaining the attitudes currently prevalent. Further, future research might also reveal whether differences between users and nonusers also hold for other concerns, such as coercion and authenticity for which data on this distinction is currently lacking.

It is important to note that the current literature focuses mostly on opinions of students, with only a few exceptions provided by studies on health care providers and the general public. Furthermore, several studies were conducted with a non-random sample of participants, or obtained a low response rate in the case of random sampling. This might have biased the results. In addition, even the studies that were conducted with random sampling of students at specific universities can create a biased population overview in our review, because differences between colleges on the use of PCE are found (e.g., McCabe et al., 2005). Furthermore, future research should provide more insight into the opinions of populations other than students, such as the general population or more specifically people active in the workforce. This would add to a more accurate picture of opinions of the general population and of potential users in those areas where use is to be expected.

Moreover, future research is called for to reveal more fine-grained differences in the public opinion for certain concerns. In the current literature, different concerns can have the same name, as is seen with fairness, while different names may also be used for the same concern, as was described for equality of opportunity. This makes it harder to draw precise conclusions on the state of research on public attitudes toward PCE and to systematically compare it with arguments from the normative debate. Although more fine-grained studies are needed to reflect the depth of the normative debate, it can be said that, thus far, concerns of the public regarding the use of PCE reflect the main issues fiercely debated in academia.

REFERENCES

*Aikins, R. D. (2011). Academic performance enhancement: a qualitative study of the perceptions and habits of prescription stimulant-using college students. *J. Coll. Stud. Dev.* 52, 560–576. doi: 10.1353/csd.2011.0064

*Asscher, E. C. A., and Schermer, M. (2013). Wish-fulfilling medicine in practice: the opinions and arguments of lay people. *J. Med. Ethics.* doi: 10.1136/medethics-2013-101480. [Epub ahead of print].

Bachman, J. G., Johnson, L. D., and O'Malley, P. M. (1998). Explaining recent increases in students' marijuana use: impacts of perceived risks and disapproval, 1976 through 1996. *Am. J. Public Health* 88, 887–892. doi: 10.2105/AJPH.88.6.887

*Ball, N., and Wolbring, G. (2014). Cognitive enhancement: perceptions among parents of children with disabilities. *Neuroethics* 1–20. doi: 10.1007/s12152-014-9201-8. [Epub ahead of print].

*Banjo, O. C., Nadler, R., and Reiner, P. B. (2010). Physician attitudes towards pharmacological cognitive enhancement: safety concerns are paramount. *PLoS ONE* 5:e14322. doi: 10.1371/journal.pone.0014322

Banks, S., Scully, J. L., and Shakespeare, T. (2006). Ordinary ethics: lay people's deliberations on social sex selection. *New Genet. Soc.* 25, 289–303. doi: 10.1080/14636770601032890

Bavarian, N., Flay, B. R., Ketcham, P. L., and Smit, E. (2013). Illicit use of prescription stimulants in a college student sample: a theory-guided analysis. *Drug Alcohol Depend.* 132, 665–673. doi: 10.1016/j.drugalcdep.2013.04.024

*Bell, S., Partridge, B., Lucke, J., and Hall, W. (2013). Australian university students' attitudes towards the acceptability and regulation of pharmaceuticals to improve academic performance. *Neuroethics* 6, 197–205. doi: 10.1007/s12152-012-9153-9

*Bergström, L. S., and Lynöe, N. (2008). Enhancing concentration, mood and memory in healthy individuals: an empirical study of attitudes among general practitioners and the general population. *Scand. J. Public Health.* 36, 532–537. doi: 10.1177/1403494807087558

*Bossaer, J. B., Gray, J. A., Miller, S. E., Enck, G., Gaddipati, V. C., and Enck, R. E. (2013). The use and misuse of prescription stimulants as "cognitive enhancers" by students at one academic health sciences center. *Acad. Med.* 88, 967–971. doi: 10.1097/Acm.0b013e318294fc7b

Bostrom, N., and Ord, T. (2006). The reversal test: eliminating status quo bias in applied ethics. *Ethics* 116, 656–679. doi: 10.1086/505233

Bostrom, N., and Sandberg, A. (2009). Cognitive enhancement: methods, ethics, regulatory challenges. *Sci. Eng. Ethics* 15, 311–341. doi: 10.1007/s11948-009-9142-5

Cabriales, J. A., Cooper, T. V., and Taylor, T. (2013). Prescription drug misuse, illicit drug use, and their potential risk and protective correlates in a Hispanic college student sample. *Exp. Clin. Psychopharmacol.* 21, 235–244. doi: 10.1037/a0031973

Cozby, P. C. (2009). *Methods in Behavioral Research.* New York, NY: McGraw-Hill.

Daniels, N. (2000). Normal functioning and the treatment-enhancement distinction. *Camb. Q. Healthc. Ethics* 9, 309–322. doi: 10.1017/S0963180100903037

Delaney, J. J., and Martin, D. P. (2011). The role of physician opinion in human enhancement. *Am. J. Bioeth.* 11, 19–20. doi: 10.1080/15265161.2010.534537

*Desantis, A. D., and Hane, A. C. (2010). "Adderall is definitely not a drug": justifications for the illegal use of ADHD stimulants. *Subst. Use Misuse* 45, 31–46. doi: 10.3109/10826080902858334

*Dodge, T., Williams, K. J., Marzell, M., and Turrisi, R. (2012). Judging cheaters: is substance misuse viewed similarly in the athletic and academic domains? *Psychol. Addict. Behav.* 26, 678–682. doi: 10.1037/A0027872

Dubljevic, V. (2013). Cognitive enhancement, rational choice and justification. *Neuroethics* 6, 179–187. doi: 10.1007/s12152-012-9173-5

*Dubljević, V., Sattler, S., and Racine, E. (2013). Cognitive enhancement and academic misconduct: a study exploring their frequency and relationship. *Ethics Behav.* doi: 10.1080/10508422.2013.869747. [Epub ahead of print].

*Eickenhorst, P., Vitzthum, K., Klapp, B. F., Groneberg, D., and Mache, S. (2012). Neuroenhancement among German university students: motives, expectations, and relationship with psychoactive lifestyle drugs. *J. Psychoactive Drugs* 44, 418–427. doi: 10.1080/02791072.2012.736845

*European Citizens' Panel. (2006). *Meeting of Minds, European Citizens' Deliberation on Brain Science.* Available online at: http://www.kbs-frb.be/otheractivity.aspx?id=193934&langtype=1033 (Accessed January 15, 2014).

Farah, M. J., Illes, J., Cook-Deegan, R., Gardner, H., Kandel, E., King, P., et al. (2004). Neurocognitive enhancement: what can we do and what should we do? *Nat. Rev. Neurosci.* 5, 421–425. doi: 10.1038/nrn1390

Farah, M. J., Smith, M. E., Ilieva, I., and Hamilton, R. H. (2014). Cognitive enhancement. *WIREs Cogn Sci.* 5, 95–103. doi: 10.1002/wcs.1250

Faulmüller, N., Maslen, H., and Santoni de Sio, F. (2013). The indirect psychological costs of cognitive enhancement. *Am. J. Bioeth.*. 13, 45–47. doi: 10.1080/15265161.2013.794880

Festinger, L. (1957). *A Theory of Cognitive Dissonance.* Stanford, CA: Stanford University Press.

Finger, G., da Silva, E. R., and Falavigna, A. (2013). Use of methylphenidate among medical students: a systematic review. *Rev. Assoc. Med. Bras.* 59, 285–289. doi: 10.1016/J.Ramb.2012.10.007

*Fitz, N. S., Nadler, R., Manogaran, P., Chong, E. W. J., and Reiner, P. B. (2013). Public attitudes toward cognitive enhancement. *Neuroethics.* doi: 10.1007/s12152-013-9190-z

*Forlini, C., and Racine, E. (2009). Autonomy and coercion in academic "Cognitive Enhancement" using methylphenidate: perspectives

of key stakeholders. *Neuroethics* 2, 163–177. doi: 10.1007/s12152-009-9043-y

*Forlini, C., and Racine, E. (2012a). Added stakeholders, added value(s) to the cognitive enhancement debate: are academic discourse and professional policies sidestepping values of stakeholders? *AJOB Prim. Res.* 3, 33–47. doi: 10.1080/21507716.2011.645116

*Forlini, C., and Racine, E. (2012b). Stakeholder perspectives and reactions to "academic" cognitive enhancement: unsuspected meaning of ambivalence and analogies. *Public Underst. Sci.* 21, 606–625. doi: 10.1177/0963662510385062

Franke, A. G., Bagusat, C., Dietz, P., Hoffmann, I., Simon, P., Ulrich, R., et al. (2013). Use of illicit and prescription drugs for cognitive or mood enhancement among surgeons. *BMC Med.* 11:102. doi: 10.1186/1741-7015-11-102

*Franke, A. G., Bonertz, C., Christmann, M., Engeser, S., and Lieb, K. (2012a). Attitudes toward cognitive enhancement in users and nonusers of stimulants for cognitive enhancement: a pilot study. *AJOB Prim. Res.* 3, 48–57. doi: 10.1080/21507716.2011.608411

*Franke, A. G., Lieb, K., and Hildt, E. (2012b). What users think about the differences between caffeine and illicit/prescription stimulants for cognitive enhancement. *PLoS ONE* 7:e40047. doi: 10.1371/journal.pone.0040047

*Franke, A. G., Papenburg, C., Schotten, E., Reiner, P. B., and Lieb, K. (2014). Attitudes towards prescribing cognitive enhancers among primary care physicians in Germany. *BMC Fam. Pract.* 15:3. doi: 10.1186/1471-2296-15-3

Goodman, R. (2010). Cognitive enhancement, cheating, and accomplishment. *Kennedy Inst. Ethics J.* 20, 145–160. doi: 10.1353/ken.0.0309

Habermas, J. (2003). *The Future of Human Nature*. Cambridge: Polity Press.

*Hotze, T. D., Shah, K., Anderson, E. E., and Wynia, M. K. (2011). "Doctor, would you prescribe a pill to help me ...?" a national survey of physicians on using medicine for human enhancement. *Am. J. Bioeth.* 11, 3–13. doi: 10.1080/15265161.2011.534957

Husain, M., and Mehta, M. A. (2011). Cognitive enhancement by drugs in health and disease. *Trends Cogn. Sci.* 15, 28–36. doi: 10.1016/j.tics.2010.11.002

Hyman, S. E. (2011). Cognitive enhancement: promises and perils. *Neuron* 69, 595–598. doi: 10.1016/j.neuron.2011.02.012

Ilieva, I., Boland, J., and Farah, M. J. (2013). Objective and subjective cognitive enhancing effects of mixed amphetamine salts in healthy people. *Neuropharmacology* 64, 496–505. doi: 10.1016/j.neuropharm.2012.07.021

*Judson, R., and Langdon, S. W. (2009). Illicit use of prescription stimulants among college students: prescription status, motives, theory of planned behaviour, knowledge and self-diagnostic tendencies. *Psychol. Health Med.* 14, 97–104. doi: 10.1080/13548500802126723

Kahneman, D., and Tversky, A. (2000). *Choices, Values, and Frames*. New York, NY: Cambridge University Press.

King, S., Griffin, S., Hodges, Z., Weatherly, H., Asseburg, C., Richardson, G., et al. (2006). A systematic review and economic model of the effectiveness and cost-effectiveness of methylphenidate, dexamfetamine and atomoxetine for the treatment of attention deficit hyperactivity disorder in children and adolescents. *Health Technol. Assess* 10, iii–iv, xiii–146.

Kociancic, T., Reed, M. D., and Findling, R. L. (2004). Evaluation of risks associated with short- and long-term psychostimulant therapy for treatment of ADHD in children. *Expert Opin. Drug Saf.* 3, 93–100. doi: 10.1517/eods.3.2.93.27337

Kroutil, L. A., Van Brunt, D. L., Herman-Stahl, M. A., Heller, D. C., Bray, R. M., and Penne, M. A. (2006). Nonmedical use of prescription stimulants in the United States. *Drug Alcohol Depend.* 84, 135–143. doi: 10.1016/j.drugalcdep.2005.12.011

*Kudlow, P. A., Treurnicht Naylor, K., Xie, B., and McIntyre, R. S. (2013). Cognitive enhancement in Canadian medical students. *J. Psychoactive Drugs*45, 360–365. doi: 10.1080/02791072.2013.825033

Maher, B. (2008). Poll results: look who's doping. *Nature* 452, 674–675. doi: 10.1038/452674a

*Maier, L. J., Liechti, M. E., Herzig, F., and Schaub, M. P. (2013). To dope or not to dope: neuroenhancement with prescription drugs and drugs of abuse among Swiss university students. *PLoS ONE* 8:e77967. doi:10.1371/journal.pone.0077967

*Maslen, H., Santoni de Sio, F., and Faulmüller, N. (in press). "With cognitive enhancement comes great responsibility?," in *Responsible Innovation*. Vol. 2, eds B. J. Koops et al. (Dordrecht: Springer).

*Mazanov, J., Dunn, M., Connor, J., and Fielding, M. L. (2013). Substance use to enhance academic performance among Australian university students. *Perform. Enhance. Health* 2, 110–118. doi: 10.1016/j.peh.2013.08.017

McCabe, S. E., Knight, J. R., Teter, C. J., and Wechsler, H. (2005). Non-medical use of prescription stimulants among US college students: prevalence and correlates from a national survey. *Addiction* 99, 96–106. doi:10.1111/j.1360-0443.2004.00944.x

*Ott, R., and Biller-Andorno, N. (2013). Neuroenhancement among Swiss students - a comparison of users and non-users. *Pharmacopsychiatry* 47, 22–28. doi: 10.1055/s-0033-1358682

*Ott, R., Lenk, C., Miller, N., Neuhaus Buhler, R., and Biller-Andorno, N. (2012). Neuroenhancement - perspectives of Swiss psychiatrists and general practitioners. *Swiss Med. Wkly.* 142, w13707. doi: 10.4414/smw.2012.13707

Parens, E. (1998). *Enhancing Human Traits: Ethical and Social Implications*. Washington, DC: Georgetown University Press.

*Partridge, B., Bell, S., Lucke, J., and Hall, W. (2013). Australian university students' attitudes towards the use of prescription stimulants as cognitive enhancers: perceived patterns of use, efficacy and safety. *Drug Alcohol Rev.* 32, 295–302. doi: 10.1111/dar.12005

*Partridge, B., Lucke, J., and Hall, W. (2012). A comparison of attitudes toward cognitive enhancement and legalized doping in sport in a community sample of Australian adults. *AJOB Prim. Res.* 3, 81–86. doi: 10.1080/21507716.2012.720639

Partridge, B., Underwood, M., Lucke, J., Bartlett, H., and Hall, W. (2009). Ethical concerns in the community about technologies to extend human life span. *Am. J. Bioeth.* 9, 68–76. doi: 10.1080/15265160903318368

President's Council on Bioethics. (2003). *Beyond Therapy. Biotechnology and the Pursuit of Happiness*. Available online at: https://bioethicsarchive.georgetown.edu/pcbe/reports/beyondtherapy/index.html (Accessed March 31, 2014).

Rawls, J. A. (1971). *A Theory of Justice*. Cambridge, MA: Harvard University Press.

Rawls, J. A. (1985). Justice as fairness: political not metaphysical. *Philos. Public Aff.* 14, 223–251.

Repantis, D., Schlattmann, P., Laisney, O., and Heuser, I. (2010). Modafinil and methylphenidate for neuroenhancement in healthy individuals: a systematic review. *Pharmacol. Res.* 62, 187–206. doi: 10.1016/j.phrs.2010.04.002

*Riis, J., Simmons, J. P., and Goodwin, G. P. (2008). Preferences for enhancement pharmaceuticals: the reluctance to enhance fundamental traits. *J. Cons. Res.* 35. doi: 10.1086/588746

*Sabini, J., and Monterosso, J. (2005). Judgments of the fairness of using performance enhancing drugs. *Ethics Behav.* 15, 81–94. doi: 10.1207/s15327019eb1501_6

*Santoni de Sio, F., Faulmüller, N., Savulescu, J., and Vincent, N. A. (in press). "Moving beyond responsibility-shifting, authenticity, and cheating, towards a nature-of-activities approach," in *Cognitive Enhancement: Ethical and Policy Implications in International Perspectives*, eds F. Jotterand, and V. Dubljevic (Oxford: Oxford University Press).

Sarewitz, D. (2010). World view: not by experts alone. *Nature* 466, 688. doi: 10.1038/466688a

*Sattler, S., Forlini, C., Racine, E., and Sauer, C. (2013a). Impact of contextual factors and substance characteristics on perspectives toward cognitive enhancement. *PLoS ONE* 8:e71452. doi: 10.1371/journal.pone.0071452

*Sattler, S., Mehlkop, G., Graeff, P., and Sauer, C. (2014). Evaluating the drivers of and obstacles to the willingness to use cognitive enhancement drugs: the influence of drug characteristics, social environment, and personal characteristics. *Subst. Abuse Treat. Prev. Policy* 9, 1–14. doi: 10.1186/1747-597X-9-8

*Sattler, S., Sauer, C., Mehlkop, G., and Graeff, P. (2013b). The rationale for consuming cognitive enhancement drugs in university students and teachers. *PLoS ONE* 8:e68821. doi: 10.1371/journal.pone.0068821

Sattler, W., and Wiegel, C. (2013). Cognitive test anxiety and cognitive enhancement: the influence of students' worries on their use of performance-enhancing drugs. *Subst. Use Misuse* 48, 220–232. doi: 10.3109/10826084.2012.751426

*Schaefer, G. O., Kahane, G., and Savulescu, J. (2013). Autonomy and enhancement. *Neuroethics*. doi: 10.1007/s12152-013-9189-5. [Epub ahead of print].

Schermer, M. (2008). Enhancements, easy shortcuts, and the richness of human activities. *Bioethics* 22, 355–363. doi: 10.1111/j.1467-8519.2008.00657.x

Schermer, M., Bolt, I., De Jongh, R., and Olivier, B. (2009). The future of psychopharmacological enhancements: expectations and policies. *Neuroethics* 2, 75–87. doi: 10.1007/s12152-009-9032-1

*Scheske, C., and Schnall, S. (2012). The ethics of 'smart drugs': moral judgments about healthy people's use of cognitive-enhancing drugs. *Basic Appl. Soc. Psych.* 34, 508–515. doi: 10.1080/01973533.2012.711692

Schicktanz, S., Schweda, M., and Wynne, B. (2012). The ethics of 'public understanding of ethics'–why and how bioethics expertise should include public and patients' voices. *Med. Health Care Philos.* 15, 129–139. doi: 10.1007/s11019-011-9321-4

*Schildmann, J., Beranek, R., and Roser, P. (2013). "Prevalence and attitudes to neurenhancement among students., results of a survey at the UAMR Universities" in *Conference Presentation* (Bochum: Ruhr University Bochum, Bochum).

Schoomaker, E. B. (2007). Military medical research on cognitive performance: the warfighter's competitive edge. *Aviat. Space Environ. Med.* 78, B4–B6.

*Schuijff, M., and Brom, F. W. A. (2013). "The dynamics of citizen deliberation regarding human enhancement in the Netherlands," in *Beyond Therapy v. Enhancement? Multidisciplinary Analysis of a Heated Debate,* ed F. Lucivero and A. Vedder (Pisa: Pisa University Press), 143–161.

Smith, M. E., and Farah, M. J. (2011). Are prescription stimulants "smart pills"? The epidemiology and cognitive neuroscience of prescription stimulant use by normal healthy individuals. *Psychol. Bull.* 137, 717–741. doi: 10.1037/a0023825

*Sweeney, S. (2010). The use of prescription drugs for academic performance enhancement in college aged students. *Social Work Theses* Paper 48.

Teter, C. J., McCabe, S. E., Cranford, J. A., Boyd, C. J., and Guthrie, S. K. (2005). Prevalence and motives for illicit use of prescription stimulants in an undergraduate student sample. *J Am. Coll. Health.* 53, 253–262. doi: 10.3200/Jach.53.6.253-262

Van Der Schaaf, M. E., Fallon, S. J., Ter Huurne, N., Buitelaar, J., and Cools, R. (2013). Working memory capacity predicts effects of methylphenidate on reversal learning. *Neuropsychopharmacology* 38, 2011–2018. doi: 10.1038/npp.2013.100

Warren, O. J., Leff, D. R., Athanasiou, T., Kennard, C., and Darzi, A. (2009). The neurocognitive enhancement of surgeons: an ethical perspective. *J. Surg. Res.* 152, 167–172. doi: 10.1016/j.jss.2007.12.761

16

Effect of biased feedback on motor imagery learning in BCI-teleoperation system

Maryam Alimardani[1,2]*, Shuichi Nishio[2] and Hiroshi Ishiguro[1,2]

[1] Department of System Innovation, Graduate school of Engineering science, Osaka University, Osaka, Japan
[2] Advanced Telecommunications Research Institute International, Kyoto, Japan

Edited by:
Mikhail Lebedev, Duke University, USA

Reviewed by:
Duk Shin, Tokyo Institute of Technology, Japan
W. Geoffrey Wright, Temple University, USA

***Correspondence:**
Maryam Alimardani, HIL, Advanced Telecommunications Research Institute International, 2-2 Hikaridai, Seika-cho, Soraku-gun, Kyoto 619-0288, Japan
e-mail: maryam@atr.jp

Feedback design is an important issue in motor imagery BCI systems. Regardless, to date it has not been reported how feedback presentation can optimize co-adaptation between a human brain and such systems. This paper assesses the effect of realistic visual feedback on users' BCI performance and motor imagery skills. We previously developed a tele-operation system for a pair of humanlike robotic hands and showed that BCI control of such hands along with first-person perspective visual feedback of movements can arouse a sense of embodiment in the operators. In the first stage of this study, we found that the intensity of this ownership illusion was associated with feedback presentation and subjects' performance during BCI motion control. In the second stage, we probed the effect of positive and negative feedback bias on subjects' BCI performance and motor imagery skills. Although the subject specific classifier, which was set up at the beginning of experiment, detected no significant change in the subjects' online performance, evaluation of brain activity patterns revealed that subjects' self-regulation of motor imagery features improved due to a positive bias of feedback and a possible occurrence of ownership illusion. Our findings suggest that in general training protocols for BCIs, manipulation of feedback can play an important role in the optimization of subjects' motor imagery skills.

Keywords: body ownership illusion, BCI-teleoperation, motor imagery learning, feedback effect, training

INTRODUCTION

Brain computer interfaces (BCIs) have widely become popular in many fields as a new communication and control channel between the human brain and an external device. However, the application of this technology is not as simple and intuitive as its concept suggests. To operate a BCI, subjects need to perform certain tasks and learn how to intentionally modulate certain characteristics of their brain activities in order to express their intentions. The motor imagery method, for instance, is one of the most commonly employed methods for BCI control of intended motions (Curran and Stokes, 2003). Subjects imagine the movement of a certain limb of their own body to induce changes in mu and beta rhythms over the corresponding sub-region of sensorimotor cortex. These changes are detected by BCI and translated into control commands. Motor imagery task requires relatively longer training compared to other BCI paradigms such as P300 or steady state visually evoked potential (SSVEP) since the mental rehearsal of a movement without actual execution is not a normal and daily practice for subjects and hence the task of motor imagery is an unfamiliar experience to most of them.

While the importance of subject's motor imagery skills in BCIs is well recognized, most studies have focused on the computer side and improving classification algorithms and very few have attended the human side and training paradigms that can facilitate the skill acquisition process for subjects (Lotte et al., 2013). As in any form of interface, users of BCIs learn to co-adapt with the system through the feedback they receive of their performance. Therefore feedback design is particularly influential in the process of motor imagery learning and performance improvement. Standard BCI protocols typically provide online visual feedback in the form of a moving cursor or target on the computer screen. Neuper et al. compared realistic presentation of feedback, in form of a grasping hand vs. abstract feedback in the form of an extending bar, on a computer screen (Neuper et al., 2009). However, they found no evidence of a significant difference between the performances of two feedback groups. In another study, the influence of motivation on BCI performance was also investigated by biasing the feedback accuracy (Barbero and Grosse-Wentrup, 2010). The results indicated that subjects with poor performance benefitted from positive biasing while those with better performance were impeded by inaccurate feedback. In a similar work (Gonzalez-Franco et al., 2011), authors provided subjects fake negative and positive feedback of their performance and reported that negative feedback had a greater learning effect on motor imagery BMIs.

Although in the above works, the effect of feedback presentation and accuracy has been probed, none of them has actually discussed the direct interaction between subject and BCI system. When performing a motor imagery task, subjects are asked to imagine their own body movements while the output is fed back in the form of movement for objects other than their own body. This mismatch and dissociation between subject's life experience and BCI task can in fact interfere with the imagination and impair the performance of motor imagery especially for novice users.

The goal of the present study is to explore the influence of feedback design on enhancement of user's performance and interaction with a BCI system. Previously we showed that BCI-operation of a pair of humanlike robotic hands by motor imagery while watching first-person perspective images of robot's movement could induce an illusion of body ownership transfer (BOT) for the operators (Alimardani et al., 2013). In post-experiment interviews, some subjects stated that when the robot moved as they intended, it felt like their own hand was moving and motor imagery became easier. We hypothesize that inducement of such feeling of ownership and the sense of agency driven toward the seen motions may have a positive loop effect on execution of motor imagery during BCI-operation. In other words, we speculate that once the thought of "I am the one moving the hands" raises the feeling of "These hands are mine," the illusion of owning hands enhances the imagery ability in subjects and boosts the inverse thought of "These are my hands so I can move them."

To that end, in this study we used the same BCI-teleoperation paradigm while exposing naïve subjects to different feedback conditions in order to probe the relationship between subject's experience of BOT and BCI-performance. Two experiments are presented. In the first experiment, by manipulating the presentation of misperformance, we surveyed how subjects' perception of their own performance could affect the intensity of BOT. In the second experiment, we then examined how this effect can be influential on subjects' real performance and trend of motor imagery learning.

Both experiments in this study were approved by the Ethics Committee of Advanced Telecommunications Research Institute International (12-506-3). All subjects read and signed a written consent form prior to experiment and received payment for their participation.

EXPERIMENT 1

This experiment was designed to investigate the inducement of body ownership illusion for a pair of BCI-operated human-like robotic hands under different presentations of feedback.

PARTICIPANTS

Forty healthy participants (26 male, 14 female, age $M = 21.13$, $SD = 1.92$) were selected for the experiment. Thirty eight participants were right-handed and 2 left-handed. All participants were naive to the research topic and received explanation prior to the experiment.

METHOD

Participants sat in a comfortable chair and were asked to remain motionless. They wore an EEG electrode cap and 27 EEG electrodes were placed over their primary sensori-motor cortex according to the international 10–20 system (FT7, FC5, FC3, FC1, FCz, FC2, FC4, FC6, FT8, T7, C5, C3, C1, Cz, C2, C4, C6, T8, TP7, CP5, CP3, CP1, CPz, CP2, CP4, CP6, TP8). A reference electrode was mounted on the right ear and a ground electrode on the forehead. Participants were asked to imagine a grasp or squeeze motion for their own hand while their cerebral activities were recorded by g.USBamp biosignal amplifiers (Guger Technologies). In an initial training session, they practiced a motor imagery task by extending a feedback bar to left or right side on a 15-inch laptop computer screen. A visual cue in the form of a horizontal pointing arrow specified the timing and the hand they were supposed to hold image for. Each trial lasted 7.5 s and started with the presentation of a fixation cross on the display. After 2 s an acoustic warning was given in the form of a "beep." From second 3 to 4.25, an arrow pointing to the left or right side randomly was shown. Depending on the arrow's direction participants were instructed to perform motor imagery. They watched the feedback bar and continued the imagery task until the fixation cross was erased. After a short pause, which took 1 second, the next trial started. The first run consisting of 40 trials (20 trials per class left/right presented in a randomized order) was conducted without feedback and lasted 5 min. The recorded brain activities in the initial non-feedback run were used to set up a subject specific classifier for the classification in the following feedback runs. In the feedback runs, participants performed similar trials but received online classification results of their performance in form of a horizontal feedback bar on the screen. Subjects' task was to extend the feedback bar in the correct direction.

The classification of recorded signals was conducted under Simulink/MATLAB (Mathworks) for offline and online parameter extraction. This process included bandpass filtering between 0.5 and 30 Hz, sampling at 128 Hz, cutting off artifacts by notch filter at 60 Hz, and adopting the Common Spatial Pattern (CSP) algorithm for discrimination of Event Related Desynchronization (ERD) and Event Related Synchronization (ERS) patterns associated with the motor imagery task (Guger et al., 2000). The classifier was trained using CSP analysis of calibration measurements. CSP found weight vectors that weighed each electrode based on its importance for the discrimination task. The spatial filters were designed such that the resulting signal had maximum variance for left trials and minimum variance for right trials. Therefore, the difference between left and right populations was maximized to show where the EEG variance fluctuated the most. Finally, when the discrimination between left and right imaginations was made, the classifier outputted a linear array signal in the range of $[-1,1]$, where -1 denotes the extreme left and 1 denotes the extreme right. Negative values were then translated as the robot's left hand grasp motions and positive values as the robot's right hand grasp motions. A threshold of ± 0.1 was considered in the system, in order to avoid multiple movements of both hands for subjects with unstable classification results.

Following training sessions the main test sessions commenced, in which subjects wore a head mounted display (Vuzix iWear VR920) and tele-operated the robot's hands using the same BCI system. They performed a motor imagery task for their right or left hand while they watched first-person images of the robot's hands performing the motions respectively (**Figure 1A**). Two LED-embedded balls were installed in the robot's grasp and provided motor imagery cues by randomly lighting. During the experiment subjects were told to look down as if they were watching their own hands and the same blankets were laid on both the robot's and participants' legs to give a similar view. Participants placed their arms in a similar position and orientation as the robot's arms. In order to measure subjects' physiological reactions to a threatening stimulus, skin conductance response (SCR)

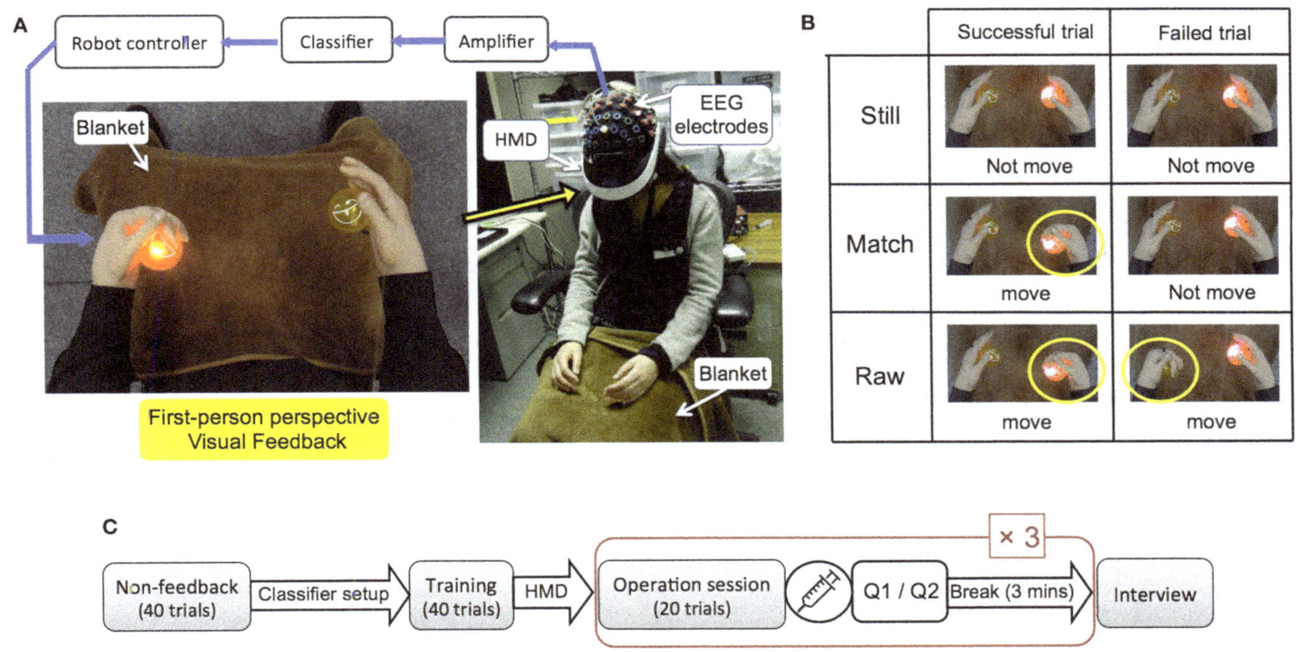

FIGURE 1 | Experiment setup. (A) EEG electrodes installed on a subject's sensorimotor cortex recorded brain activities during a motor imagery task. Subjects watched first-person images from a robot's perspective through a head mounted display. A lighting ball in front of each of the robot's hands gave motor imagery cues and subjects imagined grasping their corresponding hands. The classifier detected two classes of results (right or left) and motion command was sent to the robot's hand. **(B)** Subjects repeated the experiment under three different conditions: Still, where the robot's hand didn't move at all. Match in which the robot's hand only moved in successful trials, and Raw where the robot's hand also performed failed trials using the wrong hand. **(C)** Experimental procedure consisted of a non-feedback session for classifier setup, training sessions and three operational sessions.

electrodes were installed on their left palms. A bio-amplifier recording device (Polymate II AP216, TEAC, Japan) with sampling rate of 1000 Hz was used to record SCR measurements. Prior to the testing sessions, participants watched an act of injection via a syringe to the robot's hand (painful stimulus) through the head mounted display, which was explained to them as a necessary procedure for preparing the robot. The injection was continued until subjects' SCR responses disappeared (Armel and Ramachandran, 2003). Afterwards, testing sessions were carried out in a random order under three conditions (**Figure 1B**):

(1) Still (no feedback): The robot's hands did not move at all throughout the whole session although a subject performed motor imagery according to cues.
(2) Match (no negative feedback): The robot's hands moved only in those trials that the classification result was correct and in accordance with cue.
(3) Raw: The robot's hands moved according to the classification results in all trials. In case of wrong result that was not in accordance with cue, the robot's opposite hand moved.

Still was designed as control condition where visual images of hands without motion feedback were expected to raise no body ownership illusion. The last session is called Raw since we inputted the unprocessed values obtained from the classifier as the robot's motion parameter. In all conditions above, participants performed trials that were designed to be identical to the trials in training sessions regarding duration and stimulus timing. Each session was followed by a break of 3 min. Test sessions comprised 20 trials, lasting 2 min and 40 s each (**Figure 1C**). Following the last trial, an injection was applied to the robot's left hand to examine if the illusion of ownership could cause a response to a pain-causing stimulus (Nishio et al., 2012). Immediately after injecting the session was terminated and participants were orally asked the following questions: (Q1) When the robot's hand was injected, did it feel as if your own hand was receiving the injection? (Q2) Throughout the entire session while you were operating the robot's hands, did it feel as if they were your own hands? Participants scored Q1 and Q2 based on the seven-point Likert Scale, 1 meaning, "Didn't feel such thing at all" and 7 meaning, "Felt it very strongly." In addition to the self-assessment, we physiologically measured the body ownership illusion by recording the SCRs.

RESULT

The response variables for 40 participants were obtained from questionnaires and SCR recordings. Participants' responses in three conditions of Still, Match and Raw were averaged and compared. The mean value, standard deviation, and *p*-value are depicted on each graph (**Figure 2**).

For both Q1 and Q2, the Match condition showed a higher average value compared to the other two conditions (**Figures 2A,B**). Non-parametric statistical analysis was used

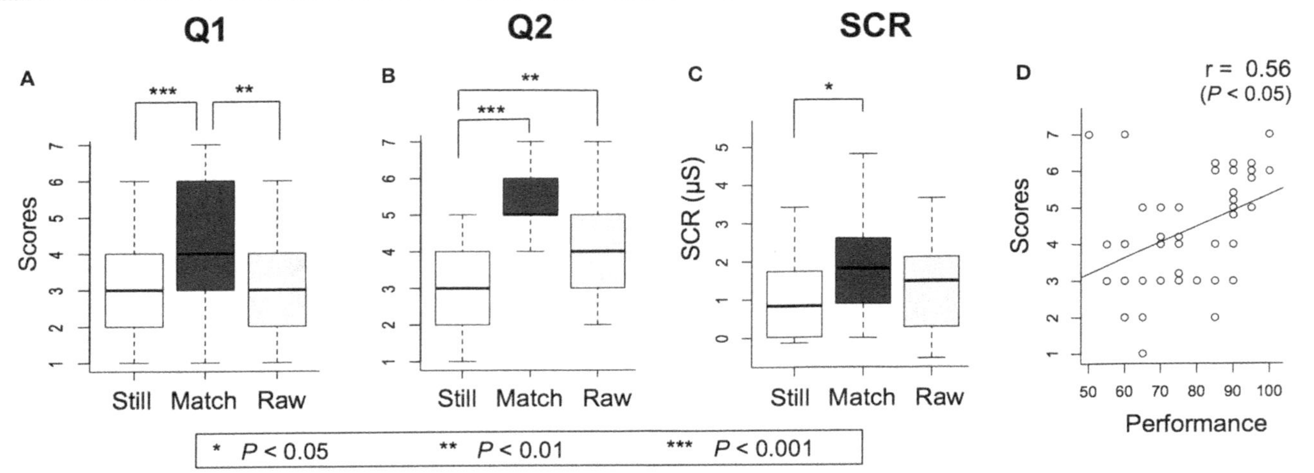

FIGURE 2 | Results for experiment 1 **(A)** Mean values and standard deviations for Q1 in each session, with Match significantly higher than Still and Raw **(B)** Mean values and standard deviations for Q2 in each session, with Match and Raw significantly higher than Still **(C)** Mean values and standard deviations of SCR values for 35 subjects, with Match associated with significantly higher responses to injection than Still **(D)** Subjects' performances vs. their scores of illusion in the Match condition. For those with the same performance and score, the score has been slightly modified to a non-integer neighbor value to avoid the overlap of the markers. A significantly positive correlation was found between BCI-performance and intensity of illusion.

to compare as Shapiro-Wilks test rejected the normal distribution for the Likert scores. Kruskal-Wallis tests showed a significant effect of BCI tele-operation on the level of BOT between the three Still, Match and Raw conditions for Q1 scores [$\chi^2_{(2)} = 19.11$, $p < 0.0001$] and for Q2 scores [$\chi^2_{(2)} = 34.52$, $p < 10^{-6}$]. *Post-hoc* Mann-Whitney *U*-tests for comparison with Bonferroni adjustment indicated that in Q1 Match ($M = 4.38$, $SD = 1.51$) raised BOT significantly higher than Still ($M = 2.83$, $SD = 1.43$); [Match > Still, $p < 0.0001$] and than Raw ($M = 3.15$, $SD = 1.57$); [Match > Raw, $p < 0.01$]. Similarly, Mann-Whitney *U*-tests with Bonferroni adjustment for Q2 scores showed significant difference between Match ($M = 5.15$, $SD = 1.10$) and Still ($M = 2.93$, $SD = 1.25$); [Match > Still, $p < 10^{-6}$] and also between Raw ($M = 4.18$, $SD = 1.38$) and Still; [Raw > Still, $p < 0.01$].

The SCR peak value within a 6-s interval (1 s after the appearance of syringe in the participant's view to 5 s after the injection) was selected as the reaction value (Alimardani et al., 2013). In this experiment, we only evaluated the response values of 35 participants, since five participants showed unchanged responses during the experiment and were excluded from analysis. Results showed a higher mean value for the Match condition compared to the other two conditions (**Figure 2C**). Due to non-normal distribution of SCR values revealed by Shapiro-Wilks test, we performed Kruskal-Wallis tests on participants' reaction values and the analysis was significant, [$\chi^2_{(2)} = 8.39$, $p < 0.01$]. *Post-hoc* comparisons by Mann-Whitney *U*-tests with Bonferroni adjustment confirmed significant differences only between Match ($M = 1.68$, $SD = 1.98$) and Still ($M = 0.90$, $SD = 1.42$); [Match > Still, $p < 0.05$]. Moreover, a significantly positive correlation was found between subjects' performances and the Q1 scores only in the Match condition (Pearson correlation coefficient $r = 0.56$, $p < 0.05$, **Figure 2D**). The term performance here refers to the rate of trials subjects could successfully grasp the lightened ball out of the total 20 trials in each run scaled in percentage.

DISCUSSION

In study 1, we investigated the inducement of body ownership illusion for a pair of BCI-operated human-like robotic hands under different feedback conditions. Results from both measurement methods (Q1 and SCR) indicated significantly high responses to the injection in the Match condition, where robot's hands moved only if the classification result was correct and same as the cue. This shows that the feeling of receiving an injection was significantly stronger when the robot's hands moved exclusively in agreement with the operator's intentions than when the robot made no motion (Still) or performed a wrong motion in the case of errors (Raw). Since this is a feeling aroused due to the illusion of ownership over robot's body, we can state that the transfer of body ownership could be evoked more reliably by precise mind-control of a robot's hands.

On the other hand, in Q2 participants directly scored their sensation of ownership for robot's body during the entire operation time. Based on participants' assessments, the feeling of ownership was significantly stronger in both the Match and Raw conditions, when the robot dynamically moved and reacted to the participant's intentions, compared to the control condition, Still, when the robot did not show any motion at all. Although Match showed a higher average response compared to Raw, no significant difference between these two conditions was confirmed in Q2. This can imply that in both the Raw and Match conditions the robot's successive motions following the participant's act of motor imagery raised a sense of agency during the session that led to a perception of owning the hands in participants.

Meanwhile, the results of this experiment showed a wide dispersion over the response values of illusion in each condition, which we presumed is due to the difference of performance level among subjects. A positive correlation was confirmed between participants' performances and their indicated scores for Q1 (**Figure 2D**), which indicates that participants with a better operational performance experienced a stronger illusion of BOT. Therefore, we can tell that subjects' skill in a motor imagery task and BCI performance are associated with the intensity of ownership illusion in such a tele-operational system.

From the obtained results in this experiment, we conclude that in a BCI-teleoperation system for humanlike hands, the feedback presentation could affect the eliciting of ownership illusion over the controlled hands; the illusion was augmented when negative feedback of subject's misperformance was eliminated. Also, a positive correlation was found between the intensity of BOT and subjects' performance, which suggests that subjects with better BCI-performance experienced a stronger illusion. Therefore BOT could be affected both by subjects' BCI-performance, and feedback design, which regulated subjects' perceptions of their own performance. On the other hand, although an intuitive conclusion of this experiment could be that better BCI-performance caused a stronger perception of illusion in subjects, the reverse thought could also be claimed; that is, higher BOT motivated subjects to perform better on the motor imagery task. Therefore, it remains to be clarified how the mutual interaction between performance and BOT is formed and how feedback design contributes to improvement of each element and their interaction (**Figure 3**). Thus, in experiment 2 we focused on the effect of feedback design on a subject's BCI-performance and examined how manipulation of subjects' perceptions of self-performance can affect the trend of their motor imagery learning and BCI-performance.

EXPERIMENT 2

From experiment 1 we found that subjects' perceptions of their own performance was important for the inducement of ownership illusion. Moreover, a close relationship between the intensity of illusion and a subject's performance was found. We were further interested in knowing how the subjects' self-evaluations and subsequent inducement of BOT can directly affect their skills in a motor imagery operational system. Therefore in this experiment, by manipulating the presentation and accuracy of subjects' performances we designed four different feedback conditions including two in which each subjects' performance was positively and negatively biased in the first half of each session. We then examined how conditioning feedback can affect the trend of learning

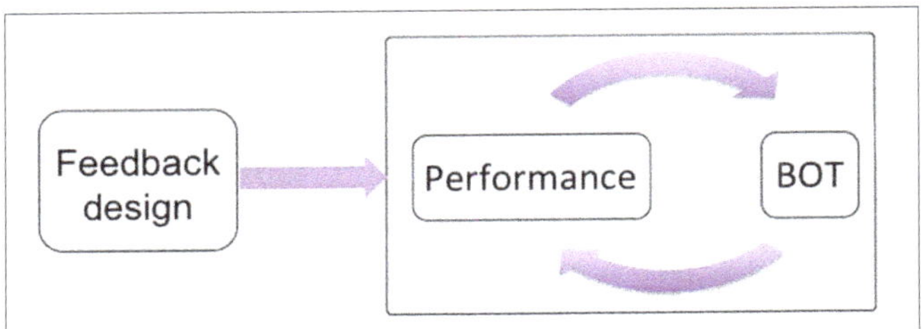

FIGURE 3 | Model diagram for effect of feedback design. Feedback bias can affect the interaction between BCI-performance and BOT illusion.

by two methods; (1) measuring subjects' online performance in the second half of sessions and (2) comparing time-variant distribution of EEG features regarding right and left hand imagery in each half of the session.

PARTICIPANTS

Sixteen healthy subjects (6 male and 10 female, age $M = 21.1$, $SD = 1.4$) participated in this experiment. 15 participants were right-handed and one left-handed. None of them had participated in our previous experiments and they were all unfamiliar with the research topic. Participants received explanation prior to the experiment.

METHOD

The BCI devices, preparation procedure and session paradigms of Experiment 2 were identical with Experiment 1, except in this experiment we used a new type of head mounted display (Sony HMZ-T1) for the real time first-person visual feedback (**Figure 1A**).

Participants performed 4 experimental sessions each consisting of 40 imagery trials which lasted 5 min. Each session was followed by a break of 3 min. The first half of each session (20 trials) was randomly conditioned as below:

(1) Raw: Participants' performance was not biased. The robot's hands grasped the ball according to the classification result.
(2) Match: Participants' performance was not biased. However, the robot's hands only grasped the lit ball when the classification results matched the cue.
(3) Positive Feedback (Fake-P): Participants' performance was biased positively. The robot's hands grasped the lit ball correctly in 90% of trials regardless of the subject's real performance.
(4) Negative Feedback (Fake-N): Participants' performance was biased negatively. The robot's hands grasped the lit ball correctly only in 20% of trials regardless of the subject's real performance.

In the first two conditions, Raw and Match (**Figure 1B**), a subject's performance was not biased although the robot's hand motion in mistaken trials differed—one with execution of wrong hand motion and one without robot motion. Raw is an equivalent feedback design of the one used in general motor imagery BCIs where subject's failure in executing motor imagery for one class results in feedbacks of the other class. However, since Raw and Match conditions previously revealed a different level of illusion (Experiment 1) we made the assumption that presentation of negative feedback affects subject's perception of self-performance and therefore influences subject's interaction with the system. To clarify this point, we respectively designed two more sessions (Fake-P and Fake-N) in which we deliberately biased feedback of performance regardless of subjects' real performance accuracy in order to extremely enhance or decrease their self-evaluation. In the second half of all sessions subjects received feedback of their real performance as they did in Raw. The goal was to seek changes in BCI-performance and motor imagery skills in the second half of each session due to the positive or negative bias of feedback. Subjects' performance in the second half of all sessions was registered.

In addition to subjects' online performance, we conducted an offline re-analysis of data to extract the feature distribution of right and left motor imagery in each session. We speculated that by receiving biased feedback or experiencing illusion, subjects may consciously or unconsciously modify the generation of their brain activity patterns throughout the experiment, although the classifier could fail to detect these changes because it did not use a learning algorithm and once the classification boundary for the two classes, Right and Left, was defined within the feature space in the initial training session, the same classifier and parameters were used to the end of the experiment. Therefore, we used the original brain signals and ran the following offline processing to seek changes in motor imagery patterns.

After artifact removal and temporal filtering (Guger et al., 2000), the features used for classification were obtained by the method of CSP. Having N channels of EEG for each left and right trial $\boldsymbol{X}$, the CSP builds an $N \times N$ projection matrix $\boldsymbol{W}$. With the projection matrix $\boldsymbol{W}$, the mapping of a trial is given as

$$Z = WX$$

The columns of $\boldsymbol{W}^{-1}$ are the CSPs and can be seen as time-invariant EEG source distribution vectors. By design the variance for imagining left hand motion is largest in the first row of $\boldsymbol{Z}$ and decreases with the increasing number of subsequent rows. To obtain reliable features, it is not necessary to calculate the variances of all N time series. The optimal number of CSPs used to build the feature vector is four (Müller-Gerking et al., 1999). Therefore, only the first and last two rows ($p = 4$) of $\boldsymbol{W}$ were used to filter data $\boldsymbol{X}$ and build a new signal $\boldsymbol{Z_p}$ ($p = 1\ldots 4$). The variance of the resulting four time series is obtained for a time window $T = (t_0, t_1)$

$$var_p = \sum_{t=t_0}^{t_1} \left(Z_{p(t)}\right)^2$$

where window length was set to be 1 s, starting 1500 ms after the presentation of the cue (Pfurtscheller and Neuper, 2001). Feature vectors were obtained after normalizing and log-transforming as following:

$$f_p = log\left(\frac{var\left(Z_p\right)}{\sum_{i=1}^{P} var\left(Z_p\right)}\right)$$

The online classifier uses each trial's feature vector $\boldsymbol{f_p}$ to categorize it into two classes of right and left. In order to estimate the goodness of this classification, we used Fisher's discriminant criterion measures in a linear discriminant analysis to observe the distribution of two classes feature vectors in a 4-dimential space. Fisher's parameter $\boldsymbol{J}$ is defined as

$$J = \frac{\left|\widetilde{\mu}_R - \widetilde{\mu}_L\right|^2}{\widetilde{s}_R^2 + \widetilde{s}_L^2}$$

where $\widetilde{\mu}_R$ and $\widetilde{\mu}_L$ are the means of feature vectors for two right and left classes and the quantity $|\widetilde{\mu}_R - \widetilde{\mu}_L|^2$ is the distance between the two classes' means. For each class $\widetilde{s}_R^2$ and $\widetilde{s}_L^2$ were defined as the scatter, an equivalent of the variance, and obtained by

$$\widetilde{s}_i^2 = \sum_{x \in f_i} \left(x - \widetilde{\mu}_i\right)^2$$

The quantity $\widetilde{s}_R^2 + \widetilde{s}_L^2$ indicates the within-class scatter. When performing motor imagery a larger $\boldsymbol{J}$ corresponds to closer dispersion of feature vectors per each class and further distance between two class means, which represents better feature distribution for classification, and therefore better execution of motor imagery task.

In each session, the $\boldsymbol{J}$ parameter for the first 20 conditioned trials (J_1) and for the second 20 test trials (J_2) was calculated. Since subjects' initial skills were diverse, and for every subject the order of sessions was considerable in the amount of motor imagery skills, the ratio $\Delta J = J_2/J_1$ was selected as a measurement of subjects' motor imagery learning in that session.

RESULT

Online performance

Performances of 16 subjects in the second half of each session were averaged and demonstrated in **Figure 4A**. The term performance refers to the percentage of successful trials among the post 20 trials. Fake-P ($M = 60.78$, $SD = 10.24$) showed the highest performance compared to Raw ($M = 49.22$, $SD = 9.07$), Match ($M = 54.37$, $SD = 10.89$) and Fake-P ($M = 50.47$, $SD = 10.58$). However, One-Way ANOVA test did not reject the null hypothesis, $[F_{(3,\ 60)} = 2.51, p = 0.07]$.

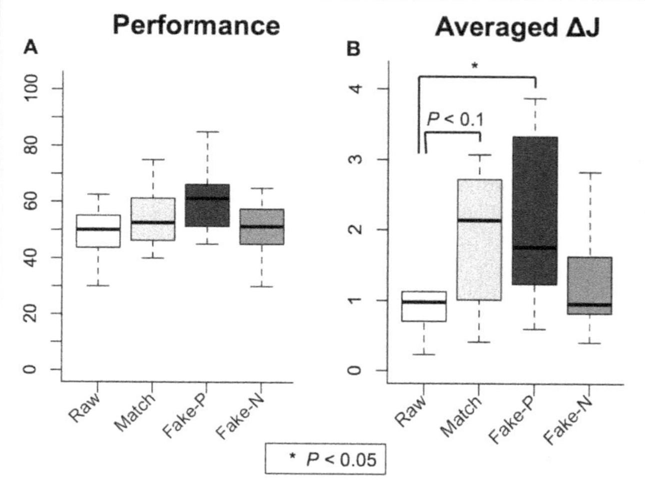

FIGURE 4 | Results for experiment 2 (A) Mean value of subjects' performances in the second half of each session is demonstrated. No significant difference was found. **(B)** Mean value of the ratio $\boldsymbol{J_2/J_1}$, an identifier of motor imagery quality, showed significantly higher values in the Fake-P and Match conditions compared to Raw.

Offline classification

We calculated ΔJ for 16 subjects. Using interquartile range (IQR) for statistical dispersion in each condition (Moore and McCabe, 1998), two outliers were detected in the Fake-N condition (S2 and S4) and one outlier was detected in the Raw condition (S15). The data of these three subjects were discarded from further analysis. The mean value of ΔJ for the remaining 13 subjects was highest in the Fake-P condition ($M = 2.12$, $SD = 1.78$) compared to the other three conditions, Raw ($M = 1.07$, $SD = 0.75$), Match ($M = 1.87$, $SD = 0.95$) and Fake-N ($M = 1.35$, $SD = 0.84$) (**Figure 4B**). A One-Way ANOVA test yielded a significant effect of feedback design for the four conditions, [$F_{(3, 48)} = 3.53$, $p < 0.05$]. Using Tukey *post-hoc* comparisons, a significance difference was obtained between Fake-P and Raw; [Fake-P > Raw, $p < 0.05$] and between Match and Raw; [Fake-P > Raw, $p = 0.08$].

DISCUSSION

In experiment 2, we biased the visual feedback of performance in a BCI-teleoperation system of a human-like robot in order to probe the effect of positive and negative feedback on subjects' BCI-performance and motor imagery skills.

Online results demonstrated no significant changes in the subjects' real time performances and the mean value of subjects' performances remained in the chance level for all conditions. On the other hand, results from offline classification revealed that the ratio J_2/J_1, an identifier of class separation between the two halves of sessions, was significantly higher in the Fake-P than in the Raw condition. This indicates that subjects could generate motor patterns that are more classifiable by CSP algorithm by receiving positive feedback of their performance in the Fake-P condition. Using a statistical significance level of 10%, a similar relation was confirmed between Match and Raw conditions, indicating that in the Match condition where subjects did not receive negative feedback of their failed performance, motor imagery improved and they could produce more separable activity patterns for two classes of right and left hand movement. Both results imply that positive bias of feedback had an enhancing effect on motor imagery learning which is consistent with some previous reports (Lotte et al., 2013). One probable cause could be the inducement of a stronger BOT due to biased feedback, which facilitated imagination of movement in motor imagery task and eventually enhanced self-regulation of brain patterns in subjects (**Figure 3**).

Unlike previous reports on biased BCI feedback, no significant improvement (Gonzalez-Franco et al., 2011) or impediment (Barbero and Grosse-Wentrup, 2010) was found in the Fake-N condition compared to other conditions. However, S2 and S4 who were discarded from analysis as outliers showed drastic ΔJ increase in Fake-N. Since subjects majorly received enhanced learning in Fake-P condition, we assume that the effect of biasing is closely relevant to the subject's personality and the influence of motivation on different individuals. While there are learners who benefit from encouragement and positive feedback of their performance, there are a few who benefit more from negative feedback and try harder when the feedback informs them that they are not performing well. In future experiments, a personality test could be used in order to categorize subjects into groups, so that results can be analyzed according to stratified personality groups.

Lastly, although in this experiment we hypothetically assume that enhancement of motor imagery learning due to positive bias of feedback was associated with ownership illusion over the controlled robot's hands (**Figure 3**), further study is required to veritably measure the intensity of illusion at the end of each conditioned section. In this experiment we suspected that pausing the sessions and asking assessment questions could shatter the illusion. In the future, comparison between human-like and non-human-like visual feedback under biased feedback is necessary to precisely verify whether illusion of body ownership influences the trend of motor imagery learning.

CONCLUSION

In this study, we designed two experiments to answer the following questions: (1) How can presentation of visual feedback affect the inducement of body ownership illusion in the BCI-operators of human-like hands, and (2) How can positively and negatively biased feedback in such a system influence operators' interaction with the system and improve their BCI performances. Results of the first experiment revealed that negative feedback of subjects' errors impeded the intensity of ownership illusion. Also BOT was correlated with subjects' performance in BCI and how well subjects felt they were in control of the hands. In the second experiment, we realized that biasing feedback could not immediately boost subjects' performance in the same session. However, the analysis of brain patterns showed that in fact it could change the trend of motor imagery learning.

In terms of feedback design for future BCI systems, it is conceivable that a more realistic feedback presentation can assist novice users to train and adapt to a system faster and more efficiently. Also, BCI users may benefit from positive bias of feedback in training sessions, although their personality should be taken into account. Meanwhile, since subjects motor imagery skills dynamically change during a session based on their state of mind, further development of sophisticated classifiers that customize classification parameters in an online session are required.

ACKNOWLEDGMENTS

This work was partially supported by JSPS KAKENHI Grant Number 25220004 and 24650114.

REFERENCES

Alimardani, M., Nishio, S., and Ishiguro, H. (2013). Humanlike robot hands controlled by brain activity arouse illusion of ownership in operators. *Sci. Rep.* 3:2396. doi: 10.1038/srep02396

Armel, K. C., and Ramachandran, V. S. (2003). Projecting sensations to external objects: evidence from skin conductance response. *Proc. Biol. Sci.* 270, 1499–1506. doi: 10.1098/rspb.2003.2364

Barbero, Á., and Grosse-Wentrup, M. (2010). Biased feedback in brain-computer interfaces. *J. Neuroeng. Rehabil.* 7, 1–4. doi: 10.1186/1743-0003-7-34

Curran, E. A., and Stokes, M. J. (2003). Learning to control brain activity: a review of the production and control of EEG components for driving brain–computer interface (BCI) systems. *Brain Cogn.* 51, 326–336. doi: 10.1016/S0278-2626(03)00036-8

Gonzalez-Franco, M., Peng, Y., Dan, Z., Bo, H., and Shangkai, G. (2011). "Motor imagery based brain-computer interface: a study of the effect of positive and negative feedback," in *Engineering in Medicine and Biology Society (EMBC), Annual International Conference of the IEEE* (Boston, MA), 6323–6326.

Guger, C., Ramoser, H., and Pfurtscheller, G. (2000). Real-time EEG analysis with subject-specific spatial patterns for a brain-computer interface (BCI). *IEEE Trans. Rehabil. Eng.* 8, 447–456. doi: 10.1109/86.895947

Lotte, F., Larrue, F., and Muhl. C. (2013). Flaws in current human training protocols for spontaneous brain-computer interfaces: lessons learned from instructional design. *Front. Hum. Neurosci.* 7:568. doi: 10.3389/fnhum.2013.00568

Moore, D. S., and McCabe, G. P. (1998). *Introduction to the Practice of Statistics, 3rd Edn*. New York, NY: W. H. Freeman.

Müller-Gerking, J., Pfurtscheller, G., and Flyvbjerg, H. (1999). Designing optimal spatial filters for single-trial EEG classification in a movement task. *Clin. Neurophysiol.* 110, 787–798. doi: 10.1016/S1388-2457(98)00038-8

Neuper, C., Scherer, R., Wriessnegger, S., and Pfurtscheller, G. (2009). Motor imagery and action observation: modulation of sensorimotor brain rhythms during mental control of a brain–computer interface. *Clin. Neurophysiol.* 120, 239–247. doi: 10.1016/j.clinph.2008.11.015

Nishio, S., Watanabe, T., Ogawa, K., and Ishiguro, H. (2012). "Body ownership transfer to teleoperated android robot," in *International Conference on Social Robotics* (*ICSR* 2012) (Chengdu), 398–407.

Pfurtscheller, G., and Neuper, C. (2001). Motor imagery and direct brain-computer communication. *Proc. IEEE* 89, 1123–1134. doi: 10.1109/5.939829

17

Screening and personalizing nootropic drugs and cognitive modulator regimens *in silico*

Leslie C. Jellen[1], Alexander Aliper[2], Anton Buzdin[3]* and Alex Zhavoronkov[2,4]*

[1] *Department of Genetics, Genomics, and Informatics, University of Tennessee Health Science Center, Memphis, TN, USA*
[2] *Aging Research, Insilico Medicine, Emerging Technology Center, Johns Hopkins University Eastern, Baltimore, MD, USA*
[3] *Personalized Medicine, Pathway Pharmaceuticals Ltd, Wan Chai, Hong Kong*
[4] *Research, Biogerontology Research Foundation, Truro, UK*

Edited by:
Ioan Opris, Wake Forest University, USA

Reviewed by:
Mikhail Lebedev, Duke University, USA
Christopher R. Madan, Boston College, USA
Stuart Richard Gilbert Calimport, Aston University, UK

***Correspondence:**
Anton Buzdin, Personalized Medicine, Pathway Pharmaceuticals Ltd, 2702-3, 56 Gloucester Road, Wan Chai, Hong Kong
e-mail: buzdin@pathway pharmaceuticals.com;
Alex Zhavoronkov, Aging Research, Insilico Medicine, Emerging Technology Center, Johns Hopkins University Eastern, B301, 1101 East 33rd Street, Baltimore, MD, USA
e-mail: alex@biogerontology.org

The go-to cognitive enhancers of today are those that are widely available rather than optimal for the user, including drugs typically prescribed for treatment of ADHD (e.g., methylphenidate) and sleep disturbances such as narcolepsy (modafinil). While highly effective in their intended therapeutic role, performance gains in healthy populations are modest at best and profoundly inconsistent across subgroups and individuals. We propose a method for *in silico* screening of possible novel cognitive enhancers followed by high-throughput *in vivo* and *in vitro* validation. The proposed method uses gene expression data to evaluate the the collection of activated or suppressed signaling pathways in tissues or neurons of the cognitively enhanced brain. An algorithm maps expression data onto signaling pathways and quantifies their individual activation strength. The collective pathways and their activation form what we term the signaling pathway cloud, a biological fingerprint of cognitive enhancement (or any other condition of interest). Drugs can then be screened and ranked based on their ability to minimize, mimic, or exaggerate pathway activation or suppression within that cloud. Using this approach, one may predict the efficacy of many drugs that may enhance various aspects of cognition before costly preclinical studies and clinical trials are undertaken.

Keywords: nootropic, cognitive enhancement, personalized medicine, drug repositioning, oncofinder, *in silico* medicine, signalome, signalome profiling

INTRODUCTION

The concept of cognitive enhancement is age-old, but despite modern advances in our understanding of the cellular and molecular bases of cognition, much remains unknown. Development of new cognitive enhancers with increased specificity, safety, and effectiveness must outpace increasing demand, particularly as off-label and illicit use of current drugs has become common in certain population subgroups (Maher, 2008) and as the aging segment of the population expands with accompanying increases in rates of cognitive decline and neurodegenerative disease (Wallace et al., 2011).

Cognition is complex and involves multiple domains, from learning and memory to attention, and cognitive enhancers can target one or more. At present, two of the most widely cited cognitive enhancers are the dopaminergic stimulants methylphenidate, prescribed for treatment of ADHD, and modafinil, prescribed for treatment of sleep disorders, such as narcolepsy. While both of these drugs can enhance memory and attention in healthy individuals (Elliott et al., 1997), their application as nootropics is secondary to their original, therapeutic purpose, and effects are disagreed upon and modest at best (Repantis et al., 2010).

A number of other potential nootropics have been developed for the treatment of cognitive deficits in aging and neurodegenerative or neuropsychiatric disease, from the FDA approved acetylcholinesterase inhibitors (e.g., donepezil) to those still under investigation: ampakines, nicotinic receptor agonists, glutamate receptor agonists, glycine inhibitors, and PDE inhibitors (for review, Wallace et al., 2011; Pieramico et al., 2014). Drugs that may play a more modulatory role target histamine, serotonin, glucocorticoid, and neuropeptide receptors and epigenetic mechanisms (Roesler and Schröder, 2011; Wallace et al., 2011). Many other drugs positioned as nootropic agents like piracetam and piracetam-like compounds are well-tolerated, but their effects and mechanisms of action are poorly understood and widely debated (Gouliaev and Senning, 1994; Gualtieri et al., 2002). While some nootropics have made it to clinical trial, others still await or have been withdrawn, and each has various drawbacks or only modest effects that are disease specific.

Development of novel nootropics is hampered by research, validation and regulatory challenges. The very definition of cognitive enhancement is difficult to pin down (Lynch et al., 2014). The road from lab to FDA approval is difficult, long, and costly. Pharmacological enhancement of healthy populations is fraught with ethical and philosophical pushback (Maslen et al., 2014). Enhancement in aging and neurodegenerative disease is less controversial, but perhaps more complex

(Pieramico et al., 2014). Moreover, therapeutic effects often contradict those in healthy populations (Kimberg et al., 1997; Belmonte and Yurgelun-Todd, 2003; Beglinger et al., 2005; Gibbs and D'Esposito, 2005, 2006; Randall et al., 2005; Frank and O'Reilly, 2006; Finke et al., 2010; Esposito et al., 2013). The U-shaped curve effect, wherein treatment effects benefit low-baseline performers but impair high-performers, is a problem with at least the dopaminergic drugs (Gibbs and D'Esposito, 2006; Finke et al., 2010; Esposito et al., 2013). Even drugs FDA-approved for therapeutic use have issues with side effects, trade-offs (one process is enhanced while another is impaired), loss of authenticity (one's true "self"), and large individual differences (Maslen et al., 2014). Long term effects are typically unknown. Finally, and most importantly, there is still much to be learned about the cellular and molecular basis for the various aspects of cognition.

For the field of neuroenhancement to advance, the benefit-to-risk ratio of pharmacological treatment must improve. This will require (a) a better understanding of the neurobiological basis of cognition; and (b) drugs with higher specificity, greater effectiveness, and fewer side effects. To this end we propose an expedited path to understanding the molecular basis of cognition and to subsequent drug discovery via a combination of advanced gene expression analysis, signaling pathway analysis, and *in silico* screening of potential nootropics. In our approach, current drugs will simply be the launching pad on the quest to find new, better performing nootropics.

SIGNALING PATHWAY ACTIVATION PROFILES AS DRUG TARGETS FOR PREDICTING NOOTROPIC EFFECTS *IN SILICO*

Enhancing cognition is a challenge as it consists of various processes each influenced by many factors and each with a distinct neurobiological framework. While single-gene studies have been an effective first step in identifying individual elements necessary for learning and memory to occur (Lee and Silva, 2009), in moving forward, integration of many other factors and influences, including the relatively few signaling pathways involved, may be more beneficial than investigating each of many potential individual network elements.

Intracellular signaling pathways show promise for complex trait analysis. At the cellular level, any two physiological states can be distinguished by changes in a set of signaling pathways, each individually activated or repressed to some extent. This collection of disturbed pathways, termed the signaling pathway cloud, is a powerful and unique biological fingerprint (Zhavoronkov and Cantor, 2011; Makarev et al., 2014; Aliper et al., 2015).

Until recently, signaling pathway analysis was impeded by the inability to quantify individual signaling pathway activation strength (PAS), owing to the complexity of protein interactions within signaling pathways and lack of experimental data to determine the importance factor for each member of a given pathway. This problem was addressed, however, with the development of Oncofinder[1], a biomathematical method that simplifies calculation of PAS and signaling pathway cloud disturbance (SPCD), as detailed below (Buzdin et al., 2014b). With the ability to calculate PAS, one can quantitatively characterize a biological condition by its associated signaling activation profile.

PAS analysis involves (1) mapping relevant pathways from the gene expression profiles for a given condition; (2) calculating individual PAS values; (3) constructing the signaling pathway cloud (net activated and repressed pathways); (4) high throughput *in silico* screening to predict and rate drugs that target these pathways, depending on the application; and (5) *in vitro* and *in vivo* validation.

The pair of conditions to be compared in signaling pathway cloud analysis is flexible. In the past, we have compared tumor biopsies to healthy tissue, revealing signaling pathway biomarkers that outperform those of single genes (Kuzmin et al., 2010; Mityaev et al., 2010; Zabolotneva et al., 2012a,b), and tissue from old vs. young patients, illustrating how this method may be useful for the screening of potential geroprotectors (Zhavoronkov and Cantor, 2011). Other applications include drug discovery and drug repurposing, as well as applications in manipulating cell differentiation.

Here, we suggest that these methods could also be applied to cognitive enhancement, first by defining what aspect of cognition is to be targeted, then by mapping signaling pathways altered in transcription profiles of the "enhanced brain" vs. control (e.g., in mouse models showing performance gains in the target cognitive domain, whether via genetic manipulation, selective breeding or inbreeding, or treatment with current nootropics) and finally by calculating disturbance of the associated signaling pathway cloud (**Figure 1**).

High throughput screening for drugs that activate or repress key pathways could then uncover drugs that replicate cloud disturbance in "enhanced" models and thus mimic or exaggerate the effects of the current drugs or genetic manipulations. These drugs could then be ranked and prioritized for validation of cognitive effects *in vivo* or *in vitro*.

These methods can be used for general screening of cognitive enhancers at present but in the future may also be used to develop personalized cognitive enhancement plans for individual patients.

The idea of using differential gene expression patterns for drug discovery is not new. The broad variability of as well as the error rates introduced by the microarray and next generation sequencing (NGS) equipment led to many early failures, impeded progress and diminished the potential of this approach. However, recent algorithmic solutions reducing complexity and smoothing variability of the gene expression mapped onto signaling pathways allow us to minimize errors and perform cross-platform analysis (Buzdin et al., 2014b). These solutions allow us to tap into legacy databases and compare hundreds of thousands of data sets in microarray and NGS repositories as well as utilize the drug effects on gene expression published in publically available databases.

STEP 1: IDENTIFYING THE PAIR OF CONDITIONS

Enhanced cognition can refer to augmented function across one or several domains and can be demonstrated in a number of highly specific paradigms or tests, thus one must first

[1] www.oncofinder.com

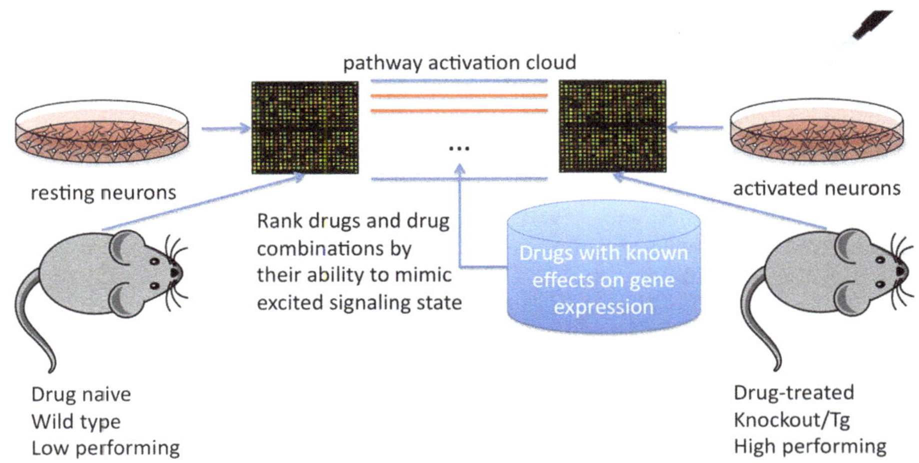

FIGURE 1 | Using differential signaling pathway activation profiles between cell/tissue culture or mice treated and untreated with known cognitive modulators or genetic models of cognitive enhancement to screen for potential nootropic compounds.

specify the goals of enhancement and choose models/tissues that demonstrate enhancement in that respect.

Ethical considerations preclude the use of human studies for this application, thus animal models would be required. Fortunately, a number of animal models are highly useful in investigating mechanisms of cognition (Roesler and Schröder, 2011). Specific aspects of attention, learning, and memory can be reliably measured in a wide variety of behavioral paradigms. Many of these have been developed for use in mice, but rats, monkeys, zebrafish, and drosophila are also potential models. For the current approach, mouse models are promising, and there are several different options within this species for comparison of the "enhanced" vs. "non-enhanced" brain.

MUTANT vs. WILD TYPE

Mice are a classic model for learning and memory and a number of models involve mutations that induce cognitive enhancement, including knockout and transgenic mutations (Lee and Silva, 2009). These model systems have revealed many genes involved in learning and memory. Hypothetically, the human orthologs of these genes would also be involved in cognition. Mutations that enhance cognition are varied in mechanism, and include enhancing excitation, dampening inhibition, regulating gene expression, regulating translation, epigenetics, microRNA biogenesis, and extracellular molecules (Lee and Silva, 2009). Generally speaking, mutations that increase the activity of cAMP response element-binding protein (CREB), a basic leucine zipper transcription factor, enhance long-term potentiation (LTP) and both long and short term memory, while those that downregulate CREB activity impair LTP and memory (Lee and Silva, 2009; Suzuki et al., 2011; Kida and Serita, 2014). In their 2009 review, Lee and Silva reported that 26 of the 29 mouse models reviewed showed enhanced LTP. In several cases, LTP was enhanced, but cognition was either not improved or was actually impaired; thus, other signaling pathways and cellular processes are involved (Lee and Silva, 2009), underscoring the potential role for signaling pathway analysis in elucidating global effects on these mice and thereby enabling pharmacological replication.

STRAIN vs. STRAIN

An alternative to single gene mutation models is selective breeding or inbreeding to exploit "natural" genetic variation among mouse strains in cognitive performance. Strains or groups of strains that perform high on paradigms of learning and memory can be compared to other low-performing strains within a genetic reference panel. The BXD strains are a good example (Williams et al., 2003). This panel of recombinant inbred strains has been extensively phenotyped for behaviors related to learning and memory and drug treatment effects as well as profiled for basal gene expression, and the data are publicly available for rapid statistical analysis on genenetwork.org (Wang et al., 2003). In minutes, known phenotypic differences can be correlated to known gene expression levels (and thus signaling pathway activation), without the unwanted or exaggerated effects of knockout or transgenic manipulation.

DRUG-TREATED vs. DRUG-NAÏVE

A third alternative for comparisons in the analysis would be *in vivo* or *in vitro* expression in organisms, tissues, or cells that have been pharmacologically treated with current nootropics vs. control. The effect of nootropics on gene expression in the brain can be large; in the case of methylphenidate treatment, over 2000 genes have been shown to be differentially expressed in the caudate putamen of mice (Adriani et al., 2006a,b). This comparison would enable screening of new nootropics that mimic current nootropics, but that are more effective, more or less specific in targeted cognitive domains, and/or have fewer side effects.

STEP 2: IDENTIFYING TARGET SIGNALING PATHWAYS

Once a specific comparison is decided upon, a predicted set of relevant pathways can be assembled from the literature or mapped from gene expression data. Here, we reviewed the literature for mouse models of cognitive enhancement, in which overexpression, knockout, loss-of-function mutation, deletion, or RNA interference of a particular gene led to significant gains in cognitive performance as measured in at least one behavioral paradigm for measuring learning and/or memory. In 2009, Lee and Silva reviewed these models and compiled list of target genes and effects of mutation. We reduced this list to only 40 genes, for which human orthologs exist. Gene set enrichment analyses of these listed entries against Insilico Cloud Intelligence signaling pathway database (Buzdin et al., 2014a) were performed using Fisher's exact test and the most enriched pathways are shown in **Table 1**. Results revealed several overrepresented signaling pathways, including IP3, IGF1R, and cAMP molecular signalization, potentially important for learning and memory in humans. Key activators/repressors of these pathways can therefore be used in further experimental assays together with the mathematical apparatus we provide in the following section.

Importantly, many of the genes and pathways identified during *in silico* screening of nootropics are also implicated in aging and longevity (Zhavoronkov and Cantor, 2011; Moskalev et al., 2014) thus suggesting that geroprotector drugs may act as nootropic agents and vice versa.

STEP 3: CALCULATING SIGNALING PATHWAY CLOUD DISTURBANCE

The work we propose involves calculating signaling activation and methods are based on our prior work with cell signaling pathways (Kiyatkin et al., 2006; Kuzmina and Borisov, 2011; Borisov et al., 2014). In the past, calculation of signaling pathway activation has been avoided because of the lack of experimental data measuring the correlation between expression and activation at the protein level. In our observation, most signal transduction proteins are far from saturation even at the peak concentrations of the activated form, in comparison with total protein abundance. From this, we suggest all activator/repressor gene products/proteins have equal importance for pathway activation/downregulation. We then arrive at the following assessment: function for overall signal pathway cloud disturbance outcome (SPCD) is proportional to the following estimator function:

$$SPCD = \frac{\prod_{i=1}^{N} [AGEL]_i}{\prod_{j=1}^{M} [RGEL]_j}$$

Here, the multiplication is performed over all possible activator and repressor proteins in the pathway, and $[AGEL]_i$ and $[RGEL]_j$ are gene expression levels of an activator i and repressor j, respectively. To obtain an additive (not multiplicative) value, one can simply switch from using absolute values of expression levels to their logarithms, arriving at the *PAS* value for each pathway

$$PAS_p = \sum_n ARR_{np} \cdot BTIF_n \cdot \lg(ECR_n)$$

In the case of cognitive enhancement, to obtain the values of *enhanced-to-control ratio (ECR)*, one divides the expression levels for a gene n in the sample taken for the enhanced group by the same average value for the normalized control group. The discrete value of activator/repressor role (ARR) is the relative strength of the target activation or repression.

The information about the activator/repressor role of a particular gene product/protein may be obtained from the analysis of open-access or customized pathway databases and from the literature. The Boolean flag of *BTIF* (beyond tolerance interval flag) equals to zero when the ECR value lies within the tolerance limit, and to one when otherwise. We determined that the ECR lies beyond the tolerance limit if it satisfies simultaneously the two criteria. First, it should be either higher than 3/2 or lower than 2/3 of the corresponding gene expression level in normal group of samples, and, second, the expression level of a gene should differ by more than two standard deviations from the average expression level for the same gene in a control group of samples.

LIMITATIONS OF DIFFERENTIAL SIGNALING PATHWAY ANALYSIS-BASED DRUG SCREENING METHODS

Acquiring gene expression data from the various regions of human brain during excitation is difficult and human data

Table 1 | Signaling pathways associated with cognitive enhancement in animal models.

Pathway name	Overlap with gene list (%)	Odds ratio	*p*-value
IP3 pathway (gene expression)	25.9	0.346	$1.53E-08$
IGF1R pathway (cell survival)	17.9	0.215	$2.39E-07$
cAMP pathway (axonal growth)	20.8	0.245	$6.88E-06$
IGF1R main pathway	6.6	0.073	$2.09E-05$
IP3 main pathway	5.2	0.058	0.000142525
IL-2 main pathway	4.4	0.044	0.002495586
Wnt main pathway	2.8	0.029	0.028947377
GPCR main pathway	2.5	0.025	0.033190669
cAMP main pathway	2.1	0.021	0.034326773

Gene set enrichment analyses of the genes implicated in cognitive performance against Insilico Cloud Intelligence signaling pathway database performed using Fisher's exact test and the most enriched pathways.

would have to be obtained from post mortem tissues or cultured cells or tissues. Gene expression data from mouse brain is easier to obtain, but further studies are required to evaluate the correlations between signaling pathway activation profiles in mice and humans. Tissue selection is also important, gene expression in one region or cell type may or may not be representative of other areas of the brain and may not capture all effects of a given condition. Also, gene expression alone may not provide the complete picture of the state of the tissue, and while the pathway activation analysis approach may be used to analyze differences in genomic DNA (Spirin et al., 2014) there may be epigenetic regulation of cognitive states that may require other analytical methods to be performed. Aside from tissue selection, the complexity of cognition presents other challenge. The proposed approach evaluates the various drugs and drug combinations that mimic or enhance the effects of already known nootropics or genetic manipulations; however, no current nootropic agents optimally enhance specific aspects of cognitive function without side effects, and even genetic models of cognitive enhancement can produce unintended impairments (Lee and Silva, 2009). In this paper, we have referred to the "enhanced" brain vs. control in describing the comparisons one would use to perform signaling pathway analysis. However, "enhanced" is a simplified, general term that does not specify effects on the various cognitive domains, and defining enhancement remains an important issue in developing new nootropics (Lynch et al., 2014).

CONCLUSION

Cognitive enhancement is in demand, whether in healthy populations or those with cognitive deficits, but current pharmacological enhancers offer only modest benefits. Testing of new cognitive enhancers is costly and time consuming. Even predicting the nootropic candidates out of the hundreds of thousands of drugs and drug combinations remains a major challenge. A screening process that would predict the efficacy of novel cognitive enhancers that may outperform current options would save time and money, both of which are limiting as the aging segment of the population explodes over the upcoming decades, with increasing rates of cognitive decline and neurodegenerative disease. Here we propose a method for *in silico* screening and ranking of drugs and other factors that act on signaling pathways involved in cognition. Predicting their efficacy would involve calculating their potential to maximize the difference in signaling pathway activation between cells or tissues of cognitively enhanced animal models, including mutant "smart" vs. wild type mice, high-performing vs. low-performing strains of mice, or drug-treated vs. drug naïve mice. This would be followed by *in vitro* and *in vivo* validation leading to a short list of promising components.

REFERENCES

Adriani, W., Leo, D., Greco, D., Rea, M., di Porzio, U., Laviola, G., et al. (2006a). Methylphenidate administration to adolescent rats determines plastic changes in reward-related behavior and striatal gene expression. *Neuropsychopharmacology* 31, 1946–1956. doi: 10.1038/sj.npp.1300962

Adriani, W., Leo, D., Guarino, M., Natoli, A., Di Consiglio, E., De Angelis, G., et al. (2006b). Short-term effects of adolescent methylphenidate exposure on brain striatal gene expression and sexual/endocrine parameters in male rats. *Ann. N Y Acad. Sci.* 1074, 52–57. doi: 10.1196/annals.1369.005

Aliper, A., Csoka, A. B., Buzdin, A., Jetka, T., Roumiantsev, S., Moskalev, A., et al. (2015). Signaling pathway activation drift during aging: Hutchinson-Gilford progeria syndrome fibroblasts are comparable to normal middle-age and old-age cells. *Aging (Albany NY)* [Epub ahead of print].

Beglinger, L. J., Tangphao-Daniels, O., Kareken, D. A., Zhang, L., Mohs, R., and Siemers, E. R. (2005). Neuropsychological test performance in healthy elderly volunteers before and after donepezil administration: a randomized, controlled study. *J. Clin. Psychopharmacol.* 25, 159–165. doi: 10.1097/01.jcp.0000155822.51962.b4

Belmonte, M. K., and Yurgelun-Todd, D. A. (2003). Functional anatomy of impaired selective attention and compensatory processing in autism. *Brain Res. Cogn. Brain Res.* 17, 651–664. doi: 10.1016/s0926-6410(03)00189-7

Borisov, N. M., Terekhanova, N. V., Aliper, A. M., Venkova, L. S., Smirnov, P. Y., Roumiantsev, S., et al. (2014). Signaling pathway activation profiles make better markers of cancer than expression of individual genes. *Oncotarget* 5, 10198–10205.

Buzdin, A. A., Zhavoronkov, A. A., Korzinkin, M. B., Roumiantsev, S. A., Aliper, A. M., Venkova, L. S., et al. (2014a). The OncoFinder algorithm for minimizing the errors introduced by the high-throughput methods of transcriptome analysis. *Front. Mol. Biosci.* 1:8. doi: 10.3389/fmolb.2014.00008

Buzdin, A. A., Zhavoronkov, A. A., Korzinkin, M. B., Vankova, L. S., Zenin, A. A., Smimov, P. Y., et al. (2014b). Oncofinder, a new method for the analysis of intracellular signaling pathway activation using transcriptomic data. *Front. Genet.* 5:55. doi: 10.3389/fgene.2014.00055

Elliott, R., Sahakian, B. J., Matthews, K., Bannerjea, A., Rimmer, J., and Robbins, T. W. (1997). Effects of methylphenidate on spatial working memory and planning in healthy young adults. *Psychopharmacology (Berl)* 131, 196–206. doi: 10.1007/s002130050284

Esposito, Pieramico, V., Ferretti, A., Macchia, A., Tommasi, M., Saggino, A., Ciavardelli, D., et al. (2013). Acute effects of modafinil on brain resting state networks in young healthy subjects. *PLoS One* 8:e69224. doi: 10.1371/journal.pone.0069224

Finke, K., Dodds, C. M., Bublak, P., Regenthal, R., Baumann, F., Manly, T., et al. (2010). Effects of modafinil and methylphenidate on visual attention capacity: a TVA-based study. *Psychopharmacology (Berl)* 210, 317–329. doi: 10.1007/s00213-010-1823-x

Frank, M. J., and O'Reilly, R. C. (2006). A mechanistic account of striatal dopamine function in human cognition: psychopharmacological studies with cabergoline and haloperidol. *Behav. Neurosci.* 120, 497–517. doi: 10.1037/0735-7044.120.3.497

Gibbs, S. E., and D'Esposito, M. (2005). Individual capacity differences predict working memory performance and prefrontal activity following dopamine receptor stimulation. *Cogn. Affect Behav. Neurosci.* 5, 212–221. doi: 10.3758/cabn.5.2.212

Gibbs, S. E., and D'Esposito, M. (2006). A functional magnetic resonance imaging study of the effects of pergolide, a dopamine receptor agonist, on component processes of working memory. *Neuroscience* 139, 359–371. doi: 10.1016/j.neuroscience.2005.11.055

Gouliaev, A. H., and Senning, A. (1994). Piracetam and other structurally related nootropics. *Brain Res. Rev.* 19, 180–222. doi: 10.1016/0165-0173(94)90011-6

Gualtieri, F., Manetti, D., Romanelli, M., and Ghelardini, C. (2002). Design and study of piracetam-like nootropics, controversial members of the problematic class of cognition-enhancing drugs. *Curr. Pharm. Des.* 8, 125–138. doi: 10.2174/1381612023396582

Kida, S., and Serita, T. (2014). Functional roles of CREB as a positive regulator in the formation and enhancement of memory. *Brain Res. Bull.* 105, 17–24. doi: 10.1016/j.brainresbull.2014.04.011

Kimberg, D. Y., D'Esposito, M., and Farah, M. J. (1997). Effects of bromocriptine on human subjects depend on working memory capacity. *Neuroreport* 8, 3581–3585. doi: 10.1097/00001756-199711100-00032

Kiyatkin, A., Aksamitiene, E., Markevich, N. I., Borisov, N. M., Hoek, J. B., and Kholodenko, B. N. (2006). Scaffolding protein Grb2-associated binder 1 sustains epidermal growth factor-induced mitogenic and survival signaling by multiple positive feedback loops. *J. Biol. Chem.* 281, 19925–19938. doi: 10.1074/jbc.m600482200

Kuzmin, D., Gogvadze, E., Kholodenko, R., Grzela, D. P., Mityaev, M., Vinogradova, T., et al. (2010). Novel strong tissue specific promoter for gene expression in human germ cells. *BMC Biotechnol.* 10:58. doi: 10.1186/1472-6750-10-58

Kuzmina, N. B., and Borisov, N. M. (2011). Handling complex rule-based models of mitogenic cell signaling (on the example of ERK activation upon EGF Stimulation). *Int. Proc. Chem. Biol. Environ. Eng.* 5, 67–82.

Lee, Y. S., and Silva, A. J. (2009). The molecular and cellular biology of enhanced cognition. *Nat. Rev. Neurosc.* 10, 126–140. doi: 10.1038/nrn2572

Lynch, G., Cox, C. D., and Gall, C. M. (2014). Pharmacological enhancement of memory or cognition in normal subjects. *Front. Syst. Neurosci.* 8:90. doi: 10.3389/fnsys.2014.00090

Maher, B. (2008). Poll results: look who's doping. *Nature* 452, 674–675. doi: 10.1038/452674a

Makarev, E., Cantor, C., Zhavoronkov, A., Buzdin, A., Aliper, A., and Csoka, A. B. (2014). Pathway activation profiling reveals new insights into age-related macular degeneration and provides avenues for therapeutic interventions. *Aging (Albany NY)* 6, 1064–1075.

Maslen, H., Faulmuller, N., and Savulescu, J. (2014). Pharmacological cognitive enhancement—how neuroscientific research could advance ethical debate. *Front. Syst. Neurosci.* 8:107. doi: 10.3389/fnsys.2014.00107

Mityaev, M. V., Kopantzev, E. P., Buzdin, A. A., Vinogradova, T. V., and Sverdlov, E. D. (2010). Enhancer element potentially involved in human survivin gene promoter regulation in lung cancer cell lines. *Biochemistry (Mosc)* 75, 182–191. doi: 10.1134/s0006297910020082

Moskalev, A. A., Aliper, A. M., Smit-McBride, Z., Buzdin, A., and Zhavoronkov, A. (2014). Genetics and epigenetics of aging and longevity. *Cell Cycle* 13, 1063–1077. doi: 10.4161/cc.28433

Pieramico, V., Esposito, R., Cesinaro, S., Frazzini, V., and Sensi, S. (2014). Effects of non-pharmacological or pharmacological interventions on cognition and brain plasticity of aging individuals. *Front. Syst. Neurosci.* 8:153. doi: 10.3389/fnsys.2014.00153

Randall, D. C., Shneerson, J. M., and File, S. E. (2005). Cognitive effects of modafinil in student volunteers may depend on IQ. *Pharmacol. Biochem. Behav.* 82, 133–139. doi: 10.1016/j.pbb.2005.07.019

Repantis, D., Schlattmann, P., Laisney, O., and Heuser, I. (2010). Modafinil and methylphenidate for neuroenhancement in healthy individuals: a systematic review. *Pharmacol. Res.* 62, 187–206. doi: 10.1016/j.phrs.2010.04.002

Roesler, R., and Schröder, N. (2011). Cognitive enhancers: focus on modulatory signaling influencing memory consolidation. *Pharmacol. Biochem. Behav.* 99, 155–163. doi: 10.1016/j.pbb.2010.12.028

Spirin, P. V., Lebedev, T. D., Orlova, N. N., Gornostaeva, A. S., Prokofjeva, M. M., Nikitenko, N. A., et al. (2014). Silencing AML1-ETO gene expression leads to simultaneous activation of both pro-apoptotic and proliferation signaling. *Leukemia* 28, 2222–2228. doi: 10.1038/leu.2014.130

Suzuki, A., Fukushima, H., Mukawa, T., Toyoda, H., Wu, L. J., Zhao, M. G., et al. (2011). Upregulation of CREB-mediated transcription enhances both short- and long-term memory. *J. Neurosci.* 31, 8786–8802. doi: 10.1523/jneurosci.3257-10.2011

Wallace, T. L., Ballard, T. M., Pouzet, B., Riedel, W. J., and Wettstein, J. G. (2011). Drug targets for cognitive enhancement in neuropsychiatric disorders. *Pharmacol. Biochem. Behav.* 99, 130–145. doi: 10.1016/j.pbb.2011.03.022

Wang, J., Williams, R. W., and Manly, K. F. (2003). WebQTL: web-based complex trait analysis. *Neuroinformatics* 1, 299–308. doi: 10.1385/ni:1:4:299

Williams, R. W., Gu, J., Qi, S., and Lu, L. (2003). The genetic structure of recombinant inbred mice: high-resolution consensus maps for complex trait analysis. *Genome Biol.* 2:RESEARCH0046. doi: 10.1186/gb-2001-2-11-research0046

Zabolotneva, A. A., Bantysh, O., Suntsova, M. V., Efimova, N., Malakhova, G. V., Schumann, G. G., et al. (2012a). Transcriptional regulation of human-specific SVAF(1) retrotransposons by cis-regulatory MAST2 sequences. *Gene* 505, 128–136. doi: 10.1016/j.gene.2012.05.016

Zabolotneva, A. A., Zhavoronkov, A., Garazha, A. V., Roumiantsev, S. A., and Buzdin, A. A. (2012b). Characteristic patterns of microRNA expression in human bladder cancer. *Front. Genet.* 3:310. doi: 10.3389/fgene.2012.00310

Zhavoronkov, A., and Cantor, C. R. (2011). Methods for structuring scientific knowledge from many areas related to aging research. *PLoS One* 6:e22597. doi: 10.1371/journal.pone.0022597

18

Partial sleep in the context of augmentation of brain function

***Ivan N. Pigarev*[1]* and Marina L. Pigareva*[2]**

[1] *Institute for Information Transmission Problems (Kharkevich Institute), Russian Academy of Sciences, Moscow, Russia*
[2] *Institute of Higher Nervous Activity and Neurophysiology, Russian Academy of Sciences, Moscow, Russia*

Edited by:
Mikhail Lebedev, Duke University, USA

Reviewed by:
Manuel Casanova, University of Louisville, USA
Mikhail Lebedev, Duke University, USA
György Benedek, Szegedi Tudományegyetem, Hungary
Elena Budkevich, North Caucasus Federal University, Russia

****Correspondence:***
Ivan N. Pigarev, Institute for Information Transmission Problems (Kharkevich Institute), Russian Academy of Sciences, Bol'shoy Karetny Lane 19, Moscow 127994, Russia
e-mail: pigarev@iitp.ru

Inability to solve complex problems or errors in decision making is often attributed to poor brain processing and raises the issue of brain augmentation. Investigation of neuronal activity in the cerebral cortex in the sleep-wake cycle offers insights into the mechanisms underlying the reduction in mental abilities for complex problem solving. Some cortical areas may transit into a sleep state while an organism is still awake. Such local sleep would reduce behavioral ability in the tasks for which the sleeping areas are crucial. The studies of this phenomenon have indicated that local sleep develops in high order cortical areas. This is why complex problem solving is mostly affected by local sleep, and prevention of local sleep might be a potential way of augmentation of brain function. For this approach to brain augmentation not to entail negative consequences for the organism, it is necessary to understand the functional role of sleep. Our studies have given an unexpected answer to this question. It was shown that cortical areas that process signals from extero- and proprioreceptors during wakefulness, switch to the processing of interoceptive information during sleep. It became clear that during sleep all "computational power" of the brain is directed to the restoration of the vital functions of internal organs. These results explain the logic behind the initiation of total and local sleep. Indeed, a mismatch between the current parameters of any visceral system and the genetically determined normal range would provide the feeling of tiredness, or sleep pressure. If an environmental situation allows falling asleep, the organism would transit to a normal total sleep in all cortical areas. However, if it is impossible to go to sleep immediately, partial sleep may develop in some cortical areas in the still behaviorally awake organism. This local sleep may reduce both the "intellectual power" and the restorative function of sleep for visceral organs.

Keywords: local sleep, cerebral cortex, slow wave sleep, sleep function, visceral control

SLEEP AND "HUMAN FACTOR"

The modern industrial style of life and necessity to live in non-natural environments often leads to dramatic errors in human behavior. Usually these errors are included in the general term "human factor" and are attributed to reduced attention, inability to predict consequences of an action in complex conditions and, finally, to reduced brain ability. Thus, the intention to augment the brain function can be considered a challenging goal for Neuroscience.

It was noticed that industrial anthropogenic disasters, traffic accidents, and medical errors often occur during the night, suggesting a probable link between sleepiness and reduced quality of brain functioning (Mitler et al., 1988; Dinges, 1995; Dinges et al., 1997; Cajochen et al., 1999; Barger et al., 2006; Akerstedt et al., 2011). Given the importance of this issue, many special studies devoted to investigation of the possible link between sleep disturbances and mental abilities were undertaken.

It was demonstrated that short-term total sleep deprivation results in cognitive impairments, especially in learning, and memory tasks (Maquet, 2001; Stickgold, 2005; Born et al., 2006; Walker, 2008, 2009; Diekelmann and Born, 2010; McCoyand and Strecker, 2011; Diekelmann et al., 2012, 2013).

In some studies, authors concluded that periods of slow wave sleep (SWS) played a particular role in these processes (Fowler et al., 1973; Plihal and Born, 1997; Diekelmann et al., 2011). Others maintained a rapid eye movement (REM) sleep dependency (Empson and Clarke, 1970), although in some studies REM sleep deprivation had no effect on different aspects of memory function (Hornung et al., 2007; Saxvig et al., 2008).

In addition to the function of memory consolidation, sleep has been proposed to benefit the encoding of new information during succeeding periods of wakefulness (McDermott et al., 2003; Yoo et al., 2007; Mander et al., 2011).

PECULIARITIES OF SLEEP DEPRIVATION EFFECTS

The impact of sleep deprivation on memory formation did not appear to be universal, but instead, differed on the basis of many factors such as the types of tasks used for learning, and personal characteristics of subjects, including their emotionality. It has been shown that sleep-dependent motor skill memory improvement was dependent on the nature of the skill to be learned (Cohen et al., 2005; Cohen and Robertson, 2007; Siengsukon and Boyd, 2008). In another study, perception, attention and memory were impaired by sleep deprivation, but visual search and logical reasoning tasks were not (Williamson et al., 2001). A deficit in perceptual classification ability in an information-integration task was observed for some, but not all, sleep-deprived individuals (Maddox et al., 2009).

In their review of the sleep deprivation literature, Harrison and Horne (2000) concluded that sleep deprivation has little effect on simple rule-following tasks, but it obstructs decision making in complex integration tasks requiring flexibility, innovation or plan revision. However, other researchers observed performance decrements in relatively simple tasks such as identification and vigilance tasks (Chee et al., 2008; Ratcliff and Van Dongen, 2009). Sleep deprived subjects exhibited decreased performance in the taking advantage task (Glass et al., 2011).

Genzel et al. (2009) used different deprivation conditions throughout the experiment and did not find that an intense decrease in the total amount of REM sleep or SWS of their volunteers led to the inhibition of learning. They even proposed that sleep-dependent memory consolidation did not rely only on intact amounts of SWS or REM sleep across a night, but required different EEG microstructures, e.g., sleep spindles, δ-waves, and PGO waves.

It was proposed that reduced visual short-term memory after sleep deprivation may be connected, not with impairment of memory consolidation mechanisms but, rather, with a decline in visual attention and/or visual processing (Chuah and Chee, 2008).

An important factor was the length of time between training and test or amount of skill practice, independent of whether there was sleep or not (Shadmehr and Brashers-Krug, 1997; Robertson et al., 2004; Keisler et al., 2007; Song et al., 2007; Criscimagna-Hemminger and Shadmehr, 2008; Doyon et al., 2009; Debas et al., 2010; Borich et al., 2011; Borich and Kimberley, 2011; Voderholzer et al., 2011; Reis et al., 2013). In a nap study (Mander et al., 2011) no differences were observed between the sleep and no sleep groups in a specific alertness control task.

Results of sleep deprivation experiments were often rather contradictory. According to Lo et al. (2012), influence of sleep deprivation depends on the task domain, prior sleep debt, circadian phase at which performance is assessed, and genetically determined subject characteristics. Degree of task difficulty and the subject's emotionality influence the outcome of experiments concerning the connection between sleep and memory (Smith, 2001; Walker and Stickgold, 2006). Small differences in test design can cause large discrepancies in the studies of sleep dependency of memory processes. This may explain why some results are regularly found only by the same groups of scientists (Genzel et al., 2009).

Even in those experiments where positive effects of sleep on memory consolidation were demonstrated, these effects were very small. It seemed unlikely to us that the only function of sleep was simply to provide such a modest improvement in memory. On the other hand, the probable connection of sleepiness with the rare but dramatic consequences of anthropogenic disasters, as well as the fantastic pictures of dreams, support the general belief that the first function of sleep is for efficient functioning of the brain.

MODERN THEORIES OF SLEEP

Several modern theories concerning the function of sleep offer hypothetical mechanisms, which could be used by the brain for this purpose, e.g., the theory of neuronal groups (Krueger and Obál, 1993; Krueger et al., 2008) or the theory of synaptic homeostasis (Tononi and Cirelli, 2003, 2006). All theories, which were based on the assumption that sleep first of all is important for efficient brain function referred to numerous studies which demonstrated, both in humans and animals, "local use dependent processes". It was shown that δ-power during the first hours of sleep is higher in those cortical areas, which were more active immediately before sleep (Kattler et al., 1994; Rector et al., 2005; Huber et al., 2006). δ-power was considered therefore as an indicator and measure of recuperative processes in the brain.

However, if to accept an idea that function of sleep is to keep the efficient brain function it would be logical to expect that the brain would be the organ most vulnerable to sleep deprivation. However, the results of fundamental studies of A. Rechtshaffen and his colleagues (Everson et al., 1989; Cirelli et al., 1999; Rechtshaffen and Bergmann, 2002) do not confirm this suggestion. Their experiments demonstrated that total sleep deprivation led first of all to multiple visceral disorders (hair loss, skin and gastro-intestinal ulcerations and so on) and, finally, to unavoidable death of animals. A striking finding was that in rats that died after several days of total sleep deprivation, the only organ, which did not have any obvious degenerative changes, was the brain (Cirelli et al., 1999). This observation is surprising, since the negative effects of sleep deprivation on mental ability are well known. However, investigation of neuronal activity in the cerebral cortex in the sleep-wake cycle offers insights into the other sleep dependent mechanisms which can explain the reduction of mental abilities for complex problem solving, even in the normally working brain.

PHENOMENON OF LOCAL (PARTIAL) SLEEP

It was generally assumed for a long time that sleep develops synchronously in all areas of the mammalian cortex. The only exception has been reported for dolphins, whose EEG show periods of deep SWS in either the right or left hemisphere alone. Such periods of unilateral sleep may last for more than 2 h. Even in dolphins, however, EEG activity in different areas of one hemisphere was always found to be synchronized, or desynchronized simultaneously (Mukhametov et al., 1977; Mukhametov, 1984).

However, later it was shown that in terrestrial animals, in particular conditions, sleep developed only in some cortical areas during behavioral wakefulness. Thus, such partial sleep might be especially dangerous, because neither the person himself nor other individuals could notice its appearance and development. At the same time, dangerous consequences of temporal disengagement of some cortical areas from the control of behavior potentially can be rather dramatic. That is why understanding the physiological mechanisms involved in initiation of sleep, and particularly of local sleep, can be considered an important element in attempts to augment brain functionality.

The phenomenon, which later was called "local sleep" was described in a study of the cat's frontal eye field (Pigarev, 1984). Neurons in this frontal cortical area strongly responded to visual stimulation only during periods of high behavioral alertness, and often became visually unresponsive during subsequent periods of quiet wakefulness. However, any sensory stimulation raising alertness (visual, auditory or olfactory), restored visual responses in this cortical area.

More detailed description of such unusual neuronal behavior in the cerebral cortex, and the term "local or partial sleep" appeared in the investigation of cortical visual area V4 in experiments with behaviorally awake monkeys (Pigarev et al., 1996, 1997; Pigarev, 1997). It was demonstrated in long-running experiments, that when a monkey had to perform a monotonic visual discrimination task, neurons became less responsive to the same visual stimuli and finally stopped responding at all, while the monkey continued to work in the task. If the task was interrupted, the monkey fell asleep for 10–20 min. After the nap, neuronal responses to visual stimuli often recovered. Neuronal background firing during such periods of temporal inactivity resembled that which these neurons demonstrated during periods of natural sleep of the animal. The monkey's performance in the visual task during periods of local sleep in the area V4 was rather high, although it was slightly reduced in comparison with that at the beginning of the experiment. Thus, one could conclude that at least visual area V1 still was working. In the same study it was noticed that, even within the area V4, local sleep developed not simultaneously but started from the periphery of the visual field. The last neurons, which were recruited in sleep, were neurons in the region of the foveal representation.

It was obvious that spread of sleep started from the "higher order" sensory areas most likely crucial for the most complicated behavioral situations. Taking all those considerations into account, one could expect to observe local sleep more often in organisms with better expressed multiple sensory representations, and most of all in primates. Indeed, the fronto-occipital trend in δ-power most pronounced during beginning of sleep was discovered in human subjects by the group of A. Borbély (Werth et al., 1996, 1997). Extensive studies of sleep spread dynamics are presented and discussed in the review of Ferrara and De Gennaro (2011).

We would like to remind here that since 1993 (Krueger and Obál, 1993; Kattler et al., 1994) the mentioned above idea concerning local use dependent sleep was widely discussed in sleep literature. Although experiments demonstrated local use dependent sleep, and observations of local sleep in behaviorally awake animals were mutually supportive, they were not absolutely identical. In the first case it was shown that in sleeping brain the depth of sleep can locally vary from region to region dependent on the previous history of activation. In the second case sleep in some cortical areas appeared during behavioral wakefulness. Namely this second case we will have in mind using the term "local sleep" in future.

Unexpected results obtained by Drummond et al. (2001, 2004) most likely were also connected with dynamics of local sleep spread over the human cerebral cortex. Investigating the effects of 35 h total sleep deprivation on memory impairments in verbal learning tasks using fMRI, these researchers demonstrated increased activity in frontal and parietal cortical regions, absent in the control non-deprived group. This can reflect partial sleep development in these high order associative cortical areas caused by sleep deprivation.

It seemed less likely that local sleep would be found in animals with more simple cortical organization and a limited number of sensory areas. However, recently, local sleep was described in behaviorally active rats, and again in the frontal cortical area (Vyazovskiy et al., 2011).

LOCAL SLEEP AND COGNITIVE IMPAIRMENTS AFTER SLEEP DEPRIVATION

Taking into account the phenomenon of local sleep, the cognitive impairments after sleep deprivation can be explained not by the general deterioration of brain efficiency, but by switching of several cortical areas from those functions, which they have to perform in wakefulness.

At first sight, the hypothesis that local sleep is responsible for a reduction of brain functionality looks similar to the proposal that after a long period of wakefulness, the brain needs recuperation during sleep. The difference is only in the temporal sequence of events. After prolonged wakefulness, all regions of the brain may fall asleep for recovery simultaneously, or certain areas may do so at first, while others remain awake for some time.

However, it is possible to consider another, fundamentally different, scenario. What if the brain, as all other visceral organs of an organism, does not need any special recuperative rest connected with total interruption of functionality? What if the brain, like a computer, can work efficiently for long periods of time, and observed "sensory isolation" of the brain during sleep just reflects switching over for processing of another flow of incoming information?

We should not forget that sleep-deprived animals die not because they become blind, deaf, have forgotten the ways to a food tray or because of serious problems with decision making. They die mainly because of multiple visceral disorders in virtually all life supporting systems, including the immune system (Rechtshaffen and Bergmann, 2002). At the same time, the brain appears to be the most resistant organ.

Our observations of the neuronal activity in the sleep-wake cycle also did not convince us that during long periods of wakefulness there were crucial pathological changes of the neuronal state, which forced a brain to switch into a sleeping "restorative" mode. Nevertheless, one can argue that it is generally recognized that the pattern of SWS EEG is very specific for this state, and differs from the pattern of EEG in wakefulness. However, interpretation of this observation also is equivocal. The EEG pattern of active SWS was usually compared with the EEG pattern in a state of very passive wakefulness, when human subjects or animals were immobile and without intensive sensory stimulation.

WHETHER CORTICAL EEG REFLECTS PECULIARITY OF BRAIN ACTIVITY IN WAKEFULNESS AND SLEEP, OR JUST PATTERN OF THE CORTICAL AFFERENT FLOW?

We proposed that difference of cortical afferentation in wakefulness and sleep might define the observed difference of neuronal activity in SWS and wakefulness. To check this proposal, general EEG and eye movements were recorded in behaviorally awake cats during SWS and active wakefulness between electrodes located over temporal and frontal cortical areas. In addition, we recorded neuronal activity and local field potentials (local EEG) from visual (**Figure 1**) and somatosensory (**Figure 2**) cortical areas using bipolar tungsten microelectrodes with distances of about 300 μm between the tips of the electrodes. During SWS the animal eyes were always deviated upward, and this allowed us to easily distinguish periods of sleep from active wakefulness in the obtained recordings. For every group of recorded neurons we applied the optimal parameters of stimulation (either visual or somatosensory), and delivered these stimuli in a rhythmic manner. We called this procedure "sleep EEG imitation in wakefulness". Using this procedure (right column), in actively awake cats, we got burst neuronal firing (not shown) and EEG slow waves, which were indistinguishable from, or even higher than, those which we had observed during the periods of natural SWS (left column). These sleep-like waves were especially well visible in the channel of the local field potentials (**Figures 1C** and **2C**, right columns) because the local EEG reflected activity of the neurons for which we used the optimal stimulation. The general EEG reflected averaged activity collected from the large cortical territory, including those neurons for which applied stimuli were not optimal. Nevertheless, some sleep-like waves were seen even in the general EEG (**Figures 1B** and **2B**, right columns). In row D in **Figures 1** and **2** we present power spectrums calculated for the 10 s fragments of the local EEG shown in row C of the corresponding column. It is seen that spectral compositions of the local EEG for SWS (left column) and imitation of sleep EEG in wakefulness (right column) were rather similar, and both differed from the usual spectrum of quiet wakefulness (central column).

The presented observations supported an idea that patterns of the cortical afferentation, rather than the state of vigilance,

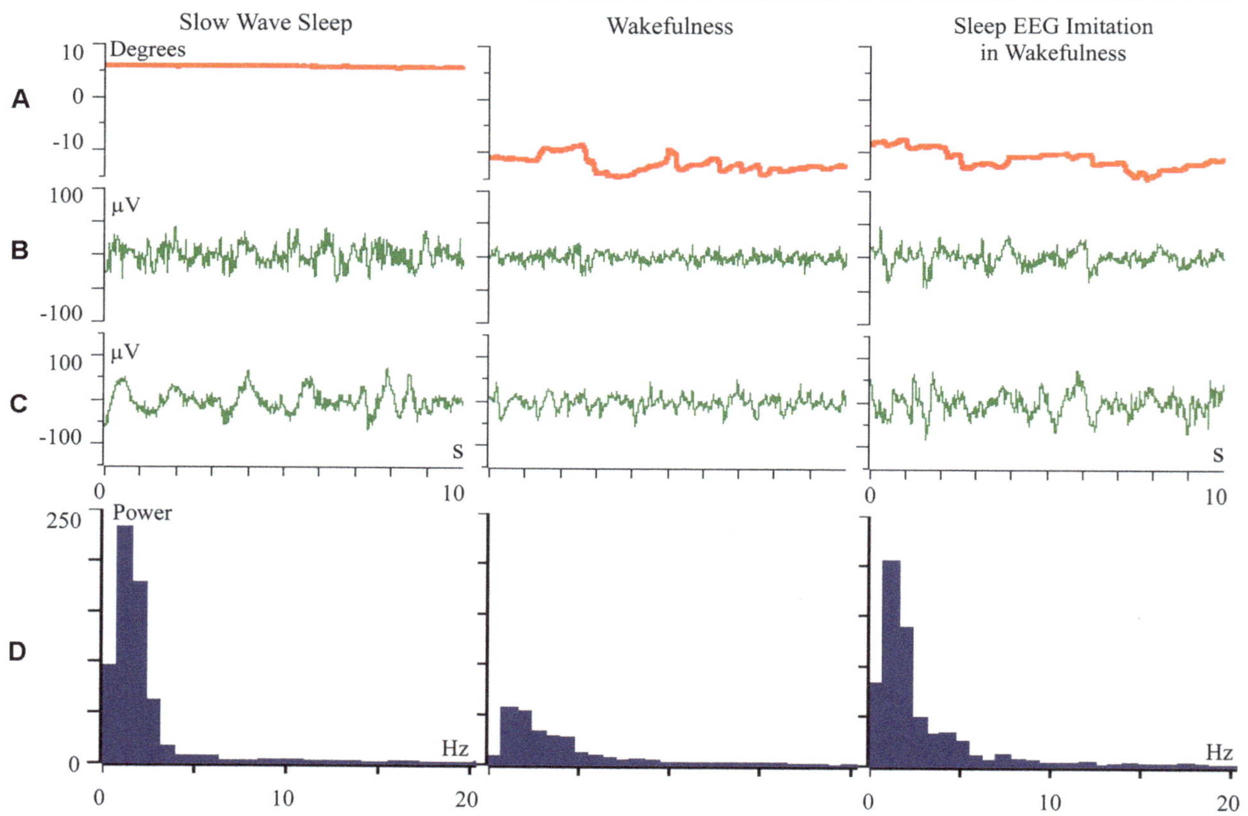

FIGURE 1 | Rhythmic stimulation by the optimal visual stimulus during wakefulness evokes sleep like slow wave activity in the cat visual cortex. The rows: **(A)** vertical component of eye movements which helps to distinguish sleep (upward deviation) from wakefulness (downward deviation); **(B)** general EEG recorded between electrodes over temporal and frontal cortical areas of the cat; **(C)** local field potentials (local EEG) recorded between two tungsten microelectrodes located 300 μm one from another within the cortical visual area V1; **(D)** power spectrum of the local EEG presented above in **panel C**. All parameters were collected during SWS (left column), during passive wakefulness (middle column), and during the procedure of "sleep EEG imitation" by visual stimulation in wakefulness, which produced strong excitation of the cortical neurons recorded by the microelectrodes (right column). Technical details of the study in Pigarev et al. (2013).

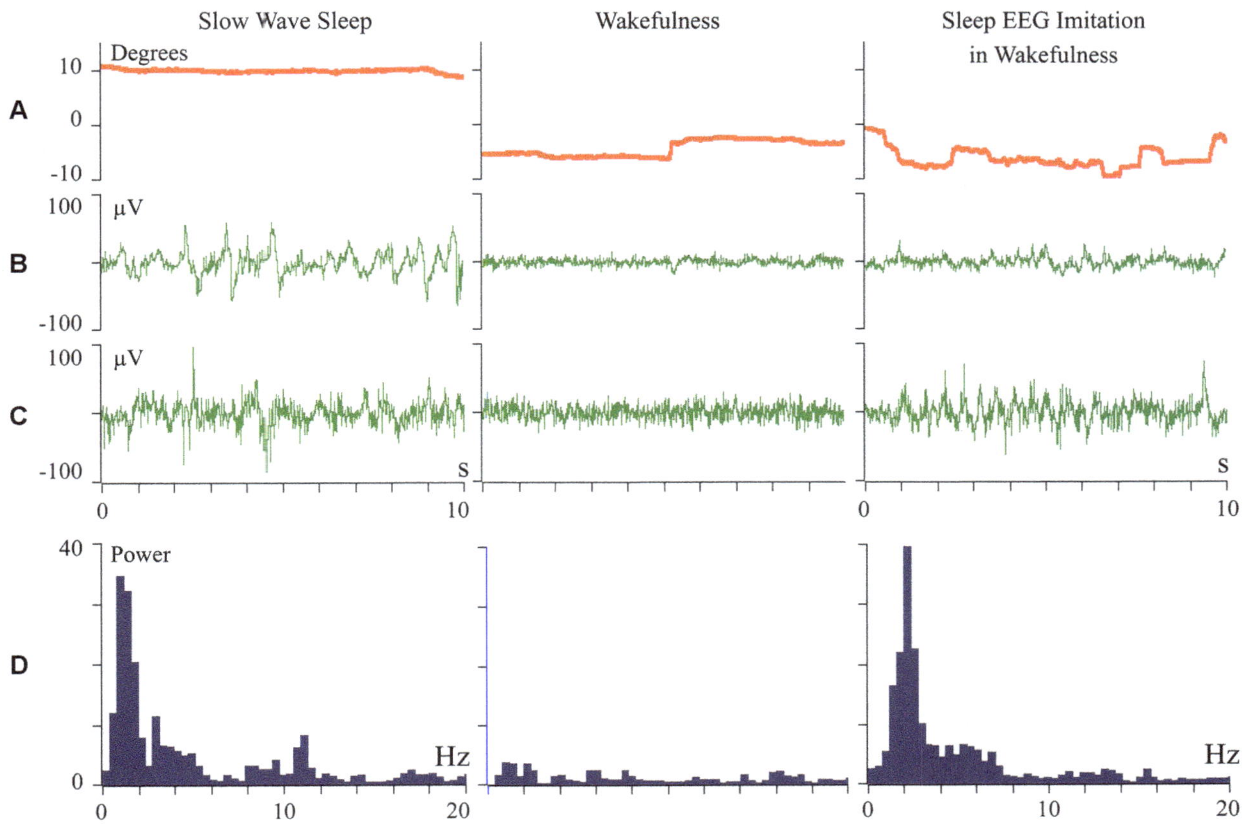

FIGURE 2 | Periodic optimal somatic stimulation during wakefulness evokes sleep like slow wave activity in the cat somatosensory cortex. The rows: **(A)** vertical component of eye movements which helps to distinguish sleep (upward deviation) from wakefulness (downward deviation); **(B)** general EEG recorded between electrodes over temporal and frontal cortical areas of the cat; **(C)** local field potentials (local EEG) recorded between two tungsten microelectrodes located 300 mm one from another within the cortical somatosensory area 5; **(D)** power spectrum of the local EEG presented above in **panel C**. All parameters were collected during SWS (left column), during passive wakefulness (middle column) and during the procedure of "sleep EEG imitation" in wakefulness by rhythmic stimulation of the contralateral forepaw, which produced strong excitation of the cortical neurons recorded by the microelectrodes. Technical details of the study in Pigarev et al. (2013).

determine the pattern of cortical activity. All above-mentioned considerations inclined us to conclude that switching to analysis of another flow of incoming information would be able to better explain the phenomenology of transition from wakefulness to sleep. The temporal organization of these incoming signals, specific for the state of sleep, will define the pattern of cortical activity during sleep.

WHICH SIGNALS COULD PROVIDE PERIODIC AND SYNCHRONOUS AFFERENTATION DURING SLEEP?

Animal physiology offered the answer on this question; that it can be periodic activity of various visceral systems, e.g., gastrointestinal peristalsis, heart and respiratory activities. We proposed that during sleep the same brain neurons that in wakefulness process exteroceptive information of various modalities switch over to the analysis of interoceptive information coming from visceral systems. Rhythmic activities of different visceral systems define this periodic afferent flow towards the cortical areas, which is reflected in cortical SWS activity. Thus, the central nervous system during sleep might be involved in the process of visceral regulation (Pigarev, 2014).

According to this proposal, periods of local sleep are not the periods when "tired" brain areas stop processing of exteroceptive information in favor of self-recuperation. During periods of local sleep, normally working brain areas respond to warning messages from the internal organs and switch to the processing of the alarming visceral afferentation. Within the frame of this hypothesis, we should "think differently" about the nature of sleep and local sleep.

This suggestion may be too fantastic for the brain paradigm generally accepted at present. This paradigm was established mainly on the basis of data collected for the state of wakefulness. On the other hand, our "fantastic" proposal opened the way for its experimental validation in simple experiments, which could not be conducted without this theoretical background. Below, we offer a short review of the experiments performed to investigate such nontrivial predictions of the visceral hypothesis of sleep.

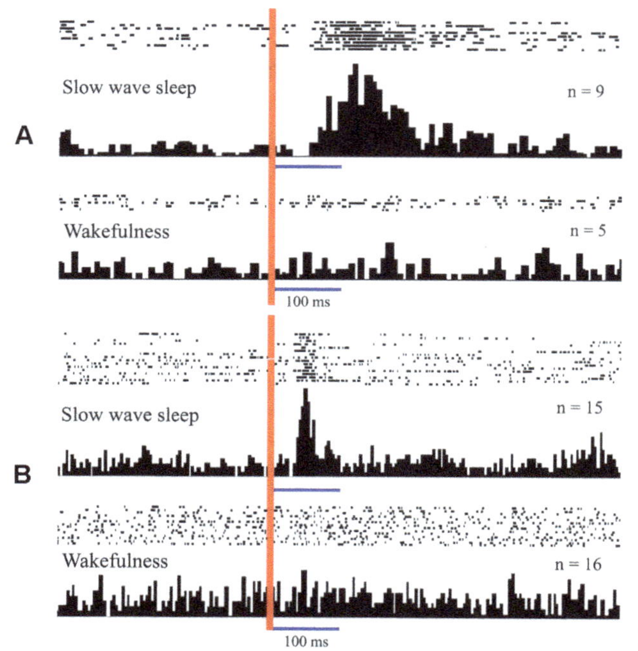

FIGURE 3 | Responses of neurons in the cat cortical visual area V1 (A) and somatosensory area 5 (B) to intraperitoneal electrical stimulation delivered in sleep and in wakefulness. Responses presented as rasters where every line corresponds to single stimulation trial. Dots represent single spikes. Below are averaged histograms. Vertical red line–moment of intraperitoneal stimulation. n—number of averaged trials. Technical details of the study in Pigarev (1994).

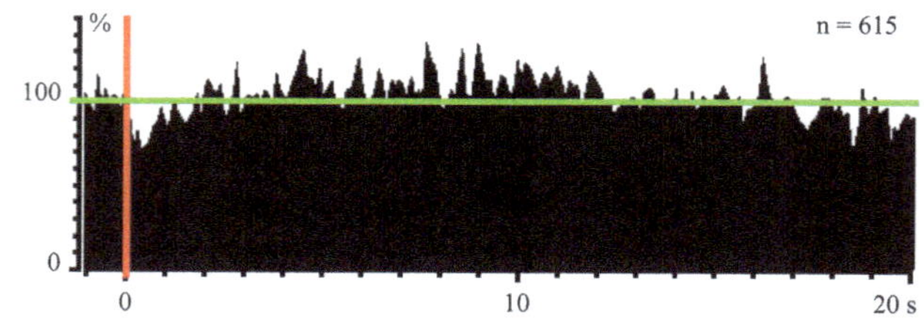

FIGURE 4 | Population response of 61 neurons (615 trials) in monkey's cortical visual area V4 to magnetic stimulation of stomach during SWS. Vertical red line–moment of stimulation. Horizontal green line indicate mean background firing rate before stimulation taken as 100%. Technical details of the study in Pigarev et al. (2008).

EXPERIMENTAL VALIDATION OF THE VISCERAL HYPOTHESIS OF SLEEP

First of all, to check this hypothesis responses of different cortical regions to extero- and interoceptive stimulation during sleep and wakefulness were compared. These experiments were started from the visual cortical areas. Visual areas were selected for these experiments because they were well studied, and it was generally recognized that in behaviorally awake animals neurons of these areas were responding exclusively to visual stimulation. In addition, one of us (Ivan N. Pigarev) had considerable experience in investigation of various visual areas in behaviorally awake animals. Later, similar experiments were conducted with neurons not only in occipital, but also in frontal and parietal cortical areas.

In **Figure 3** (adopted from Pigarev, 1994; Pigarev and Pigareva, 2012) we show responses of complex neurons in visual cortical area V1 (**panel A**) and somatosensory area 5 (**panel B**) of cats to electrical intraperitoneal stimulation delivered in SWS and in wakefulness. These neurons in the state of wakefulness responded to visual and somatosensory stimuli respectively. During SWS both neurons responded to electrical stimulation of the area of the small intestine, and these apparent responses immediately disappeared in REM sleep and after awakening.

Similar experiments were conducted with monkeys, where evoked responses to intraperitoneal electrical stimulation were recorded above the cortical visual area V1 (Pigarev et al., 2006). Evoked responses were again obtained only during SWS, and disappeared during REM sleep and in the state of wakefulness.

In experiments with one monkey we used magnetic stimulation, with the coil located close to the surface of the monkey's stomach. In response to magnetic pulses, which did not wake the animal, we obtained cortical evoked responses, recorded by the electrodes above the occipital pole of the skull. These responses were observed again only during SWS (Pigarev et al., 2008). Simultaneous recording of the neuronal activity in the visual area V4 revealed a strong short latency inhibition in response to these magnetic pulses, which was obviously visible even in the population response of 61 neurons (**Figure 4**). After this short latency inhibition, the delayed (5–15 s) activation of the background firing took place. This result deserves attention because receptive fields in area V4 had small excitatory areas and huge inhibitory surrounds. The applied magnetic pulses could activate those parts of visceral organs, which projected to this huge inhibitory periphery of the studied receptive fields. On the other hand, after some delay, peristaltic waves provoked by the stimulation could reach regions, which projected to the central excitatory part of the receptive fields, causing the observed delayed activation. All these responses to magnetic stimulation again disappeared in wakefulness.

In experiments with rabbits (Pigarev et al., 2004), we also recorded evoked responses to electrical intraperitoneal stimulation in visual and somatosensory cortical areas, which appeared again exclusively during SWS.

It has been argued that electrical and magnetic stimuli are not natural, and that observed effects could have a non-specific origin. Although the main information concerning organization of the nervous system was obtained using electrical stimulation, it would be much more important to demonstrate a functional link between visceral organs and cortical areas during sleep in natural conditions, without any artificial stimulation.

Such experiments were conducted with the help of our colleagues from the Pavlov Institute of Physiology (St. Petersburg), prof. V. A. Bagaev and I. I. Busigina. Recording electrodes were implanted in the walls of the small intestine and stomach of cats, together with stomach fistula. With this approach, in addition to cortical neuronal activity, EEG, and ocular movements we could record myoelectrical activity of small intestine and stomach, and to change intragastric contents.

In **Figure 5** we present a spectrogram of cat cortical EEG (A) recorded simultaneously with myoelectrical activity of the stomach (B) during an episode of SWS. In the spectrogram, yellow colors indicate higher power, and periodic vertical blue fragments indicate moments of short desynchronizations connected with lack of low frequency components. These desynchronized intervals are well known to anybody who has recorded EEG during SWS. It was previously demonstrated (Oniani et al., 1974) that, behaviorally, sleep was not interrupted during these periods, and thresholds for awakening during such short desynchronizations still were very high. What was new in the presented figure was a surprising coincidence of these EEG desynchronizations with the appearance of periodic migrating myoelectrical complexes in the stomach (short vertical inclinations in B). There was no need for any special analysis in order to notice such coincidence. Simultaneous appearance of the migrating myoelectrical complexes in stomach activity and short desynchronizations in the cortical EEG usually happened during intervals of 10–20 min of SWS. The observed coincidence of these effects can disappear for a while and appear again later. This was a very robust effect, observed in most of our sleep recordings, which included the periods of corresponding stomach activity.

More impressive were results of those experiments where we have studied interaction of the neuronal activity in various cortical visual areas and myoelectrical activity from the wall of the duodenum (Pigarev et al., 2013). It was demonstrated that about one third of more than 200 of the studied cortical neurons during SWS established a causal relationship with the activity of the duodenum during SWS. Even more, these neurons demonstrated selectivity to particular types of duodenal rhythmicity. Some neurons preferred simple duodenal waves, and others responded only to waves with spike potentials. Such a relationship was never observed in wakefulness.

Finally it was found that changes of the intragastric medium (water infusion via fistula into the stomach) performed in the period of SWS lead to changes in the EEG pattern and temporal reorganization of the background neuronal spiking, revealed by Fano factor analysis (Pigarev et al., 2010).

We do not imply that only the structures of the digestive system are represented in the cerebral cortex during sleep. In other experiments we recorded evoked responses to heartbeats during sleep (Pigarev and Feodorov, 2012). An example of neuronal firing and local field potentials in the visual area V1, which synchronized with respiration during SWS, is shown in **Figure 6**. Dr. M. Lebedev, during experiments with monkeys under anesthesia, also observed unexpected neuronal activity synchronized with respiration in somatosensory cortical areas within the representation of the hind paw (personal communication).

THE VISCERAL SLEEP THEORY AND OBSERVATIONS OF "SLOW WAVE" ACTIVITY IN THE CORTICAL SLABS AND SLICES

According to the visceral sleep theory, patterns of periodic activation coming from the visceral organs determine the oscillating picture of cortical activity during SWS. The desynchronized pattern of cortical EEG during REM sleep can be connected with afferentation coming to the cerebral cortex from visceral systems lacking obvious rhythmic activity, e.g., liver, kidneys, reproductive organs and, finally, the brain itself. The brain's status within this theory is obviously dual. On the one hand, the brain is the central processor which controls behavior in the environment during wakefulness and defines recovery of all visceral organs during sleep. However, on the other hand, the brain itself is an enormously complicated visceral organ, which certainly should be in need of service. How and when such brain self-service is realized is a challenging question. It may happen, for example, during particular phases of REM or SWS, or it may be organized as a permanent service, e.g., by glial cells. The recently discovered "glymphatic" mechanism may reflect elements of such brain self-servicing (Nedergaard, 2013; Xie et al., 2013). Various other options can be offered, but that is a topic for future studies.

Our approach to sleep function supposes that cortical activity during sleep is defined by the afferent flow coming to the cerebral cortex from various visceral organs. On the other hand, there is substantial evidence that sleep-like activity can be generated in cortical slabs (Timofeev et al., 2000) and isolated cortical slices (Sanchez-Vives and McCormick, 2000) without any interoceptive inputs. However, we do not think that these observations are inconsistent with our theoretical proposal. Of relevance is the

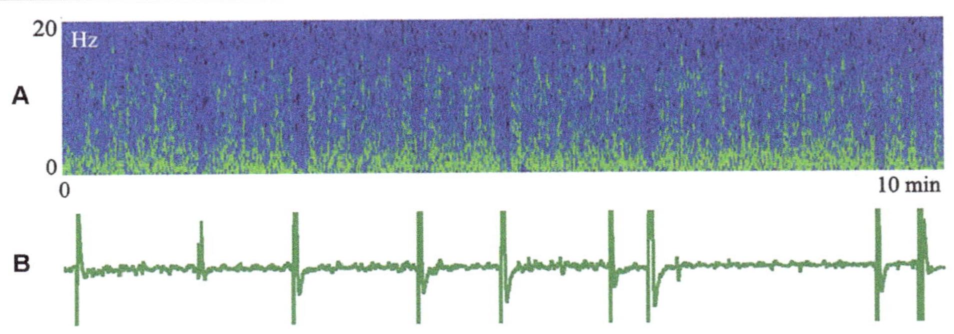

FIGURE 5 | Episode of SWS. (A) Spectrogram of the cat cortical EEG. Yellow color indicates higher power. **(B)** Myoelectrical activity of stomach. Technical details of the study in Pigarev et al. (2013).

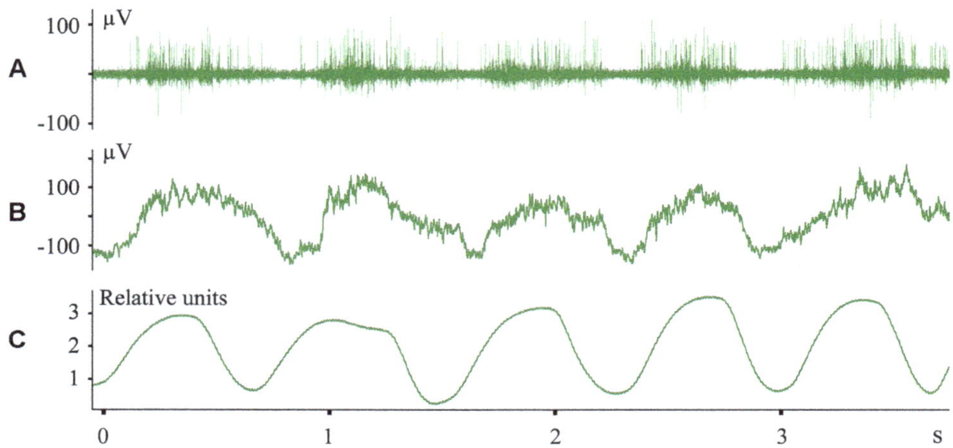

FIGURE 6 | Neuronal activity in the cat primary visual cortex synchronized with respiration during SWS. (A) Multiunit activity; **(B)** local field potentials (local EEG); **(C)** nasal air flow in relative units. Technical details of the study in Pigarev et al. (2013).

important discovery of Steriade et al. (2001), who performed the first intracellular recordings of neuronal cortical activity in naturally sleeping cats. They found that waves of hyperpolarization reflected as periodic silent pauses in neuronal firing during SWS were connected not with active inhibition, but with disfacilitation caused by the lack of excitatory inputs to these cortical neurons. At the time of their study it was generally recognized that, during sleep, the cerebral cortex was disconnected from any afferent inputs, and they had to conclude that, "during SWS, neocortical neurons may be engaged in information processing of internally generated signals...", which provided such excitatory inputs. As a source of such "internally generated signals" they considered intracortical excitation (Steriade et al., 2001).

The studies performed on the isolated cortical slices demonstrated that, in certain conditions, it was possible to evoke periodic neuronal discharges, which had some features of similarity with real SWS oscillations. Later it was shown in experiments on thalamo-cortical slices that activation of the thalamo-cortical neurons dominates in triggering such cortical oscillations (Contreras and Steriade, 1995; Rigas and Castro-Alamancos, 2007). In a review (Crunelli and Hughes, 2010) it was recognized that most likely several mechanisms might elicit the cortical slow waves. We propose that "internally generated signals", which define cortical waves during SWS, are actually coming from various visceral systems using the same thalamo-cortical pathways, which activate cortical neurons during wakefulness.

THE PATHWAYS FOR THE VISCERAL AFFERENTATION TO THE CEREBRAL CORTEX DURING SLEEP

One may inquire about the ways by which the information from various visceral systems may reach "the same thalamo-cortical pathways". For the somatosensory system it is well investigated. It is known since early anatomical studies in the 19th century (Head, 1896), that visceral and somatosensory afferents terminate at the same neurons in the spinal cord, and thus visceral information may travel to the cerebral cortex through the fibers of the somatosensory columns. The fact of such combined projections was confirmed in many studies (e.g., Kuo et al., 1981; Cervero, 1983; Cervero et al., 1984; Akeyson and Schramm, 1994; Perry and Lawson, 1998) and this overlap is regarded as the most probable mechanism of the referred pains (Head, 1896; Arendt-Nielsen and Svensson, 2001; Peles et al., 2004; Hobson et al., 2010).

However, this overlap created a yet unresolved problem–how the central nervous system manages to distinguish spikes coming by a single fiber from so different sources. Our hypothesis offers a solution to this problem. The transmission of the somatosensory information happens during wakefulness, while visceral information is transmitted to the central nervous system during sleep, when muscles are relaxed and movements are excluded.

To our knowledge, pathways of the visceral information to the visual cortical areas have never been investigated. Here we offer only some considerations. It is well known that, in the main thalamic visual relay (lateral geniculate nucleus), retinal synaptic terminals form only one third of all synaptic terminals. Another third of terminals belong to backward cortico-thalamic projections. The remaining one third of terminals is of non-visual origin, and come from the pontine and the brain stem regions (Hughes and Mullikin, 1984). Activation from pontine nuclei reaches the lateral geniculate nucleus during sleep, especially during REM sleep, and reflects in the visual cortical areas as well known ponto-geniculo-occipital waves (Brooks and Bizzi, 1963). The origin of this pontine activity has not yet been investigated. On the other hand, pontine and brain stem projections to the lateral geniculate nucleus come from the regions of entering and passage of various visceral nerves. Therefore, their link with visceral information is very probable.

K-COMPLEXES AND VISCERAL AFFERENTATION, USE DEPENDENCY AND SLEEP HOMEOSTASIS

In discussions of cortical visceral activation during sleep, one often argues that these visceral responses can be of nonspecific origin, resembling sensory-triggered K-complexes. This topic was investigated in detail in our special study (Pigarev et al., 2011). It was shown that visually induced K-complexes had absolutely specific origin. Even more, K-complexes could be induced by sensory stimuli only during short intervals of developing sleep. In contrast, cortical visceral responses could be recorded during periods of deep SWS, when K-complexes could not be induced by any sensory stimulation. In addition, we presented arguments indicating that visually induced K-complexes were also of visceral origin.

The attempts to link various visceral events with the elements of EEG recorded during sleep, e.g., K-complexes, has been undertaken in many studies (Pampiglione and Ackner, 1958; Johnson and Karpan, 1968; Halász et al., 1985; Heald et al., 1989; Hornyak et al., 1991; Okada et al., 1991; Niiyama et al., 1996; Monstad and Guilleminault, 1999; Tank et al., 2003). The same idea was expressed in a study of Cash et al. (2009), where it was suggested that spontaneous K-complexes appearing in the EEG during transition from wakefulness to sleep could be induced by a "sensory stimulus occult to the investigator (e.g., gastric)".

In the middle of the previous century, cortical responses to the stimulation of various visceral nerves were described and intensively investigated in several laboratories (e.g., Bailey and Bremer, 1938; Amassian, 1951; Patton and Amassian, 1952; Gardner et al., 1955; Chernigovskiy, 1960). These studies were performed in acute experiments under anesthesia. However, in later experiments without anesthesia, these results could not be reproduced. In wakefulness, neurons in these areas responded only to visual or somatosensory stimulation. Thus, cortical responses to visceral stimulation were regarded as probable artifacts of anesthesia.

In our studies we have demonstrated that without any anesthesia, in natural conditions, cortical areas do establish connections with visceral organs, but this link is functionally active only during sleep. Involvement of the highest levels of the central nervous system, up to the cerebral cortex in mammals, in the processing of visceral information during periods of sleep may be the main, if not the exclusive, function of sleep.

Here we should come back to the above-mentioned effect of "use dependency", which is widely explored now as an experimental argument in favor of the concepts that sleep is necessary for brain recovery (Kattler et al., 1994; Rector et al., 2005; Huber et al., 2006). This effect can also be explained by the visceral sleep theory. High activation of some cortical areas by intensive exteroceptive stimulation during wakefulness will lower the neuronal thresholds of the neurons in these areas (e.g., due to the LTP mechanism). As a result, during sleep, these neurons will respond more strongly to visceral stimulation, coming to the same neurons through the same synaptic connections. Consequently the δ-power of the EEG will grow.

Discussing the visceral sleep theory we would like to draw attention to the distinguished theory of A. Borbély—the two-process model of sleep regulation (Borbély, 1982; Borbély and Achermann, 1999). This model proposes that sleep is regulated by the interaction of two processes—homeostatic and circadian. The homeostatic process allows for a constant amount of sleep during 24 h. Visceral sleep theory offers the physiological framework of this homeostatic mechanism. Homeostasis of all visceral systems is supported during sleep due to the involvement of all the cerebral cortex in the processing of information from internal organs. These informational processes define the total length of sleep.

MECHANISM OF SLEEP INITIATION AND FEATURES OF LOCAL SLEEP

The visceral sleep theory explains the logic behind the initiation of sleep. Indeed, a mismatch between the current parameters of any visceral system and the genetically determined range for these parameters would provide the feeling of tiredness, or sleep pressure. If an environmental situation allows sleep, an organism would transit to normal total sleep in all cortical areas. Actually the chain of events for sleep initiation is more complicated. Evaluation of the visceral problems may need engagement of the mechanisms of emotions and such structures as hippocampus, amygdala and prefrontal cortex. All those questions were discussed in our recent article (Pigarev and Pigareva, 2013), and we will not continue this topic here. Now we would like to go back to the phenomenon of local sleep and to discuss it within the frame of the presented visceral sleep theory.

In the cases when, because of visceral problems, the need for sleep is dramatically increased, but environmental conditions do not allow sleep to occur, sleep may progress only in some cortical areas in still behaviorally active organisms. According to the information cited above, the development of sleep starts from the most recent, "high order" cortical areas. The proportion of such areas is highest in the frontal pole of the brain. This might underlie the reported fronto-occipital trend in the development of sleep.

It is logical to propose that those behavioral tasks, which do not need engagement of the highest cortical resources would be normally realized even in conditions when part of the brain is sleeping. However, in the situation when all cortical computational ability is required for decision making in a complicated problem, local sleep may lead to severe and often dramatic behavioral errors.

Conditions of local sleep development indicate that local sleep is very probable when it is necessary to remain awake during periods of high (natural) sleep pressure. For humans this might happen during work at the time of the maximal sleepiness. For rats, local sleep can accompany experiments during the light phase of the day, if the rats are caged in animal houses with non-inverted conditions of illumination.

People with habitual or forced short length of night sleep are at permanent risk of partial sleep development. For some professions partial sleep provoked by such chronic sleep deprivation may not cause any troubles. However, for professions connected with responsible and complex decision making, especially during night shifts, the dangerous consequences of local sleep are very high. For these professions, any visceral disorders, especially in the gastro-intestinal system, may dramatically increase the risk of wrong decisions.

Besides the negative effects of partial sleep for mental ability due to the disengagement of some cortical areas from the intellectual work, one should also not neglect the possible negative consequences of this phenomenon for the visceral health of an organism. As participation of all cortical areas in information processing is essential for the efficient solution of complex problems in wakefulness, for efficient management of visceral systems, all cortical areas should be involved into the processing of visceral information. Appearance of local sleep during wakefulness means that the length of total sleep during the nighttime was not sufficient, and may indicate hidden problems in some visceral systems.

CONCLUSION

The detailed investigation of brain involvement in the regulation of the various visceral systems during sleep is a goal for further studies. At present, following the visceral theory of sleep, we can state that efficient and sufficient sleep, together with visceral health, might be the cheapest, safest and most pleasant way to augment brain function.

AUTHOR CONTRIBUTIONS

Both co-authors have equal contribution to all steps of preparation of this article and both approved the version to be published.

ACKNOWLEDGMENTS

We are very thankful to Dr. Denys Garden for critical reading of the manuscript and many helpful comments. The study was supported by Russian Foundation for Basic Researches grants 13-04-00941 and 13-04-00741.

REFERENCES

Akerstedt, T., Philip, P., Capelli, A., and Kecklun, G. (2011). Sleep loss and accidents–work hours, life style and sleep pathology. *Prog. Brain Res.* 190, 169–188. doi: 10.1016/b978-0-444-53817-8.00011-6

Akeyson, E. W., and Schramm, L. P. (1994). Splanchnic and somatic afferent convergence on cervical spinal neurons of the rat. *Am. J. Physiol.* 266(Suppl. 1), R268–R276.

Amassian, V. E. (1951). Cortical representation of visceral afferents. *J. Neurophysiol.* 14, 435–446.

Arendt-Nielsen, L., and Svensson, P. (2001). Referred muscle pain: basic and clinical findings. *Clin. J. Pain* 17, 11–19. doi: 10.1097/00002508-200103000-00003

Bailey, P., and Bremer, F. (1938). A sensory cortical representation of the vagus nerve. With a note on the effects of low blood pressure on the cortical electrogramm. *J. Neurophysiol.* 1, 405–414.

Barger, L. K., Ayas, N. T., Cade, B. E., Cronin, J. W., Rosner, B., Speizer, F. E., et al. (2006). Impact of extended-duration shifts on medical errors, adverse events and attentional failures. *PLoS Med.* 3:e487. doi: 10.1371/journal.pmed.0030487

Borbély, A. A., and Achermann, P. (1999). Sleep homeostasis and models of sleep regulation. *J. Biol. Rhythms* 14, 557–568.

Borbély, A. A. (1982). A two process model of sleep regulation. *Hum. Neurobiol.* 1, 195–204. doi: 10.1007/978-3-540-29678-2_6166

Borich, M., Furlong, M., Holsman, D., and Kimberley, T. J. (2011). Goal-directed visuomotor skill learning: off-line enhancement and the importance of the primary motor cortex. *Restor. Neurol. Neurosci.* 29, 105–113. doi: 10.3233/RNN-2011-0584

Borich, M. R., and Kimberley, T. J. (2011). Both sleep and wakefulness support consolidation of continuous, goal-directed, visuomotor skill. *Exp. Brain Res.* 214, 619–630. doi: 10.1007/s00221-011-2863-0

Born, J., Rasch, B., and Gais, S. (2006). Sleep to remember. *Neuroscientist* 12, 410–424. doi: 10.1177/1073858406292647

Brooks, D. C., and Bizzi, E. (1963). Brain stem electrical activity during deep sleep. *Arch. Ital. Biol.* 101, 648–665.

Cajochen, C., Foy, R., and Dijk, D. J. (1999). Frontal predominance of a relative increase in sleep delta and theta EEG activity after sleep loss in humans. *Sleep Res. Online* 2, 65–69.

Cash, S. S., Halgren, E., Dehghani, N., Rossetti, A. O., Thesen, T., Wang, C., et al. (2009). The human K-complex represents an isolated cortical down-state. *Science* 324, 1084–1087. doi: 10.1126/science.1169626

Cervero, F. (1983). Somatic and visceral inputs to the thoracic spinal cord of the cat: effects of noxious stimulation of the biliary system. *J. Physiol.* 337, 51–67.

Cervero, F., Connell, L. A., and Lawson, S. N. (1984). Somatic and visceral primary afferents in the lower thoracic dorsal root ganglia of the cat. *J. Comp. Neurol.* 228, 422–431. doi: 10.1002/cne.902280309

Chee, M. W., Tan, J. C., Zheng, H., Parimal, S., Weissman, D. H., Zagorodnov, V., et al. (2008). Lapsing during sleep deprivation is associated with distributed changes in brain activation. *J. Neurosci.* 28, 5519–5528. doi: 10.1523/jneurosci.0733-08.2008

Chernigovskiy, V. N. (1960). *Interoceptors.* Moscow: Medgiz. 650.

Chuah, L. Y., and Chee, M. W. (2008). Cholinergic augmentation modulates visual task performance in sleep-deprived young adults. *J. Neurosci.* 28, 11369–11377. doi: 10.1523/jneurosci.4045-08.2008

Cirelli, C., Shaw, P. J., Rechtschaffen, A., and Tononi, G. (1999). No evidence of brain cell degeneration after long-term sleep deprivation in rats. *Brain Res.* 840, 184–193. doi: 10.1016/s0006-8993(99)01768-0

Cohen, D. A., Pascual-Leone, A., Press, D. Z., and Robertson, E. M. (2005). Off-line learning of motor skill memory: a double dissociation of goal and movement. *Proc. Nat. Acad. Sci. U S A* 102, 18237–18241. doi: 10.1073/pnas.0506072102

Cohen, D. A., and Robertson, E. M. (2007). Motor sequence consolidation: constrained by critical time windows or competing components. *Exp. Brain Res.* 177, 440–446. doi: 10.1007/s00221-006-0701-6

Contreras, D., and Steriade, M. (1995). Cellular basis of EEG slow rhythms: a study of dynamic cortico-thalamic relationships. *J. Neurosci.* 15, 604–622.

Criscimagna-Hemminger, S. E., and Shadmehr, R. (2008). Consolidation patterns of human motor memory. *J. Neurosci.* 28, 9610–9618. doi: 10.1523/jneurosci.3071-08.2008

Crunelli, V., and Hughes, S. W. (2010). The slow (<1 Hz) rhythm of non-REM sleep: a dialogue between three cardinal oscillators. *Nat. Neurosci.* 13, 9–17. doi: 10.1038/nn.2445

Debas, K., Carrier, J., Orban, P., Barakat, M., Lungu, O., Vandewalle, G., et al. (2010). Brain plasticity related to the consolidation of motor sequence learning and motor adaptation. *Proc. Natl. Acad. Sci. U S A* 107, 17839–17844. doi: 10.1073/pnas.1013176107

Diekelmann, S., and Born, J. (2010). The memory function of sleep. *Nat. Rev. Neurosci.* 11, 114–126. doi: 10.1038/nrn2762

Diekelmann, S., Biggel, S., Rasch, B., and Born, J. (2012). Offline consolidation of memory varies with time in slow wave sleep and can be accelerated by cuing memory reactivations. *Neurobiol. Learn. Mem.* 98, 103–111. doi: 10.1016/j.nlm.2012.07.002

Diekelmann, S., Büchel, C., Born, J., and Rasch, B. (2011). Labile or stable: opposing consequences for memory when reactivated during waking and sleep. *Nat. Neurosci.* 14, 381–386. doi: 10.1038/nn.2744

Diekelmann, S., Wilhelm, I., Wagner, U., and Born, J. (2013). Sleep to implement an intention. *Sleep* 36, 149–153. doi: 10.5665/sleep.2322

Dinges, D. F. (1995). An overview of sleepiness and accidents. *J. Sleep Res.* 4, 4–14. doi: 10.1111/j.1365-2869.1995.tb00220.x

Dinges, D. F., Pack, F., Williams, K., Gillen, K. A., Powell, J. W., Ott, G. E., et al. (1997). Cumulative sleepiness, mood disturbance and psychomotor vigilance performance decrements during a week of sleep restricted to 4–5 hours per night. *Sleep* 20, 267–277.

Doyon, J., Korman, M., Morin, A., Dostie, V., Hadj Tahar, A., Benali, H., et al. (2009). Contribution of night and day sleep vs. simple passage of time to the consolidation of motor sequence and visuomotor adaptation learning. *Exp. Brain Res.* 195, 15–26. doi: 10.1007/s00221-009-1748-y

Drummond, S. P., Brown, G. G., Salamat, J. S., and Gillin, J. C. (2004). Increasing task difficulty facilitates the cerebral compensatory response to total sleep deprivation. *Sleep* 27, 445–451.

Drummond, S. P. A., Gillin, J. C., and Brown, G. G. (2001). Increased cerebral response during divided attention task following sleep deprivation. *J. Sleep Res.* 10, 85–92. doi: 10.1046/j.1365-2869.2001.00245.x

Empson, J. A. C., and Clarke, P. (1970). Rapid eye movements and remembering. *Nature* 227, 287–288. doi: 10.1038/227287a0

Everson, C. A., Bergmann, B. M., and Rechtschaffen, A. (1989). Sleep deprivation in the rat. III. Total sleep deprivation. *Sleep* 12, 13–21.

Ferrara, M., and De Gennaro, L. (2011). Going local: insights from EEG and stereo-EEG studies of the human sleep-wake cycle. *Curr. Top. Med. Chem.* 11, 2423–2437. doi: 10.2174/156802611797470268

Fowler, M., Sullivan, M., and Ekstrand, B. (1973). Sleep and memory. *Science* 179, 302–304. doi: 10.1126/science.179.4070.302

Gardner, E. D., Thomas, L. M., and Morin, F. (1955). Cortical projections of fast visceral afferents in the cat and monkey. *Am. J. Physiol.* 183, 438–444.

Genzel, L., Dresler, M., Wehrle, R., Grözinger, M., and Steiger, A. (2009). Slow wave sleep and REM sleep awakenings do not affect sleep dependent memory consolidation. *Sleep* 32, 302–310

Glass, B. D., Maddox, W. T., Bowen, C., Savarie, Z. R., Mattews, M. D., Markman, A. B., et al. (2011). The effects of 24-hour sleep deprivation on the exploration-exploitation trade-off. *Biol. Rhythm Res.* 42, 99–110. doi: 10.1080/09291011003726532

Halász, P., Pál, I., and Rajna, P. (1985). K-complex formation of the EEG in sleep. A survey and new examinations. *Acta Physiol. Hung.* 65, 3–35.

Harrison, Y., and Horne, J. A. (2000). The impact of sleep deprivation on decision making: a review. *J. Exp. Psychol. Appl.* 6, 236–249. doi: 10.1037/1076-898x.6.3.236

Head, H. (1896). On disturbances of sensation with especial reference to the pain of visceral disease. *Brain* 19, 211–276. doi: 10.1093/brain/19.2-3.153

Heald, S., Siebers, R. W., and Maling, T. J. (1989). K-complex vasoconstrictor response: evidence for central vasomotor downregulation in borderline hypertension. *J. Hypertens. Suppl.* 7, S28–S29. doi: 10.1097/00004872-198900076-00011

Hobson, A. R., Chizh, B., Hicks, K., Aziz, Q., Worthen, S., Lawrence, P., et al. (2010). Neurophysiological evaluation of convergent afferents innervating the human esophagus and area of referred pain on the anterior chest wall. *Am. J. Physiol. Gastrointest. Liver Physiol.* 298, G31–G36. doi 10.1152/ajpgi.00288.2009

Hornung, O. P., Regen, F., Danker-Hopfe, H., Schredl, M., and Heuser, I. (2007). The relationship between REM sleep and memory consolidation in old age and effects of cholinergic medication. *Biol. Psychiatry* 61, 750–757. doi: 10.1016/j.biopsych.2006.08.034

Hornyak, M., Cejnar, M., Elam, M., Matousek, M., and Wallin, B. G. (1991). Sympathetic muscle nerve activity during sleep in man. *Brain* 114, 1281–1295. doi: 10.1093/brain/114.3.1281

Huber, R., Ghilardi, M. F., Massimini, M., Ferrarelli, F., Riedner, B. A., Peterson, M. J., et al. (2006). Arm immobilization causes cortical plastic changes and locally decreases sleep slow wave activity. *Nat. Neurosci.* 9, 1169–1176. doi: 10.1038/nn1758

Hughes, H. C., and Mullikin, W. H. (1984). Brainstem afferents to the lateral geniculate nucleus of the cat. *Exp. Brain Res.* 54, 253–258. doi: 10 1007/bf00236224

Johnson, L. C., and Karpan, W. E. (1968). Autonomic correlates of the spontaneous K-complex. *Psychophysiology* 4, 444–452. doi: 10.1111/j.1469-8986.1968.tb02785.x

Kattler, H., Dijk, D. J., and Borbély, A. A. (1994). Effect of unilateral somatosensory stimulation prior to sleep on the sleep EEG in humans. *J. Sleep Res.* 3, 159–164. doi: 10.1111/j.1365-2869.1994.tb00123.x

Keisler, A., Ashe, J., and Willingham, D. T. (2007). Time of day accounts for overnight improvement in sequence learning. *Learn. Mem.* 14, 669–672. doi: 10.1101/lm.751807

Krueger, J. M., and Obál, F. (1993). A neuronal group theory of sleep function. *J. Sleep Res.* 2, 63–69. doi: 10.1111/j.1365-2869.1993.tb00064.x

Krueger, J. M., Rector, D. M., Roy, S., Van Dongen, H. P., Belenky, G., and Panksepp, J. (2008). Sleep as a fundamental property of neuronal assemblies. *Nat. Rev. Neurosci.* 9, 910–919. doi: 10.1038/nrn2521

Kuo, D. C., Krauthamer, G. M., and Yamasaki, D. S. (1981). The organization of visceral sensory neurons in thoracic dorsal root ganglia (DRG) of the cat studied by horseradish peroxidase (HRP) reaction using the cryostat. *Brain Res.* 208, 187–191. doi: 10.1016/0006-8993(81)90630-2

Lo, J. C., Groeger, J. A., Santhi, N., Arbon, E. L., Lazar, A. S., Hasan, S., et al. (2012). Effects of partial and acute total sleep deprivation on performance across cognitive domains, individuals and circadian phase. *PLoS One* 7:e45987. doi: 10.1371/journal.pone.0045987

Maddox, W. T., Glass, B. D., Wolosin, S. M., Savarie, Z. R., Bowen, C., Matthews, M. D., et al. (2009). The effects of sleep deprivation on information-integration categorization performance. *Sleep* 32, 1439–1448.

Mander, B. A., Santhanam, S., Saletin, J. M., and Walker, M. P. (2011). Wake deterioration and sleep restoration of human learning. *Curr. Biol.* 21, R183–R184. doi: 10.1016/j.cub.2011.01.019

Maquet, P. (2001). The role of sleep in learning and memory. *Science* 294, 1048–1052. doi: 10.1126/science.1062856

McCoyand, G., and Strecker, R. E. (2011). The cognitive cost of sleep lost. *Neurobiol. Learn. Mem.* 96, 564–582. doi: 10.1016/j.nlm.2011.07.004

McDermott, C. M., LaHoste, G. J., Chen, C., Musto, A., Bazan, N. G., and Magee, J. C. (2003). Sleep deprivation causes behavioral, synaptic and membrane excitability alterations in hippocampal neurons. *J. Neurosci.* 23, 9687–9695.

Mitler, M. M., Carskadon, M. A., Czeisler, C. A., Dement, W. C., Dinges, D. F., and Graeber, R. C. (1988). Catastrophes, sleep, and public policy: consensus report. *Sleep* 11, 100–109.

Monstad, P., and Guilleminault, C. (1999). Cardiovascular changes associated with spontaneous and evoked K-complexes. *Neurosci. Lett.* 263, 211–213. doi: 10.1016/s0304-3940(99)00142-1

Mukhametov, L. M. (1984). Sleep in marine mammals. *Exp. Brain Res.* 8, 227–238. doi: 10.1007/978-3-642-69554-4_17

Mukhametov, L. M., Supin, A. Y., and Polyakova, I. G. (1977). Interhemispheric asymmetry of the electroencephalographic sleep patterns in dolphins. *Brain Res.* 134, 581–584. doi: 10.1016/0006-8993(77)90835-6

Nedergaard, M. (2013). Garbage truck of the brain. *Science* 340, 1529–1530. doi: 10.1126/science.1240514

Niiyama, Y., Sato, N., Katsuzava, O., and Hishikawa, Y. (1996). Electrophysiological evidence suggesting that sensory stimuli of unknown origin induced spontaneous K-complexes. *Electroencephalogr. Clin. Neurophysiol.* 98, 394–400. doi: 10.1016/0013-4694(96)95103-2

Okada, H., Iwase, S., Mano, T., Sugiyama, Y., and Watanabe, T. (1991). Changes in muscle sympathetic nerve activity during sleep in humans. *Neurology* 41, 1961–1966. doi: 10.1212/wnl.41.12.1961

Oniani, T. N., Koridze, M. G., Kavkasidze, M. G., and Gvetadze, L. B. (1974). "The dynamics in excitability of various brain structures during different phases of wakefulness-sleep cycle," in *Neirofiziologia Emotsii I Tsikla Bodrstvovanie-Son*, ed T. N. Oniani (Tbilisi: Metsniereba), 120–159.

Pampiglione, G., and Ackner, B. (1958). The effects of repeated stimuli upon EEG and vasomotor activity during sleep in man. *Brain* 81, 64–74. doi: 10.1093/brain/81.1.64

Patton, H. D., and Amassian, V. E. (1952). Cortical projection zone of chorda tympany nerve in cat. *J. Neurophysiol.* 15, 245–254.

Peles, S. H., Miranda, A., Shaker, R., and Sengupta, J. N. (2004). Acute nociceptive somatic stimulus sensitizes neurones in the spinal cord to colonic distension in the rat. *J. Physiol.* 560, 291–302. doi: 10.1113/jphysiol.2004.069070

Perry, M. J., and Lawson, S. N. (1998). Differences in expression of oligosaccharides, neuropeptides, carbonic anhydrase and neurofilament in rat primary afferent neurons retrogradely labelled via skin, muscle or visceral nerves. *Neuroscience* 85, 293–310. doi: 10.1016/s0306-4522(97)00629-5

Pigarev, I. N., Almirall, H., Marimon, J., and Pigareva, M. L. (2004). Dynamic pattern of the viscero-cortical projections during sleep. Study in New Zealand rabbits. *J. Sleep Res.* 13(Suppl. 1), 574–575.

Pigarev, I. N. (1984). New visual area on the inferior bank of the cruciate sulcus of the cat brain. *Neirofiziologiia* 16, 766–773.

Pigarev, I. N. (1994). Neurons of visual cortex respond to visceral stimulation during slow wave sleep. *Neuroscience* 62, 1237–1243. doi: 10.1016/0306-4522(94)90355-7

Pigarev, I. N. (1997). Partial sleep in cortical areas. *WFSRS Newsletters* 5, 7–8.

Pigarev, I. N. (2014). The visceral theory of sleep. *Neurosci. Behav. Physiol.* 44, 421–434. doi: 10.1007/s11055-014-9928-z

Pigarev, I. N., Almirall, H., and Pigareva, M. L. (2008). Cortical evoked responses to magnetic stimulation of macaque's abdominal wall in sleep-wake cycle. *Acta Neurobiol. Exp. (Wars)* 68, 91–96.

Pigarev, I. N., Almirall, H., Pigareva, M. L., Bautista, V., Sánchez-Bahillo, A., Barcia, C., et al. (2006). Visceral signals reach visual cortex during slow wave sleep: study in monkeys. *Acta Neurobiol. Exp. (Wars)* 66, 69–73.

Pigarev, I. N., Bagaev, V. A., Busigina, I. I., and Bibikov, N. G. (2010). "The state of sleep – period of the cortical control of the visceral functions," in *The Regulation of Physiological Functions During Adaptation to Environmental Changes*, (St.-Petersburg: I.P. Pavlov Institute of Physiology), 228.

Pigarev, I. N., Bagaev, V. A., Levichkina, E. V., Fedorov, G. O., and Busigina, I. I. (2013). Cortical visual areas process intestinal information during the periods slow-wave sleep. *Neurogastroenterol. Motil.* 25, 268–275, e169. doi: 10.1111/nmo.12052

Pigarev, I. N., Fedorov, G. O., Levichkina, E. V., Marimon, J. M., Pigareva, M. L., and Almirall, H. (2011). Visually triggered K-complexes: a study in New Zealand rabbits. *Exp. Brain Res.* 210, 131–142. doi: 10.1007/s00221-011-2606-2

Pigarev, I. N., and Feodorov, G. O. (2012). "Reflection of the heart beats in the cortical electrical activity during sleep," in *Physiology of the Visceral Systems*, eds E. L. Poliakov and V. N. Shouvaeva (S.-Petersbourg: Pavlov Inst. Physiology Press), 182.

Pigarev, I. N., Nothdurft, H.-Ch., Rodionova, E. I., and Kastner, S. (1996). Asynchronous sleep development in cortical areas. *J. Sleep Res.* 5(Suppl. 1), 176.

Pigarev, I. N., Nothdurft, H.-Ch., and Kastner, S. (1997). Evidence for asynchronous development of sleep in cortical areas. *Neuroreport* 8, 2557–2560. doi: 10.1097/00001756-199707280-00027

Pigarev, I. N., and Pigareva, M. L. (2013). Sleep, emotions and visceral control. *Hum. Physiol.* 39, 590–601. doi: 10.1134/s036211971306008x

Pigarev, I. N., and Pigareva, M. L. (2012). Sleep and control of visceral functions. *Neurosci. Behav. Physiol.* 42, 948–956. doi: 10.1007/s11055-012-9661-4

Plihal, W., and Born, J. (1997). Effects of early and late nocturnal sleep on declarative and procedural memory. *J. Cogn. Neurosci.* 9, 534–547. doi: 10.1162/jocn.1997.9.4.534

Ratcliff, R., and Van Dongen, H. P. A. (2009). Sleep deprivation affects multiple distinct cognitive processes. *Psychon. Bull. Rev.* 16, 742–751. doi: 10.3758/pbr.16.4.742

Rechtshaffen, A., and Bergmann, B. M. (2002). Sleep deprivation in the rat: an update of the 1989 paper. *Sleep* 25, 18–24.

Rector, D. M., Topchiy, I. A., Carter, K. M., and Rojas, M. J. (2005). Local functional state differences between rat cortical columns. *Brain Res.* 1047, 45–55. doi: 10.1016/j.brainres.2005.04.002

Reis, J., Fischer, J. T., Prichard, G., Weiller, C., Cohen, L. G., and Fritsch, B. (2013). Time–but not sleep-dependent consolidation of tDCS-enhanced visuomotor skills. *Cereb. Cortex* doi: 10.4324/9780080473321. [Epub ahead of print].

Rigas, P., and Castro-Alamancos, M. A. (2007). Thalamo-cortical Up states: different effects of intrinsic and extrinsic cortical inputs on persistent activity. *J. Neurosci.* 27, 4261–4272. doi: 10.1523/jneurosci.0003-07.2007

Robertson, E. M., Pascual-Leone, A., and Press, D. Z. (2004). Awareness modifies the skill-learning benefits of sleep. *Curr. Biol.* 14, 208–212. doi: 10.1016/s0960-9822(04)00039-9

Sanchez-Vives, M. V., and McCormick, D. A. (2000). Cellular and network mechanisms of rhythmic recurrent activity in neocortex. *Nat. Neurosci.* 3, 1027–1034. doi: 10.1038/79848

Saxvig, I. W., Lundervold, A. J., Gronli, J., Ursin, R., Bjorvatn, B., and Portas, C. M. (2008). The effect of a REM sleep deprivation procedure on different aspects of memory function in humans. *Psychophysiology* 45, 309–317. doi: 10.1111/j.1469-8986.2007.00623.x

Shadmehr, R., and Brashers-Krug, T. (1997). Functional stages in the formation of human long-term motor memory. *J. Neurosci.* 17, 409–419.

Siengsukon, C. F., and Boyd, L. A. (2008). Sleep enhances implicit motor skill learning in individuals poststroke. *Top. Stroke Rehabil.* 15, 1–12. doi: 10.1310/tsr1501-1

Smith, C. (2001). Sleep states and memory processes in humans: procedural versus declarative memory systems. *Sleep Med. Rev.* 5, 491–506. doi: 10.1053/smrv.2001.0164

Song, S., Howard, J. H., and Howard, D. V. (2007). Sleep does not benefit probabilistic motor sequence learning. *J. Neurosci.* 27, 12475–12483. doi: 10.1523/jneurosci.2062-07.2007

Steriade, M., Timofeev, I., and Grenier, F. (2001). Natural waking and sleep states: a view from inside neocortical neurons. *J. Neurophysiol.* 85, 1969–1985.

Stickgold, R. (2005). Sleep-dependent memory consolidation. *Nature* 437, 1272–1278. doi: 10.1038/nature04286

Tank, J., Diedrich, A., Hale, N., Niaz, F. E., Furlan, R., Robertson, R. M., et al. (2003). Relationship between blood pressure, sleep K-complexes and muscle sympathetic nerve activity in humans. *Am. J. Physiol. Regul. Integr. Comp. Physiol.* 285, R208–R214.

Timofeev, I., Grenier, F., and Bazhenov, M. (2000). Origin of slow cortical oscillations in deafferented cortical slabs. *Cereb. Cortex* 10, 1185–1199. doi: 10.1093/cercor/10.12.1185

Tononi, G., and Cirelli, C. (2003). Sleep and synaptic homeostasis: a hypothesis. *Brain Res. Bull.* 62, 143–150. doi: 10.1016/j.brainresbull.2003.09.004

Tononi, G., and Cirelli, C. (2006). Sleep function and synaptic homeostasis. *Sleep Med. Rev.* 10, 49–62. doi: 10.1016/j.smrv.2005.05.002

Voderholzer, U., Piosczyk, H., Holz, J., Landmann, N., Feige, B., Loessl, B., et al. (2011). Sleep restriction over several days does not affect long-term recall of declarative and procedural memories in adolescents. *Sleep Med.* 12, 170–178. doi: 10.1016/j.sleep.2010.07.017

Vyazovskiy, V. V., Olcese, U., Hanlon, E. C., Nir, Y., Cirelli, C., and Tononi, G. (2011). Local sleep in awake rats. *Nature* 472, 443–447. doi: 10.1038/nature10009

Walker, M. P. (2008). Cognitive consequences of sleep and sleep loss. *Sleep Med.* 9, S29–S34. doi: 10.1016/s1389-9457(08)70014-5

Walker, M. P. (2009). The role of sleep in cognition and emotion. *Ann. N Y Acad. Sci.* 1156, 168–197. doi: 10.1111/j.1749-6632.2009.04416.x

Walker, M. P., and Stickgold, R. (2006). Sleep, memory, and plasticity. *Annu. Rev. Psychol.* 57, 139–166. doi: 10.1146/annurev.psych.56.091103.070307

Werth, E., Achermann, P., and Borbely, A. A. (1996). Brain topography of the human sleep EEG: antero-posterior shifts of spectral power. *Neuroreport* 8, 123–127. doi: 10.1097/00001756-199612200-00025

Werth, E., Achermann, P., and Borbely, A. A. (1997). Fronto-occipital EEG power gradients on human sleep. *J. Sleep Res.* 6, 102–112. doi: 10.1046/j.1365-2869.1997.d01-36.x

Williamson, A. M., Feyer, A., Mattick, R. P., Friswell, R., and Finlay-Brown, S. (2001). Developing measures of fatigue using an alcohol comparison to validate the effects of fatigue on performance. *Accid. Anal. Prev.* 33, 313–326. doi: 10.1016/s0001-4575(00)00045-2

Xie, L., Kang, H., Xu, Q., Chen, M. J., Liao, Y., Thiyagarajan, M., et al. (2013). Sleep drives metabolite clearance from the adult brain. *Science* 342, 373–377. doi: 10.1126/science.1241224

Yoo, S. S., Hu, P. T., Gujar, N., Jolesz, F. A., and Walker, M. P. (2007). A deficit in the ability to form new human memories without sleep. *Nat. Neurosci.* 10, 385–392. doi: 10.1038/nn1851

19

What do temporal lobe epilepsy and progressive mild cognitive impairment have in common?

Yvonne Höller* and Eugen Trinka

Department of Neurology, Christian Doppler Medical Centre and Centre for Cognitive Neuroscience, Paracelsus Medical University, Salzburg, Austria

Edited by:
Mikhail Lebedev, Duke University, USA

Reviewed by:
João P. Leite, University of São Paulo School of Medicine at Ribeirão Preto, Brazil
Mikhail Lebedev, Duke University, USA
Amara Gul, The Islamia University of Bahawalpur, Pakistan

****Correspondence:***
Yvonne Höller, Department of Neurology, Christian Doppler Medical Centre and Centre for Cognitive Neuroscience, Paracelsus Medical University, Ignaz-Harrer-Str. 79, 5020 Salzburg, Austria
e-mail: yvonne.hoeller@pmu.ac.at

Temporal lobe epilepsy (TLE) and mild cognitive impairment (MCI) are both subject to intensive memory research. Memory problems are a core characteristic of both conditions and we wonder if there are analogies which would enrich the two distinct research communities. In this review we focus on memory decline in both conditions, that is, the most feared psychosocial effect. While it is clear that memory decline in MCI is highly likely and would lead to the more severe diagnosis of Alzheimer's disease, it is a debate if TLE is a dementing disease or not. As such, like for MCI, one can differentiate progressive from stable TLE subtypes, mainly depending on the age of onset. Neuroimaging techniques such as volumetric analysis of the hippocampus, entorhinal, and perirhinal cortex show evidence of pathological changes in TLE and are predictive for memory decline in MCI. Several studies emphasize that it is necessary to extend the region of interest—even whole-brain characteristics can be predictive for conversion from MCI to Alzheimer's disease. Electroencephalography is increasingly subject to computational neuroscience, revealing new approaches for analyzing frequency, spatial synchronization, and information content of the signals. These methods together with event-related designs that assess memory functions are highly promising for understanding the mechanisms of memory decline in both TLE and MCI populations. Finally, there is evidence that the potential of such markers for memory decline is far from being exhausted. Similar structural and neurophysiological characteristics are linked to memory decline in TLE and MCI. We raise the hope that interdisciplinary research and cross-talk between fields such as research on epilepsy and dementia, will shed further light on the dementing characteristics of the pathological basis of MCI and TLE and support the development of new memory enhancing treatment strategies.

Keywords: epilepsy, mild cognitive impairment, subjective cognitive complaints, memory decline, neuroimaging, neurophysiology

1. INTRODUCTION

Memory problems are a core symptom of amnestic mild cognitive impairment (MCI) (Stewart, 2012a), but are also one of the chief complaints of patients with temporal lobe epilepsy (TLE) (Helmstädter, 2002; Butler and Zeman, 2008). Even worse, quality of life is negatively influenced by memory impairment (Fisher et al., 2000). This superficial analogy is not only a possible link between TLE and MCI but can serve as starting point from which researchers in each field may add innovative aspects to their respective research areas. Detection of early prognostic markers of memory deficits in MCI and TLE would obviously pave the way for new therapeutic programs, for memory augmentation, and treatment of memory deficits, possibly reducing the overall prevalence of memory disorders and improving quality of life in these patients (DeKosky and Marek, 2003; Geda, 2012).

Current research endeavors are focused on early diagnosis of MCI and TLE. In the case of MCI it is clear that neuropsychological tests alone are not sufficient, since they are not sensitive enough for patients with subjective complaints and no significant and clinically detectable deficits (Stewart, 2012b). Analogously, electroencephalographic assessment and imaging may lead to dubious findings, or no findings at all, in the epileptogenesis or latency period of epilepsy (Engel et al., 2013). Because of the various aetiologies and pathologic processes that may lead to memory impairment, it is suggested that a combination of several biomarkers is necessary to provide an early diagnosis with reliable prognostic validity (DeKosky and Marek, 2003). In this review, we want to highlight promising biomarkers from a pool of structural and electroencephalographical measures for which prognostic validity was evidenced for one of the two clinical groups with similar cognitive impairments, TLE and MCI. While prediction of memory decline and conversion to Alzheimer's disease is an established field of research, prognosis of memory decline in TLE mainly focuses on the prediction of post-surgical memory impairment and only rarely on the prediction of change over the course of the disorder; in this review, we focus on the latter case. As such, we identify commonalities between the two disorders, which could give rise to new approaches in research.

2. NEUROPSYCHOLOGY AND PROGNOSIS

TLE is most often associated with impaired long-term memory (Hermann et al., 1997). In addition to problematic long-term memory, MCI is especially annoying for patients because of impairment of prospective memory (van den Berg et al., 2012). Patients with epilepsy rank cognitive dysfunction highest among the problems experienced (Fisher et al., 2000). However, in many cases such impairments are not detected by standard neuropsychological tests of memory functions, so that complaints about memory decline commonly mismatch with test performance (Butler and Zeman, 2008). Specifically, standard test intervals ranging from some hours to days are too short to detect impaired long-term memory. Indeed, it is the episodic memory which is affected in TLE (Helmstädter, 2002). In addition, it seems difficult to tell from neuropsychological tests alone if patients are already impaired during encoding or if they just fail to retrieve learned information. Similarly, it is necessary to distinguish free recall of memories from recognition. Thus, research should take into consideration the existence of inter-individual differences with respect to the type of impairment, i.e., encoding or retrieval, recall or recognition, within the specific pathologies.

Epileptic seizures might trigger neurodegenerative changes leading eventually to memory impairments (Helmstädter, 2002; Stefan and Pauli, 2008). However, the question whether TLE is a dementing disease due to seizure activity is under debate (Helmstaedter and Elger, 1999, 2009; Jokeit and Ebner, 1999, 2002; Dodrill, 2004; Elger et al., 2004; Mantoan et al., 2009; Gonzalez et al., 2012). The typical course of epilepsy includes in the early phase a long silent period after the brain insult before recurrent seizures start, which then allows an accurate diagnosis (see Najm et al., 2001, for a review on epidemiology and risk factors). The early evolution is often caused by a structural lesion, that is, the epileptogenic lesion (Rosenow and Lüders, 2001). In fact, memory deficits correlate well with the age of the early precipitating event. This might produce an artificial correlation of memory impairment with the duration of epilepsy (Kaaden and Helmstaedter, 2009). For example, no difference between the extent of memory deficits at the time of the first diagnosis and a 5-year follow up was found (Äikiä et al., 2001), suggesting a non-progressive course of memory deficits in TLE. In fact, Helmstaedter and co-workers found that memory decline which is specific to TLE occurs in childhood and early adolescence, while a further progress of loss of memory functions runs in parallel with normal aging (Helmstaedter and Elger, 2009). On the other hand, deficits are more severe in patients with chronic TLE as compared with newly diagnosed patients (Äikiä et al., 2001). Similarly, there is a correlation between time and severity of memory impairments for patients with long chronic course (>27 years) but only for those with more than 10 secondarily generalized seizures per year, and not for complex-partial seizures (Stefan and Pauli, 2002). There are further studies suggesting that patients with a longer duration of refractory TLE exhibit more severe cognitive impairments (Hattiangady and Shetty, 2008; Stefan and Pauli, 2008; Mantoan et al., 2009). However, a longitudinal study over at least 10 years at the stage of severe, chronic and intractable epilepsy showed that duration has less influence on cognitive decline than what was found in cross-sectional studies (Thompson and Duncan, 2005). Most importantly, in this study it was demonstrated that in refractory epilepsy a high frequency of tonic-clonic seizures was the strongest predictor for cognitive decline. However, it is necessary to disentangle the influence of the underlying causes, such as mitochondrial dysfunction or inflammatory causes from seizure activity (Helmstaedter, 2007). It is obvious that progressive brain diseases, such as a malignant brain tumor, lead to a progressive pathology of memory function and it is therefore important to provide an accurate diagnosis which allows identification of progressive comorbidity.

Epileptic seizures can occur also at the stage of MCI or early Alzheimer's disease (Vossel et al., 2013) and the initial diagnosis of late-onset TLE, more specifically the epileptic amnesic syndrome, can be indicative for development of MCI and Alzheimer's disease (Cretin et al., 2012). Most interestingly, Vossel and coworkers reported that cognitive decline is detectable in patients with amnestic MCI or Alzheimer's disease on average 6.8 (MCI) or 5.5 (Alzheimer's disease) years earlier in the case of comorbid epilepsy (Vossel et al., 2013). It is important to note that epileptic symptoms predated memory symptoms or at least showed up contemporaneously.

Finally, memory deficits in TLE may be caused by clinical or subclinical seizure activity, structural, or other underlying brain pathology, adverse effects of anticonvulsant medication, and psychological mechanisms (Butler and Zeman, 2008; Hermann et al., 2010). Helmstaedter suggests that assessing two types of patients could explain contributory mechanisms of memory decline (Helmstädter, 2002). The first type includes newly diagnosed TLE patients at first presentation, i.e., after experiencing first seizures. The second type includes TLE patients with chronic course and drug resistant seizures. A follow-up measurement of memory performance should help to answer the question whether memory deficits are progressive or not. However, examining newly diagnosed TLE patients is a challenge. After the first or second seizure, a patient is usually not subjected to cost-intensive, extensive examinations, such as long-term video-monitoring which is the gold standard to reliably establish a diagnosis. Instead, in clinical practice an appropriate first line medication is chosen in order to control seizures, even if the type of epilepsy is not fully elucidated. Again, simple and reliable biomarkers to ascertain diagnosis at this early stage are highly warranted. For example, in a large multicenter study, hippocampal T2 hyperintensity and impaired hippocampal growth were found to be an early biomarker for epilepsy after febrile status epilepticus in children (Lewis et al., 2013).

A similar challenge is met by family doctors with respect to MCI. The first examination in primary care needs to reliably distinguish between age-associated memory impairment (Hänninen and Soininen, 1997), subjective memory complaints, and MCI (Stewart, 2012a,b). Classification is performed according to the global deterioration scale for aging and dementia (Reisberg et al., 1982). This scale stages individuals into Level 1, being free of both subjective and objective clinical deficits, Level 2, having subjective deficits only, Level 3, having subtle deficits in cognition and some impairments in executive functioning, affecting complex occupational and social activities, and finally Level 4, having clear deficits in cognition and functioning with reduced performance in instrumental activities of daily life (Gauthier et al., 2006). Thus, patients which present memory complaints in primary care without fulfilling the criteria for MCI are considered to suffer from so-called subjective memory complaints. These complaints are not related to significant deficits on neuropsychological scales but could still be an early form of a neurodegenerative disorder since this diagnosis implies high risk to experience further decline toward MCI (Reisberg et al., 2010). It contrast, it is possible that a patient who is diagnosed as suffering from subjective cognitive complaints has simply detected an age-associated memory impairment, which can be a symptom of normal aging. As such, subjective complaints do not necessarily correlate with progress of decline (Förstl et al., 1995). However, the diagnosis of age-associated memory impairment does not imply that the patient's memory performance is normal (Goldman and Morris, 2001). A normal test-performance can still be seen after a significant decline when the patient's starting level of memory was high. As such, neuropsychological tests cannot identify progressive memory decline alone.

If a patient has ascertained the diagnosis of MCI, the diagnosis can be further refined into amnestic, multi-domain and single, non-memory-domain subtypes (Winblad et al., 2004), as well as into a stable and a progressive group. While 30–50% of newly diagnosed MCI patients do not experience further decline of cognitive functions over 3–5 years, or even return to normal, the residual 50–70% show progress toward a more severe form of impairment (Rossini et al., 2007). This broad range of progression rates results from a large number of studies, in which inclusion and exclusion criteria varied to some degree. It is possible that correlating neuropsychological progression to specific biomarkers could yield less variable estimations of conversion rates. Therefore, the following sections of this review are dedicated to promising biomarkers in the fields of neuroimaging and neurophysiology. Finally, we close with an outlook on possible strategies for augmentation of memory function with respect to the discussed biomarkers.

3. NEUROIMAGING

Neuroimaging is of high value for diagnosis and prognosis of neurodegenerative diseases (Borghesani et al., 2010) such as MCI (Winblad et al., 2004). A characteristic symptom in MCI is atrophy of the medial temporal lobe, including memory related structures such as the hippocampus. Brain atrophy correlates with the progression of cognitive decline at the stage of subjective cognitive complaints (Förstl et al., 1995). More specifically, medial temporal lobe atrophy is able to predict progression to dementia in patients with MCI (Korf et al., 2004) with a reasonable predictive value (positive and negative predictive values 0.44 and 0.91, respectively Geroldi et al., 2006).

Decreased volumes of hippocampal formations are also a common finding in TLE patients. There is a relation between degree of memory impairment and seizure frequency, but it is suggested that structural pathologies in the temporal lobe rather than seizures cause memory difficulties (Butler and Zeman, 2008). However, these pathologies may be the consequence as well as the cause of seizures (Mathern et al., 2002a) and there are controversial findings in these respects. While neuronal cell loss in the hippocampus is not related to duration of the epilepsy, decreased neuronal density in the dentate gyrus evidenced by histology correlates positively with memory impairment in patients with TLE (Pauli et al., 2006). In addition, TLE is also associated with reduced neurogenesis in this region, further contributing to the decreased neuronal density (Mathern et al., 2002b). Neurogenesis of functional granule cells in the dentate gyrus of the hippocampus might facilitate hippocampal-dependent learning and episodic memory (Hattiangady and Shetty, 2008; Kuruba et al., 2009). On the other hand, some studies have indicated a correlation between epilepsy duration and neuronal loss (Mathern et al., 1995, 2002a). In other words, reduced neurogenesis and/or neuronal loss in this region in the chronic stage of TLE may be closely related to impairments in learning, memory, and other cognitive functions. In fact, it seems that the origin of memory problems in TLE is in childhood or adolescence (Helmstaedter and Elger, 2009). Well in line with this, hippocampal sclerosis is associated with poorer performance independent of age. However, temporal lobe atrophy is not present in all TLE patients. (Bernasconi et al., 2000) averaged six slices containing the head, body, and tail of the hippocampus. They found that the obtained hippocampal T2 relaxation times better predicted the epileptic focus than analyzing atrophy. Most interestingly, in addition to hippocampal damage, entorhinal lesions seem to play a special role in memory impairment in TLE. Especially lesions in layer III which are frequently found in TLE (Schwarcz and Witter, 2002). These findings and the importance of the rhinal cortex for memory consolidation (Axmacher et al., 2008) suggest that extracting biomarkers of the rhinal cortex may shed further light on memory problems in TLE. Thus, it is very likely that also other characteristics and other regions need to be addressed in the debate of whether memory decline in TLE is progressive or not.

Since hippocampal volumes discriminate patients with Alzheimer's disease and correlate with episodic memory performance, the volume and shape of this structure has the potential for a valid biomarker (Mueller et al., 2012). However, the hippocampus is not the only relevant structure in memory deficits. Research in MCI and Alzheimer's disease suggests that it is possibly not even the most relevant one. Volumetry of the hippocampal formation with Magnetic Resonance Imaging (MRI) revealed a relative risk of 0.69 for transition from MCI to Alzheimer's disease (Jack et al., 1999). A recent review suggests that perirhinal lesions have a stronger impact on memory functions than hippocampal lesions (Salig, 2009). Thus, atrophy of both structures, hippocampus and entorhinal cortex, may be a better marker for MCI, than either one of these alone (Winblad et al., 2004). Similarly, for TLE patients, entorhinal and perirhinal cortices are reduced in volume. Atrophy of the entorhinal cortex ipsilateral to the seizure onset zone is only found in patients with TLE, but not in other forms of epilepsy (Bernasconi et al., 2003). In addition, there is evidence that a global cortical atrophy marker such as widening of cerebrospinal fluid spaces might also be predictive for conversion from MCI to Alzheimer's disease (Teipel et al., 2007). Well in line with this, in MCI and Alzheimer's disease brain atrophy is prominent in the medial temporal lobe but also widespread over posterior cingulate and neocortical temporoparietal regions (Fox et al., 2001). Similarly, gray-matter decrease in the hippocampal area, inferior and middle temporal gyrus, posterior cingulate, and precuneus is greater in patients who convert from MCI to Alzheimer's disease than in non-converters (Chételat et al., 2005). Moreover, entorhinal and perirhinal cortices reveal reduced numbers of cells before the hippocampus is affected by degeneration (Dickerson and Sperling, 2008). The special role of the enthorinal cortex is further supported by a study which revealed that best classification accuracy of MCI was based on enthorinal cortex volume and best classification accuracy of Alzheimer's disease was based on hippocampal volume (Pennanen et al., 2004). Similarly, enthorinal cortex thickness was found to predict further memory decline in established Alzheimer's disease (Velayudhan et al., 2013). Thus, it would be worth analyzing more globally defined markers for atrophy or different combinations of regions, depending on the questions being asked.

However, by interpreting the role of hippocampal volumetry for predicting memory decline we have to consider the large variation between protocols for the delineation of the hippocampus in MR images. Up to date, there is no consistently applied standard which would allow comparing results of different studies to each other. Major differences refer to inclusion and exclusion of hippocampal white matter, definition of the anterior hippocampal—amygdala border, definition of the posterior border, and the extent to which the hippocampal tail is included, definition of the inferior medial border of the hippocampus, and use of varying arbitrary lines (Konrad et al., 2008). Therefore, it is difficult to estimate the real validity of volumetry in predicting memory decline. Alternatively, hippocampal shape features may be used instead of hippocampal volumetry. (Gerardin et al., 2009) utilized these shape features to train a support vector machine in order to perform multidimensional classification. The resulting classification rates were 94% for patients with Alzheimer's disease and 83% for MCI patients. Regarding the entorhinal cortex, reliable findings support stability of cortical thickness, volume, and surface area in normal aging (Lemaitre et al., 2012). The average cortical thickness over a region is a feature which is mostly independent from defined borders. Finally, to account for global atrophy, measures of intensity and deformation were of high predictive value for memory decline (Duchesne et al., 2010). Similarly, whole brain atrophy measures are predictive for conversion from MCI to Alzheimer's disease (Jack et al., 2005; Spulber et al., 2010).

Another promising MR technique is Diffusion Tensor Imaging (DTI). The potential of DTI for diagnosing MCI and its ability to predict further decline might have been underestimated so far, possibly due to a higher variability of fractional anisotropy than volumetric measures (Mueller et al., 2012). Indeed, DTI has been shown to be superior to hippocampal volumetry in distinguishing MCI from healthy controls (Muller et al., 2007). Hippocampal diffusivity predicts conversion from amnestic MCI to Alzheimer's disease at least as well as hippocampal atrophy (Kantarci et al., 2005; Fellgiebel et al., 2006).

4. NEUROPHYSIOLOGY

Clinical EEG is the standard neurophysiological test in patients with epilepsy, with a high positive and low negative predictive value of epileptiform discharges, such as spikes and sharp waves in routine recordings. While the literature on EEG-biomarker for localization of the seizure-onset zone is overwhelming, the information about memory-relevant biomarkers is scarce, and there is even less literature about prediction of memory decline.

Analysis of peak-frequency showed that poorer memory performance coincides with lower alpha peak (Ripper et al., 2001). Similarly, in children with epilepsy the differential activation of memory-resources has been documented with event-related power changes in the theta and lower-alpha range (Krause et al., 2008). Thus, assessing frequency properties of the EEG in TLE patients may reveal memory-relevant features. As such, using the rat pilocarpine model of TLE, it was found that spatial memory declines soon after status epilepticus and that these deficits correlate with a decrease of theta power but not with interictal-like activity in the hippocampus (Chauviere et al., 2009). Similarly to results from cross-sectional studies in humans (Helmstaedter and Elger, 2009), the loss of spatial memory ability is stable and not progressive in this model.

Intracranial EEG is only used in presurgical assessment to better delineate the seizure onset zone (Foldvary-Schaefer, 2004) and cannot be applied in the early stages of TLE. Indeed, neurophysiological parameters have been underutilized to assess the functional deficit zone, including memory deficits in patients with TLE (Grunwald and Vannucci, 2004). Event related designs, assessing brain signals in response to items that have to be memorized and recalled, are well suited to identify abnormal patterns in the surface and intracranial EEG of patients. We suggest that it would be of interest if such designs could help identifying abnormal changes over time in patients with TLE.

Despite the fact that the use of EEG for diagnosis of Alzheimer's disease or MCI is not a standard in clinical practice, a large number of studies succeeded in identifying markers that distinguish patients with Alzheimer's disease from MCI. EEG-biomarkers also successfully differentiated MCI from healthy subjects (see Rossini et al., 2007, for a review). Dauwels et al. (2010) summarize characteristics of the EEG in these clinical groups. First, the EEG is dominated by slower frequencies (Bonanni et al., 2008). Fast Fourier Transformations (FFTs) show a relative increase of activity below 8 Hz and decrease above this range. This characteristic was the first measure used in quantitative EEG-evaluation in MCI patients (Prichep et al., 1994) and therefore probably the most well known in the field. However, this slowing is possibly caused by perturbations in synchronization and decreased neural complexity (Cantero et al., 2009), representing two characteristic features of EEG in MCI. Synchrony can be expressed as Pearson's correlation coefficient, coherence, Granger causality, information-theoretic and state space based synchrony measures, phase synchrony indices, stochastic event synchrony, spatial distribution of phase synchrony, and small world network characteristics, among others (see Dauwels et al., 2010, for a review). Different measures of synchronization may be increased or decreased in MCI depending on frequency range, type of analysis, and regions being assessed (Jelic et al., 2000; Stam et al., 2003; Pijnenburg et al., 2004; Koenig et al., 2005; Babiloni et al., 2006). In addition, analysis of complexity of EEG signals is a valuable approach for resting EEG (Stam, 2005). Therefore, we suggest to apply complexity analysis for prognostic assessments. For example one could use approximate entropy, auto mutual information, sample entropy, multiscale entropy, Lempel-Ziv complexity, Hjorth parameters, Petrosian fractal dimension, or Higuchi fractal dimension (see also Bao et al., 2009; Dauwels et al., 2010).

It is remarkable that assessing frequency characteristics of MCI patients differentiates progressive from stable patients. It was found that a reduction of alpha power over posterior leads is characteristic for the progressive subgroup (Luckhaus et al., 2008). Despite this success, it is acknowledged that markers of resting EEG largely overlap between progressive MCI and stable MCI (Giannakopoulos et al., 2009). For example, it was shown that measures based on frequency analysis are valuable approaches for diagnosis and they change over the course of progression, but have no prognostic validity at baseline (Jelic et al., 2000). Thus, such markers (i.e., theta and beta power) have to be recorded longitudinally to detect changes which correlate with cognitive decline. It is suggested to use event-related EEG dynamic analysis to examine neocortical circuits and neuronal networks in order to predict memory decline (Giannakopoulos et al., 2009). The major advantage of doing memory research using event related designs in the EEG is the high temporal resolution, showing immediately pathologically delayed responses. In fact, it was found that delayed components of the event-related potential differ between stable and progressive MCI (Missonier et al., 2007). As such, it is highly likely that the combination of frequency, complexity, and synchrony characteristics in event-related EEG can shed further light on the progressive nature of MCI and eventually also of memory characteristics in TLE.

Since both TLE and MCI have impaired long-term memory, it is reasonable compare the mechanisms of successful and non-successful memory formation. A large number of studies have aimed at identifying the markers in the event related potential. The studies looked at efficient encoding which was recorded during the patient's learning of items. This was compared to the patient's recall performance in a later session (Fernández et al., 2002; Voss and Paller, 2007). Another approach refers to the dual route theory of recognition, that is, familiarity and recollection components (see Rugg and Curran, 2007, for a review). Familiarity is impaired in Alzheimer's disease but to some extent preserved in amnestic MCI while recollection is impaired in both clinical groups (Ally et al., 2009). However, other research groups report that familiarity is preserved in Alzheimer's disease and MCI for pictures (Westerberg et al., 2006), and that familiarity is impaired to at least the same extent as recollection in amnestic MCI, distinguishing MCI from normal aging population but not from Alzheimer's disease (Wolk et al., 2008). These findings from functional research are well in line with decreased volume of the perirhinal cortex and the hippocampus. While the perirhinal cortex mediates familiarity, the hippocampus is considered a core region for recollection (Turriziani et al., 2008; Brown et al., 2010). Thus, when designing event-related EEG studies the dimensions of familiarity and recollection, as well as encoding and retrieval, have to be addressed.

5. AUGMENTATION OF MEMORY FUNCTION

There are several strategies to augment human memory, and some of these are candidates for future treatment strategies in the here discussed patient populations. Madan (2014) discusses nootropic agents, brain stimulation, mnemonic strategies, and external aids as possible approaches to support memory. These strategies include common ones such as caffeine and notes, but also implanted devices which stimulate deep brain structures electrically. The hippocampus is an obvious target for memory stimulation. For example, it was found that working memory in rats could be transferred from one animal to the other by applying hippocampal firing patterns via electrical stimulation (Deadwyler et al., 2013). Deep brain stimulation in the entorhinal cortex of epilepsy patients enhanced spatial memory (Suthana et al., 2012). Similarly, in-phase stimulation during long-term encoding in the rhinal cortex and the hippocampus of epileptic patients modulated memory performance (Fell et al., 2013) and stimulation in the fornix of Alzheimer's patients activated entorhinal and hippocampal regions, which lead to improved memory (Laxton et al., 2010). Thus, it is not surprising that Alzheimer's disease and temporal lobe epilepsy were mentioned as possible target for deep brain stimulation and memory enhancement (Suthana and Fried, 2014).

However, these stimulation techniques are still at an experimental stage and can't be used in every single patient. Specifically, most stimulation studies were performed in epilepsy patients with intracranial electrodes implanted for pre-surgical evaluation. In contrast, cognitive intervention is an established strategy for memory augmentation in MCI (Rapp et al., 2002; Simon et al., 2012). The changes are not only measurable by the assessment of memory function, but also with fMRI (Simon et al., 2012), and can be enhanced by incorporating emotional content into the training (Broster et al., 2012). While there have been several endeavors to support the validity of cognitive training in MCI or dementia, there is still room for research in temporal lobe epilepsy.

6. CONCLUSIONS

Even if the debate of whether TLE is a dementing disease or if there are just a few subtypes with progressive course is still ongoing, there is a lot of literature about structural markers for impaired memory whereas the literature about EEG-markers is scarce. Valid biomarkers, which can reliably predict conversion from MCI to Alzheimer's disease, could shed new light on the question of whether TLE is a disorder with progressive memory decline. It is likely that memory decline occurs in TLE patients with early onset but after a certain age does not result in a progressive course. There may be elderly patients with MCI-like symptoms who instead suffer from late-onset epilepsy and could be misdiagnosed. The biomarkers summarized in this review could help determine the mechanisms of memory loss at early-onset of TLE and, most importantly, identify patients with late-onset TLE.

Prediction of conversion from MCI to Alzheimer's disease has been paid much attention so far, but TLE research and specifically intracranial recordings in presurgical evaluations may help to find new biomarkers for both disorders. For example, the importance of the rhinal cortex for memory consolidation has been shown by use of intracranial EEG in TLE research and can be translated into prediction of memory loss in MCI by use of structural imaging. As such, functional EEG is a promising approach which should be paid more attention in the future, since it allows one to combine the strength of neuropsychological assessments and the physiological assessment of brain function at a high temporal resolution.

Finally, the mentioned structures could be target for stimulating interventions such as deep brain stimulation in the rhinal, entorhinal, and hippocampal regions. The basis for these stimulation studies are the knowledge about the functional relevance of the mentioned structures but also about the involved EEG-oscillations. While deep brain stimulation is at an experimental stage we should not forget about the good effects of cognitive intervention, being established in MCI and having the potential of enhancing memory function in TLE patients.

AUTHOR CONTRIBUTIONS

Conception, decision on which references to include, revising, and approving of this work was carried out by all authors. The first author wrote the manuscript in accordance with the intellectual input of all authors. All authors agree to be accountable for all aspects of the work in ensuring that questions related to the accuracy or integrity of any part of the work are appropriately investigated and resolved.

ACKNOWLEDGMENTS

We thank Amy Melissa Lett for language editing and Jonas Potthoff for help in retrieving literature.

REFERENCES

Äikiä, M., Salmenperä, T., Partanen, K., and Kälviäinen, R. (2001). Verbal memory in newly diagnosed patients and patients with chronic left temporal lobe epilepsy. *Epilepsy Behav.* 2, 20–27. doi: 10.1006/ebeh.2000.0140

Ally, B., Gold, C., and Budson, A. (2009). An evaluation of recollection and familiarity in alzheimer's disease and mild cognitive impairment using receiver operating characteristics. *Brain Cogn.* 69, 504–513. doi: 10.1016/j.bandc.2008.11.003

Axmacher, N., Elger, C., and Fell, J. (2008). Ripples in the medial temporal lobe are relevant for human memory consolidation. *Brain* 131, 1806–1817. doi: 10.1093/brain/awn103

Babiloni, C., Ferri, R., Binetti, G., Cassarino, A., Forno, G. D., Ercolani, M., et al. (2006). Fronto-parietal coupling of brain rhythms in mild cognitive impairment: a multicentric eeg study. *Brain Res. Bull.* 69, 63–73. doi: 10.1016/j.brainresbull.2005.10.013

Bao, F., Gao, J., Hu, J., Lie, D., Zhang, Y., and Oommen, K. (2009). Automated epilepsy diagnosis using interictal scalp EEG. *CoRR* abs/0904.3808.

Bernasconi, A., Bernasconi, N., Caramanos, Z., Reutens, D., Andermann, F., Dubeau, F., et al. (2000). T2 relaxometry can lateralize mesial temporal lobe epilepsy in patients with normal MRI. *Neuroimage* 12, 739–746. doi: 10.1006/nimg.2000.0724

Bernasconi, N., Andermann, F., Arnold, D., and Bernasconi, A. (2003). Entorhinal cortex MRI assessment in temporal, extratemporal, and idiopathic generalized epilepsy. *Epilepsia* 44, 1070–1074. doi: 10.1046/j.1528-1157.2003.64802.x

Bonanni, L., Thomas, A., Tiraboschi, P., Perfetti, B., Varanese, S., and Onofrj, M. (2008). EEG comparisons in early Alzheimer's disease, dementia with Lewy bodies and Parkinson's disease with dementia patients with a 2-year follow-up. *Brain* 131, 690–705. doi: 10.1093/brain/awm322

Borghesani, P., DeMers, S., Manchanda, V., Pruthi, S., Lewis, D., and Borson, S. (2010). Neuroimaging in the clinical diagnosis of dementia: observations from a memory disorders clinic. *JAGS* 58, 1453–1458. doi: 10.1111/j.1532-5415.2010.02975.x

Broster, L., Blonder, L., and Jiang, Y. (2012). Does emotional memory enhancement assist the memory-impaired? *Front. Aging Neurosci.* 4:2. doi: 10.3389/fnagi.2012.00002

Brown, M., Warburton, E., and Aggleton, J. (2010). Recognition memory: material, processes, and substrates. *Hippocampus* 20, 1228-1244. doi: 10.1002/hipo.20858

Butler, C., and Zeman, A. (2008). Recent insights into the impairment of memory in epilepsy: transient epileptic amnesia, accelerated long-term forgetting and remote memory impairment. *Brain* 131, 2243–2263. doi: 10.1093/brain/awn127

Cantero, J. L., Atienza, M., Cruz-Vadell, A., Suarez-Gonzalez, A., and Gil-Neciga, E. (2009). Increased synchronization and decreased neural complexity underlie thalamocortical oscillatory dynamics in mild cognitive impairment. *Neuroimage* 46, 938–948. doi: 10.1016/j.neuroimage.2009.03.018

Chauviere, L., Rafrafi, N., Thinus-Blanc, C., Bartolomei, F., Esclapez, M., and Bernard, C. (2009). Early deficits in spatial memory and theta rhythm in experimental temporal lobe epilepsy. *J. Neurosci.* 29, 5402–5410. doi: 10.1523/JNEUROSCI.4699-08.2009

Chételat, G., Landeau, B., Eustache, F., Mézenge, F., Viader, F., de la Sayette, V., et al. (2005). Using voxel-based morphometry to map the structural changes associated with rapid conversion in MCI: a longitudinal MRI study. *Neuroimage* 27, 934–946. doi: 10.1016/j.neuroimage.2005.05.015

Cretin, B., Blanc, F., Gaultier, C., and Sellal, F. (2012). Epileptic amnesic syndrome revealing alzheimer's disease. *Epilepsy Res.* 102, 206–209. doi: 10.1016/j.eplepsyres.2012.08.002

Dauwels, J., Vialatte, F., and Cichocki, A. (2010). Diagnosis of alzheimer's disease from EEG signals: where are we standing? *Curr. Alzheimer Res.* 7, 487–505. doi: 10.2174/156720510792231720

Deadwyler, S., Berger, T., Sweatt, A., Song, D., Chan, R., Opris, I., et al. (2013). Donor/recipient enhancement of memory in rat hippocampus. *Front. Syst. Neurosci.* 7:120. doi: 10.3389/fnsys.2013.00120

DeKosky, S., and Marek, K. (2003). Looking backward to move forward: early detection of neurodegenerative disorders. *Science* 302, 830–834. doi: 10.1126/science.1090349

Dickerson, B., and Sperling, R. (2008). Functional abnormalities of the medial temporal lobe memory system in mild cognitive impairment and alzheimers disease: insights from functional MRI studies. *Neuropsychologia* 46, 1624–1635. doi: 10.1016/j.neuropsychologia.2007.11.030

Dodrill, C. (2004). Neuropsychological effects of seizures. *Epilepsy Behav.* 5, 21–24. doi: 10.1016/j.yebeh.2003.11.004

Duchesne, S., Bocti, C., K., D., Frisoni, G., Chertkow, H., and Collins, D. (2010). Amnestic MCI future clinical status prediction using baseline MRI features. *Neurobiol. Aging* 31, 1606–1617. doi: 10.1016/j.neurobiolaging.2008.09.003

Elger, C., Helmstaedter, C., and Kurthen, M. (2004). Chronic epilepsy and cognition. *Lancet Neurol.* 3, 663–672. doi: 10.1016/S1474-4422(04)00906-8

Engel, J., Pitkänen, A., Loeb, J., Dudek, F., EH, B., Cole, A., et al. (2013). Epilepsy biomarkers. *Epilepsia* 54, 61–69. doi: 10.1111/epi.12299

Fell, J., Staresina, B., Do Lam, A., Widman, G., Helmstaedter, C., Elger, C., et al. (2013). Memory modulation by weak synchronous deep brain stimulation: a pilot study. *Brain Stimul.* 6, 270–273. doi: 10.1016/j.brs.2012.08.001

Fellgiebel, A., Dellani, P., Greverus, D., Scheurich, A., Stoeter, P., and Müller, M. (2006). Predicting conversion to dementia in mild cognitive impairment by volumetric and diffusivity measurements of the hippocampus. *Psychiatry Res.* 146, 283–287. doi: 10.1016/j.pscychresns.2006.01.006

Fernández, G., Klaver, P., Fell, J., Grunwald, T., and Elger, C. (2002). Human declarative memory formation: segregating rhinal and hippocampal contributions. *Hippocampus* 12, 514–519. doi: 10.1002/hipo.10050

Fisher, R., Vickrey, B., Gibson, P., Hermann, B., Penovich, P., Scherer, A., et al. (2000). The impact of epilepsy from the patient's perspective i. Descriptions and subjective perceptions. *Epilepsy Res.* 41, 39–51. doi: 10.1016/S0920-1211(00)00128-5

Foldvary-Schaefer, N. (2004). "Noninvasive EEG in the definition of the seizure-onset zone," in *Presurgical Assessment of the Epilepsies with Clinical Neurophysiology and Functional Imaging.* Handbook of clinical neurophysiology, Vol. 3, eds F. Rosenow and H. Lüders (Amsterdam, The Netherlands: Elsevier), 85–96. doi: 10.1016/S1567-4231(03)03007-7

Förstl, H., Hentschel, F., Sattel, H., Geiger-Kabisch, C., Besthorn, C., Czech, C., et al. (1995). Age-associated memory impairment and early alzheimer's disease. Only time will tell the difference. *Arzneimittelforschung* 45, 394–397.

Fox, N., Crum, W., Scahill, R., Stevens, J., Janssen, J., and Rossor, M. (2001). Imaging of onset and progression of alzheimer's disease with voxel-compression mapping of serial magnetic resonance images. *Lancet* 385, 201–205. doi: 10.1016/S0140-6736(01)05408-3

Gauthier, S., Reisberg, B., Zaudig, M., Petersen, R., Ritchie, K. Broich, K., et al. (2006). Mild cognitive impairment. *Lancet* 367, 1262–1270. doi: 10.1016/S0140-6736(06)68542-5

Geda, Y. (2012). Mild cognitive impairment in older adults. *Curr. Psychiatry Rep.* 14, 320–327. doi: 10.1007/s11920-012-0291-x

Gerardin, E., Chéetlat, G., Chubin, M., Cuingnet, R., Desgranges, B., Kim, H., et al. (2009). Multidimensional classification of hippocampal shape features discriminates Alzheimer's disease and mild cognitive impairment from normal aging. *Neuroimage* 47, 1476–1486. doi: 10.1016/S1053-8119(09)70228-9

Geroldi, C., Rossi, R., Calvagna, C., Testa, C., Bresciani, L., Binetti, G., et al. (2006). Medial temporal atrophy but not memory deficits predict progression to dementia in patients with mild cognitive impairment. *J. Neurol. Neurosurg. Psychiatry* 77, 1219–1222. doi: 10.1136/jnnp.2005.082651

Giannakopoulos, P., Missonnier, P., Kŝvari, E., Gold, G., and Michon, A. (2009). Electrophysiological markers of rapid cognitive decline in mild cognitive impairment. *Front. Neurol. Neurosci.* 24, 39–46. doi: 10.1159/000197898

Goldman, W., and Morris, J. (2001) Evidence that age-associated memory impairment is not a normal variant of aging. *Alzheimer Dis. Assoc. Disord.* 15, 72–79. doi: 10.1097/00002093-200104000-00006

Gonzalez, L., Mahdavi, N., Anderson, V., and Harvey, A. (2012). Changes in memory function in children and young adults with temporal lobe epilepsy: a follow-up study. *Epilepsy Behav.* 23, 213–219. doi: 10 1016/j.yebeh.2011.11.017

Grunwald, T., and Vannucci, M. (2004). "Cognition-related potentials in the definition of functional-deficit zones," in *Presurgical Assessment of the Epilepsies with Clinical Neurophysiology and Functional imaging.* Handbook of clinical neurophysiology, Vol. 3, eds F. Rosenow and H. Lüders (Amsterdam, The Netherlands: Elsevier), 501–511. doi: 10.1016/S1567-4231(03)03038-7

Hänninen, T., and Soininen, H. (1997). Age-associated memory impairment. Normal aging or warning of dementia? *Drugs Aging* 11, 480–489. doi: 10.2165/00002512-199711060-00007

Hattiangady, B., and Shetty, A. (2008). Implications of decreased hippocampal neurogenesis in chronic temporal lobe epilepsy. *Epilepsia* 49, 26–41. doi: 10.1111/j.1528-1167.2008.01635.x

Helmstädter, C. (2002). Effects of chronic epilepsy on declarative memory systems. *Prog. Brain Res.* 135, 439–453. doi: 10.1016/S0079-6123(02)35041-6

Helmstaedter, C. (2007). Cognitive outcome of status epilepticus in adults. *Epilepsia* 48, 85–90. doi: 10.1111/j.1528-1167.2007.01360.x

Helmstaedter, C., and Elger, C. (1999). The phantom of progressive dementia in epilepsy. *Lancet* 354, 2133–2134. doi: 10.1016/S0140-6736(99)03542-4

Helmstaedter, C., and Elger, C. (2009). Chronic temporal lobe epilepsy: a neurodevelopmental or progressively dementing disease? *Brain* 132, 2822–2830. doi: 10.1093/brain/awp182

Hermann, B., Meador, K., Gaillard, W., and Cramer, J. (2010). Cognition across the lifespan: antiepileptic drugs, epilepsy, or both? *Epilepsy Behav.* 17, 1–5. doi: 10.1016/j.yebeh.2009.10.019

Hermann, B., Seidenberg, M., Schoenfeld, J., and Davies, K. (1997). Neuropsychological characteristics of the syndrome of mesial temporal lobe epilepsy. *Arch. Neurol.* 54, 369–376. doi: 10.1001/archneur.1997.00550160019010

Jack, C., Petersen, R., Xu, Y., O'Brien, P., Smith, G., Ivnik, R., et al. (1999). Prediction of AD with MRI-based hippocampal volume in mild cognitive impairment. *Neurology* 352, 1397–1403. doi: 10.1212/WNL.52.7.1397

Jack, C., Shiung, M., Weigand, S., O'Brien, P., Gunter, J., Boeve, B., et al. (2005). Brain atrophy rates predict subsequent clinical conversion in normal elderly and amnestic MCI. *Neurology* 65, 1227–1231. doi: 10.1212/01.wnl.0000180958.22678.91

Jelic, V., Johansson, S., Almkvist, O., Shigeta, M., Julin, P., Nordberg, A., et al. (2000). Quantitative electroencephalography in mild cognitive impairment: longitudinal changes and possible prediction of alzheimer's disease. *Neurobiol. Aging* 21, 533–540. doi: 10.1016/S0197-4580(00)00153-6

Jokeit, H., and Ebner, A. (1999). Long term effects of refractory temporal lobe epilepsy on cognitive abilities: a cross sectional study. *J. Neurol. Neurosurg. Psychiat.* 67, 44–50. doi: 10.1136/jnnp.67.1.44

Jokeit, H., and Ebner, A. (2002). Effects of chronic epilepsy on intellectual functions. *Prog. Brain Res.* 135, 455–463. doi: 10.1016/S0079-6123(02)35042-8

Kaaden, S., and Helmstaedter, C. (2009). Age at onset of epilepsy as a determinant of intellectual impairment in temporal lobe epilepsy. *Epilepsy Behav.* 15, 213–217. doi: 10.1016/j.yebeh.2009.03.027

Kantarci, K., Petersen, R., Boeve, B., Knopman, D., Weigand, S., O'Brien, P., et al. (2005). DWI predicts future progression to alzheimer disease in amnestic mild cognitive impairment. *Neurology* 64, 902–904. doi: 10.1212/01.WNL.0000153076.46126.E9

Koenig, T., Prichep, L., Dierks, T., Hubl, D., Wahlund, L. O., John, E. R., et al. (2005). Decreased eeg synchronization in alzheimer's disease and mild cognitive impairment. *Neurobiol. Aging* 26, 165–171. doi: 10.1016/j.neurobiolaging.2004.03.008

Konrad, C., Ukas, T., Nebel, C., Arolt, V., Toga, A., and Narr, K. (2008). Defining the human hippocampus in cerebral magnetic resonance images - an overview of current segmentation protocols. *Neuroimage* 47, 1185–1195. doi: 10.1016/j.neuroimage.2009.05.019

Korf, E., Wahlund, L., Visser, P., and Scheltens, P. (2004). Medial temporal lobe atrophy on mri predicts dementia in patients with mild cognitive impairment. *Neurology* 63, 94–100. Cited By (since 1996) 115. doi: 10.1212/01.WNL.0000133114.92694.93

Krause, C., Boman, P., L., S., Varho, T., and Holopainen, I. (2008). Brain oscillatory EEG event-related desynchronization (ERD) and -synchronization (ERS) responses during an auditory memory task are altered in children with epilepsy. *Seizure* 17, 1–10. doi: 10.1016/j.seizure.2007.05.015

Kuruba, R., Hattiangady, B., and Shetty, A. (2009). Hippocampal neurogenesis and neural stem cells in temporal lobe epilepsy. *Epilepsy Behav.* 14, 65–73. doi: 10.1016/j.yebeh.2008.08.020

Laxton, A., Tang-Wai, D., McAndrews, M., Zumsteg, D., Wennberg, R., Keren, R., et al. (2010). A phase i trial of deep brain stimulation of memory circuits in alzheimer's disease. *Ann. Neurol.* 68, 521–534. doi: 10.1002/ana.22089

Lemaitre, H., Goldman, A., Samataro, F., Verchinski, B., Meyer-Lindenberg, A., Weinberger, D., et al. (2012). Normal age-related brain morphometric changes: nonuniformity across cortical thickness, surface area and gray matter volume? *Neurobiol. Aging* 33, 617.e1–617.e9. doi: 10.1016/j.neurobiolaging.2010.07.013

Lewis, D., Shinnar, S., Hesdorffer, D., Bagiella, E., Bello, J., Chan, S., et al. (2013). Hippocampal sclerosis after febrile status epilepticus: the FEBSTAT study. *Ann. Neurol.* 75, 178–185. doi: 10.1002/ana.24081

Luckhaus, C., Grass-Kapanke, B., Blaeser, I., Ihl, R., Supprian, T., Winterer, G., et al. (2008). Quantitative EEG in progressive vs stable mild cognitive impairment (MCI): results of a 1-year follow-up study. *Int. J. Geriatr. Psychiatry* 23, 1148–1155. doi: 10.1002/gps.2042

Madan, C. (2014). Augmented memory: a survey of the approaches to remembering more. *Front. Syst. Neurosci.* 8:30. doi: 10.3389/fnsys.2014.00030

Mantoan, M. A., Caboclo, L. O., de Figueiredo Ferreira Guilhoto, L. M., Lin, K., da Silva Noffs, M. H., de Souza Silva Tudesco, I., et al. (2009). Correlation between memory, proton magnetic resonance spectroscopy, and interictal epileptiform discharges in temporal lobe epilepsy related to mesial temporal sclerosis. *Epilepsy Behav.* 16, 447–453. doi: 10.1016/j.yebeh.2009.08.032

Mathern, G., Adelson, P., Cahan, L., and Leite, J. (2002a). Hippocampal neuron damage in human epilepsy: Meyer's hypothesis revisited. *Prog. Brain Res.* 135, 237–251. doi: 10.1016/S0079-6123(02)35023-4

Mathern, G., Babb, T., Pretorius, J., Melendez, M., and Lévesque, M. (1995). The pathophysiologic relationships between lesion pathology, intracranial ictal EEG onsets, and hippocampal neuron losses in temporal lobe epilepsy. *Epilepsy Res.* 21, 133–147. doi: 10.1016/0920-1211(95)00014-2

Mathern, G., Leiphart, J., De Vera, A., Adelson, P., Seki, T., Neder, L., et al. (2002b). Seizures decrease postnatal neurogenesis and granule cell development in the human fascia dentata. *Epilepsia* 43, 68–73. doi: 10.1046/j.1528-1157.43.s.5.28.x

Missonier, P., Deiber, M., Gold, G., Herrmann, F., Millet, P., Michon, A., et al. (2007). Working memory load-related electroencephalographic parameters can differentiate progressive from stable mild cognitive impairment. *Neuroscience* 150, 346–356. doi: 10.1016/j.neuroscience.2007.09.009

Mueller, S., Keeser, D., Reiser, M., Teipel, S., and Meindl, T. (2012). Functional and structural MR imaging in neuropsychiatric disorders, part 1: imaging techniques and their application in mild cognitive impairment and alzheimer disease. *AJNR Am. J. Neuroradiol.* 33, 1845–1850. doi: 10.3174/ajnr.A2799

Muller, M., Greverus, D., Weibrich, C., Dellani, P., Scheurich, A., Stoeter, P., et al. (2007). Diagnostic utility of hippocampal size and mean diffusivity in amnestic MCI. *Neurobiol. Aging* 28, 398–403. doi: 10.1016/j.neurobiolaging.2006.01.009

Najm, I., Babb, T., Mohamed, A., Diehl, B., Ng, T., Bingaman, W., et al. (2001). "Mesial temporal lobe sclerosis," in *Magnetic Resonance in Epilepsy. Neuroimaging Techniques*, 2nd Edn, eds H. Lüders and Y. Comair (Philadelphia, PA: Lippincott Williams & Wilkins), 95–103.

Pauli, E., Hildebrandt, M., and Romstck, J. E. A. (2006). Deficient memory acquisition in temporal lobe epilepsy is predicted by hippocampal granule cell loss. *Neurology* 67, 1383–1389. doi: 10.1212/01.wnl.0000239828.36651.73

Pennanen, C., Kivipelto, M., Tuomainen, S., Hartikainen, P., Hänninen, T., Laakso, M., et al. (2004). Hippocampus and entorhinal cortex in mild cognitive impairment and early AD. *Neurobiol. Aging* 25, 303–310. doi: 10.1016/S0197-4580(03)00084-8

Pijnenburg, Y. A. L., vd Made, Y., van Cappellen van Walsum, A. M., Knol, D. L., Scheltens, P., and Stam, C. J. (2004). Eeg synchronization likelihood in mild cognitive impairment and alzheimer's disease during a working memory task. *Clin. Neurophysiol.* 115, 1332–1339. doi: 10.1016/j.clinph.2003.12.029

Prichep, L., John, E., Ferris, S., Reisberg, B., Almas, M., Alper, K., et al. (1994). Quantitative EEG correlates of cognitive deterioriation in the elderly. *Neurobiol. Aging* 15, 85–90. doi: 10.1016/0197-4580(94)90147-3

Rapp, S., Brenes, G., and Marsh, A. (2002). Memory enhancement training for older adults with mild cognitive impairment: a preliminary study. *Aging Ment. Health* 6, 5–11. doi: 10.1080/13607860120101077

Reisberg, B., Ferris, S., de Leon, M., and Crook, T. (1982). The global deterioration scale for assessment of primary degenerative dementia. *Am. J. Psychiatry* 139, 1136–1139.

Reisberg, B., Shulman, M., Torossian, C., Leng, L., and Zhu, W. (2010). Outcome over seven years of healthy adults with and without subjective cognitive impairment. *Alzheimers Dement.* 6, 11–24. doi: 10.1016/j.jalz.2009.10.002

Ripper, B., Trinka, E., Schimke, H., Wranek, U., and Ladurner, G. (2001). Temporallappenepilepsie: EEG-Alphafrequenz, Gedächtnisleistung und Lokalisation von Läsionen. *Klin. Neurophysiol.* 1, 16–32. doi: 10.1055/s-2001-15410

Rosenow, F., and Lüders, H. (2001). Presurgical evaluation of epilepsy. *Brain* 124, 1683–1700. doi: 10.1093/brain/124.9.1683

Rossini, P., Rossi, S., Babiloni, C., and Polich, J. (2007). Clinical neurophysiology of aging brain: from normal aging to neurodegeneration. *Prog. Neurobiol.* 83, 375–400. doi: 10.1016/j.pneurobio.2007.07.010

Rugg, M., and Curran, T. (2007). Event-related potentials and recognition memory. *Trends Cogn. Sci.* 11, 251–257. doi: 10.1016/j.tics.2007.04.004

Salig, M. (2009). Verbal memory in mesial temporal lobe epilepsy: beyond material specifity. *Brain* 132, 570–582. doi: 10.1093/brain/awp012

Schwarcz, R., and Witter, M. (2002). Memory impairment in temporal lobe epilepsy: the role of entorhinal lesions. *Epilepsy Res.* 50, 161–177. doi: 10.1016/S0920-1211(02)00077-3

Simon, S., Yokomizo, J., and Bottino, C. (2012). Cognitive intervention in amnestic mild cognitive impairment: a systematic review. *Neurosci. Biobehav. Rev.* 36, 1163–1178. doi: 10.1016/j.neubiorev.2012.01.007

Spulber, G., Niskanen, E., MacDonald, S., Smilovici, O., Chen, K., Reiman, E., et al. (2010). Whole brain atrophy rate predicts progression from MCI to Alzheimer's disease. *Neurobiol. Aging* 31, 1601–1605. doi: 10.1016/j.neurobiolaging.2008.08.018

Stam, C. (2005). Nonlinear dynamical analysis of EEG and MEG: review of an emerging field. *Clin. Neurophys.* 116, 2266–2301. doi: 10.1016/j.clinph.2005.06.011

Stam, C., Van Der Made, Y., Pijnenburg, Y., and Scheltens, P. (2003). EEG synchronization in mild cognitive impairment and alzheimer's disease. *Acta Neurol. Scand.* 108, 90–96. doi: 10.1034/j.1600-0404.2003.02067.x

Stefan, H., and Pauli, E. (2002). Progressive cognitive decline in epilepsy: an indication of ongoing plasticity. *Prog. Brain Res.* 135, 409–417. doi: 10.1016/S0079-6123(02)35038-6

Stefan, H., and Pauli, E. (2008). Kognition und epilepsien. *Nervenarzt* 79, 77–92. doi: 10.1007/s00115-008-2463-9

Stewart, R. (2012a). Mild cognitive impairment-the continuing challenge of its "real-world" detection and diagnosis. *Arch. Med. Res.* 43, 609–614. doi: 10.1016/j.arcmed.2012.10.011

Stewart, R. (2012b). Subjective cognitive impairment. *Curr. Opin. Psychiatry* 25, 445–450. doi: 10.1097/YCO.0b013e3283586fd8

Suthana, N., and Fried, I. (2014). Deep brain stimulation for enhancement of learning and memory. *Neuroimage* 85, 996–1002. doi: 10.1016/j.neuroimage.2013.07.066

Suthana, N., Haneef, Z., Stern, J., Mukamel, R., Behnke, E., Knowlton, B., et al. (2012). Memory enhancement and deep-brain stimulation of the entorhinal area. *N. Engl. J. Med.* 366, 502–510. doi: 10.1056/NEJMoa1107212

Teipel, S., Born, C., Ewers, M., Bokde, A., Reiser, M., Möller, H., et al. (2007). Multivariate deformation-based analysis of brain atrophy to predict Alzheimer's disease in mild cognitive impairment. *Neuroimage* 38, 13–24. doi: 10.1016/j.neuroimage.2007.07.008

Thompson, P., and Duncan, J. (2005). Cognitive decline in severe intractable epilepsy. *Epilepsia* 46, 1780–1787. doi: 10.1111/j.1528-1167.2005.00279.x

Turriziani, P., Serra, L., Fadda, L., Caltagirone, C., and Carlesimo, G. (2008). Recollection and familiarity in hippocampal amnesia. *Hippocampus* 18, 469–480. doi: 10.1002/hipo.20412

van den Berg, E., Kant, N., and Postma, A. (2012). Remember to buy milk on the way home! a meta-analytic review of prospective memory in mild cognitive impairment and dementia. *J. Int. Neuropsychol. Soc.* 18, 706–716. doi: 10.1017/S1355617712000331

Velayudhan, L., Proitsi, P., Westman, E., Muehlboeck, J., Mecocci, P., Vellas, B., et al. (2013). Entorhinal cortex thickness predicts cognitive decline in Alzheimer's disease. *J. Alzheimers Dis.* 33, 755–766. doi: 10.3233/JAD-2012-121408

Voss, J., and Paller, K. (2007). Brain substrates of implicit and explicit memory: the importance of concurrently acquired neural signals of both memory types. *Neuropsychologia* 46, 3021–3029. doi: 10.1016/j.neuropsychologia.2008.07.010

Vossel, K., Beagle, A., Rabinovici, G., Shu, H., Lee, S., Naasan, G., et al. (2013). Seizures and epileptiform activity in the early stages of Alzheimer disease. *JAMA Neurol.* 70, 1158–1166. doi: 10.1001/jamaneurol.2013.136

Westerberg, C., Paller, K., Weintraub, S., Mesulam, M., Holdstock, J., Mayes, A., et al. (2006). When memory does not fail: familiarity-based recognition in mild cognitive impairment and alzheimer's disease. *Neuropsychology* 20, 193–205. doi: 10.1037/0894-4105.20.2.193

Winblad, B., Palmer, K., Kivipelto, M., Jelic, V., Fratiglioni, L., Wahlund, L., et al. (2004). Mild cognitive impairment - beyond controversies, towards a consensus: report of the International Working Group on Mild Cognitive Impairment. *J. Intern. Med.* 256, 240–246. doi: 10.1111/j.1365-2796.2004.01380.x

Wolk, D., Signoff, E., and DeKosky, S. (2008). Recollection and familiarity in amnestic mild cognitive impairment: a global decline in recognition memory. *Neuropsychologia* 46, 1965–1978. doi: 10.1016/j.neuropsychologia.2008.01.017

20

Environmental enrichment and the sensory brain: the role of enrichment in remediating brain injury

Dasuni S. Alwis and Ramesh Rajan*

Department of Physiology, Monash University, Clayton, VIC, Australia

Edited by:
Mikhail Lebedev, Duke University, USA

Reviewed by:
James W. Grau, Texas A&M University, USA
Robert N. S. Sachdev, Yale University, USA

****Correspondence:***
Ramesh Rajan, Department of Physiology, Monash University, Building 13F, Wellington Road, Clayton, VIC 3800, Australia
e-mail: ramesh.rajan@monash.edu

The brain's life-long capacity for experience-dependent plasticity allows adaptation to new environments or to changes in the environment, and to changes in internal brain states such as occurs in brain damage. Since the initial discovery by Hebb (1947) that environmental enrichment (EE) was able to confer improvements in cognitive behavior, EE has been investigated as a powerful form of experience-dependent plasticity. Animal studies have shown that exposure to EE results in a number of molecular and morphological alterations, which are thought to underpin changes in neuronal function and ultimately, behavior. These consequences of EE make it ideally suited for investigation into its use as a potential therapy after neurological disorders, such as traumatic brain injury (TBI). In this review, we aim to first briefly discuss the effects of EE on behavior and neuronal function, followed by a review of the underlying molecular and structural changes that account for EE-dependent plasticity in the normal (uninjured) adult brain. We then extend this review to specifically address the role of EE in the treatment of experimental TBI, where we will discuss the demonstrated sensorimotor and cognitive benefits associated with exposure to EE, and their possible mechanisms. Finally, we will explore the use of EE-based rehabilitation in the treatment of human TBI patients, highlighting the remaining questions regarding the effects of EE.

Keywords: EE, sensory cortices, traumatic brain injury, neuronal excitability

Experience-dependent plasticity encompasses a vast number of paradigms that range from deprivation to alterations and enrichments in the environment, and has been investigated in great detail across development through to adulthood (see reviews by Hubel and Wiesel, 1970; Hubel, 1978; Kaas, 1991; Klintsova and Greenough, 1999; Sur and Leamey, 2001; De Villers-Sidani and Merzenich, 2011; Bengoetxea et al., 2012). For the purposes of the present review, we chose to focus on plasticity conferred by global changes to the environment, termed environmental enrichment (EE). We will focus only on the changes evoked by this manipulation when applied in adulthood as our final aim is to demonstrate that it represents an exciting potential therapy in adult traumatic brain injury (TBI). As we shall review, EE alters neuronal function through a range of morphological and molecular interactions, which lead to alterations in sensorimotor and cognitive behavior. These changes make EE an ideal candidate in the treatment of TBI. To lead to this thesis, we first commence with a review of EE's capacity to evoke plasticity in the uninjured brain, to provide the context in which we will cast the role of EE in TBI. We focus here on EE-induced changes in sensory cortices due to the demonstrated effects of TBI on altering neuronal function in sensory cortices (Hall and Lifshitz, 2010; Ding et al., 2011; Alwis et al., 2012; Johnstone et al., 2013); it is also our view that changes in neuronal activity in sensory cortices after injury must underlie a significant portion of the persistent cognitive deficits found in TBI (Caeyenberghs et al., 2009; Davis and Dean, 2010; Lew et al., 2010; Folmer et al., 2011). The review of EE effects in the normal brain is also necessary to understand the mechanisms whereby EE produces changes in neuronal function in the normal brain, before we can begin to hypothesize about how EE exerts its beneficial effects after brain injury. Finally, we discuss the current literature regarding the use of EE as a potential therapy post-TBI, in animal studies with induced TBI, and in studies of human rehabilitation after injury.

WHAT IS EE?

EE refers to an experimental paradigm in which laboratory animals are housed in an environment allowing cognitive, motor and sensory stimulation at levels much greater than those which occur under standard laboratory housing conditions (Hebb, 1947, 1949; Van Praag et al., 2000). Early studies in animals have shown that the enhanced stimulation from EE produces many remarkable benefits at anatomical, molecular and behavioral levels (Hebb, 1947; Bennett et al., 1969; Diamond et al., 1972, 1976; Greenough and Volkmar, 1973; Torasdotter et al., 1998), with numerous studies following on from this work to further characterize the effects of EE (see reviews by Van Praag et al., 2000; Nithianantharajah and Hannan, 2006). In EE, the housing environment is modified by providing a larger enclosure, natural bedding and a variety of novel objects, in the expectation that this will promote greater physical activity in exploration and interaction with a novel and complex environment (Benaroya-Milshtein et al., 2004; Zebunke et al., 2013). Social enrichment in the EE environment, involving housing animals with multiple cagemates to encourage complex social interactions (Rosenzweig et al., 1978; Mesa-Gresa et al., 2013), is also believed to contribute to an enhanced sensorimotor and cognitive experience. Enhanced physical activity and enhanced social interaction each provide benefits to the brain; physical activity on its own improves cognitive performance in parallel with a range of neural changes including enhanced neurogenesis and increased levels of neurotrophic growth factors and increased neurotransmitter subunit expression (Van Praag et al., 1999; Farmer et al., 2004; Erickson et al., 2011), while social enrichment on its own has been shown to result in an increase in brain weight (Rosenzweig et al., 1978). When the two are combined in an appropriately enriched environment, a much more extensive set of cerebral changes occurs (Rosenzweig et al., 1978; Johansson and Ohlsson, 1996; Sozda et al., 2010).

The combination of social, physical and cognitive stimulation is most often used in studies of EE and we term this "generic" EE, wherein the whole environment is non-selectively enriched. However, in some instances, in what we term "specific" EE, enrichment has been targeted to affect a specific system, e.g., auditory-specific enrichment (Engineer et al., 2004; Percaccio et al., 2005, 2007; Jakkamsetti et al., 2012) consisting of components of generic EE in combination with systems designed to produce a variety of salient sounds; or tactile-specific enrichment (Bourgeon et al., 2004; Xerri et al., 2005) where rats were raised in an environment consisting of objects with various textures. Differences in generic and specific EE will be highlighted further, in the context of EE effects on neuronal function in the cortex.

BENEFICIAL EFFECTS OF EE ON BEHAVIOR

EE exposure results in a range of sensorimotor and cognitive benefits in laboratory animals, which we only briefly summarize as these have been well reviewed elsewhere (Van Praag et al., 2000; Nithianantharajah and Hannan, 2006; Simpson and Kelly, 2011). In normal animals, EE significantly improves spatial and non-spatial learning and memory, novel object discrimination, increases the speed of spatial learning and enhances spatial searching strategies (Van Praag et al., 2000; Schrijver et al., 2002; Nithianantharajah and Hannan, 2006; Kulesskaya et al., 2011; Vedovelli et al., 2011; Leger et al., 2012). EE appears to decrease anxiety, as evidenced in a variety of tests (Fernandez-Teruel et al., 2002; Larsson et al., 2002; Galani et al., 2007; Harati et al., 2013). EE also improves task-learning, and recent and remote memory retrieval (Harati et al., 2013), likely due to a greater ability to consolidate and retain information because of social enrichment (Gardner et al., 1975). However, effects are not all positive and studies have shown both increases and decreases in aggressive social behavior after EE (Abou-Ismail, 2011; Workman et al., 2011; McQuaid et al., 2012; Mesa-Gresa et al., 2013), possibly due to factors such as differences in EE housing conditions, strain differences, and experimental design.

In a similar vein, the consensus (Nithianantharajah and Hannan, 2006; Kazlauckas et al., 2011; Landers et al., 2011) is that EE encourages activity and exploratory behavior though there are some inconsistencies: some studies show increased activity in novel environments (Benaroya-Milshtein et al., 2004), and others show faster habituation and less activity (Zimmermann et al., 2001; Schrijver et al., 2002; Elliott and Grunberg, 2005), when compared with animals housed in standard or impoverished environments (Varty et al., 2000; Zimmermann et al., 2001). Recently, Zebunke et al. (2013) showed a decrease in general activity during an open field test, with an increase in duration of exploration of novel objects by pigs exposed to cognitive enrichment. Similarly, Mesa-Gresa et al. (2013) also found that EE rats exhibited longer durations of novel object exploration, while Schrijver et al. (2002) found an increase in activity in a light/dark box in EE rats. Bruel-Jungerman et al. (2005) have also reported that EE animals were capable of retaining memory during a novel object recognition test for up to 48 h after initial exposure, despite a lower object exploration time during the learning phase of the test.

Among the most robust of findings is that EE and sensory training/learning improves stimulus discrimination (Gibson, 1953; Kendrick et al., 1992; Recanzone et al., 1993). Mandairon et al. (2006a,b) have shown that olfactory enrichment results in an improved ability to discriminate between odor pairs, likely due to changes in neuronal response properties (Buonviso and Chaput, 2000; Fletcher and Wilson, 2003). Similarly, EE enhances spatial discrimination of sound source, with faster reaction times and improved discrimination accuracy (Cai et al., 2009). Bourgeon et al. (2004) reported that while EE housing did not affect an animal's tactile ability to discriminate between textured surfaces, enriched animals did learn to perform the discrimination task faster. The changes in behavior reported above must occur as a consequence of the effects of EE on neuronal function, which in turn, occur as a result of the various molecular and morphological changes mediated by EE.

NEURONAL FUNCTIONAL CHANGES ASSOCIATED WITH EXPOSURE TO EE

The EE-induced changes in behavior can be linked to specific changes in neuronal functionality. This has been studied in best detail for behavior associated with hippocampal function (Van Praag et al., 2000; Eckert and Abraham, 2013) and we briefly describe these as a prelude to describing the changes seen in adult sensory cortices, the particular brain regions of interest here in the context of our over-arching thesis (Alwis et al., 2012) that many persistent cognitive and motor deficits in TBI have sensory deficits as an underlying cause. The studies discussed below have used electrophysiological techniques such as *in vivo* and *in vitro* intra and extracellular recordings to specifically investigate EE-induced changes in neuronal function.

EE-induced improvements in hippocampal-dependent memory function have been linked to experience-dependent changes in hippocampal synaptic strength (Kempermann et al., 1997; Schrijver et al., 2002; Vedovelli et al., 2011), with reports of increases in excitatory post-synaptic potential (EPSP) amplitudes and evoked population spikes in rats exposed to generic EE, both in *in vivo* studies (Sharp et al., 1985; Irvine and Abraham, 2005; Irvine et al., 2006) and in *in vitro* studies of slices from the dentate gyrus (Green and Greenough, 1986; Foster et al., 1996) or the CA3-CA1 pathway (Foster and Dumas, 2001; Malik and Chattarji, 2012). The enhanced synaptic efficacy in dentate gyrus appears likely to act through AMPA and NMDA receptor mediated mechanisms (Foster et al., 1996). Interestingly, these increases did not outlast the termination of EE housing

(Green and Greenough, 1986), even though EE-induced changes in behavior and morphology persist after discontinuation of EE (Camel et al., 1986; Cheng et al., 2012), suggesting that information stored in the dentate gyrus may be related to more transient behavioral effects of EE. However, there is also contradiction in studies of EE-induced long-term hippocampal plasticity. Eckert and Abraham (2010) reported that long-term exposure to EE did not result in enhanced synaptic transmission in the hippocampus, both *in vivo* and *in vitro*, suggesting that the variability in these studies may have be due to different EE paradigms, or to homeostatic mechanisms to re-establish normal synaptic transmission (Turrigiano, 1999, 2008). Foster and colleagues (Foster et al., 1996; Foster and Dumas, 2001) demonstrated that EE housing inhibits LTP induction in the perforant pathway, suggesting that both experience-dependent synaptic plasticity and LTP expression share similar yet-unknown underlying mechanisms. Conversely, increased LTP expression has been reported after EE exposure (Duffy et al., 2001; Artola et al., 2006; Eckert and Abraham, 2010; Malik and Chattarji, 2012). One resolution for these effects, other than differences in the EE conditions, is that LTP induction after EE may be differentially regulated in different regions of the hippocampus.

It is worth noting here that short-term plasticity in the hippocampus has not been shown to be affected by EE (Foster et al., 1996; Foster and Dumas, 2001; Eckert and Abraham, 2010; Malik and Chattarji, 2012).

In contrast to the hippocampus, little is known about EE-induced changes in neuronal functionality in cortex. What changes there are in cortical neuronal function have mainly been examined at the level of the sensory cortices and we discuss these studies in detail below. EE-induced changes in neuronal function in the normal (uninjured) sensory cortices are particularly salient to our thesis and may provide us with insights into the role of EE on neuronal function after brain injury, of which nothing is known as yet.

EE AND SENSORY CORTICES

The effects of EE have been studied most extensively in auditory cortex, in some detail in somatosensory cortex, and only to a limited degree in visual cortex.

In auditory cortex, the effect of EE has been studied at levels ranging from brain slices through to extracellular recordings from neurons in anaesthetized animals. In the investigation of the effects of EE on the auditory cortex, studies have used enriched environments that include specific auditory enrichment in the form of playback of various sounds within the housing environment (Engineer et al., 2004; Percaccio et al., 2005, 2007; Nichols et al., 2007). Many studies report effects that mirror those seen in the hippocampus, of increased synaptic efficiency. Thus, auditory cortex slices show that specific EE induces an increase in excitatory post-synaptic current (EPSC) amplitudes, coupled with a decrease in current rise-times in supragranular cortical layers and no changes in infragranular layer V (Nichols et al., 2007). *In vivo* recordings from the anaesthetized rat, primarily from Layers 4/5 of adult primary auditory cortex after specific auditory EE, have demonstrated an increase in cortical responsiveness (both spontaneous and stimulus-evoked), decreased response latencies, and an increase in frequency selectivity (Engineer et al., 2004; Percaccio et al., 2005; Cai et al., 2009). Percaccio et al. (2005, 2007) also found that EE increased paired pulse depression (PPD) in the rat auditory cortex, indicating an increased probability of synaptic transmitter release and thus, enhanced synaptic transmission. Other studies in auditory cortex found EE could cause reorganization of the cortical tonotopic map (Norena et al., 2006; Pienkowski and Eggermont, 2009; Zhou et al., 2011; Kim and Bao, 2013), and alterations in stimulus frequency selectivity over either a range of frequencies (Zhou et al., 2011) or for frequencies specific to those used as a part of the enrichment condition (Norena et al., 2006; Pienkowski and Eggermont, 2009).

The effects of auditory enrichment are not restricted to primary auditory cortex, and Jakkamsetti et al. (2012) have reported that responses in posterior auditory field (PAF) are also increased when compared with animals housed in standard environments. These increased firing rates were accompanied by decreases in response latency and duration, and a reduction in receptive field size, as seen in primary auditory cortex (Engineer et al., 2004; Zhou et al., 2011; Jakkamsetti et al., 2012).

Unlike the above-noted reports, some studies do not report increased neuronal responsiveness and sharper frequency tuning after exposure to auditory enrichment (Condon and Weinberger, 1991; Bao et al., 2003). Instead, these studies found that a repeated auditory stimulus decreased responsiveness to frequencies used in the stimulus (Condon and Weinberger, 1991), and exposure to noise burst trains produced broadly tuned receptive fields (Bao et al., 2003). Percaccio et al. (2007) have suggested that a critical variable in eliciting EE effects in auditory cortex is the nature of the enrichment, i.e., how engaging or complex the stimuli are. This would explain the increased neuronal responsiveness reported by Percaccio et al. (2007) in rats receiving even passive exposure to specific auditory EE, which included situation-dependent stimuli from the environment and from cagemates, as opposed to simple, less behaviorally relevant stimuli.

Similar to studies in auditory cortex, generic EE (i.e., non-specific enrichment) results in reorganized cortical topographic maps, decreased receptive field sizes, increased response selectivity and increased sensory evoked potentials in the somatosensory cortex (Xerri et al., 1996; Coq and Xerri, 1998; Polley et al., 2004; Devonshire et al., 2010). One interesting effect demonstrated here is that EE effects on receptive field sizes and responses to stimulation of the main topographic input to the neurons may be laminar selective (an effect that does not appear to have been explored in auditory cortex). Thus, in the rodent barrel cortex that receives tactile input from the mystacial whiskers, EE caused a decrease in receptive field size and in neuronal responses evoked by stimulation of the "Principal Whisker" (the topographically matched whisker providing the main input to a group of neurons in the barrel cortex) in supragranular cortical Layers 2/3, but there were no changes in response strength or receptive field size in input Layer 4 (Polley et al., 2004). It is worth noting that Guic et al. (2008) found that EE caused an increase in cortical representational area in Layer 4. However, these effects were seen after stimulation of only a few selective whiskers, while other whiskers were trimmed whereas Polley et al. (2004) used a non-deprived paradigm where all whiskers remained untrimmed.

These different effects are likely a reflection of variations in experimental design of the EE conditions, consistent with the conclusions drawn from studies in auditory cortex that the nature of EE conditions influences neuronal outcomes.

These studies, where the emphasis was on measuring receptive field sizes and responses only to simple input from the main topographically-matched region of the body, indicated laminar specificity of effects. However, when neuronal encoding of sophisticated sensory input is the metric, the effects of generic EE occur globally across all cortical layers. Thus, in our own studies, 8–10 weeks of EE exposure increased neuronal firing rates globally across all layers 2–5 of the rat barrel cortex, and did so in response to both simple stimuli and a variety of complex, naturalistic stimuli (Alwis and Rajan, 2013). It is interesting to note that these effects occur even to the complex stimuli as our previous work on TBI (Alwis et al., 2012) had suggested that the complex stimuli may engage a diversity of intra-cortical processing mechanisms not seen with the simple stimuli. These effects occurred without any change in response latency, suggesting that the effects were specific to cortex and not due to changes at lower levels of the somatic pathways to cortex.

Although not often studied on its own in somatosensory cortex, recently EE has been combined with another manipulation that induces experience-dependent plasticity in barrel cortex, viz. whisker trimming and/or stimulation (Armstrong-James et al., 1992; Diamond et al., 1993, 1994; Rema et al., 2006; Guic et al., 2008; Megevand et al., 2009). Here the picture is rather murky, with one study suggesting that EE operates through different mechanisms than other plasticity mechanisms in barrel cortex, but another suggesting that it operates through the same mechanisms. The first seems to apply in the case of whisker trimming: when whisker pairing (all whiskers on one side of the face trimmed except for a pair of adjacent whiskers) is coupled with short (15 h) generic EE exposure, there is an accentuation of the effects induced by whisker trimming alone: a faster shift of receptive field bias toward the untrimmed whiskers, stronger evoked responses to the intact paired whisker than to deprived whiskers, and increased spontaneous activity in supra-granular and granular layers (Rema et al., 2006). In contrast EE may operate through the same mechanisms as some other plasticity cases. Thus, a short duration of whisker stimulation at a frequency often used during exploratory whisking behavior increases stimulus evoked potentials in both supra-granular and granular barrel cortex layers (Megevand et al., 2009)—but, addition of EE to the whisker stimulation paradigm does *not* further potentiate responses (Megevand et al., 2009).

Finally, only a limited number of studies have examined the effects of EE in the normal visual cortex. In area 17 of the adult visual cortex, similar to effects seen in the auditory cortex, generic EE results in sharper bandwidths in orientation tuned cells, increased neuronal responses to light stimuli, increased visual acuity, as well as increased stimulus contrast and temporal selectivity (Beaulieu and Cynader, 1990a,b; Mainardi et al., 2010). In addition to these effects in normal adult visual cortex, studies of EE-induced plasticity in the adult visual cortex have also examined effects in the context of monocular deprivation (MD) and amblyopia. MD during developmentally critical periods induces a shift in ocular dominance (OD) so that more neurons respond to stimulation of the open eye (Frenkel and Bear, 2004; Mrsic-Flogel et al., 2007). Such plasticity is normally not seen when MD is started in adulthood, but EE housing for 3 weeks re-activates cortical plasticity in supragranular layers of adult visual cortex such that OD changes are possible again and visual evoked potentials (VEPs) elicited by stimulation of the deprived eye are greatly depressed (Baroncelli et al., 2010b). In amblyopia, individual components of EE such as motor and visual stimulation, as well as the combination of these components, also recover visual acuity and restore OD plasticity and binocularity in supragranular layers of adult visual cortex (Sale et al., 2007; Baroncelli et al., 2012; Tognini et al., 2012).

Taken together, these studies of EE effects in sensory cortices show that generic EE is potent at producing many changes in neuronal responses, such as stronger responses and greater stimulus selectivity; that the receptive field effects may be laminar-selective and depend on the type of enrichment but that effects on more sophisticated neuronal processing, particularly of naturalistic stimuli that mimic everyday events, occur across all cortical laminae; and finally, that EE may operate independent of some other mechanisms of cortical plasticity.

MECHANISMS UNDERLYING EE-INDUCED CHANGES IN NEURONAL FUNCTION

There are numerous well-documented structural and biochemical consequences of EE which may underlie the effects of EE on neuronal function. We broadly review these changes with EE (summarized in **Figure 1**). It must be noted that in most cases, we do not know how these structural and molecular changes contribute to EE-induced changes in neuronal function: to date, there has been very limited attempt only to directly manipulate these fine-scale changes to determine to what extent they cause EE-related changes in neuronal functionality.

MORPHOLOGICAL CHANGES

It was very early recognized that exposure to complex, enriched environments causes gross morphological changes in an overall increase in brain weight, particularly in cortical and hippocampal weight and thickness (Bennett et al., 1969; Walsh et al., 1969; Diamond et al., 1972, 1976). The factors contributing to these gross morphological changes include increased neuronal density and size, increased dendritic branching and length, increased dendritic spine density, and increased turnover in pyramidal and stellate cells (Holloway, 1966; Diamond et al., 1967; Volkmar and Greenough, 1972; Globus et al., 1973; Greenough and Volkmar, 1973; Greenough et al., 1973; Uylings et al., 1978; Connor et al., 1982; Turner and Greenough, 1985; Kempermann et al., 1997; Leggio et al., 2005; Jung and Herms, 2012). Unsurprisingly, the changes in dendritic morphology are accompanied by synaptic alterations, with EE resulting in increased numbers of synapses and synaptic contacts (Jones et al., 1997; Briones et al., 2004; Landers et al., 2011), which could enhance cortical synaptic transmission and hence, alter cortical excitation/inhibition balances.

One particularly notable EE-induced change is neurogenesis, which may contribute to enhanced cognitive performance

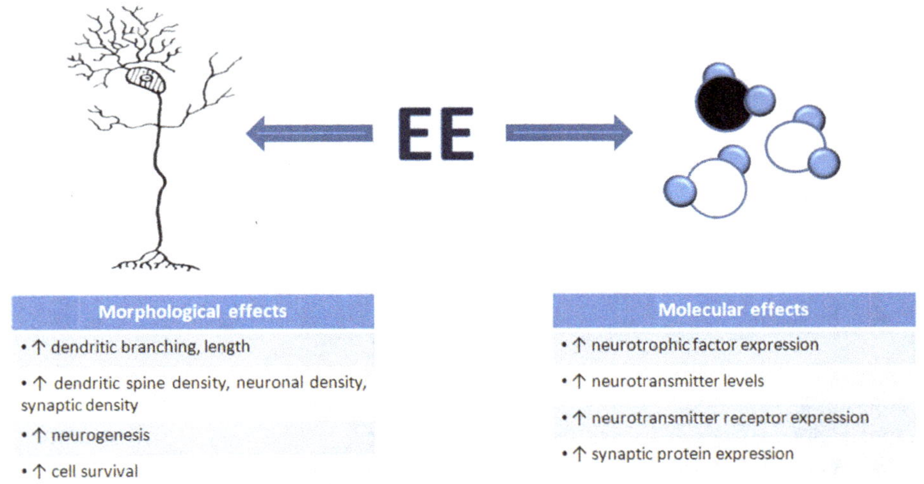

FIGURE 1 | Environmental enrichment induces morphological and molecular changes in the brain. An overview of the number of structural and molecular mechanisms that contribute to the changes in neuronal function, and ultimately, changes in behavior, seen after EE exposure. These mechanisms are thought to underlie EE-induced neural plasticity.

(Kempermann et al., 1997, 1998; Nilsson et al., 1999; Bruel-Jungerman et al., 2005). Cell proliferation, improved neuronal survival and functional integration of new neurons have all been demonstrated to occur in the adult dentate gyrus after EE (Kempermann et al., 1997, 1998; Van Praag et al., 2000; Lu et al., 2003; Bruel-Jungerman et al., 2005) and pharmacological inhibition of cell proliferation during EE prevented hippocampal neurogenesis and any improvement in a hippocampal-based memory task (Bruel-Jungerman et al., 2005). Decreased neurogenesis has been linked to cognitive decline (Drapeau et al., 2003, 2007), and restoration of neuronal proliferation and survival leads to an improvement in cognitive behavior (Kempermann, 2002).

The enhanced hippocampal neurogenesis, improved neuronal cell survival, increased synaptic density and dendritic branching (Kempermann et al., 1997, 1998; Bruel-Jungerman et al., 2005), and the growth factor up-regulation that is discussed below, have all been suggested to be responsible for EE-induced improvements in spatial and non-spatial learning and memory and enhanced spatial searching strategies (Van Praag et al., 2000; Schrijver et al., 2002; Nithianantharajah and Hannan, 2006; Kulesskaya et al., 2011; Vedovelli et al., 2011; Leger et al., 2012). Increased habituation to novel objects has also been attributed to a decrease in activation of hippocampal neurons during novel object exposure in enriched animals, in contrast to the increased activation seen in animals housed in standard conditions when exposed to objects in novel environments (Zhu et al., 1997; Leger et al., 2012). These results support the idea that EE-induced morphological changes contribute to alterations in behavior, through changes in overall neuronal function.

It must be noted here that similar neurogenesis has not been demonstrated to occur in cortex after EE, but this may be for a want of study not for an absence of the effect. In the absence of this effect, it is difficult to speculate to what extent neurogenesis contributes to EE-induced changes in cortical neuronal functionality or cortex-based processes. We will argue below that, in any case, neurogenesis is not required to occur in cortex to produce the EE-induced changes in responses and in functionality and that those changes can be produced by alterations in the balance between excitation/inhibition interplay that shapes neuronal responses and function.

MOLECULAR CHANGES

The EE-induced structural and functional changes described above occur through molecular cascades that involve increases in neurotrophic factor and neurotransmitter levels (Van Praag et al., 2000; Mohammed et al., 2002; Will et al., 2004; Nithianantharajah and Hannan, 2006), and increased expression of regulatory proteins that enhance the number and stability of synapses, increase cell proliferation, and promote neurotransmitter release (Rampon et al., 2000; Frick and Fernandez, 2003; Nithianantharajah et al., 2004).

Neurotrophic factors of particular importance to EE include brain derived neurotrophic factor (BDNF) and nerve growth factor (NGF), with levels of both increasing following exposure to exercise and EE (Pham et al., 1999; Birch et al., 2013) in brain regions including cortex, hippocampus and cerebellum (Torasdotter et al., 1998; Angelucci et al., 2009). In the adult brain, BDNF and NGF promote experience-dependent plasticity by enhancing synaptic plasticity, signaling, learning and memory (Kang and Schuman, 1995; Torasdotter et al., 1998; Pham et al., 1999; Bekinschtein et al., 2011). Increases in neurotrophins appear to underlie improved motor and cognitive function after EE (Falkenberg et al., 1992; Henriksson et al., 1992; Linnarsson et al., 1997; Bekinschtein et al., 2011; Gelfo et al., 2011; Bechara and Kelly, 2013; Birch et al., 2013) since suppression of BDNF levels causes deficits in neurogenesis, learning behavior and memory (Linnarsson et al., 1997; Minichiello et al., 1999; Rossi et al., 2006; Heldt et al., 2007; Furini et al., 2010).

Similarly, neurotransmitter levels are also affected by exposure to EE, suggesting a role in the mediation of brain plasticity. Serotonin is important in promoting neuroplasticity (Maya Vetencourt et al., 2008; Baroncelli et al., 2010a), and EE induces an increase in serotonin receptor expression and in serotonin levels (Rasmuson et al., 1998; Koh et al., 2007; Baroncelli et al., 2010a). Levels of other neurotransmitters associated with synaptic plasticity, such as acetylcholine and noradrenaline, also increase following EE (Por et al., 1982; Galani et al., 2007; Brenes et al., 2009). Increased cortical responsiveness may then be attributed to increases in synaptic transmission efficacy and synaptic strength (Mainardi et al., 2010) brought about by EE-induced molecular changes.

In conjunction with these changes in neurotransmitter levels, excitatory activity also shifts following EE housing, with increases in hippocampal extracellular glutamate levels coupled with an enhanced expression of AMPA and NMDA receptors (Tang et al., 2001; Naka et al., 2005; Segovia et al., 2006). Changes in hippocampal field potentials have been attributed to factors that include increased AMPA receptor-mediated transmitter binding, increased expression of AMPA and NMDA receptor subunits, increased dendritic spine density and upregulation of growth factors (Sharp et al., 1985; Green and Greenough, 1986; Foster and Dumas, 2001; Eckert and Abraham, 2010). There is also evidence of synaptic plasticity, in the form of increased dentate gyrus LTP, in the hippocampus after physical activity, which is an important component of the EE experience (Van Praag et al., 1999). The role of these changes in excitation will be discussed in greater detail below where we argue that a principal mechanism through which EE alters brain function and behavior is by promoting a shift toward excitation in neuronal responses.

ROLE OF CHANGES IN CORTICAL EXCITATION/INHIBITION BALANCE IN EE-INDUCED CHANGES IN NEURONAL FUNCTIONALITY

As shown above, EE-induced brain plasticity is likely to occur through the combination of structural and biochemical changes that can impact on neuronal functionality. We believe that there is substantive evidence that one particularly important end-effect through which EE alters neuronal function is alterations in the balance between excitation and inhibition in cortex (Engineer et al., 2004; Percaccio et al., 2005, 2007). This E/I balance is a critical factor in regulating cortical neuronal functionality and critical periods of cortical plasticity which occur throughout development are governed by this E/I balance (Hensch and Fagiolini, 2005; Levelt and Hubener, 2012) whereby immaturity of cortical inhibition promotes plasticity while maturation of inhibitory circuits results in the decrease in plasticity associated with cortical maturation (Huang et al., 1999; Fagiolini and Hensch, 2000). Shifts in this E/I balance may also play a major role in the experience-dependent cortical plasticity, which includes plasticity induced by EE or deprivation, that occurs outside developmental critical periods (Hensch and Fagiolini, 2005; Sale et al., 2007; Benali et al., 2008; Maya Vetencourt et al., 2008; Megevand et al., 2009; Baroncelli et al., 2010b, 2011; Luz and Shamir, 2012; Maya-Vetencourt et al., 2012). Changes in neuronal function in the adult brain suggest that EE exposure causes a reactivation of forms of neuronal plasticity generally seen only in the developing, immature brain (Chang and Merzenich, 2003; Chang et al., 2005) in which inhibitory mechanisms are immature.

Experience-dependent changes in response strength and sensitivity in adult sensory cortices have been attributed to decreased levels of cortical inhibition (Buonomano and Merzenich, 1998; Baroncelli et al., 2011), which shift cortical E/I ratios to favor excitation. Studies have demonstrated the importance of GABA synthesis in promoting plasticity (Hensch et al., 1998; Harauzov et al., 2010) after MD, and disruption of GABA-ergic inhibition through pharmacological treatments or EE reinstates plasticity to restore OD plasticity in adult visual cortex (Sale et al., 2007; Maya Vetencourt et al., 2008; Harauzov et al., 2010; Zhou et al., 2011; Maya-Vetencourt et al., 2012). Similarly, Zhou et al. (2011) found that EE-induced plasticity in auditory cortex was accompanied by a decrease in GABA receptor subunit expression. Sale et al. (2007) have also shown that EE exposure results in a decrease in basal extracellular GABA levels in the visual cortex, and that EE-induced plasticity can be countered by pharmacologically increasing inhibitory activity. EE-induced decreases in cortical inhibition have been demonstrated in studies of auditory and visual cortex, through decreases in GABA receptor subunit expression, inhibitory synapse density and basal levels of GABA (Beaulieu and Colonnier, 1987; Zhou et al., 2011; Jakkamsetti et al., 2012), while GAD67 expression has also been shown to decrease following exposure to EE (Scali et al., 2012; Tognini et al., 2012).

However, decreased inhibition may just be one mechanism underlying EE-induced plasticity via shifts in the excitation/inhibition balance, with studies also suggesting an increase in cortical excitation with EE. Nichols et al. (2007) have shown that exposure to EE induces an AMPA-receptor mediated increase in EPSC amplitudes in supragranular layers of the auditory cortex, with no changes in GABA-ergic transmission, while the increase in PPD after EE demonstrated by Percaccio et al. (2005) suggests an increase in the transmitter release probability of excitatory synapses.

Taken together, the results presented in this section suggest that EE exerts its effects through molecular changes, which in turn support changes in morphology and neuronal function. These results also suggest that in conditions such as brain injury, which result in abnormal neuronal activity, EE-induced plasticity may have the potential as a therapy to steer neuronal activity toward a more functionally relevant state. This is particularly the case when it is considered that excitation/inhibition shifts may also occur in brain injury (Ding et al., 2008; Alwis et al., 2012; Johnstone et al., 2013).

EE AND THE DAMAGED BRAIN

Considering that the brain plasticity evoked by EE results in various behavioral benefits, it is hardly surprising that EE (and specifically the form we have termed "generic" EE) has been proposed as a putative therapy for neurological conditions ranging from Alzheimer's disease through to ischemia/stroke (Faherty et al., 2005; Jadavji et al., 2006; Buchhold et al., 2007; Nithianantharajah et al., 2008; Wang et al., 2008; Hu et al., 2010; Valero et al., 2011; Du et al., 2012). Indeed, EE ameliorates the behavioral and pathological deficits associated with many of these conditions:

for example, in models of Alzheimer's disease, EE enhances neuronal proliferation, survival and maturation, leading to improved cognition (Hu et al., 2010; Valero et al., 2011), while in studies of stroke/ischemia, EE improves sensorimotor function, such as impaired gait and limb placement (Buchhold et al., 2007; Wang et al., 2008).

Our focus in this review is on the potential role of EE as a therapy for TBI, based on its known effects on brain changes induced by TBI, especially in the sensory cortices. For this consideration, it is necessary to first define some of the basic features of TBI and its effects on brain and behavior. There are two major forms of TBI—focal and diffuse. Focal brain injury is caused by direct, localized damage to the brain, while diffuse injury is most commonly caused by indirect forces, such as during rapid acceleration/deceleration of the head (Andriessen et al., 2010; Alwis et al., 2013). TBI affects approximately 2 million individuals every year in the US alone (Faul et al., 2010) and has been shown to result in a number of persistent sensory deficits, which are thought to underlie TBI-associated cognitive disabilities (Caeyenberghs et al., 2009; Davis and Dean, 2010; Lew et al., 2010; Folmer et al., 2011). People with mild to moderate diffuse TBI usually recover motor skills fully, but have other prolonged deficits, including cognitive deficits and memory loss, likely from axonal injury (Strich, 1956; Adams et al., 1999; Graham et al., 2000; Little et al., 2010).

In TBI there are often substantial and prolonged functional deficits in cognition, memory and movement (Gagnon et al., 1998; Draper and Ponsford, 2008; Park et al., 2008; Faul et al., 2010; Risdall and Menon, 2011) and these are invariably viewed as resulting from damage to brain areas specific to those functions. What has been consistently overlooked is that most TBI sufferers show deficits in how they process sensory information. What we see, hear, touch is used to understand the world and guide complex behaviors like thinking, movement, or memory; sensory processing deficits easily affect these behaviors. It has been recognized that at least some impairments may involve disruption of the integration of sensory input (Brosseau-Lachaine et al., 2008; Patel et al., 2011). In humans, speeded motor tasks and response time tasks are also affected in mild/moderate TBI (Bawden et al., 1985; Haaland et al., 1994), and animal studies have shown persistent abnormal sensory behavior (McNamara et al., 2010), again suggesting disturbances in sensorimotor processing, and there are many long-lasting sensory and cognitive impairments even after motor function has recovered (Narayan et al., 2002; Draper and Ponsford, 2009; Faul et al., 2010; Risdall and Menon, 2011).

Consistent with this hypothesis of a sensory cortices basis for persistent cognitive, memory and motor deficits in TBI, experimental TBI causes significant time-dependent changes in neuronal excitability in sensory cortices (Hall and Lifshitz, 2010; Ding et al., 2011; Alwis et al., 2012). In the immediate post-TBI period, changes in neuronal activity occur across all cortical layers, and consist in a depth-dependent (from the cortical surface) suppression of responses to all types of simple and complex naturalistic stimuli (Johnstone et al., 2013; Yan et al., 2013). However, by the long-term (8–10 weeks post-TBI), effects are found only in the upper cortical layers, layers 2 and upper layer 3, and decrease with cortical depth such that there are no long-term changes in input layer 4 (Alwis et al., 2012); further the changes in the upper layers are no longer a suppression of responses but, rather, a hyper-excitation (Alwis et al., 2012). These persistent effects are consistent with an imbalance in cortical excitation/inhibition (Ding et al., 2011; Alwis et al., 2012).

Given the known effects of EE on the E/I balance in cortex, we believe that there is potential for EE to remediate TBI-induced changes in neuronal function by restoring the cortical excitation/inhibition balance, to improve sensorimotor and cognitive behavior. However, there is no current literature probing the effects of EE specifically on neuronal function post-TBI, highlighting the need for studies examining the mechanisms underlying the EE-induced functional improvements that have been reported in the literature. Hence, in the following section of the review, we will first consolidate and discuss studies that have examined the effects of EE after experimental brain injury, which have focussed on mainly behavioral effects. We will then discuss possible mechanisms through which EE acts to improve functional outcomes post-injury, based on the known mechanisms underlying the effects of EE (as discussed above). Finally, we will review the implementation and efficacy of EE as a therapeutic option to remediate brain injury in a clinical setting.

THE BENEFICIAL EFFECTS OF EE POST-TBI

Only a few studies have investigated the effects of EE on functional recovery post-experimental TBI and shown that exposure to EE ameliorates motor and cognitive deficits and TBI-induced histopathologies (Hamm et al., 1996; Passineau et al., 2001; Hicks et al., 2002; Sozda et al., 2010; De Witt et al., 2011; Matter et al., 2011; Monaco et al., 2013; Bondi et al., 2014), with some very limited work on the effect of EE on TBI-induced sensory morbidities. These studies have predominantly studied the use of generic EE in the treatment of TBI, except for some work that has included the use of multi-modal sensory stimulation with generic EE (discussed further below).

EE improves TBI-induced cellular histopathologies: EE-treated animals show decreases in lesion volume, increased neuronal survival, and reduced neuronal degeneration in cortex (Passineau et al., 2001; Lippert-Gruner et al., 2007; Monaco et al., 2013). Muthuraju et al. (2012) recently reported an EE-mediated decrease in cell death, in conjunction with an increase in neurogenesis in the striatum, post-TBI. Additionally, in correlation with the positive effects on motor and cognitive function, decreased apoptosis and lesion volume have also been shown using a combination of multi-modal sensory stimulation and EE (Maegele et al., 2005a; Lippert-Gruner et al., 2007). These effects suggest that EE may be able to ameliorate or attenuate damage caused by secondary injury processes, which are often complex and dynamic in nature.

The effects of EE on motor and cognitive function after TBI have only been investigated in TBI models that cause a mixture of focal and diffuse TBI (Hamm et al., 1996; Passineau et al., 2001; Hicks et al., 2002; Hoffman et al., 2008; Sozda et al., 2010; De Witt et al., 2011; Matter et al., 2011; Monaco et al., 2013), and to date, no studies have examined the effect of EE after a purely diffuse model of TBI. The studies of EE effects in mixed model TBI have demonstrated positive effects of EE on neuromotor and cognitive function, especially for spatial navigation and memory. Hamm et al. (1996) found that at 11–15 days after mixed-model TBI, animals exposed to generic EE displayed elevated spatial memory function in the Morris Water Maze (MWM) test, when compared with TBI animals housed in standard conditions. EE housing also improved cognitive functioning to levels comparable to those of sham controls (Hamm et al., 1996). These findings are similar to reports demonstrating EE-induced recovery of spatial navigation and spatial memory after hippocampal/cortical lesions (Will et al., 1977; Einon et al., 1980; Whishaw et al., 1984). EE-induced improvements in spatial navigation, increases in spatial acquisition task rate, as well as improved spatial memory, have been demonstrated in other experimental models of mixed-model TBI (Passineau et al., 2001; Hicks et al., 2002; Wagner et al., 2002; De Witt et al., 2011; Matter et al., 2011; Monaco et al., 2013). EE-mediated recovery of locomotor activity and motor function in beam-walking and rotatod tasks has also been documented post-TBI (Wagner et al., 2002; De Witt et al., 2011; Matter et al., 2011; Monaco et al., 2013), while EE exposure also improved recovery time of forelimb function after CCI (controlled cortical impact) injury (Smith et al., 2007).

While EE on its own has all of these benefits for motor and cognitive function, there is also evidence that the use of additional multi-modal sensorimotor stimulation together with EE can improve cognitive and motor function (Maegele et al., 2005b; Lippert-Gruener et al., 2007; Lippert-Gruner et al., 2007, 2011) at both acute (7 and 15d; Maegele et al., 2005a,b; Lippert-Gruner et al., 2007), and chronic (30d; Lippert-Gruener et al., 2007) time-points post-injury. Such enhanced stimulation is thought to better mimic rehabilitation paradigms used in clinical settings in the treatment of brain injury. Maegele et al. (2005a) have demonstrated that enhanced sensory stimulation in combination with EE improves behavioral outcomes more than the use of EE on its own (Maegele et al., 2005a), suggesting that any neuroplasticity conferred by increased stimulation may be therapeutically relevant.

Only a very few studies have examined the efficacy of EE in ameliorating sensory deficits after TBI, with only one study (Johnson et al., 2013) reporting that EE exposure completely recovers TBI-induced sensory neglect, a condition where there is a reduction in responsiveness to sensorimotor stimuli (Kim et al., 1999). Conversely, in a unilateral cortical lesion model of brain injury, Rose et al. (1987) found that EE did not facilitate recovery from sensory neglect post-lesion. These contradictory results may be explained by differences in the nature of injury, or even the timing of EE exposure: in the Johnson et al. (2013) study, 15 days of EE exposure occurred immediately *prior* to TBI, whilst Rose et al. (1987) examined the effects of 6 weeks of EE exposure commencing 10–12 days post-lesion. We will demonstrate below that the timing of the application of EE is absolutely critical for ameliorating TBI-induced behavior deficits.

In most of these studies, the type of EE applied has been what we have termed "generic" EE. Whether fortuitous or planned, this form of EE, which must engage a range of sensory, motor, cognitive and social behaviors, appears to greatly improve recovery post-TBI. Thus, Hoffman et al. (2008) indicate that EE-induced functional recovery may depend on task-specific experience: post-TBI, animals show enhanced recovery of motor function (e.g., beam traversing and balancing) and spatial learning and memory (decreased latency to locate a platform in the MWM), when exposed to both EE *and* task-specific training for the motor and cognitive tests. They also suggest that the enhanced motor, social and cognitive stimulation provided by housing in EE conditions could, in themselves, contribute to the improved motor and cognitive they observed. It is possible that exposure to general EE vs. specific EE dictates the level of functionality that is conferred; although it is true that often studies using specific EE focus on tasks related to the aspect of EE that they enhance. Considering the ambiguity that remains concerning this issue, further investigations are required to determine whether exposure to task-specific experience or specific EE can improve overall functionality in a range of tasks.

It has been suggested that improved sensorimotor function after brain injury may actually be attributed to behavioral compensation rather than functional recovery; improvements on multi-sensory tasks, such as a MWM test, could be due to the use of cues from alternate (presumably undamaged) modalities (Finger, 1978; Rose et al., 1987, 1993; Kolb et al., 1996). This view receives support from studies that show that EE has much more limited or negligible benefit in tasks involving a single sensory modality (Rose et al., 1987, 1988). However, there is also no reason why the two effects could not o-exist and in keeping with this possibility, studies have shown a degree of EE-induced functional recovery after cortical injury, accompanied by an observed difference in the movements of the animals during task performance such as skilled reaching post-injury (Whishaw et al., 1991; Rowntree and Kolb, 1997; Kolb, 1999), suggesting that perhaps both recovery and compensation may account for improved functional outcomes after injury, possibly through the recruitment of uninjured cortical circuits (Kolb, 1999). We therefore turn now to a consideration of the potential mechanisms whereby EE could improve outcomes after TBI.

MECHANISMS PROMOTING IMPROVED BEHAVIORAL AND PATHOLOGICAL RECOVERY

To understand how EE could promote recovery after TBI, it is necessary to understand some of the mechanisms underlying TBI. This is not a simple endeavor since neurodegeneration caused by TBI occurs as a result of a number of complex and dynamic inter-related mechanisms (Smith et al., 1991; Hicks et al., 1993; Pierce et al., 1998; Hall and Lifshitz, 2010; McNamara et al., 2010). Only a few studies have examined how EE impacts on these complex molecular and anatomical factors affected in TBI or any other form of brain injury. Thus, ideas of how EE might produce improvements in sensorimotor and cognitive behavior after TBI or any brain injury are often based on extrapolations of the known actions of EE in the normal brain.

In uninjured animals, EE enhances neurogenesis, improves neuronal survival, and decreases apoptotic cell death (Kempermann et al., 1997; Van Praag et al., 2000; Lu et al., 2003; Bruel-Jungerman et al., 2005), all of which have been linked to improved behavioral recovery after TBI (Passineau et al., 2001; Gaulke et al., 2005; Sozda et al., 2010; Monaco et al., 2013). Additionally, Miller et al. (2013) have also recently demonstrated a decrease in hippocampal volume loss in TBI patients, with increased engagement with cognitively, physically and socially demanding activities, supporting the role of EE in directly preventing neuronal death.

Post-injury EE housing has been shown to decrease injury-induced lesion volume, increase synaptic density, increase post-synaptic density (PSD) thickness, increase dendritic spine density and dendritic branching in supragranular and infragranular layers of injured cortex (Biernaskie and Corbett, 2001; Ip et al., 2002; Johansson and Belichenko, 2002; Xu et al., 2009a,b). Such structural changes may lead to EE-enabled compensation and recovery of function after injury (Rose et al., 1987; Kolb and Gibb, 1991; Whishaw et al., 1991; Passineau et al., 2001; Will et al., 2004). Under uninjured conditions, EE-induced structural changes are thought to occur due to upregulation of trophic factors such as VEGF and BDNF which promote cell survival and plasticity, and an increase in activation of transcription factors of proteins mediating plasticity (Young et al., 1999; Rampon et al., 2000; Keyvani et al., 2004; Will et al., 2004; Gaulke et al., 2005; Hoffman et al., 2008; Sozda et al., 2010; Monaco et al., 2013; Ortuzar et al., 2013). Interestingly, studies have reported an increase in BDNF expression after TBI (Hicks et al., 1997; Chen et al., 2005), with no further increase following exposure to EE (Chen et al., 2005) suggesting that EE-induced benefits for recovery after TBI may not depend on increasing the levels of trophic factors.

The effects of TBI may also be exerted through inflammatory processes: as we have noted previously (Alwis et al., 2013), activation of inflammatory cascades as part of the normal cellular response to injury can cause further injury to the already damaged brain (Menge et al., 2001; Morganti-Kossmann et al., 2002). The inflammatory response in TBI involves production of pro-inflammatory cytokines like interleukin-1 (IL-1), IL-6 and tumor necrosis factor (TNF-a), and anti-inflammatory cytokines such as IL-10 and IL-12, all of which are seen in the cerebrospinal fluid of TBI patients within a few hours of the primary injury. Inflammatory cytokines IL-1a, IL-1b, and IL-18 are also increased after TBI (Menge et al., 2001; Morganti-Kossmann et al., 2002). Interestingly, EE is able to decrease levels of pro-inflammatory molecules such as tumor necrosis factor alpha (TNF-α) and interleukin 1b (IL-1b; Briones et al., 2013) in the cortex and hippocampus post-injury. Given the up-regulation of these factors by TBI, the EE effect may attenuate secondary-injury related damage.

EE also induces an increase in neurotransmitter levels such as noradrenaline and dopamine, NMDA receptor expression, and brain metabolic activity, all of which are altered in TBI and have been implicated in impairment of motor and cognitive function; thus, exposure to EE could possibly regulate TBI-induced changes in these factors (Brenner et al., 1983; Boyeson and Feeney, 1990; Liljequist et al., 1993; Dietrich et al., 1994; Hamm et al., 1996).

We noted above that some work indicates that EE in animal models of epilepsy attenuates onset of seizures, a functional consequence of aberrant neuronal excitability after TBI (Pitkanen and McIntosh, 2006; Hunt et al., 2013; Shultz et al., 2013). While the exact mechanisms underlying this protective effect are unknown, it is thought to occur through an EE-induced enhancement of trophic support, changes in receptor expression and enhanced neurogenesis (as previously described; Liu et al., 1993; Cheng et al., 1995; Young et al., 1999; Reibel et al., 2000; Korbey et al., 2008).

This review shows that overall, there are insufficient data available to decide if EE effects on all of the TBI-induced molecular events noted above are all (or any of them) involved in the beneficial effects of EE in TBI. Given the limited amount of knowledge of the effects of EE specifically in TBI, it is worth also considering how EE acts therapeutically in other neurological disorders. The general trend of how EE has benefits in other brain disorders is summarized in **Table 1**, where it can be seen that EE acts to increase neurogenesis, dendritic branching and spine density, and increase the expression of growth factors (Johansson and Ohlsson, 1996; Young et al., 1999; Jadavji et al., 2006; Pereira et al., 2007; Gelfo et al., 2011; Valero et al., 2011). Similarly, recent work by Koopmans et al. (2012) has also demonstrated increased spinal cord progenitor cell differentiation and increased serotonergic innervation after experimental SCI, while others have shown increased dendritic spine density in the motor cortex (Kim et al., 2008) and increased BDNF levels (Berrocal et al., 2007). These studies, as well as those focussing on TBI, show that EE appears to be a promising post-injury treatment to improve sensorimotor and cognitive function in brain injury, most likely due to similar underlying structural and molecular mechanisms. Due to the wide and inter-connected nature of the effects of EE, it is likely that a combination of both molecular and morphological changes needs to occur in order to see improvements in neuronal function and behavior.

TIMING OF THE USE OF EE AS A THERAPY AFTER TBI

Some clues as to the potential mechanism by which EE could rescue brain function in TBI comes from the finding that the timing and duration of EE are important factors governing motor and cognitive recovery post-TBI (**Figure 2**; Hoffman et al., 2008; De Witt et al., 2011; Matter et al., 2011; Cheng et al., 2012). Thus, Hoffman et al. (2008) reported that recovery of motor and cognitive function, such as beam-walking and spatial learning and memory, depended on an optimal time and length of EE exposure relative to time after injury. After mixed focal-diffuse TBI, even a short period of EE exposure (6 h) was sufficient to improve motor and cognitive behavior to a level comparable to the enhanced performance seen after much longer (3 weeks), continuous exposure to EE (Hoffman et al., 2008; De Witt et al., 2011; Matter et al., 2011). The benefits of EE were not dose-dependent, however, as task performance in animals exposed to shorter periods of EE (2 and 4 h) did not differ significantly from those of injured animals housed in standard conditions, suggesting a minimal threshold of EE exposure is needed for beneficial effects (De Witt et al., 2011). EE-induced plasticity has persisting effects such that even limited exposure (3 weeks) to EE post-TBI can result in long-term protection from memory deficits, as assessed by the MWM task, for up to 6 months after animals are withdrawn from EE conditions (Cheng et al., 2012), making it an ideal candidate for therapy post-TBI.

Recent studies have also demonstrated that even pre-injury exposure to EE is neuroprotective (Kozlowski et al., 2004; Johnson et al., 2013). Kozlowski et al. (2004) showed that brief (15d) EE

Table 1 | Behavioral, morphological, and molecular effects of EE in various neurological disease conditions.

Neurological disorder	Behavioral effects	Morphological effects	Molecular effects	References
Stroke/hypoxia-ischemia	Improved motor function (reaching, beam-walk, rotating pole) Improved declarative memory (Novel object recognition test) Improved spatial learning and memory (Morris water maze, Radial arm maze)	Increased dendritic length and branching in cortex Preserved dendritic spine density loss/increased spine density in hippocampus, cortex Decreased cortical infarct volume Enhances cell proliferation	Increased growth factor expression	Ohlsson and Johansson, 1995; Johansson and Ohlsson, 1996; Biernaskie and Corbett, 2001; Johansson and Belichenko, 2002; Risedal et al., 2002; Dahlqvist et al., 2004; Gobbo and O'Mara, 2004; Komitova et al., 2006; Buchhold et al., 2007; Pereira et al., 2007; Rojas et al., 2013
Lesions	Improved motor function (posture, ladder climb) Improved spatial learning and memory (Morris water maze)	Increased dendritic length in cerebellum Increased dendritic branching and spine density in hippocampus, cortex	Increased growth factor expression	Kelche and Will, 1982; Held et al., 1985; Kolb and Gibb, 1991; Bindu et al., 2007; Frechette et al., 2009; De Bartolo et al., 2011; Gelfo et al., 2011
Epilepsy	Increased seizure resistance Increased exploratory activity (Open field) Improved spatial learning (Morris water maze)	Decreased hippocampal cell death Increased neurogenesis	Increased growth factor expression Enhanced expression of neuronal and synaptic plasticity mediators	Young et al., 1999; Auvergne et al., 2002; Faverjon et al., 2002; Rutten et al., 2002; Koh et al., 2007; Korbey et al., 2008
Huntington's disease	Delayed onset of motor deficits Improved spatial memory (Barnes maze, Morris water maze)	Delays degenerative loss of cerebral volume Attenuates deficits in hippocampal neurogenesis Reduced aggregation of huntingtin protein fragments	Increased growth factor expression Increased synaptic protein expression	Van Dellen et al., 2000; Hockly et al., 2002; Spires et al., 2004; Lazic et al., 2006; Nithianantharajah et al., 2008; Wood et al., 2010
Alzheimer's disease	Improved spatial learning and memory (Morris water maze, Barnes maze) Improved working memory (Radial arm water maze)	Increased/decreased Aβ and amyloid deposition Increased neuronal progenitor cell proliferation Increased/decreased neurogenesis Decreased progenitor cell survival	Increased growth factor expression Increased synaptophysin expression	Jankowsky et al., 2003, 2005; Levi et al., 2003; Arendash et al., 2004; Wen et al., 2004; Lazarov et al., 2005; Berardi et al., 2007; Cracchiolo et al., 2007; Levi and Michaelson, 2007; Valero et al., 2011
Parkinson's disease	Improved motor function (skilled reaching task)	Decreased dopaminergic neuron and transporter loss Decreased cell death	Increased growth factor expression	Bezard et al., 2003; Faherty et al., 2005; Jadavji et al., 2006

Summary of findings from studies that have investigated the effects of EE after various neurological conditions.

exposure in immature rats at p21, prior to TBI in adulthood (approximately 3 months old), results in a paradoxical increase in cortical lesion volume, but coupled with faster recovery of forelimb function, assessed by foot fault and asymmetry tests. Similarly, exposure to 15 days of EE immediately pre-TBI attenuates spatial and long-term memory deficits in the MWM task, in a manner similar to that seen after post-injury EE exposure (Johnson et al., 2013). However, the relevance of such a model in a clinical setting is limited. It is however, likely that, in accord with the Hebbian theory of plasticity, pre-injury exposure to EE acts mainly to strengthen existing connections in the uninjured brain, which may carry forward post-injury. This is likely to occur through the upregulation of trophic factors such as BDNF, which are shown to increase after exposure to motor enrichment before and after injury (Kleim et al., 2003). In contrast, post-injury EE exposure acts mainly to develop and strengthen new/previously silent/remaining connections to compensate for the damage in existing pathways (Taub et al., 2002), while elevated growth factor expression acts to limit the spread of damage (Kleim et al., 2003). This would suggest that although pre- and post-injury EE-exposure is beneficial for protection and/or recovery from injury, the underlying mechanisms may be different.

The fact that even pre-injury exposure to EE can ameliorate the effects of TBI may be taken to indicate that the benefits of EE are independent of the TBI-induced molecular and structural changes that cause deficits to brain and behavior. However, this is, as yet, an unsafe assumption for the reasons that brain processes are so highly inter-linked and often use common pathways. For example, as noted above, TBI increases inflammatory cascades while EE reduces many of the same cascades; thus

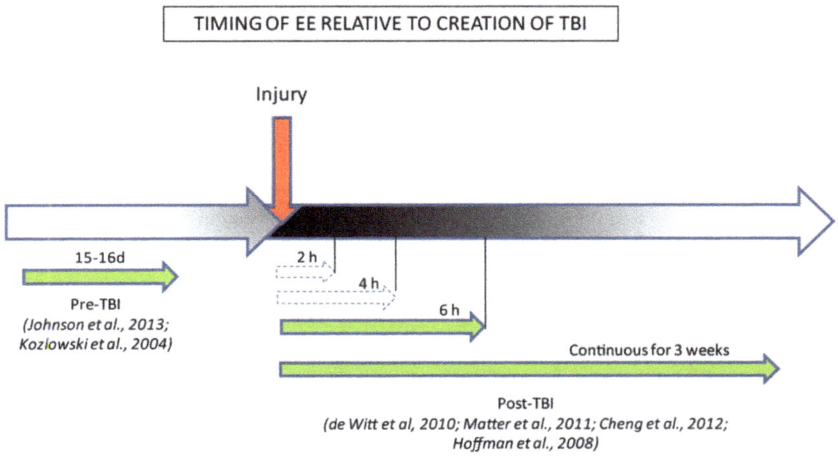

FIGURE 2 | Behavioral benefits conferred by the timing/duration of EE relative to creation of TBI. The efficacy of EE treatment when administered pre/post-injury is represented by green full-line arrows which indicate EE timing conditions that ameliorated behaviors, while white dashed arrows indicate EE timing conditions that failed to ameliorate behaviors.

down-regulation of these cascades by pre-exposure to EE may reduce subsequent TBI-induced activation of the inflammatory mechanisms and thereby reduce secondary injury processes, producing neuroprotection.

BEYOND THE BENCH

The current body of literature on the effects of EE in neurological disease indicates that EE represents significant therapeutic potential, on its own and in combination with pharmacological treatments (Kline et al., 2007, 2010, 2012), by inducing neuroprotective mechanisms involving molecular, structural, and functional processes to improve histopathologies and behavioral outcomes. Considering the many positive effects of EE demonstrated after experimental brain injury, it would be logical to try to aid recovery by applying EE in a clinical setting. Certainly, intellectually, physically and socially active lifestyles (that are akin to EE) have been linked to improved cognitive function and lower incidences of cognitive impairment, particularly in older, uninjured adults (Seeman et al., 2001; Scarmeas and Stern, 2003; Wilson et al., 2003; Newson and Kemps, 2005; Fujiwara et al., 2009; Voss et al., 2011). Similarly, cognitive enrichment early in life has also been linked to improved cognitive abilities in later life (Milgram et al., 2006), while Kramer et al. (2004) have suggested that enhanced cognitive enrichment results in improved crystallized intelligence.

Indeed, the use of EE as a rehabilitative treatment for humans post-TBI has been suggested to be effective in positively influencing long-term outcomes. However, the concept of EE for humans is more complex to define than what constitutes as EE for animals, as factors such as engagement and motivation play a role in classifying the level of enrichment an individual receives. In a clinical setting, EE can be broadly classified as a paradigm that specifically enhances and promotes engagement with cognitive, social and physical stimulation. An important caveat to the discussion about the role of EE in the treatment of TBI is that post-TBI rehabilitation programs are widely considered to be comparable to enriched environments, in that these programs often comprise of multiple components that are considered hallmarks of EE, which include physical and cognitive therapy, multi-modal stimulation, novelty, duration, functional relevance, and social integration. It has to be noted, however, that specific skill rehabilitation paradigms often do not result in improved general performance in the post-discharge environment, and instead act to improve task-specific performance (Sohlberg et al., 2000; Park and Ingles, 2001). It has instead been suggested that a more generalized treatment would be beneficial in improving overall function (Toglia, 1991; Toglia et al., 2010). Rehabilitation paradigms treating brain injury are often implemented in the acute stages post-injury, in an in-patient hospital setting. Rehabilitation based on EE principles in TBI patients results in better general functional outcomes, such as improved cognitive and motor skills (Willer et al., 1999; Powell et al., 2002; Cifu et al., 2003; Boman et al., 2004; Hayden et al., 2013), and better community integration (Zhu et al., 2001; Cicerone et al., 2004). A number of studies have also shown that increasing the duration and intensity of exposure to rehabilitative therapy results in improved recovery times (Blackerby, 1990; Spivack et al., 1992; Shiel et al., 2001; Zhu et al., 2001, 2007; Slade et al., 2002; Cifu et al., 2003; Cicerone et al., 2004).

It has also been suggested that a lack or an absence of EE is linked to cognitive decline post-injury (Till et al., 2008; Frasca et al., 2013), demonstrating the importance of continued exposure to EE in the post-discharge stages after brain injury. In that sense, a number of factors could contribute to the provision of an appropriate level of enrichment once a patient has left an intensive rehabilitative environment. These factors include ease of access to activities and resources that are cognitively, physically and socially stimulating, as well as support that encourages participation and integration with these environments (Frasca et al., 2013). Frasca et al. (2013) have also suggested that although patients eventually return to an environment that could be considered enriched post-TBI, interactions with these environments may be restricted due to limitations in cognitive and/or physical deficits. This is especially relevant during the transition from the in-patient rehabilitation environment, to post-discharge home environments, where complexity of, and engagement with environments may reduce. A reduction in enrichment in the post-acute period could be detrimental to recovery as studies have shown that functions gained during stimulation of neural pathways (such as during rehabilitation) can be lost through under-use (Rubinov et al., 2009; Warraich and Kleim, 2010; Frasca et al., 2013). Post-discharge, the major forms of therapy mapped onto EE principles include community-based and home-based rehabilitation, with the aim that these programs would aid in improving behaviors and skills required for everyday functioning, improving community integration, and preventing cognitive decline (Fryer and Haffey, 1987; Frasca et al., 2013). Studies have shown that continued enrichment in the form of cognitive rehabilitation in the post-discharge setting (i.e., domestic or vocational environments) increases neuropsychological function, learning and memory (Willer et al., 1999; Boman et al., 2004).

Given the complexity and ethics of manipulations of the environment in humans recovering from TBI, in addition to the difficulties in accurately comparing the effectiveness of various rehabilitation paradigms, questions of the correlation between these effects and EE-induced functional changes remain. Injury heterogeneity also raises challenges in defining exactly what level of enrichment is optimal and beneficial. However, the findings presented in this section strongly suggest that EE or EE-based therapy tailored to the patient's needs could significantly improve outcomes when applied in both the in-patient, acute and post-discharge, chronic settings.

CONCLUSION

The studies described here well support the use of EE as a therapeutic paradigm in the treatment of TBI. However, while the results of these studies all show promise in improving TBI-induced histopathologies and sensorimotor and cognitive deficits, there is still much work to be done to clarify our understanding of how EE exerts its effects in disease conditions. Paramount to the understanding of how EE improves behavioral outcomes after injury is the investigation of how EE changes neuronal function post-TBI, of which we know nothing. Only once these effects are unveiled will we be able to implement EE as a treatment option post-injury at its maximum potential.

It is also worth adding the caution that while EE holds promise in its application as a therapeutic tool after brain injury in humans, the complex nature of utilizing EE in a clinical setting makes it difficult to standardize treatment and compare outcomes. It is also true that EE as an experimental paradigm in animal studies has yet to be standardized, with housing conditions, environmental stimuli, number of animals per cage, age of animals at onset of enrichment, as well as the duration of enrichment, varying markedly between studies. The extent of contribution of these factors is particularly relevant when considering the demonstrated neuroprotective effects of EE in neurological disease states, where little is known about how improved functional outcomes relate to changes in neuronal function. Using experimental models that are easily controlled and manipulated, however, would provide us with valuable insight into the therapeutic potential of EE, both in laboratory and clinical settings.

REFERENCES

Abou-Ismail, U. A. (2011). The effects of cage enrichment on agonistic behaviour and dominance in male laboratory rats (Rattus norvegicus). *Res. Vet. Sci.* 90, 346–351. doi: 10.1016/j.rvsc.2010.06.010

Adams, J. H., Jennett, B., Mclellan, D. R., Murray, L. S., and Graham, D. I. (1999). The neuropathology of the vegetative state after head injury. *J. Clin. Pathol.* 52, 804–806. doi: 10.1136/jcp.52.11.804

Alwis, D., Yan, E. B., Morganti-Kossmann, M. C., and Rajan, R. (2012). Sensory cortex underpinnings of traumatic brain injury deficits. *PLoS ONE* 7:e52169. doi: 10.1371/journal.pone.0052169

Alwis, D. S., Johnstone, V., Yan, E., and Rajan, R. (2013). Diffuse traumatic brain injury and the sensory brain. *Clin. Exp. Pharmacol. Physiol.* 40, 473–483. doi: 10.1111/1440-1681.12100

Alwis, D. S., and Rajan, R. (2013). Environmental enrichment causes a global potentiation of neuronal responses across stimulus complexity and lamina of sensory cortex. *Front. Cell. Neurosci.* 7:124. doi: 10.3389/fncel.2013.00124

Andriessen, T. M., Jacobs, B., and Vos, P. E. (2010). Clinical characteristics and pathophysiological mechanisms of focal and diffuse traumatic brain injury. *J. Cell. Mol. Med.* 14, 2381–2392. doi: 10.1111/j.1582-4934.2010.01164.x

Angelucci, F., De Bartolo, P., Gelfo, F., Foti, F., Cutuli, D., Bossu, P., et al. (2009). Increased concentrations of nerve growth factor and brain-derived neurotrophic factor in the rat cerebellum after exposure to environmental enrichment. *Cerebellum* 8, 499–506. doi: 10.1007/s12311-009-0129-1

Arendash, G. W., Garcia, M. F., Costa, D. A., Cracchiolo, J. R., Wefes, I. M., and Potter, H. (2004). Environmental enrichment improves cognition in aged Alzheimer's transgenic mice despite stable beta-amyloid deposition. *Neuroreport* 15, 1751–1754. doi: 10.1097/01.wnr.0000137183.68847.4e

Armstrong-James, M., Fox, K., and Das-Gupta, A. (1992). Flow of excitation within rat barrel cortex on striking a single vibrissa. *J. Neurophysiol.* 68, 1345–1358.

Artola, A., Von Frijtag, J. C., Fermont, P. C., Gispen, W. H., Schrama, L. H., Kamal, A., et al. (2006). Long-lasting modulation of the induction of LTD and LTP in rat hippocampal CA1 by behavioural stress and environmental enrichment. *Eur. J. Neurosci.* 23, 261–272. doi: 10.1111/j.1460-9568.2005.04552.x

Auvergne, R., Lere, C., El Bahh, B., Arthaud, S., Lespinet, V., Rougier, A., et al. (2002). Delayed kindling epileptogenesis and increased neurogenesis in adult rats housed in an enriched environment. *Brain Res.* 954, 277–285. doi: 10.1016/S0006-8993(02)03355-3

Bao, S., Chang, E. F., Davis, J. D., Gobeske, K. T., and Merzenich, M. M. (2003). Progressive degradation and subsequent refinement of acoustic representations in the adult auditory cortex. *J. Neurosci.* 23, 10765–10775.

Baroncelli, L., Bonaccorsi, J., Milanese, M., Bonifacino, T., Giribaldi, F., Manno, I., et al. (2012). Enriched experience and recovery from amblyopia in adult rats: impact of motor, social and sensory components. *Neuropharmacology* 62, 2388–2397. doi: 10.1016/j.neuropharm.2012.02.010

Baroncelli, L., Braschi, C., Spolidoro, M., Begenisic, T., Maffei, L., and Sale, A. (2011). Brain plasticity and disease: a matter of inhibition. *Neural Plast.* 2011, 286073. doi: 10.1155/2011/286073

Baroncelli, L., Braschi, C., Spolidoro, M., Begenisic, T., Sale, A., and Maffei, L. (2010a). Nurturing brain plasticity: impact of environmental enrichment. *Cell Death Differ.* 17, 1092–1103. doi: 10.1038/cdd.2009.193

Baroncelli, L., Sale, A., Viegi, A., Maya Vetencourt, J. F., De Pasquale, R., Baldini, S., et al. (2010b). Experience-dependent reactivation of ocular dominance plasticity in the adult visual cortex. *Exp. Neurol.* 226, 100–109. doi: 10.1016/j.expneurol.2010.08.009

Bawden, H. N., Knights, R. M., and Winogron, H. W. (1985). Speeded performance following head injury in children. *J. Clin. Exp. Neuropsychol.* 7, 39–54. doi: 10.1080/01688638508401241

Beaulieu, C., and Colonnier, M. (1987). Effect of the richness of the environment on the cat visual cortex. *J. Comp. Neurol.* 266, 478–494. doi: 10.1002/cne.902660404

Beaulieu, C., and Cynader, M. (1990a). Effect of the richness of the environment on neurons in cat visual cortex. I. Receptive field properties. *Brain Res. Dev. Brain Res.* 53, 71–81.

Beaulieu, C., and Cynader, M. (1990b). Effect of the richness of the environment on neurons in cat visual cortex. II. Spatial and temporal frequency characteristics. *Brain Res. Dev. Brain Res.* 53, 82–88.

Bechara, R. G., and Kelly, A. M. (2013). Exercise improves object recognition memory and induces BDNF expression and cell proliferation in cognitively enriched rats. *Behav. Brain Res.* 245, 96–100. doi: 10.1016/j.bbr.2013.02.018

Bekinschtein, P., Oomen, C. A., Saksida, L. M., and Bussey, T. J. (2011). Effects of environmental enrichment and voluntary exercise on neurogenesis, learning and memory, and pattern separation: BDNF as a critical variable? *Semin. Cell Dev. Biol.* 22, 536–542. doi: 10.1016/j.semcdb.2011.07.002

Benali, A., Weiler, E., Benali, Y., Dinse, H. R., and Eysel, U. T. (2008). Excitation and inhibition jointly regulate cortical reorganization in adult rats. *J. Neurosci.* 28, 12284–12293. doi: 10.1523/JNEUROSCI.1952-08.2008

Benaroya-Milshtein, N., Hollander, N., Apter, A., Kukulansky, T., Raz, N., Wilf, A., et al. (2004). Environmental enrichment in mice decreases anxiety, attenuates stress responses and enhances natural killer cell activity. *Eur. J. Neurosci.* 20, 1341–1347. doi: 10.1111/j.1460-9568.2004.03587.x

Bengoetxea, H., Ortuzar, N., Bulnes, S., Rico-Barrio, I., Lafuente, J. V., and Argandona, E. G. (2012). Enriched and deprived sensory experience induces structural changes and rewires connectivity during the postnatal development of the brain. *Neural Plast.* 2012:305693. doi: 10.1155/2012/305693

Bennett, E. L., Rosenzweig, M. R., and Diamond, M. C. (1969). Rat brain: effects of environmental enrichment on wet and dry weights. *Science* 163, 825–826. doi: 10.1126/science.163.3869.825

Berardi, N., Braschi, C., Capsoni, S., Cattaneo, A., and Maffei, L. (2007). Environmental enrichment delays the onset of memory deficits and reduces neuropathological hallmarks in a mouse model of Alzheimer-like neurodegeneration. *J. Alzheimers Dis.* 11, 359–370.

Berrocal, Y., Pearse, D. D., Singh, A., Andrade, C. M., Mcbroom, J. S., Puentes, R., et al. (2007). Social and environmental enrichment improves sensory and motor recovery after severe contusive spinal cord injury in the rat. *J. Neurotrauma* 24, 1761–1772. doi: 10.1089/neu.2007.0327

Bezard, E., Dovero, S., Belin, D., Duconger, S., Jackson-Lewis, V., Przedborski, S., et al. (2003). Enriched environment confers resistance to 1-methyl-4-phenyl-1,2,3,6-tetrahydropyridine and cocaine: involvement of dopamine transporter and trophic factors. *J. Neurosci.* 23, 10999–11007.

Biernaskie, J., and Corbett, D. (2001). Enriched rehabilitative training promotes improved forelimb motor function and enhanced dendritic growth after focal ischemic injury. *J. Neurosci.* 21, 5272–5280.

Bindu, B., Alladi, P. A., Mansooralikhan, B. M., Srikumar, B. N., Raju, T. R., and Kutty, B. M. (2007). Short-term exposure to an enriched environment enhances dendritic branching but not brain-derived neurotrophic factor expression in the hippocampus of rats with ventral subicular lesions. *Neuroscience* 144, 412–423. doi: 10.1016/j.neuroscience.2006.09.057

Birch, A. M., Mcgarry, N. B., and Kelly, A. M. (2013). Short-term environmental enrichment, in the absence of exercise, improves memory, and increases NGF concentration, early neuronal survival, and synaptogenesis in the dentate gyrus in a time-dependent manner. *Hippocampus* 23, 437–450. doi: 10.1002/hipo.22103

Blackerby, W. F. (1990). Intensity of rehabilitation and length of stay. *Brain Inj.* 4, 167–173. doi: 10.3109/02699059009026162

Boman, I. L., Lindstedt, M., Hemmingsson, H., and Bartfai, A. (2004). Cognitive training in home environment. *Brain Inj.* 18, 985–995. doi: 10.1080/02699050410001672396

Bondi, C. O., Klitsch, K. C., Leary, J. B., and Kline, A. E. (2014). Environmental enrichment as a viable neurorehabilitation strategy for experimental traumatic brain injury. *J. Neurotrauma* 31, 873–888. doi: 10.1089/neu.2014.3328

Bourgeon, S., Xerri, C., and Coq, J. O. (2004). Abilities in tactile discrimination of textures in adult rats exposed to enriched or impoverished environments. *Behav. Brain Res.* 153, 217–231. doi: 10.1016/j.bbr.2003.12.002

Boyeson, M. G., and Feeney, D. M. (1990). Intraventricular norepinephrine facilitates motor recovery following sensorimotor cortex injury. *Pharmacol. Biochem. Behav.* 35, 497–501. doi: 10.1016/0091-3057(90)90279-Q

Brenes, J. C., Padilla, M., and Fornaguera, J. (2009). A detailed analysis of open-field habituation and behavioral and neurochemical antidepressant-like effects in postweaning enriched rats. *Behav. Brain Res.* 197, 125–137. doi: 10.1016/j.bbr.2008.08.014

Brenner, E., Mirmiran, M., Uylings, H. B., and Van Der Gugten, J. (1983). Impaired growth of the cerebral cortex of rats treated neonatally with 6-hydroxydopamine under different environmental conditions. *Neurosci. Lett.* 42, 13–17. doi: 10.1016/0304-3940(83)90414-7

Briones, T. L., Klintsova, A. Y., and Greenough, W. T. (2004). Stability of synaptic plasticity in the adult rat visual cortex induced by complex environment exposure. *Brain Res.* 1018, 130–135. doi: 10.1016/j.brainres.2004.06.001

Briones, T. L., Woods, J., and Rogozinska, M. (2013). Decreased neuroinflammation and increased brain energy homeostasis following environmental enrichment after mild traumatic brain injury is associated with improvement in cognitive function. *Acta Neuropathol. Commun.* 1, 57. doi: 10.1186/2051-5960-1-57

Brosseau-Lachaine, O., Gagnon, I., Forget, R., and Faubert, J. (2008). Mild traumatic brain injury induces prolonged visual processing deficits in children. *Brain Inj.* 22, 657–668. doi: 10.1080/02699050802203353

Bruel-Jungerman, E., Laroche, S., and Rampon, C. (2005). New neurons in the dentate gyrus are involved in the expression of enhanced long-term memory following environmental enrichment. *Eur. J. Neurosci.* 21, 513–521. doi: 10.1111/j.1460-9568.2005.03875.x

Buchhold, B., Mogoanta, L., Suofu, Y., Hamm, A., Walker, L., Kessler, C., et al. (2007). Environmental enrichment improves functional and neuropathological indices following stroke in young and aged rats. *Restor. Neurol. Neurosci.* 25, 467–484.

Buonomano, D. V., and Merzenich, M. M. (1998). Cortical plasticity: from synapses to maps. *Annu. Rev. Neurosci.* 21, 149–186. doi: 10.1146/annurev.neuro.21.1.149

Buonviso, N., and Chaput, M. (2000). Olfactory experience decreases responsiveness of the olfactory bulb in the adult rat. *Neuroscience* 95, 325–332. doi: 10.1016/S0306-4522(99)00450-9

Caeyenberghs, K., Wenderoth, N., Smits-Engelsman, B. C., Sunaert, S., and Swinnen, S. P. (2009). Neural correlates of motor dysfunction in children with traumatic brain injury: exploration of compensatory recruitment patterns. *Brain* 132, 684–694. doi: 10.1093/brain/awn344

Cai, R., Guo, F., Zhang, J., Xu, J., Cui, Y., and Sun, X. (2009). Environmental enrichment improves behavioral performance and auditory spatial representation of primary auditory cortical neurons in rat. *Neurobiol. Learn. Mem.* 91, 366–376. doi: 10.1016/j.nlm.2009.01.005

Camel, J. E., Withers, G. S., and Greenough, W. T. (1986). Persistence of visual cortex dendritic alterations induced by postweaning exposure to a "superenriched" environment in rats. *Behav. Neurosci.* 100, 810–813. doi: 10.1037/0735-7044.100.6.810

Chang, E. F., Bao, S., Imaizumi, K., Schreiner, C. E., and Merzenich, M. M. (2005). Development of spectral and temporal response selectivity in the auditory cortex. *Proc. Natl. Acad. Sci. U.S.A.* 102, 16460–16465. doi: 10.1073/pnas.0508239102

Chang, E. F., and Merzenich, M. M. (2003). Environmental noise retards auditory cortical development. *Science* 300, 498–502. doi: 10.1126/science.1082163

Chen, X., Li, Y., Kline, A. E., Dixon, C. E., Zafonte, R. D., and Wagner, A. K. (2005). Gender and environmental effects on regional brain-derived neurotrophic factor expression after experimental traumatic brain injury. *Neuroscience* 135, 11–17. doi: 10.1016/j.neuroscience.2005.05.041

Cheng, B., Furukawa, K., O'Keefe, J. A., Goodman, Y., Kihiko, M., Fabian, T., et al. (1995). Basic fibroblast growth factor selectively increases AMPA-receptor subunit GluR1 protein level and differentially modulates Ca2+ responses to AMPA and NMDA in hippocampal neurons. *J. Neurochem.* 65, 2525–2536. doi: 10.1046/j.1471-4159.1995.65062525.x

Cheng, J. P., Shaw, K. E., Monaco, C. M., Hoffman, A. N., Sozda, C. N., Olsen, A. S., et al. (2012). A relatively brief exposure to environmental enrichment after experimental traumatic brain injury confers long-term cognitive benefits. *J. Neurotrauma* 29, 2684–2688. doi: 10.1089/neu.2012.2560

Cicerone, K. D., Mott, T., Azulay, J., and Friel, J. C. (2004). Community integration and satisfaction with functioning after intensive cognitive rehabilitation for traumatic brain injury. *Arch. Phys. Med. Rehabil.* 85, 943–950. doi: 10.1016/j.apmr.2003.07.019

Cifu, D. X., Kreutzer, J. S., Kolakowsky-Hayner, S. A., Marwitz, J. H., and Englander, J. (2003). The relationship between therapy intensity and rehabilitative outcomes after traumatic brain injury: a multicenter analysis. *Arch. Phys. Med. Rehabil.* 84, 1441–1448. doi: 10.1016/S0003-9993(03)00272-7

Condon, C. D., and Weinberger, N. M. (1991). Habituation produces frequency-specific plasticity of receptive fields in the auditory cortex. *Behav. Neurosci.* 105, 416–430. doi: 10.1037/0735-7044.105.3.416

Connor, J. R., Wang, E. C., and Diamond, M. C. (1982). Increased length of terminal dendritic segments in old adult rats' somatosensory cortex:

an environmentally induced response. *Exp. Neurol.* 78, 466–470. doi: 10.1016/0014-4886(82)90064-4

Coq, J. O., and Xerri, C. (1998). Environmental enrichment alters organizational features of the forepaw representation in the primary somatosensory cortex of adult rats. *Exp. Brain Res.* 121, 191–204. doi: 10.1007/s002210050452

Cracchiolo, J. R., Mori, T., Nazian, S. J., Tan, J., Potter, H., and Arendash, G. W. (2007). Enhanced cognitive activity–over and above social or physical activity–is required to protect Alzheimer's mice against cognitive impairment, reduce Abeta deposition, and increase synaptic immunoreactivity. *Neurobiol. Learn. Mem.* 88, 277–294. doi: 10.1016/j.nlm.2007.07.007

Dahlqvist, P., Ronnback, A., Bergstrom, S. A., Soderstrom, I., and Olsson, T. (2004). Environmental enrichment reverses learning impairment in the Morris water maze after focal cerebral ischemia in rats. *Eur. J. Neurosci.* 19, 2288–2298. doi: 10.1111/j.0953-816X.2004.03248.x

Davis, A. S., and Dean, R. S. (2010). Assessing sensory-motor deficits in pediatric traumatic brain injury. *Appl. Neuropsychol.* 17, 104–109. doi: 10.1080/09084281003708951

De Bartolo, P., Gelfo, F., Burello, L., De Giorgio, A., Petrosini, L., and Granato, A. (2011). Plastic changes in striatal fast-spiking interneurons following hemicerebellectomy and environmental enrichment. *Cerebellum* 10, 624–632. doi: 10.1007/s12311-011-0275-0

De Villers-Sidani, E., and Merzenich, M. M. (2011). Lifelong plasticity in the rat auditory cortex: basic mechanisms and role of sensory experience. *Prog. Brain Res.* 191, 119–131. doi: 10.1016/B978-0-444-53752-2.00009-6

Devonshire, I. M., Dommett, E. J., Grandy, T. H., Halliday, A. C., and Greenfield, S. A. (2010). Environmental enrichment differentially modifies specific components of sensory-evoked activity in rat barrel cortex as revealed by simultaneous electrophysiological recordings and optical imaging *in vivo*. *Neuroscience* 170, 662–669. doi: 10.1016/j.neuroscience.2010.07.029

De Witt, B. W., Ehrenberg, K. M., Mcaloon, R. L., Panos, A. H., Shaw, K. E., Raghavan, P. V., et al. (2011). Abbreviated environmental enrichment enhances neurobehavioral recovery comparably to continuous exposure after traumatic brain injury. *Neurorehabil. Neural Repair* 25, 343–350. doi: 10.1177/1545968310390520

Diamond, M. C., Ingham, C. A., Johnson, R. E., Bennett, E. L., and Rosenzweig, M. R. (1976). Effects of environment on morphology of rat cerebral cortex and hippocampus. *J. Neurobiol.* 7, 75–85. doi: 10.1002/neu.480070108

Diamond, M. C., Lindner, B., and Raymond, A. (1967). Extensive cortical depth measurements and neuron size increases in the cortex of environmentally enriched rats. *J. Comp. Neurol.* 131, 357–364. doi: 10.1002/cne.901310305

Diamond, M. C., Rosenzweig, M. R., Bennett, E. L., Lindner, B., and Lyon, L. (1972). Effects of environmental enrichment and impoverishment on rat cerebral cortex. *J. Neurobiol.* 3, 47–64. doi: 10.1002/neu.480030105

Diamond, M. E., Armstrong-James, M., and Ebner, F. F. (1993). Experience-dependent plasticity in adult rat barrel cortex. *Proc. Natl. Acad. Sci. U.S.A.* 90, 2082–2086. doi: 10.1073/pnas.90.5.2082

Diamond, M. E., Huang, W., and Ebner, F. F. (1994). Laminar comparison of somatosensory cortical plasticity. *Science* 265, 1885–1888. doi: 10.1126/science.8091215

Dietrich, W. D., Alonso, O., Busto, R., and Ginsberg, M. D. (1994). Widespread metabolic depression and reduced somatosensory circuit activation following traumatic brain injury in rats. *J. Neurotrauma* 11, 629–640. doi: 10.1089/neu.1994.11.629

Ding, M. C., Lo, E. H., and Stanley, G. B. (2008). Sustained focal cortical compression reduces electrically-induced seizure threshold. *Neuroscience* 154, 551–555. doi: 10.1016/j.neuroscience.2008.03.088

Ding, M. C., Wang, Q., Lo, E. H., and Stanley, G. B. (2011). Cortical excitation and inhibition following focal traumatic brain injury. *J. Neurosci.* 31, 14085–14094. doi: 10.1523/JNEUROSCI.3572-11.2011

Drapeau, E., Mayo, W., Aurousseau, C., Le Moal, M., Piazza, P. V., and Abrous, D. N. (2003). Spatial memory performances of aged rats in the water maze predict levels of hippocampal neurogenesis. *Proc. Natl. Acad. Sci. U.S.A.* 100, 14385–14390. doi: 10.1073/pnas.2334169100

Drapeau, E., Montaron, M. F., Aguerre, S., and Abrous, D. N. (2007). Learning-induced survival of new neurons depends on the cognitive status of aged rats. *J. Neurosci.* 27, 6037–6044. doi: 10.1523/JNEUROSCI.1031-07.2007

Draper, K., and Ponsford, J. (2008). Cognitive functioning ten years following traumatic brain injury and rehabilitation. *Neuropsychology* 22, 618–625. doi: 10.1037/0894-4105.22.5.618

Draper, K., and Ponsford, J. (2009). Long-term outcome following traumatic brain injury: a comparison of subjective reports by those injured and their relatives. *Neuropsychol. Rehabil.* 19, 645–661. doi: 10.1080/17405620802613935

Du, X., Leang, L., Mustafa, T., Renoir, T., Pang, T. Y., and Hannan, A. J. (2012). Environmental enrichment rescues female-specific hyperactivity of the hypothalamic-pituitary-adrenal axis in a model of Huntington's disease. *Transl. Psychiatry* 2, e133. doi: 10.1038/tp.2012.58

Duffy, S. N., Craddock, K. J., Abel, T., and Nguyen, P. V. (2001). Environmental enrichment modifies the PKA-dependence of hippocampal LTP and improves hippocampus-dependent memory. *Learn. Mem.* 8, 26–34. doi: 10.1101/lm.36301

Eckert, M. J., and Abraham, W. C. (2010). Physiological effects of enriched environment exposure and LTP induction in the hippocampus *in vivo* do not transfer faithfully to *in vitro* slices. *Learn. Mem.* 17, 480–484. doi: 10.1101/lm.1822610

Eckert, M. J., and Abraham, W. C. (2013). Effects of environmental enrichment exposure on synaptic transmission and plasticity in the hippocampus. *Curr. Top. Behav. Neurosci.* 15, 165–187. doi: 10.1007/7854_2012_215

Einon, D. F., Morgan, M. J., and Will, B. E. (1980). Effects of post-operative environment on recovery from dorsal hippocampal lesions in young rats: tests of spatial memory and motor transfer. *Q. J. Exp. Psychol.* 32, 137–148. doi: 10.1080/00335558008248239

Elliott, B. M., and Grunberg, N. E. (2005). Effects of social and physical enrichment on open field activity differ in male and female Sprague-Dawley rats. *Behav. Brain Res.* 165, 187–196. doi: 10.1016/j.bbr.2005.06.025

Engineer, N. D., Percaccio, C. R., Pandya, P. K., Moucha, R., Rathbun, D. L., and Kilgard, M. P. (2004). Environmental enrichment improves response strength, threshold, selectivity, and latency of auditory cortex neurons. *J. Neurophysiol.* 92, 73–82. doi: 10.1152/jn.00059.2004

Erickson, K. I., Voss, M. W., Prakash, R. S., Basak, C., Szabo, A., Chaddock, L., et al. (2011). Exercise training increases size of hippocampus and improves memory. *Proc. Natl. Acad. Sci. U.S.A.* 108, 3017–3022. doi: 10.1073/pnas.1015950108

Fagiolini, M., and Hensch, T. K. (2000). Inhibitory threshold for critical-period activation in primary visual cortex. *Nature* 404, 183–186. doi: 10.1038/35004582

Faherty, C. J., Raviie Shepherd, K., Herasimtschuk, A., and Smeyne, R. J. (2005). Environmental enrichment in adulthood eliminates neuronal death in experimental Parkinsonism. *Brain Res. Mol. Brain Res.* 134, 170–179. doi: 10.1016/j.molbrainres.2004.08.008

Falkenberg, T., Mohammed, A. K., Henriksson, B., Persson, H., Winblad, B., and Lindefors, N. (1992). Increased expression of brain-derived neurotrophic factor mRNA in rat hippocampus is associated with improved spatial memory and enriched environment. *Neurosci. Lett.* 138, 153–156. doi: 10.1016/0304-3940(92)90494-R

Farmer, J., Zhao, X., Van Praag, H., Wodtke, K., Gage, F. H., and Christie, B. R. (2004). Effects of voluntary exercise on synaptic plasticity and gene expression in the dentate gyrus of adult male Sprague-Dawley rats *in vivo*. *Neuroscience* 124, 71–79. doi: 10.1016/j.neuroscience.2003.09.029

Faul, M., Xu, L., Wald, M. M., and Coronado, V. G. (2010). *Traumatic Brain Injury in the United States: Emergency Department Visits, Hospitalizations, and Deaths 2002-2006.* Atlanta, GA: Centers for Disease Control and Prevention; National Center for Injury Prevention and Control.

Faverjon, S., Silveira, D. C., Fu, D. D., Cha, B. H., Akman, C., Hu, Y., et al. (2002). Beneficial effects of enriched environment following status epilepticus in immature rats. *Neurology* 59, 1356–1364. doi: 10.1212/01.WNL.0000033588.59005.55

Fernandez-Teruel, A., Gimenez-Llort, L., Escorihuela, R. M., Gil, L., Aguilar, R., Steimer, T., et al. (2002). Early-life handling stimulation and environmental enrichment: are some of their effects mediated by similar neural mechanisms? *Pharmacol. Biochem. Behav.* 73, 233–245. doi: 10.1016/S0091-3057(02)00787-6

Finger, S. (1978). *Environmental Attenuation of Brain Lesion Symptoms.* London: Plenum Press.

Fletcher, M. L., and Wilson, D. A. (2003). Olfactory bulb mitral-tufted cell plasticity: odorant-specific tuning reflects previous odorant exposure. *J. Neurosci.* 23, 6946–6955.

Folmer, R. L., Billings, C. J., Diedesch-Rouse, A. C., Gallun, F. J., and Lew, H. L. (2011). Electrophysiological assessments of cognition and sensory processing in TBI: applications for diagnosis, prognosis and rehabilitation. *Int. J. Psychophysiol.* 82, 4–15. doi: 10.1016/j.ijpsycho.2011.03.005

Foster, T. C., and Dumas, T. C. (2001). Mechanism for increased hippocampal synaptic strength following differential experience. *J. Neurophysiol.* 85, 1377–1383.

Foster, T. C., Gagne, J., and Massicotte, G. (1996). Mechanism of altered synaptic strength due to experience: relation to long-term potentiation. *Brain Res.* 736, 243–250.

Frasca, D., Tomaszczyk, J., McFadyen, B. J., and Green, R. E. (2013). Traumatic brain injury and post-acute decline: what role does environmental enrichment play? A scoping review. *Front. Hum. Neurosci.* 7:31. doi: 10.3389/fnhum.2013.00031

Frechette, M., Rennie, K., and Pappas, B. A. (2009). Developmental forebrain cholinergic lesion and environmental enrichment: behaviour, CA1 cytoarchitecture and neurogenesis. *Brain Res.* 1252, 172–182. doi: 10.1016/j.brainres.2008.11.082

Frenkel, M. Y., and Bear, M. F. (2004). How monocular deprivation shifts ocular dominance in visual cortex of young mice. *Neuron* 44, 917–923. doi: 10.1016/j.neuron.2004.12.003

Frick, K. M., and Fernandez, S. M. (2003). Enrichment enhances spatial memory and increases synaptophysin levels in aged female mice. *Neurobiol. Aging* 24, 615–626. doi: 10.1016/S0197-4580(02)00138-0

Fryer, L. J., and Haffey, W. J. (1987). Cognitive rehabilitation and community readaptation: outcomes from two program models. *J. Head Trauma Rehabil.* 2, 51–63. doi: 10.1097/00001199-198709000-00007

Fujiwara, Y., Chaves, P. H., Yoshida, H., Amano, H., Fukaya, T., Watanabe, N., et al. (2009). Intellectual activity and likelihood of subsequently improving or maintaining instrumental activities of daily living functioning in community-dwelling older Japanese: a longitudinal study. *Int. J. Geriatr. Psychiatry* 24, 547–555. doi: 10.1002/gps.2148

Furini, C. R., Rossato, J. I., Bitencourt, L. L., Medina, J. H., Izquierdo, I., and Cammarota, M. (2010). Beta-adrenergic receptors link NO/sGC/PKG signaling to BDNF expression during the consolidation of object recognition long-term memory. *Hippocampus* 20, 672–683. doi: 10.1002/hipo.20656

Gagnon, I., Forget, R., Sullivan, S. J., and Friedman, D. (1998). Motor performance following a mild traumatic brain injury in children: an exploratory study. *Brain Inj.* 12, 843–853. doi: 10.1080/026990598122070

Galani, R., Berthel, M. C., Lazarus, C., Majchrzak, M., Barbelivien, A., Kelche, C., et al. (2007). The behavioral effects of enriched housing are not altered by serotonin depletion but enrichment alters hippocampal neurochemistry. *Neurobiol. Learn. Mem.* 88, 1–10. doi: 10.1016/j.nlm.2007.03.009

Gardner, E. B., Boitano, J. J., Mancino, N. S., and D'amico, D. P. (1975). Environmental enrichment and deprivation: effects on learning, memory and exploration. *Physiol. Behav.* 14, 321–327. doi: 10.1016/0031-9384(75)90040-2

Gaulke, L. J., Horner, P. J., Fink, A. J., Mcnamara, C. L., and Hicks, R. R. (2005). Environmental enrichment increases progenitor cell survival in the dentate gyrus following lateral fluid percussion injury. *Brain Res. Mol. Brain Res.* 141, 138–150. doi: 10.1016/j.molbrainres.2005.08.011

Gelfo, F., Cutuli, D., Foti, F., Laricchiuta, D., De Bartolo, P., Caltagirone, C., et al. (2011). Enriched environment improves motor function and increases neurotrophins in hemicerebellar lesioned rats. *Neurorehabil. Neural Repair* 25, 243–252. doi: 10.1177/1545968310380926

Gibson, E. J. (1953). Improvement in perceptual judgments as a function of controlled practice or training. *Psychol. Bull.* 50, 401–431. doi: 10.1037/h0055517

Globus, A., Rosenzweig, M. R., Bennett, E. L., and Diamond, M. C. (1973). Effects of differential experience on dendritic spine counts in rat cerebral cortex. *J. Comp. Physiol. Psychol.* 82, 175–181. doi: 10.1037/h0033910

Gobbo, O. L., and O'Mara, S. M. (2004). Impact of enriched-environment housing on brain-derived neurotrophic factor and on cognitive performance after a transient global ischemia. *Behav. Brain Res.* 152, 231–241. doi: 10.1016/j.bbr.2003.10.017

Graham, D. I., Mcintosh, T. K., Maxwell, W. L., and Nicoll, J. A. (2000). Recent advances in neurotrauma. *J. Neuropathol. Exp. Neurol.* 59, 641–651.

Green, E. J., and Greenough, W. T. (1986). Altered synaptic transmission in dentate gyrus of rats reared in complex environments: evidence from hippocampal slices maintained *in vitro*. *J. Neurophysiol.* 55, 739–750.

Greenough, W. T., and Volkmar, F. R. (1973). Pattern of dendritic branching in occipital cortex of rats reared in complex environments. *Exp. Neurol.* 40, 491–504. doi: 10.1016/0014-4886(73)90090-3

Greenough, W. T., Volkmar, F. R., and Juraska, J. M. (1973). Effects of rearing complexity on dendritic branching in frontolateral and temporal cortex of the rat. *Exp. Neurol.* 41, 371–378. doi: 10.1016/0014-4886(73)90278-1

Guic, E., Carrasco, X., Rodriguez, E., Robles, I., and Merzenich, M. M. (2008). Plasticity in primary somatosensory cortex resulting from environmentally enriched stimulation and sensory discrimination training. *Biol. Res.* 41, 425–437. doi: 10.4067/S0716-97602008000400008

Haaland, K. Y., Temkin, N., Randahl, G., and Dikmen, S. (1994). Recovery of simple motor skills after head injury. *J. Clin. Exp. Neuropsychol.* 16, 448–456. doi: 10.1080/01688639408402655

Hall, K. D., and Lifshitz, J. (2010). Diffuse traumatic brain injury initially attenuates and later expands activation of the rat somatosensory whisker circuit concomitant with neuroplastic responses. *Brain Res.* 1323, 161–173. doi: 10.1016/j.brainres.2010.01.067

Hamm, R. J., Temple, M. D., O'Dell, D. M., Pike, B. R., and Lyeth, B. G. (1996). Exposure to environmental complexity promotes recovery of cognitive function after traumatic brain injury. *J. Neurotrauma* 13, 41–47. doi: 10.1089/neu.1996.13.41

Harati, H., Barbelivien, A., Herbeaux, K., Muller, M. A., Engeln, M., Kelche, C., et al. (2013). Lifelong environmental enrichment in rats: impact on emotional behavior, spatial memory vividness, and cholinergic neurons over the lifespan. *Age (Dordr).* 35, 1027–1043. doi: 10.1007/s11357-012-9424-8

Harauzov, A., Spolidoro, M., Dicristo, G., De Pasquale, R., Cancedda, L., Pizzorusso, T., et al. (2010). Reducing intracortical inhibition in the adult visual cortex promotes ocular dominance plasticity. *J. Neurosci.* 30, 361–371. doi: 10.1523/JNEUROSCI.2233-09.2010

Hayden, M. E., Plenger, P., Bison, K., Kowalske, K., Masel, B., and Qualls, D. (2013). Treatment effect versus pretreatment recovery in persons with traumatic brain injury: a study regarding the effectiveness of postacute rehabilitation. *PM R* 5, 319–327; quiz 327. doi: 10.1016/j.pmrj.2012.12.005

Hebb, D. O. (1947). The effects of early experience on problem-solving at maturity. *Am. Psychol.* 2, 306–307.

Hebb, D. O. (1949). *The Organization of Behaviour.* New York, NY: Wiley.

Held, J. M., Gordon, J., and Gentile, A. M. (1985). Environmental influences on locomotor recovery following cortical lesions in rats. *Behav. Neurosci.* 99, 678–690. doi: 10.1037/0735-7044.99.4.678

Heldt, S. A., Stanek, L., Chhatwal, J. P., and Ressler, K. J. (2007). Hippocampus-specific deletion of BDNF in adult mice impairs spatial memory and extinction of aversive memories. *Mol. Psychiatry* 12, 656–670. doi: 10.1038/sj.mp.4001957

Henriksson, B. G., Soderstrom, S., Gower, A. J., Ebendal, T., Winblad, B., and Mohammed, A. H. (1992). Hippocampal nerve growth factor levels are related to spatial learning ability in aged rats. *Behav. Brain Res.* 48, 15–20. doi: 10.1016/S0166-4328(05)80134-2

Hensch, T. K., and Fagiolini, M. (2005). Excitatory-inhibitory balance and critical period plasticity in developing visual cortex. *Prog. Brain Res.* 147, 115–124. doi: 10.1016/S0079-6123(04)47009-5

Hensch, T. K., Fagiolini, M., Mataga, N., Stryker, M. P., Baekkeskov, S., and Kash, S. F. (1998). Local GABA circuit control of experience-dependent plasticity in developing visual cortex. *Science* 282, 1504–1508. doi: 10.1126/science.282.5393.1504

Hicks, R. R., Numan, S., Dhillon, H. S., Prasad, M. R., and Seroogy, K. B. (1997). Alterations in BDNF and NT-3 mRNAs in rat hippocampus after experimental brain trauma. *Brain Res. Mol. Brain Res.* 48, 401–406. doi: 10.1016/S0169-328X(97)00158-7

Hicks, R. R., Smith, D. H., Lowenstein, D. H., Saint Marie, R., and Mcintosh, T. K. (1993). Mild experimental brain injury in the rat induces cognitive deficits associated with regional neuronal loss in the hippocampus. *J. Neurotrauma* 10, 405–414. doi: 10.1089/neu.1993.10.405

Hicks, R. R., Zhang, L., Atkinson, A., Stevenon, M., Veneracion, M., and Seroogy, K. B. (2002). Environmental enrichment attenuates cognitive deficits, but does not alter neurotrophin gene expression in the hippocampus following lateral fluid percussion brain injury. *Neuroscience* 112, 631–637. doi: 10.1016/S0306-4522(02)00104-5

Hockly, E., Cordery, P. M., Woodman, B., Mahal, A., Van Dellen, A., Blakemore, C., et al. (2002). Environmental enrichment slows disease progression in R6/2 Huntington's disease mice. *Ann. Neurol.* 51, 235–242. doi: 10.1002/ana.10094

Hoffman, A. N., Malena, R. R., Westergom, B. P., Luthra, P., Cheng, J. P., Aslam, H. A., et al. (2008). Environmental enrichment-mediated functional improvement after experimental traumatic brain injury is contingent on task-specific neurobehavioral experience. *Neurosci. Lett.* 431, 226–230. doi: 10.1016/j.neulet.2007.11.042

Holloway, R. L. Jr. (1966). Dendritic branching: some preliminary results of training and complexity in rat visual cortex. *Brain Res.* 2, 393–396.

Hu, Y. S., Xu, P., Pigino, G., Brady, S. T., Larson, J., and Lazarov, O. (2010). Complex environment experience rescues impaired neurogenesis, enhances synaptic plasticity, and attenuates neuropathology in familial Alzheimer's disease-linked APPswe/PS1DeltaE9 mice. *FASEB J.* 24, 1667–1681. doi: 10.1096/fj.09-136945

Huang, Z. J., Kirkwood, A., Pizzorusso, T., Porciatti, V., Morales, B., Bear, M. F., et al. (1999). BDNF regulates the maturation of inhibition and the critical period of plasticity in mouse visual cortex. *Cell* 98, 739–755. doi: 10.1016/S0092-8674(00)81509-3

Hubel, D. H. (1978). Effects of deprivation on the visual cortex of cat and monkey. *Harvey Lect.* 72, 1–51.

Hubel, D. H., and Wiesel, T. N. (1970). The period of susceptibility to the physiological effects of unilateral eye closure in kittens. *J. Physiol.* 206, 419–436.

Hunt, R. F., Boychuk, J. A., and Smith, B. N. (2013). Neural circuit mechanisms of post-traumatic epilepsy. *Front. Cell. Neurosci.* 7:89. doi: 10.3389/fncel.2013.00089

Ip, E. Y., Giza, C. C., Griesbach, G. S., and Hovda, D. A. (2002). Effects of enriched environment and fluid percussion injury on dendritic arborization within the cerebral cortex of the developing rat. *J. Neurotrauma* 19, 573–585. doi: 10.1089/089771502753754055

Irvine, G. I., and Abraham, W. C. (2005). Enriched environment exposure alters the input-output dynamics of synaptic transmission in area CA1 of freely moving rats. *Neurosci. Lett.* 391, 32–37. doi: 10.1016/j.neulet.2005.08.031

Irvine, G. I., Logan, B., Eckert, M., and Abraham, W. C. (2006). Enriched environment exposure regulates excitability, synaptic transmission, and LTP in the dentate gyrus of freely moving rats. *Hippocampus* 16, 149–160. doi: 10.1002/hipo.20142

Jadavji, N. M., Kolb, B., and Metz, G. A. (2006). Enriched environment improves motor function in intact and unilateral dopamine-depleted rats. *Neuroscience* 140, 1127–1138. doi: 10.1016/j.neuroscience.2006.03.027

Jakkamsetti, V., Chang, K. Q., and Kilgard, M. P. (2012). Reorganization in processing of spectral and temporal input in the rat posterior auditory field induced by environmental enrichment. *J. Neurophysiol.* 107, 1457–1475. doi: 10.1152/jn.01057.2010

Jankowsky, J. L., Melnikova, T., Fadale, D. J., Xu, G. M., Slunt, H. H., Gonzales, V., et al. (2005). Environmental enrichment mitigates cognitive deficits in a mouse model of Alzheimer's disease. *J. Neurosci.* 25, 5217–5224. doi: 10.1523/JNEUROSCI.5080-04.2005

Jankowsky, J. L., Xu, G., Fromholt, D., Gonzales, V., and Borchelt, D. R. (2003). Environmental enrichment exacerbates amyloid plaque formation in a transgenic mouse model of Alzheimer disease. *J. Neuropathol. Exp. Neurol.* 62, 1220–1227.

Johansson, B. B., and Belichenko, P. V. (2002). Neuronal plasticity and dendritic spines: effect of environmental enrichment on intact and postischemic rat brain. *J. Cereb. Blood Flow Metab.* 22, 89–96. doi: 10.1097/00004647-200201000-00011

Johansson, B. B., and Ohlsson, A. L. (1996). Environment, social interaction, and physical activity as determinants of functional outcome after cerebral infarction in the rat. *Exp. Neurol.* 139, 322–327. doi: 10.1006/exnr.1996.0106

Johnson, E. M., Traver, K. L., Hoffman, S. W., Harrison, C. R., and Herman, J. P. (2013). Environmental enrichment protects against functional deficits caused by traumatic brain injury. *Front. Behav. Neurosci.* 7:44. doi: 10.3389/fnbeh.2013.00044

Johnstone, V. P., Yan, E. B., Alwis, D. S., and Rajan, R. (2013). Cortical hypoexcitation defines neuronal responses in the immediate aftermath of traumatic brain injury. *PLoS ONE* 8:e63454. doi: 10.1371/journal.pone.0063454

Jones, T. A., Klintsova, A. Y., Kilman, V. L., Sirevaag, A. M., and Greenough, W. T. (1997). Induction of multiple synapses by experience in the visual cortex of adult rats. *Neurobiol. Learn. Mem.* 68, 13–20. doi: 10.1006/nlme.1997.3774

Jung, C. K., and Herms, J. (2012). Structural dynamics of dendritic spines are influenced by an environmental enrichment: an *in vivo* imaging study. *Cereb. Cortex* 24, 377–384. doi: 10.1093/cercor/bhs31

Kaas, J. H. (1991). Plasticity of sensory and motor maps in adult mammals. *Annu. Rev. Neurosci.* 14, 137–167. doi: 10.1146/annurev.ne.14.030191.001033

Kang, H., and Schuman, E. M. (1995). Long-lasting neurotrophin-induced enhancement of synaptic transmission in the adult hippocampus. *Science* 267, 1658–1662. doi: 10.1126/science.7886457

Kazlauckas, V., Pagnussat, N., Mioranzza, S., Kalinine, E., Nunes, F., Pettenuzzo, L., et al. (2011). Enriched environment effects on behavior, memory and BDNF in low and high exploratory mice. *Physiol. Behav.* 102, 475–480. doi: 10.1016/j.physbeh.2010.12.025

Kelche, C., and Will, B. (1982). Effects of postoperative environments following dorsal hippocampal lesions on dendritic branching and spines in rat occipital cortex. *Brain Res.* 245, 107–115.

Kempermann, G. (2002). Why new neurons? Possible functions for adult hippocampal neurogenesis. *J. Neurosci.* 22, 635–638.

Kempermann, G., Kuhn, H. G., and Gage, F. H. (1997). More hippocampal neurons in adult mice living in an enriched environment. *Nature* 386, 493–495. doi: 10.1038/386493a0

Kempermann, G., Kuhn, H. G., and Gage, F. H. (1998). Experience-induced neurogenesis in the senescent dentate gyrus. *J. Neurosci.* 18, 3206–3212.

Kendrick, K. M., Levy, F., and Keverne, E. B. (1992). Changes in the sensory processing of olfactory signals induced by birth in sheep. *Science* 256, 833–836. doi: 10.1126/science.1589766

Keyvani, K., Sachser, N., Witte, O. W., and Paulus, W. (2004). Gene expression profiling in the intact and injured brain following environmental enrichment. *J. Neuropathol. Exp. Neurol.* 63, 598–609.

Kim, B. G., Dai, H. N., Mcatee, M., and Bregman, B. S. (2008). Modulation of dendritic spine remodeling in the motor cortex following spinal cord injury: effects of environmental enrichment and combinatorial treatment with transplants and neurotrophin-3. *J. Comp. Neurol.* 508, 473–486. doi: 10.1002/cne.21686

Kim, H., and Bao, S. (2013). Experience-dependent over-representation of ultrasonic vocalization frequencies in the rat primary auditory cortex. *J. Neurophysiol.* 110, 1087–1096. doi: 10.1152/jn.00230.2013

Kim, M., Na, D. L., Kim, G. M., Adair, J. C., Lee, K. H., and Heilman, K. M. (1999). Ipsilesional neglect: behavioural and anatomical features. *J. Neurol. Neurosurg. Psychiatr.* 67, 35–38. doi: 10.1136/jnnp.67.1.35

Kleim, J. A., Jones, T. A., and Schallert, T. (2003). Motor enrichment and the induction of plasticity before or after brain injury. *Neurochem. Res.* 28, 1757–1769. doi: 10.1023/A:1026025408742

Kline, A. E., Mcaloon, R. L., Henderson, K. A., Bansal, U. K., Ganti, B. M., Ahmed, R. H., et al. (2010). Evaluation of a combined therapeutic regimen of 8-OH-DPAT and environmental enrichment after experimental traumatic brain injury. *J. Neurotrauma* 27, 2021–2032. doi: 10.1089/neu.2010.1535

Kline, A. E., Olsen, A. S., Sozda, C. N., Hoffman, A. N., and Cheng, J. P. (2012). Evaluation of a combined treatment paradigm consisting of environmental enrichment and the 5-HT1A receptor agonist buspirone after experimental traumatic brain injury. *J. Neurotrauma* 29, 1960–1969. doi: 10.1089/neu.2012.2385

Kline, A. E., Wagner, A. K., Westergom, B. P., Malena, R. R., Zafonte, R. D., Olsen, A. S., et al. (2007). Acute treatment with the 5-HT(1A) receptor agonist 8-OH-DPAT and chronic environmental enrichment confer neurobehavioral benefit after experimental brain trauma. *Behav. Brain Res.* 177, 186–194. doi: 10.1016/j.bbr.2006.11.036

Klintsova, A. Y., and Greenough, W. T. (1999). Synaptic plasticity in cortical systems. *Curr. Opin. Neurobiol.* 9, 203–208. doi: 10.1016/S0959-4388(99)80028-2

Koh, S., Magid, R., Chung, H., Stine, C. D., and Wilson, D. N. (2007). Depressive behavior and selective down-regulation of serotonin receptor expression after early-life seizures: reversal by environmental enrichment. *Epilepsy Behav.* 10, 26–31. doi: 10.1016/j.yebeh.2006.11.008

Kolb, B. (1999). Synaptic plasticity and the organization of behaviour after early and late brain injury. *Can. J. Exp. Psychol.* 53, 62–76. doi: 10.1037/h0087300

Kolb, B., and Gibb, R. (1991). Environmental enrichment and cortical injury: behavioral and anatomical consequences of frontal cortex lesions. *Cereb. Cortex* 1, 189–198. doi: 10.1093/cercor/1.2.189

Kolb, B., Ladowski, R., Gibb, R., and Gorny, G. (1996). Does dendritic growth underly recovery from neonatal occipital lesions in rats. *Behav. Brain Res.* 77, 125–133. doi: 10.1016/0166-4328(95)00208-1

Komitova, M., Perfilieva, E., Mattsson, B., Eriksson, P. S., and Johansson, B. B. (2006). Enriched environment after focal cortical ischemia enhances the generation of astroglia and NG2 positive polydendrocytes in adult rat neocortex. *Exp. Neurol.* 199, 113–121. doi: 10.1016/j.expneurol.2005.12.007

Koopmans, G. C., Deumens, R., Honig, W. M., Hamers, F. P., Mey, J., Van Kleef, M., et al. (2012). Functional recovery, serotonergic sprouting, and endogenous progenitor fates in response to delayed environmental enrichment after spinal cord injury. *J. Neurotrauma* 29, 514–527. doi: 10.1089/neu.2011.1949

Korbey, S. M., Heinrichs, S. C., and Leussis, M. P. (2008). Seizure susceptibility and locus ceruleus activation are reduced following environmental enrichment in an animal model of epilepsy. *Epilepsy Behav.* 12, 30–38. doi: 10.1016/j.yebeh.2007.09.013

Kozlowski, D. A., Nahed, B. V., Hovda, D. A., and Lee, S. M. (2004). Paradoxical effects of cortical impact injury on environmentally enriched rats. *J. Neurotrauma* 21, 513–519. doi: 10.1089/089771504774129856

Kramer, A. F., Bherer, L., Colcombe, S. J., Dong, W., and Greenough, W. T. (2004). Environmental influences on cognitive and brain plasticity during aging. *J. Gerontol. A Biol. Sci. Med. Sci.* 59, M940–M957. doi: 10.1093/gerona/59.9.M940

Kulesskaya, N., Rauvala, H., and Voikar, V. (2011). Evaluation of social and physical enrichment in modulation of behavioural phenotype in C57BL/6J female mice. *PLoS ONE* 6:e24755. doi: 10.1371/journal.pone.0024755

Landers, M. S., Knott, G. W., Lipp, H. P., Poletaeva, I., and Welker, E. (2011). Synapse formation in adult barrel cortex following naturalistic environmental enrichment. *Neuroscience* 199, 143–152. doi: 10.1016/j.neuroscience.2011.10.040

Larsson, F., Winblad, B., and Mohammed, A. H. (2002). Psychological stress and environmental adaptation in enriched vs. impoverished housed rats. *Pharmacol. Biochem. Behav.* 73, 193–207. doi: 10.1016/S0091-3057(02)00782-7

Lazarov, O., Robinson, J., Tang, Y. P., Hairston, I. S., Korade-Mirnics, Z., Lee, V. M., et al. (2005). Environmental enrichment reduces Abeta levels and amyloid deposition in transgenic mice. *Cell* 120, 701–713. doi: 10.1016/j.cell.2005.01.015

Lazic, S. E., Grote, H. E., Blakemore, C., Hannan, A. J., Van Dellen, A., Phillips, W., et al. (2006). Neurogenesis in the R6/1 transgenic mouse model of Huntington's disease: effects of environmental enrichment. *Eur. J. Neurosci.* 23, 1829–1838. doi: 10.1111/j.1460-9568.2006.04715.x

Leger, M., Quiedeville, A., Paizanis, E., Natkunarajah, S., Freret, T., Boulouard, M., et al. (2012). Environmental enrichment enhances episodic-like memory in association with a modified neuronal activation profile in adult mice. *PLoS ONE* 7:e48043. doi: 10.1371/journal.pone.0048043

Leggio, M. G., Mandolesi, L., Federico, F., Spirito, F., Ricci, B., Gelfo, F., et al. (2005). Environmental enrichment promotes improved spatial abilities and enhanced dendritic growth in the rat. *Behav. Brain Res.* 163, 78–90. doi: 10.1016/j.bbr.2005.04.009

Levelt, C. N., and Hubener, M. (2012). Critical-period plasticity in the visual cortex. *Annu. Rev. Neurosci.* 35, 309–330. doi: 10.1146/annurev-neuro-061010-113813

Levi, O., Jongen-Relo, A. L., Feldon, J., Roses, A. D., and Michaelson, D. M. (2003). ApoE4 impairs hippocampal plasticity isoform-specifically and blocks the environmental stimulation of synaptogenesis and memory. *Neurobiol. Dis.* 13, 273–282. doi: 10.1016/S0969-9961(03)00045-7

Levi, O., and Michaelson, D. M. (2007). Environmental enrichment stimulates neurogenesis in apolipoprotein E3 and neuronal apoptosis in apolipoprotein E4 transgenic mice. *J. Neurochem.* 100, 202–210. doi: 10.1111/j.1471-4159.2006.04189.x

Lew, H. L., Weihing, J., Myers, P. J., Pogoda, T. K., and Goodrich, G. L. (2010). Dual sensory impairment (DSI) in traumatic brain injury (TBI)–An emerging interdisciplinary challenge. *Neurorehabilitation* 26, 213–222. doi: 10.3233/NRE-2010-0557

Liljequist, R., Henriksson, B. G., Latif, N., Pham, T., Winblad, B., and Mohammed, A. H. (1993). Subchronic MK-801 treatment to juvenile rats attenuates environmental effects on adult spatial learning. *Behav. Brain Res.* 56, 107–114. doi: 10.1016/0166-4328(93)90027-N

Linnarsson, S., Bjorklund, A., and Ernfors, P. (1997). Learning deficit in BDNF mutant mice. *Eur. J. Neurosci.* 9, 2581–2587. doi: 10.1111/j.1460-9568.1997.tb01687.x

Lippert-Gruener, M., Maegele, M., Garbe, J., and Angelov, D. N. (2007). Late effects of enriched environment (EE) plus multimodal early onset stimulation (MEOS) after traumatic brain injury in rats: ongoing improvement of neuromotor function despite sustained volume of the CNS lesion. *Exp. Neurol.* 203, 82–94. doi: 10.1016/j.expneurol.2006.07.025

Lippert-Gruner, M., Maegele, M., Pokorny, J., Angelov, D. N., Svestkova, O., Wittner, M., et al. (2007). Early rehabilitation model shows positive effects on neural degeneration and recovery from neuromotor deficits following traumatic brain injury. *Physiol. Res.* 56, 359–368.

Lippert-Gruner, M., Magele, M., Svestkova, O., Angerova, Y., Ester-Bode, T., and Angelov, D. N. (2011). Rehabilitation intervention in animal model can improve neuromotor and cognitive functions after traumatic brain injury: pilot study. *Physiol. Res.* 60, 367–375.

Little, D. M., Kraus, M. F., Joseph, J., Geary, E. K., Susmaras, T., Zhou, X. J., et al. (2010). Thalamic integrity underlies executive dysfunction in traumatic brain injury. *Neurology* 74, 558–564. doi: 10.1212/WNL.0b013e3181cff5d5

Liu, Z., D'amore, P. A., Mikati, M., Gatt, A., and Holmes, G. L. (1993). Neuroprotective effect of chronic infusion of basic fibroblast growth factor on seizure-associated hippocampal damage. *Brain Res.* 626, 335–338.

Lu, L., Bao, G., Chen, H., Xia, P., Fan, X., Zhang, J., et al. (2003). Modification of hippocampal neurogenesis and neuroplasticity by social environments. *Exp. Neurol.* 183, 600–609. doi: 10.1016/S0014-4886(03)00248-6

Luz, Y., and Shamir, M. (2012). Balancing feed-forward excitation and inhibition via Hebbian inhibitory synaptic plasticity. *PLoS Comput. Biol.* 8:e1002334. doi: 10.1371/journal.pcbi.1002334

Maegele, M., Lippert-Gruener, M., Ester-Bode, T., Garbe, J., Bouillon, B., Neugebauer, E., et al. (2005a). Multimodal early onset stimulation combined with enriched environment is associated with reduced CNS lesion volume and enhanced reversal of neuromotor dysfunction after traumatic brain injury in rats. *Eur. J. Neurosci.* 21, 2406–2418. doi: 10.1111/j.1460-9568.2005.04070.x

Maegele, M., Lippert-Gruener, M., Ester-Bode, T., Sauerland, S., Schafer, U., Molcanyi, M., et al. (2005b). Reversal of neuromotor and cognitive dysfunction in an enriched environment combined with multimodal early onset stimulation after traumatic brain injury in rats. *J. Neurotrauma* 22, 772–782. doi: 10.1089/neu.2005.22.772

Mainardi, M., Landi, S., Gianfranceschi, L., Baldini, S., De Pasquale, R., Berardi, N., et al. (2010). Environmental enrichment potentiates thalamocortical transmission and plasticity in the adult rat visual cortex. *J. Neurosci. Res.* 88, 3048–3059. doi: 10.1002/jnr.22461

Malik, R., and Chattarji, S. (2012). Enhanced intrinsic excitability and EPSP-spike coupling accompany enriched environment-induced facilitation of LTP in hippocampal CA1 pyramidal neurons. *J. Neurophysiol.* 107, 1366–1378. doi: 10.1152/jn.01009.2011

Mandairon, N., Stack, C., Kiselycznyk, C., and Linster, C. (2006a). Enrichment to odors improves olfactory discrimination in adult rats. *Behav. Neurosci.* 120, 173–179. doi: 10.1037/0735-7044.120.1.173

Mandairon, N., Stack, C., and Linster, C. (2006b). Olfactory enrichment improves the recognition of individual components in mixtures. *Physiol. Behav.* 89, 379–384. doi: 10.1016/j.physbeh.2006.07.013

Matter, A. M., Folweiler, K. A., Curatolo, L. M., and Kline, A. E. (2011). Temporal effects of environmental enrichment-mediated functional improvement after experimental traumatic brain injury in rats. *Neurorehabil. Neural Repair* 25, 558–564. doi: 10.1177/1545968310397206

Maya-Vetencourt, J. F., Baroncelli, L., Viegi, A., Tiraboschi, E., Castren, E., Cattaneo, A., et al. (2012). IGF-1 restores visual cortex plasticity in adult life by reducing local GABA levels. *Neural Plast.* 2012:250421. doi: 10.1155/2012/250421

Maya Vetencourt, J. F., Sale, A., Viegi, A., Baroncelli, L., De Pasquale, R., O'Leary, O. F., et al. (2008). The antidepressant fluoxetine restores plasticity in the adult visual cortex. *Science* 320, 385–388. doi: 10.1126/science.1150516

McNamara, K. C. S., Lisembee, A. M., and Lifshitz, J. (2010). The whisker nuisance task identifies a late-onset, persistent sensory sensitivity in diffuse brain-injured rats. *J. Neurotrauma* 27, 695–706. doi: 10.1089/neu.2009.1237

McQuaid, R. J., Audet, M. C., and Anisman, H. (2012). Environmental enrichment in male CD-1 mice promotes aggressive behaviors and elevated corticosterone and brain norepinephrine activity in response to a mild stressor. *Stress* 15, 354–360. doi: 10.3109/10253890.2011.623249

Megevand, P., Troncoso, E., Quairiaux, C., Muller, D., Michel, C. M., and Kiss, J. Z. (2009). Long-term plasticity in mouse sensorimotor circuits after rhythmic whisker stimulation. *J. Neurosci.* 29, 5326–5335. doi: 10.1523/JNEUROSCI.5965-08.2009

Menge, T., Jander, S., and Stoll, G. (2001). Induction of the proinflammatory cytokine interleukin-18 by axonal injury. *J. Neurosci. Res.* 65, 332–339. doi: 10.1002/jnr.1158

Mesa-Gresa, P., Perez-Martinez, A., and Redolat, R. (2013). Environmental enrichment improves novel object recognition and enhances agonistic behavior in male mice. *Aggress. Behav.* 39, 269–279. doi: 10.1002/ab.21481

Milgram, N. W., Siwak-Tapp, C. T., Araujo, J., and Head, E. (2006). Neuroprotective effects of cognitive enrichment. *Ageing Res. Rev.* 5, 354–369. doi: 10.1016/j.arr.2006.04.004

Miller, L. S., Colella, B., Mikulis, D., Maller, J., and Green, R. E. (2013). Environmental enrichment may protect against hippocampal atrophy in the chronic stages of traumatic brain injury. *Front. Hum. Neurosci.* 7:506. doi: 10.3389/fnhum.2013.00506

Minichiello, L., Korte, M., Wolfer, D., Kuhn, R., Unsicker, K., Cestari, V., et al. (1999). Essential role for TrkB receptors in hippocampus-mediated learning. *Neuron* 24, 401–414. doi: 10.1016/S0896-6273(00)80853-3

Mohammed, A. H., Zhu, S. W., Darmopil, S., Hjerling-Leffler, J., Ernfors, P., Winblad, B., et al. (2002). Environmental enrichment and the brain. *Prog. Brain Res.* 138, 109–133. doi: 10.1016/S0079-6123(02)38074-9

Monaco, C. M., Mattiola, V. V., Folweiler, K. A., Tay, J. K., Yelleswarapu, N. K., Curatolo, L. M., et al. (2013). Environmental enrichment promotes robust functional and histological benefits in female rats after controlled cortical impact injury. *Exp. Neurol.* 247, 410–418. doi: 10.1016/j.expneurol.2013.01.007

Morganti-Kossmann, M. C., Rancan, M., Stahel, P. F., and Kossmann, T. (2002). Inflammatory response in acute traumatic brain injury: a double-edged sword. *Curr. Opin. Crit. Care* 8, 101–105. doi: 10.1097/00075198-200204000-00002

Mrsic-Flogel, T. D., Hofer, S. B., Ohki, K., Reid, R. C., Bonhoeffer, T., and Hubener, M. (2007). Homeostatic regulation of eye-specific responses in visual cortex during ocular dominance plasticity. *Neuron* 54, 961–972. doi: 10.1016/j.neuron.2007.05.028

Muthuraju, S., Pati, S., Rafiqul, M., Abdullah, J. M., and Jaafar, H. (2012). IntelliCage provides voluntary exercise and an enriched environment, improving locomotive activity in mice following fluid percussion injury. *Basal Ganglia* 2, 143–151. doi: 10.1016/j.baga.2012.06.004

Naka, F., Narita, N., Okado, N., and Narita, M. (2005). Modification of AMPA receptor properties following environmental enrichment. *Brain Dev.* 27, 275–278. doi: 10.1016/j.braindev.2004.07.006

Narayan, R. K., Michel, M. E., Ansell, B., Baethmann, A., Biegon, A., Bracken, M. B., et al. (2002). Clinical trials in head injury. *J. Neurotrauma* 19, 503–557. doi: 10.1089/089771502753754037

Newson, R. S., and Kemps, E. B. (2005). General lifestyle activities as a predictor of current cognition and cognitive change in older adults: a cross-sectional and longitudinal examination. *J. Gerontol. B Psychol. Sci. Soc. Sci.* 60, P113–P120. doi: 10.1093/geronb/60.3.P113

Nichols, J. A., Jakkamsetti, V. P., Salgado, H., Dinh, L., Kilgard, M. P., and Atzori, M. (2007). Environmental enrichment selectively increases glutamatergic responses in layer II/III of the auditory cortex of the rat. *Neuroscience* 145, 832–840. doi: 10.1016/j.neuroscience.2006.12.061

Nilsson, M., Perfilieva, E., Johansson, U., Orwar, O., and Eriksson, P. S. (1999). Enriched environment increases neurogenesis in the adult rat dentate gyrus and improves spatial memory. *J. Neurobiol.* 39, 569–578.

Nithianantharajah, J., Barkus, C., Murphy, M., and Hannan, A. J. (2008). Gene-environment interactions modulating cognitive function and molecular correlates of synaptic plasticity in Huntington's disease transgenic mice. *Neurobiol. Dis.* 29, 490–504. doi: 10.1016/j.nbd.2007.11.006

Nithianantharajah, J., and Hannan, A. J. (2006). Enriched environments, experience-dependent plasticity and disorders of the nervous system. *Nat. Rev. Neurosci.* 7, 697–709. doi: 10.1038/nrn1970

Nithianantharajah, J., Levis, H., and Murphy, M. (2004). Environmental enrichment results in cortical and subcortical changes in levels of synaptophysin and PSD-95 proteins. *Neurobiol. Learn. Mem.* 81, 200–210. doi: 10.1016/j.nlm.2004.02.002

Norena, A. J., Gourevitch, B., Aizawa, N., and Eggermont, J. J. (2006). Spectrally enhanced acoustic environment disrupts frequency representation in cat auditory cortex. *Nat. Neurosci.* 9, 932–939. doi: 10.1038/nn1720

Ohlsson, A. L., and Johansson, B. B. (1995). Environment influences functional outcome of cerebral infarction in rats. *Stroke* 26, 644–649. doi: 10.1161/01.STR.26.4.644

Ortuzar, N., Rico-Barrio, I., Bengoetxea, H., Argandona, E. G., and Lafuente, J. V. (2013). VEGF reverts the cognitive impairment induced by a focal traumatic brain injury during the development of rats raised under environmental enrichment. *Behav. Brain Res.* 246, 36–46. doi: 10.1016/j.bbr.2013.02.036

Park, E., Bell, J. D., and Baker, A. J. (2008). Traumatic brain injury: can the consequences be stopped? *CMAJ* 178, 1163–1170. doi: 10.1503/cmaj.080282

Park, N. W., and Ingles, J. L. (2001). Effectiveness of attention rehabilitation after an acquired brain injury: a meta-analysis. *Neuropsychology* 15, 199–210. doi: 10.1037/0894-4105.15.2.199

Passineau, M. J., Green, E. J., and Dietrich, W. D. (2001). Therapeutic effects of environmental enrichment on cognitive function and tissue integrity following severe traumatic brain injury in rats. *Exp. Neurol.* 168, 373–384. doi: 10.1006/exnr.2000.7623

Patel, R., Ciuffreda, K. J., Tannen, B., and Kapoor, N. (2011). Elevated coherent motion thresholds in mild traumatic brain injury. *Optometry* 82, 284–289. doi: 10.1016/j.optm.2010.10.012

Percaccio, C. R., Engineer, N. D., Pruette, A. L., Pandya, P. K., Moucha, R., Rathbun, D. L., et al. (2005). Environmental enrichment increases paired-pulse depression in rat auditory cortex. *J. Neurophysiol.* 94, 3590–3600. doi: 10.1152/jn.00433.2005

Percaccio, C. R., Pruette, A. L., Mistry, S. T., Chen, Y. H., and Kilgard, M. P. (2007). Sensory experience determines enrichment-induced plasticity in rat auditory cortex. *Brain Res.* 1174, 76–91. doi: 10.1016/j.brainres.2007.07.062

Pereira, L. O., Arteni, N. S., Petersen, R. C., Da Rocha, A. P., Achaval, M., and Netto, C. A. (2007). Effects of daily environmental enrichment on memory deficits and brain injury following neonatal hypoxia-ischemia in the rat. *Neurobiol. Learn. Mem.* 87, 101–108. doi: 10.1016/j.nlm.2006.07.003

Pham, T. M., Ickes, B., Albeck, D., Soderstrom, S., Granholm, A. C., and Mohammed, A. H. (1999). Changes in brain nerve growth factor levels and nerve growth factor receptors in rats exposed to environmental enrichment for one year. *Neuroscience* 94, 279–286. doi: 10.1016/S0306-4522(99)00316-4

Pienkowski, M., and Eggermont, J. J. (2009). Long-term, partially-reversible reorganization of frequency tuning in mature cat primary auditory cortex can be induced by passive exposure to moderate-level sounds. *Hear. Res.* 257, 24–40. doi: 10.1016/j.heares.2009.07.011

Pierce, J. E., Smith, D. H., Trojanowski, J. Q., and McIntosh, T. K. (1998). Enduring cognitive, neurobehavioral and histopathological changes persist for up to one year following severe experimental brain injury in rats. *Neuroscience* 87, 359–369. doi: 10.1016/S0306-4522(98)00142-0

Pitkanen, A., and McIntosh, T. K. (2006). Animal models of post-traumatic epilepsy. *J. Neurotrauma* 23, 241–261. doi: 10.1089/neu.2006.23.241

Polley, D. B., Kvasnak, E., and Frostig, R. D. (2004). Naturalistic experience transforms sensory maps in the adult cortex of caged animals. *Nature* 429, 67–71. doi: 10.1038/nature02469

Por, S. B., Bennett, E. L., and Bondy, S. C. (1982). Environmental enrichment and neurotransmitter receptors. *Behav. Neural Biol.* 34, 132–140. doi: 10.1016/S0163-1047(82)91514-X

Powell, J., Heslin, J., and Greenwood, R. (2002). Community based rehabilitation after severe traumatic brain injury: a randomised controlled trial. *J. Neurol. Neurosurg. Psychiatry* 72, 193–202. doi: 10.1136/jnnp.72.2.193

Rampon, C., Jiang, C. H., Dong, H., Tang, Y. P., Lockhart, D. J., Schultz, P. G., et al. (2000). Effects of environmental enrichment on gene expression in the brain. *Proc. Natl. Acad. Sci. U.S.A.* 97, 12880–12884. doi: 10.1073/pnas.97.23.12880

Rasmuson, S., Olsson, T., Henriksson, B. G., Kelly, P. A., Holmes, M. C., Seckl, J. R., et al. (1998). Environmental enrichment selectively increases 5-HT1A receptor mRNA expression and binding in the rat hippocampus. *Brain Res. Mol. Brain Res.* 53, 285–290.

Recanzone, G. H., Schreiner, C. E., and Merzenich, M. M. (1993). Plasticity in the frequency representation of primary auditory cortex following discrimination training in adult owl monkeys. *J. Neurosci.* 13, 87–103.

Reibel, S., Larmet, Y., Le, B. T., Carnahan, J., Marescaux, C., and Depaulis, A. (2000). Brain-derived neurotrophic factor delays hippocampal kindling in the rat. *Neuroscience* 100, 777–788. doi: 10.1016/S0306-4522(00)00351-1

Rema, V., Armstrong-James, M., Jenkinson, N., and Ebner, F. F. (2006). Short exposure to an enriched environment accelerates plasticity in the barrel cortex of adult rats. *Neuroscience* 140, 659–672. doi: 10.1016/j.neuroscience.2006.02.043

Risdall, J. E., and Menon, D. K. (2011). Traumatic brain injury. *Philos. Trans. R. Soc. Lond. B. Biol. Sci.* 366, 241–250. doi: 10.1098/rstb.2010.0230

Risedal, A., Mattsson, B., Dahlqvist, P., Nordborg, C., Olsson, T., and Johansson, B. B. (2002). Environmental influences on functional outcome after a cortical infarct in the rat. *Brain Res. Bull.* 58, 315–321. doi: 10.1016/S0361-9230(02)00796-7

Rojas, J. J., Deniz, B. F., Miguel, P. M., Diaz, R., Hermel Edo, E., Achaval, M., et al. (2013). Effects of daily environmental enrichment on behavior and dendritic spine density in hippocampus following neonatal hypoxia-ischemia in the rat. *Exp. Neurol.* 241, 25–33. doi: 10.1016/j.expneurol.2012.11.026

Rose, F. D., Al-Khamees, K., Davey, M. J., and Attree, E. A. (1993). Environmental enrichment following brain damage: an aid to recovery or compensation? *Behav. Brain Res.* 56, 93–100.

Rose, F. D., Davey, M. J., Love, S., and Dell, P. A. (1987). Environmental enrichment and recovery from contralateral sensory neglect in rats with large unilateral neocortical lesions. *Behav. Brain Res.* 24, 195–202. doi: 10.1016/0166-4328(87)90057-X

Rose, F. D., Dell, P. A., Love, S., and Davey, M. J. (1988). Environmental enrichment and recovery from a complex Go/No-Go reversal deficit in rats following large unilateral neocortical lesions. *Behav. Brain Res.* 31, 37–45. doi: 10.1016/0166-4328(88)90156-8

Rosenzweig, M. R., Bennett, E. L., Hebert, M., and Morimoto, H. (1978). Social grouping cannot account for cerebral effects of enriched environments. *Brain Res.* 153, 563–576.

Rossi, C., Angelucci, A., Costantin, L., Braschi, C., Mazzantini, M., Babbini, F., et al. (2006). Brain-derived neurotrophic factor (BDNF) is required for the enhancement of hippocampal neurogenesis following environmental enrichment. *Eur. J. Neurosci.* 24, 1850–1856. doi: 10.1111/j.1460-9568.2006.05059.x

Rowntree, S., and Kolb, B. (1997). Blockade of basic fibroblast growth factor retards recovery from motor cortex injury in rats. *Eur. J. Neurosci.* 9, 2432–2441. doi: 10.1111/j.1460-9568.1997.tb01660.x

Rubinov, M., McIntosh, A. R., Valenzuela, M. J., and Breakspear, M. (2009). Simulation of neuronal death and network recovery in a computational model of distributed cortical activity. *Am. J. Geriatr. Psychiatry* 17, 210–217. doi: 10.1097/JGP.0b013e318187137a

Rutten, A., Van Albada, M., Silveira, D. C., Cha, B. H., Liu, X., Hu, Y. N., et al. (2002). Memory impairment following status epilepticus in immature rats: time-course and environmental effects. *Eur. J. Neurosci.* 16, 501–513. doi: 10.1046/j.1460-9568.2002.02103.x

Sale, A., Maya Vetencourt, J. F., Medini, P., Cenni, M. C., Baroncelli, L., De Pasquale, R., et al. (2007). Environmental enrichment in adulthood promotes amblyopia recovery through a reduction of intracortical inhibition. *Nat. Neurosci.* 10, 679–681. doi: 10.1038/nn1899

Scali, M., Baroncelli, L., Cenni, M. C., Sale, A., and Maffei, L. (2012). A rich environmental experience reactivates visual cortex plasticity in aged rats. *Exp. Gerontol.* 47, 337–341. doi: 10.1016/j.exger.2012.01.007

Scarmeas, N., and Stern, Y. (2003). Cognitive reserve and lifestyle. *J. Clin. Exp. Neuropsychol.* 25, 625–633. doi: 10.1076/jcen.25.5.625.14576

Schrijver, N. C., Bahr, N. I., Weiss, I. C., and Wurbel, H. (2002). Dissociable effects of isolation rearing and environmental enrichment on exploration, spatial learning and HPA activity in adult rats. *Pharmacol. Biochem. Behav.* 73, 209–224. doi: 10.1016/S0091-3057(02)00790-6

Seeman, T. E., Lusignolo, T. M., Albert, M., and Berkman, L. (2001). Social relationships, social support, and patterns of cognitive aging in healthy, high-functioning older adults: MacArthur studies of successful aging. *Health Psychol.* 20, 243–255. doi: 10.1037/0278-6133.20.4.243

Segovia, G., Yague, A. G., Garcia-Verdugo, J. M., and Mora, F. (2006). Environmental enrichment promotes neurogenesis and changes the extracellular concentrations of glutamate and GABA in the hippocampus of aged rats. *Brain Res. Bull.* 70, 8–14. doi: 10.1016/j.brainresbull.2005.11.005

Sharp, P. E., McNaughton, B. L., and Barnes, C. A. (1985). Enhancement of hippocampal field potentials in rats exposed to a novel, complex environment. *Brain Res.* 339, 361–365.

Shiel, A., Burn, J. P., Henry, D., Clark, J., Wilson, B. A., Burnett, M. E., et al. (2001). The effects of increased rehabilitation therapy after brain injury: results of a prospective controlled trial. *Clin. Rehabil.* 15, 501–514. doi: 10.1191/026921501680425225

Shultz, S. R., Cardamone, L., Liu, Y. R., Hogan, R. E., Maccotta, L., Wright, D. K., et al. (2013). Can structural or functional changes following traumatic brain injury in the rat predict epileptic outcome? *Epilepsia* 54, 1240–1250. doi: 10.1111/epi.12223

Simpson, J., and Kelly, J. P. (2011). The impact of environmental enrichment in laboratory rats–behavioural and neurochemical aspects. *Behav. Brain Res.* 222, 246–264. doi: 10.1016/j.bbr.2011.04.002

Slade, A., Tennant, A., and Chamberlain, M. A. (2002). A randomised controlled trial to determine the effect of intensity of therapy upon length of stay in a neurological rehabilitation setting. *J. Rehabil. Med.* 34, 260–266. doi: 10.1080/165019702760390347

Smith, D. H., Okiyama, K., Thomas, M. J., Claussen, B., and McIntosh, T. K. (1991). Evaluation of memory dysfunction following experimental brain injury using the Morris water maze. *J. Neurotrauma* 8, 259–269. doi: 10.1089/neu.1991.8.259

Smith, J. M., Lunga, P., Story, D., Harris, N., Le Belle, J., James, M. F., et al. (2007). Inosine promotes recovery of skilled motor function in a model of focal brain injury. *Brain* 130, 915–925. doi: 10.1093/brain/awl393

Sohlberg, M. M., McLaughlin, K. A., Pavese, A., Heidrich, A., and Posner, M. I. (2000). Evaluation of attention process training and brain injury education in persons with acquired brain injury. *J. Clin. Exp. Neuropsychol.* 22, 656–676. doi: 10.1076/1380-3395(200010)22:5;1-9;FT656

Sozda, C. N., Hoffman, A. N., Olsen, A. S., Cheng, J. P., Zafonte, R. D., and Kline, A. E. (2010). Empirical comparison of typical and atypical environmental enrichment paradigms on functional and histological outcome after experimental traumatic brain injury. *J. Neurotrauma* 27, 1047–1057. doi: 10.1089/neu.2010.1313

Spires, T. L., Grote, H. E., Varshney, N. K., Cordery, P. M., Van Dellen, A., Blakemore, C., et al. (2004). Environmental enrichment rescues protein deficits in a mouse model of Huntington's disease, indicating a possible disease mechanism. *J. Neurosci.* 24, 2270–2276. doi: 10.1523/JNEUROSCI.1658-03.2004

Spivack, G., Spettell, C. M., Ellis, D. W., and Ross, S. E. (1992). Effects of intensity of treatment and length of stay on rehabilitation outcomes. *Brain Inj.* 6, 419–434. doi: 10.3109/02699059209008138

Strich, S. J. (1956). Diffuse degeneration of the cerebral white matter in severe dementia following head injury. *J. Neurol. Neurosurg. Psychiatry* 19, 163–185. doi: 10.1136/jnnp.19.3.163

Sur, M., and Leamey, C. A. (2001). Development and plasticity of cortical areas and networks. *Nat. Rev. Neurosci.* 2, 251–262. doi: 10.1038/35067562

Tang, Y. P., Wang, H., Feng, R., Kyin, M., and Tsien, J. Z. (2001). Differential effects of enrichment on learning and memory function in NR2B transgenic mice. *Neuropharmacology* 41, 779–790. doi: 10.1016/S0028-3908(01)00122-8

Taub, E., Uswatte, G., and Elbert, T. (2002). New treatments in neurorehabilitation founded on basic research. *Nat. Rev. Neurosci.* 3, 228–236. doi: 10.1038/nrn754

Till, C., Colella, B., Verwegen, J., and Green, R. E. (2008). Postrecovery cognitive decline in adults with traumatic brain injury. *Arch. Phys. Med. Rehabil.* 89, S25–S34. doi: 10.1016/j.apmr.2008.07.004

Toglia, J., Johnston, M. V., Goverover, Y., and Dain, B. (2010). A multicontext approach to promoting transfer of strategy use and self regulation after brain injury: an exploratory study. *Brain Inj.* 24, 664–677. doi: 10.3109/02699051003610474

Toglia, J. P. (1991). Generalization of treatment: a multicontext approach to cognitive perceptual impairment in adults with brain injury. *Am. J. Occup. Ther.* 45, 505–516. doi: 10.5014/ajot.45.6.505

Tognini, P., Manno, I., Bonaccorsi, J., Cenni, M. C., Sale, A., and Maffei, L. (2012). Environmental enrichment promotes plasticity and visual acuity recovery in adult monocular amblyopic rats. *PLoS ONE* 7:e34815. doi: 10.1371/journal.pone.0034815

Torasdotter, M., Metsis, M., Henriksson, B. G., Winblad, B., and Mohammed, A. H. (1998). Environmental enrichment results in higher levels of nerve growth factor mRNA in the rat visual cortex and hippocampus. *Behav. Brain Res.* 93, 83–90. doi: 10.1016/S0166-4328(97)00142-3

Turner, A. M., and Greenough, W. T. (1985). Differential rearing effects on rat visual cortex synapses. I. Synaptic and neuronal density and synapses per neuron. *Brain Res.* 329, 195–203.

Turrigiano, G. G. (1999). Homeostatic plasticity in neuronal networks: the more things change, the more they stay the same. *Trends Neurosci.* 22, 221–227. doi: 10.1016/S0166-2236(98)01341-1

Turrigiano, G. G. (2008). The self-tuning neuron: synaptic scaling of excitatory synapses. *Cell* 135, 422–435. doi: 10.1016/j.cell.2008.10.008

Uylings, H. B., Kuypers, K., Diamond, M. C., and Veltman, W. A. (1978). Effects of differential environments on plasticity of dendrites of cortical pyramidal neurons in adult rats. *Exp. Neurol.* 62, 658–677. doi: 10.1016/0014-4886(78)90276-5

Valero, J., Espana, J., Parra-Damas, A., Martin, E., Rodriguez-Alvarez, J., and Saura, C. A. (2011). Short-term environmental enrichment rescues adult neurogenesis and memory deficits in APP(Sw,Ind) transgenic mice. *PLoS ONE* 6:e16832. doi: 10.1371/journal.pone.0016832

Van Dellen, A., Blakemore, C., Deacon, R., York, D., and Hannan, A. J. (2000). Delaying the onset of Huntington's in mice. *Nature* 404, 721–722. doi: 10.1038/35008142

Van Praag, H., Christie, B. R., Sejnowski, T. J., and Gage, F. H. (1999). Running enhances neurogenesis, learning, and long-term potentiation in mice. *Proc. Natl. Acad. Sci. U.S.A.* 96, 13427–13431. doi: 10.1073/pnas.96.23.13427

Van Praag, H., Kempermann, G., and Gage, F. H. (2000). Neural consequences of environmental enrichment. *Nat. Rev. Neurosci.* 1, 191–198. doi: 10.1038/35044558

Varty, G. B., Paulus, M. P., Braff, D. L., and Geyer, M. A. (2000). Environmental enrichment and isolation rearing in the rat: effects on locomotor behavior and startle response plasticity. *Biol. Psychiatry* 47, 864–873. doi: 10.1016/S0006-3223(99)00269-3

Vedovelli, K., Silveira, E., Velho, E., Stertz, L., Kapczinski, F., Schroder, N., et al. (2011). Effects of increased opportunity for physical exercise and learning experiences on recognition memory and brain-derived neurotrophic factor levels in brain and serum of rats. *Neuroscience* 199, 284–291. doi: 10.1016/j.neuroscience.2011.08.012

Volkmar, F. R., and Greenough, W. T. (1972). Rearing complexity affects branching of dendrites in the visual cortex of the rat. *Science* 176, 1445–1447. doi: 10.1126/science.176.4042.1445

Voss, M. W., Nagamatsu, L. S., Liu-Ambrose, T., and Kramer, A. F. (2011). Exercise, brain, and cognition across the life span. *J. Appl. Physiol. (1985)* 111, 1505–1513. doi: 10.1152/japplphysiol.00210.2011

Wagner, A. K., Kline, A. E., Sokoloski, J., Zafonte, R. D., Capulong, E., and Dixon, C. E. (2002). Intervention with environmental enrichment after experimental brain trauma enhances cognitive recovery in male but not female rats. *Neurosci. Lett.* 334, 165–168. doi: 10.1016/S0304-3940(02)01103-5

Walsh, R. N., Budtz-Olsen, O. E., Penny, J. E., and Cummins, R. A. (1969). The effects of environmental complexity on the histology of the rat hippocampus. *J. Comp. Neurol.* 137, 361–366. doi: 10.1002/cne.901370309

Wang, Y., Bontempi, B., Hong, S. M., Mehta, K., Weinstein, P. R., Abrams, G. M., et al. (2008). A comprehensive analysis of gait impairment after experimental stroke and the therapeutic effect of environmental enrichment in rats. *J. Cereb. Blood Flow Metab.* 28, 1936–1950. doi: 10.1038/jcbfm.2008.82

Warraich, Z., and Kleim, J. A. (2010). Neural plasticity: the biological substrate for neurorehabilitation. *PM R* 2, S208–S219. doi: 10.1016/j.pmrj.2010.10.016

Wen, P. H., Hof, P. R., Chen, X., Gluck, K., Austin, G., Younkin, S. G., et al. (2004). The presenilin-1 familial Alzheimer disease mutant P117L impairs neurogenesis in the hippocampus of adult mice. *Exp. Neurol.* 188, 224–237. doi: 10.1016/j.expneurol.2004.04.002

Whishaw, I. Q., Pellis, S. M., Gorny, B. P., and Pellis, V. C. (1991). The impairments in reaching and the movements of compensation in rats with motor cortex lesions: an endpoint, videorecording, and movement notation analysis. *Behav. Brain Res.* 42, 77–91. doi: 10.1016/S0166-4328(05)80042-7

Whishaw, I. Q., Zaborowski, J. A., and Kolb, B. (1984). Postsurgical enrichment aids adult hemidecorticate rats on a spatial navigation task. *Behav. Neural Biol.* 42, 183–190. doi: 10.1016/S0163-1047(84)91046-X

Will, B., Galani, R., Kelche, C., and Rosenzweig, M. R. (2004). Recovery from brain injury in animals: relative efficacy of environmental enrichment, physical exercise or formal training (1990-2002). *Prog. Neurobiol.* 72, 167–182. doi: 10.1016/j.pneurobio.2004.03.001

Will, B. E., Rosenzweig, M. R., Bennett, E. L., Hebert, M., and Morimoto, H. (1977). Relatively brief environmental enrichment aids recovery of learning capacity and alters brain measures after postweaning brain lesions in rats. *J. Comp. Physiol. Psychol.* 91, 33–50. doi: 10.1037/h0077306

Willer, B., Button, J., and Rempel, R. (1999). Residential and home-based postacute rehabilitation of individuals with traumatic brain injury: a case control study. *Arch. Phys. Med. Rehabil.* 80, 399–406. doi: 10.1016/S0003-9993(99)90276-9

Wilson, R., Barnes, L., and Bennett, D. (2003). Assessment of lifetime participation in cognitively stimulating activities. *J. Clin. Exp. Neuropsychol.* 25, 634–642. doi: 10.1076/jcen.25.5.634.14572

Wood, N. I., Carta, V., Milde, S., Skillings, E. A., McAllister, C. J., Ang, Y. L., et al. (2010). Responses to environmental enrichment differ with sex and genotype in a transgenic mouse model of Huntington's disease. *PLoS ONE* 5:e9077. doi: 10.1371/journal.pone.0009077

Workman, J. L., Fonken, L. K., Gusfa, J., Kassouf, K. M., and Nelson, R. J. (2011). Post-weaning environmental enrichment alters affective responses and interacts with behavioral testing to alter nNOS immunoreactivity. *Pharmacol. Biochem. Behav.* 100, 25–32. doi: 10.1016/j.pbb.2011.07.008

Xerri, C., Bourgeon, S., and Coq, J. O. (2005). Perceptual context-dependent remodeling of the forepaw map in the SI cortex of rats trained on tactile discrimination. *Behav. Brain Res.* 162, 207–221. doi: 10.1016/j.bbr.2005.03.003

Xerri, C., Coq, J. O., Merzenich, M. M., and Jenkins, W. M. (1996). Experience-induced plasticity of cutaneous maps in the primary somatosensory cortex of adult monkeys and rats. *J. Physiol. Paris* 90, 277–287. doi: 10.1016/S0928-4257(97)81438-6

Xu, T., Yu, X., Perlik, A. J., Tobin, W. F., Zweig, J. A., Tennant, K., et al. (2009a). Rapid formation and selective stabilization of synapses for enduring motor memories. *Nature* 462, 915–919. doi: 10.1038/nature08389

Xu, X., Ye, L., and Ruan, Q. (2009b). Environmental enrichment induces synaptic structural modification after transient focal cerebral ischemia in rats. *Exp. Biol. Med. (Maywood)* 234, 296–305. doi: 10.3181/0804-RM-128

Yan, E. B., Johnstone, V. P., Alwis, D. S., Morganti-Kossmann, M. C., and Rajan, R. (2013). Characterising effects of impact velocity on brain and behaviour in a model of diffuse traumatic axonal injury. *Neuroscience* 248C, 17–29. doi: 10.1016/j.neuroscience.2013.05.045

Young, D., Lawlor, P. A., Leone, P., Dragunow, M., and During, M. J. (1999). Environmental enrichment inhibits spontaneous apoptosis, prevents seizures and is neuroprotective. *Nat. Med.* 5, 448–453. doi: 10.1038/7449

Zebunke, M., Puppe, B., and Langbein, J. (2013). Effects of cognitive enrichment on behavioural and physiological reactions of pigs. *Physiol. Behav.* 118, 70–79. doi: 10.1016/j.physbeh.2013.05.005

Zhou, X., Panizzutti, R., De Villers-Sidani, E., Madeira, C., and Merzenich, M. M. (2011). Natural restoration of critical period plasticity in the juvenile and adult primary auditory cortex. *J. Neurosci.* 31, 5625–5634. doi: 10.1523/JNEUROSCI.6470-10.2011

Zhu, X. L., Poon, W. S., Chan, C. C., and Chan, S. S. (2007). Does intensive rehabilitation improve the functional outcome of patients with traumatic brain injury (TBI)? A randomized controlled trial. *Brain Inj.* 21, 681–690. doi: 10.1080/02699050701468941

Zhu, X. L., Poon, W. S., Chan, C. H., and Chan, S. H. (2001). Does intensive rehabilitation improve the functional outcome of patients with traumatic brain injury? Interim result of a randomized controlled trial. *Br. J. Neurosurg.* 15, 464–473. doi: 10.1080/02688690120097688

Zhu, X. O., McCabe, B. J., Aggleton, J. P., and Brown, M. W. (1997). Differential activation of the rat hippocampus and perirhinal cortex by novel visual stimuli and a novel environment. *Neurosci. Lett.* 229, 141–143. doi: 10.1016/S0304-3940(97)00437-0

Zimmermann, A., Stauffacher, M., Langhans, W., and Wurbel, H. (2001). Enrichment-dependent differences in novelty exploration in rats can be explained by habituation. *Behav. Brain Res.* 121, 11–20. doi: 10.1016/S0166-4328(00)00377-6

Decoding the ERD/ERS: influence of afferent input induced by a leg assistive robot

Giuseppe Lisi[1,2]*, Tomoyuki Noda[1] and Jun Morimoto[1]

[1] ATR Computational Neuroscience Laboratories, Department of Brain Robot Interface, ATR, Kyoto, Japan
[2] Mathematical Informatics Laboratory, Department of Information Science, Nara Institute of Science and Technology, Nara, Japan

Edited by:
Mikhail Lebedev, Duke University, USA

Reviewed by:
Yuri P. Ivanenko, IRCCS Fondazione Santa Lucia, Italy
Marta Gandolla, Politecnico di Milano, Italy

***Correspondence:**
Giuseppe Lisi, ATR Computational Neuroscience Laboratories, Department of Brain Robot Interface, ATR, 2-2-2 Hikaridai, Seika-cho, Soraku-gun, Kyoto, 619-0288, Japan
e-mail: beppelisi@gmail.com

This paper investigates the influence of the leg afferent input, induced by a leg assistive robot, on the decoding performance of a BMI system. Specifically, it focuses on a decoder based on the event-related (de)synchronization (ERD/ERS) of the sensorimotor area. The EEG experiment, performed with healthy subjects, is structured as a 3 × 2 factorial design, consisting of two factors: "finger tapping task" and "leg condition." The former is divided into three levels (BMI classes), being left hand finger tapping, right hand finger tapping and no movement (Idle); while the latter is composed by two levels: leg perturbed (*Pert*) and leg not perturbed (*NoPert*). Specifically, the subjects' leg was periodically perturbed by an assistive robot in 5 out of 10 sessions of the experiment and not moved in the remaining sessions. The aim of this study is to verify that the decoding performance of the finger tapping task is comparable between the two conditions *NoPert* and *Pert*. Accordingly, a classifier is trained to output the class of the finger tapping, given as input the features associated with the ERD/ERS. Individually for each subject, the decoding performance is statistically compared between the *NoPert* and *Pert* conditions. Results show that the decoding performance is notably above chance, for all the subjects, under both conditions. Moreover, the statistical comparison do not highlight a significant difference between *NoPert* and *Pert* in any subject, which is confirmed by feature visualization.

Keywords: brain robot interface, assistive exoskeleton robot, ERD/ERS of the sensorimotor hand area, lower limb afferent input, ICA/CSP, wavelet, PCA/LDA, sparse logistic regression

1. INTRODUCTION

Brain-machine interfaces (BMI) have recently raised much interest in that they can help improve the quality of life of people with severe motor disabilities. In previous studies, the brain signal has been used to control devices that affect the surrounding environment such as wheelchairs or neuroprosthesis (Mussa-Ivaldi, 2000; Daly and Wolpaw, 2008; Pfurtscheller and Solis-Escalante, 2008). Regarding the nature of ERD/ERS, movement or preparation for movement is typically accompanied by a decrease in mu and beta rhythms, particularly contralateral to the movement (Wolpaw et al., 2002). This phenomenon has been named event-related desynchronization or ERD (Babiloni et al., 1999). Its opposite, rhythm increase, or event-related synchronization (ERS), occurs after movement and with relaxation (Pfurtscheller and Lopes da Silva, 1999). To note that similar ERD/ERS patterns in the sensorimotor area can be elicited also by motor imagery (Pfurtscheller and Neuper, 1997; Pfurtscheller and Lopes da Silva, 1999; McFarland et al., 2000). These features make it possible to use a BMI system based on ERD/ERS for the control of an external device (Pfurtscheller et al., 2000b; Wolpaw et al., 2003; Babiloni et al., 2007). If this is done irrespectively of any system cues, the control paradigm is called asynchronous and allows the subject to make self-paced decisions (Müller-Putz et al., 2006; Zhao et al., 2009; Solis-Escalante et al., 2010).

A similar control paradigm has yet to be carefully investigated for a lower limb exoskeleton robot. Of particular interest would be a BMI system, based on the ERD/ERS of the sensorimotor area, able to control an assistive robot (downward arrow of **Figure 1**). Similarly, Tsui et al. (2011); Huang et al. (2012) have succeeded in controlling a wheelchair by means of a BMI based on event-related (de)synchronization (ERD/ERS). Nonetheless, one of the differences between a wheelchair and a lower limb assistive robot is that the latter induces movements of the legs. In this context, the ERD/ERS phenomenon is not only related to active movements or motor imagery, but also to passive movements (upward arrow of **Figure 1**; Cassim et al., 2001; Müller et al., 2003; Müller-Putz et al., 2007; Wagner et al., 2012). Especially, Müller-Putz et al. (2007) highlighted that passive movements of the feet produce a significant ERD/ERS not only at the vertex, but over the whole sensorimotor cortex. This raises the question whether the somatosensory afferent input, induced by the periodic leg perturbation, interferes with the decoding ability of a BMI system based on the ERD/ERS of the sensorimotor hand area (horizontal arrow of **Figure 1**).

Specifically, in this paper, we investigate whether the periodic perturbation of lower limbs produces a significant decrease in the classification performance of actual right and left hand finger movements. The reason for decoding the right and left sensorimotor hand area stands in the reliability of the contralateral ERD/ERS spatial distribution (Wang et al., 2007) and in the fact that this approach is exhaustively discussed in literature (Guger et al., 2000; Pfurtscheller et al., 2000b; Blankertz et al.,

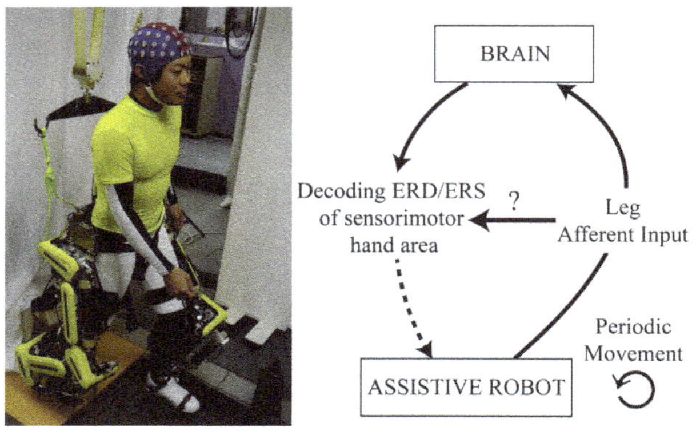

FIGURE 1 | Conceptual representation of the problem. Understanding how the leg afferent input, induced by a leg assistive robot, influences the decoding of the ERD/ERS of the sensorimotor hand area. The paper focuses on the concepts represented by the solid arrows of this figure.

2008a). Moreover, the *Idle* class is considered in order to simulate the behavior of the system in an online asynchronous setup (Müller-Putz et al., 2006).

Furthermore, the motivation for using real movements instead of motor imagery, is that the latter cannot be mechanically measured nor visually assessed by the experiment operator. As such, in case of misclassification, there is no certainty about whether the subject failed in generating a significant ERD/ERS by motor imagery or if the somatosensory afferent input of the leg actually affected the decoding. On the other hand, for real upper limb movements, the motor output is visible; therefore, we are certain that the motor cortex has produced a control command.

To note that even though patterns of mu and beta de/synchronization associated with actual movements are similar to those with motor imagery, they differ in magnitude (McFarland et al., 2000). Specifically, the spectral perturbations associated with motor imagery are considerably smaller than the ones of actual movements (Solis-Escalante et al., 2010). Nonetheless, according to Pfurtscheller et al. (1998), the beta ERS is significantly larger with hand as compared to finger movement. Therefore, the latter is chosen in this experiment, so as to deal with a spectral perturbation that is as close as possible to the one associated with motor imagery, while preserving the necessary property of objective measurability by the experiment operator.

Previous studies have dealt with EEG-based neuroprosthesis control (Pfurtscheller et al., 2000a; Müller-Putz et al., 2005, 2006, 2009), but to our knowledge this is the first time that the possibility of interference between the rhythms associated with passive and active movements is investigated.

2. METHODS

Five healthy subjects were asked to perform real right/left-hand brisk finger tapping, or not to move (idle), while their brain activity was recorded by EEG. Each task lasted 2 s and was instructed by visual cues, interleaved by periods of rest of 8 s. Simultaneously, the subjects' leg was *perturbed by a periodic swing movement of a lower limb assistive robot* in 5 out of 10 sessions of the experiment. In this way, the experiment is characterized by two conditions: leg perturbed (*Pert*) and leg not perturbed (*NoPert*).

Therefore, the main question regarding the influence of the leg afferent input on the decoding of the sensorimotor area ERD/ERS can be stated as follows: *is the performance of finger tapping decoding significantly different between the NoPert and Pert conditions, for one or more subjects?* To answer this question, a classifier is trained to output the class of the finger tapping (*Idle, Left, Right*), given as input the features associated with the ERD/ERS. Cross-validated Kappa score (see section 2.3) is used to assess the decoding performance separately for *NoPert* and *Pert*. Then, individually for each subject, the Kappa scores of the two conditions are statistically compared by the Z-test (see Appendix). Moreover, it is important to perform an analysis that is as independent as possible from the characteristics of a specific decoder. For this reason, two types of feature extraction methods are used separately: *Unsupervised feature extraction* (ICA, Wavelet and PCA) and *Supervised feature extraction* (CSP, Wavelet, LDA).

As discussed in the introduction, actual left/right hand finger tapping and idle were chosen because of the following reasons:

1. the contralateral ERD/ERS spatial distribution associated with left or right hand movements can be reliably decoded;
2. actual movements are observable by the experiment operator, or mechanically measurable, therefore we are certain that an ERD/ERS activation must have been elicited by the motor task (with motor imagery the subject may fail to produce ERD/ERS);
3. finger movements are characterized by a significantly smaller ERS as compared to hand movements (Pfurtscheller et al., 1998), which makes the task as close as possible to a motor imagery one, while preserving the properties at point 1 and 2;
4. the idle class is used to simulate an online asynchronous setup.

2.1. EXPERIMENTAL SETUP

2.1.1. Assistive robot specifications

Our custom made one degree of freedom robot (oneDOF, Noda et al., 2012) was used as assistive robot (**Figure 2A**). OneDOF is actuated using a pneumatic-electric hybrid strategy. In detail, two antagonistic pneumatic artificial muscles (PAM) generate large force by converting pressured gas energy into contraction force through their rubber tube. The advantage of using a PAM is that it can exert very large torques (maximal 70 Nm), while generating insignificant electromagnetic noise from the point of view of the EEG system. Moreover, an electric motor generates parallel small torque (maximal 5 Nm) in order to make fast and precise corrections to the torque generated by PAM. This strategy allows for both a powerful and precise actuation of the robot.

For this specific experiment, OneDOF was mounted on a custom made support in order to allow subjects to sit near to the robot (**Figure 2B**). Moreover a leg-shaped thermoplastic polymer was anchored to OneDOF in order to secure the subject's leg (**Figure 2C**).

2.1.2. Data acquisition

The experiment, which was carried out with five healthy subjects aged 23–27, can be represented by a 3×2 factorial design

(**Figure 3**) consisting of two factors: "finger tapping task" and "leg condition." The former is divided into three levels, being left tapping, right tapping and idle; while the latter is composed by two levels: *NoPert* and *Pert*.

With regard to the "leg condition" factor, five sessions of the experiment were performed while the assistive robot was stopped (*NoPert*) and other five while the robot continuously swung up and down at a frequency of 0.5 Hz between 5° and 50° of the knee joint (*Pert*).

During all the 10 sessions of the experiment the finger tapping task was carried out as follows: an hyphen was shown on the screen for 8 s to indicate that the subject should not move (rest). After this period, a left or right arrow randomly appeared, or the hyphen was maintained on the screen, for 2 s, indicating respectively that the subject should perform left or right hand brisk continuous finger tapping, or keep not moving (idle). Within one session, each of the three tasks, Left/Right tapping and Idle, was performed 10 times, resulting in 30 trials per session. After each session, subjects rested for about 5 min. Moreover, the EEG signal was recorded at a sampling rate of 2048 Hz with a 64-electrode cap and a Biosemi Active Two system for amplification and analog-to-digital conversion.

In order to confirm that to each visual cue corresponds a motor action, the finger tapping performance was visually

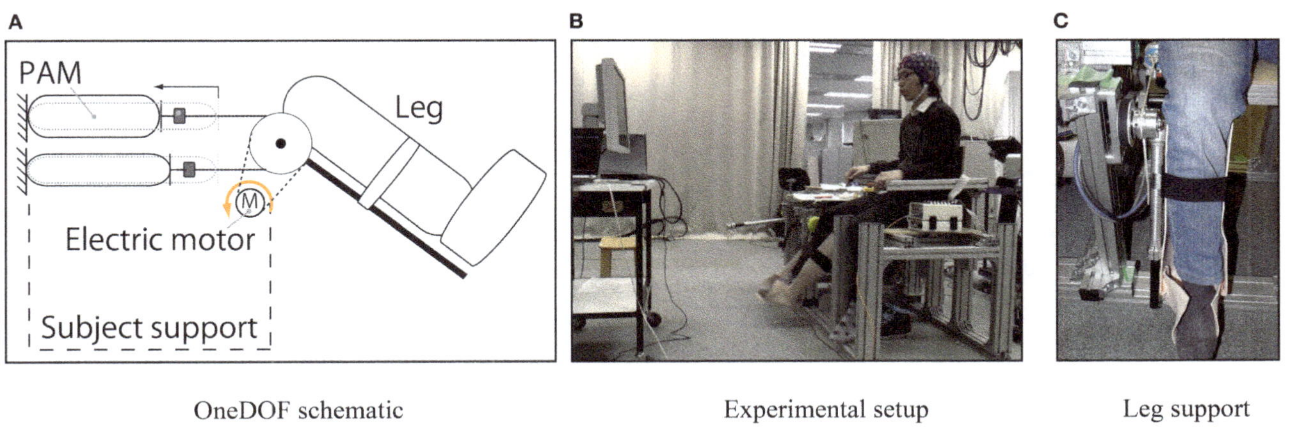

FIGURE 2 | Robot used during the experiment. (A) PAM and electric actuators can exert parallel torques to move the leg. **(B)** Representation of the experimental setup. **(C)** Representation of the thermoplastic polymer leg support anchored to the robot and holding up the subject's leg.

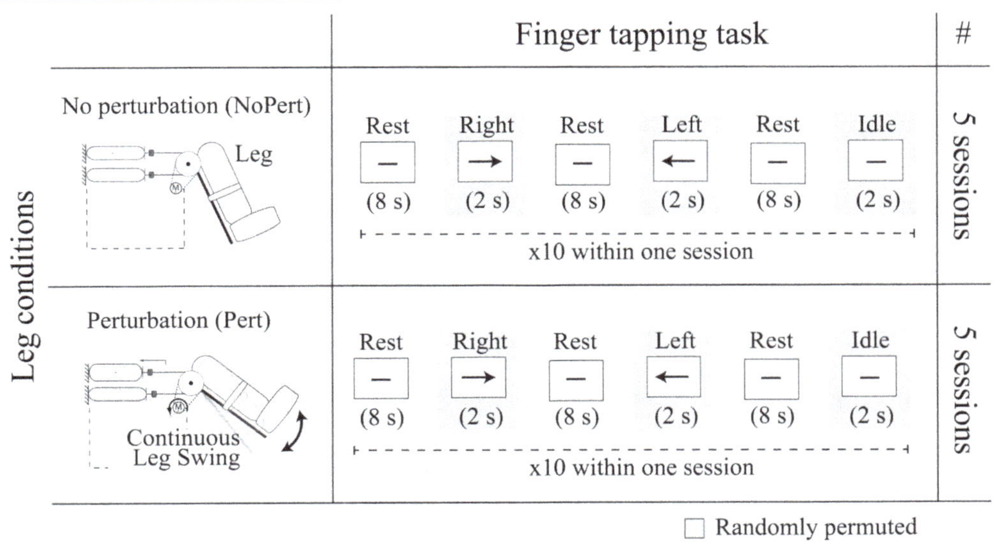

FIGURE 3 | Experimental design. The experiment is structured as a 3 × 2 factorial design, consisting of two factors "finger tapping task" and "leg condition." The former is divided into three levels, being left hand finger tapping (Left), right hand finger tapping (Right) and Idle, whose temporal representation is visualized in the "Finger tapping task" column. The "leg condition" factor is divided into two levels *NoPert* and *Pert*, which are represented, respectively, in the first and second rows of the table. To note that *Rest* is the resting period between tasks and that the visual cues of the tasks are randomly permuted within a session. Moreover, in the last column, the number of sessions performed for each experimental condition are visualized.

observed by the experiment operator. Moreover, for the first three subjects the experiment was recorded on video, while for the other two subjects the index finger angle was measured by means of a goniometer sensor (Biometrics Ltd).

Subjects gave written informed consent for the experimental procedures, which were approved by the ATR Human Subject Review Committee.

2.2. DECODER TRAINING

In this section, we introduce the methodology to train and test the decoder that is used in the cross-validation procedure described in section 2.3. Moreover, we refer to "training set" and "test set," detailed as well in section 2.3, but for the time being it is sufficient to think of them as two independent datasets that are used to, respectively, fit the parameters of a model (decoder) and evaluate the predictive power of the trained (fitted) model.

The six steps of the training algorithm (**Figure 4**) are: *1. preprocessing* (section 2.2.1), *2. spatial filter identification* (section 2.2.2), *3. wavelet transform for time-frequency feature extraction* (section 2.2.3), *4. spatial filter selection* (section 2.2.4), *5. feature dimensionality reduction* (section 2.2.5) and *6. training of a classifier* (section 2.2.6). In order to produce results that are independent from the characteristics of a specific feature extraction method, two types of decoder are used separately:

- *Unsupervised feature extraction*-based: the spatial filter identification step is performed by Independent Component Analysis (ICA) and feature dimensionality reduction by Principal Component Analysis (PCA);
- *Supervised feature extraction*-based: the spatial filter identification is carried out by Common Spatial Patterns (CSP) and feature dimensionality reduction by Linear Discriminant Analysis (LDA).

It is important to stress that the *Unsupervised feature extraction*-based decoder is trained and tested independently from the *Supervised feature extraction*-based one.

2.2.1. Preprocessing

This step is common to both the *Unsupervised* and *Supervised feature extraction*-based decoders. Only a subset of 35 electrodes, centered at the motor cortex, is used: all the electrodes positioned within the ranges F5-F6, FC5-FC6, C5-C6, CP5-CP6, P5-P6. The training and test sets are resampled at 128 Hz and bandpass filtered (FIR filter implemented in EEGLAB, Delorme and Makeig, 2004) in the range from 8 to 30 Hz, encompassing the mu and beta frequency bands, which have been shown to be most important for movement classification. Epochs are extracted with respect to the visual cues presented to the subjects. In particular, the epoch starts 0.5 s before the cue onset and ends 2.5 s after the offset, for a total of 5 s. The time window after the movement offset is needed to capture completely the ERS, also considering that, sometimes, this is slightly delayed due to the subject's reaction time. In the following subsections $\mathbf{E}_j \in \mathbb{R}^{c \times t}$ represents the single-trial EEG signals of the training set, where c is the number of channels, t is the number of time samples and $j = 1 \ldots n$ where n is the number of training trials.

2.2.2. Spatial filter identification (ICA and CSP)

Previous studies have demonstrated that spatial filters are useful in single-trial analysis, in order to improve the signal-to-noise ratio (Blankertz et al., 2008b). For this purpose, Independent Component Analysis (ICA) is implemented in the *Unsupervised feature extraction*-based decoder, while Common Spatial Patterns (CSP) is used in the *Supervised feature extraction*-based one. Both ICA and CSP transform the observed EEG signals as:

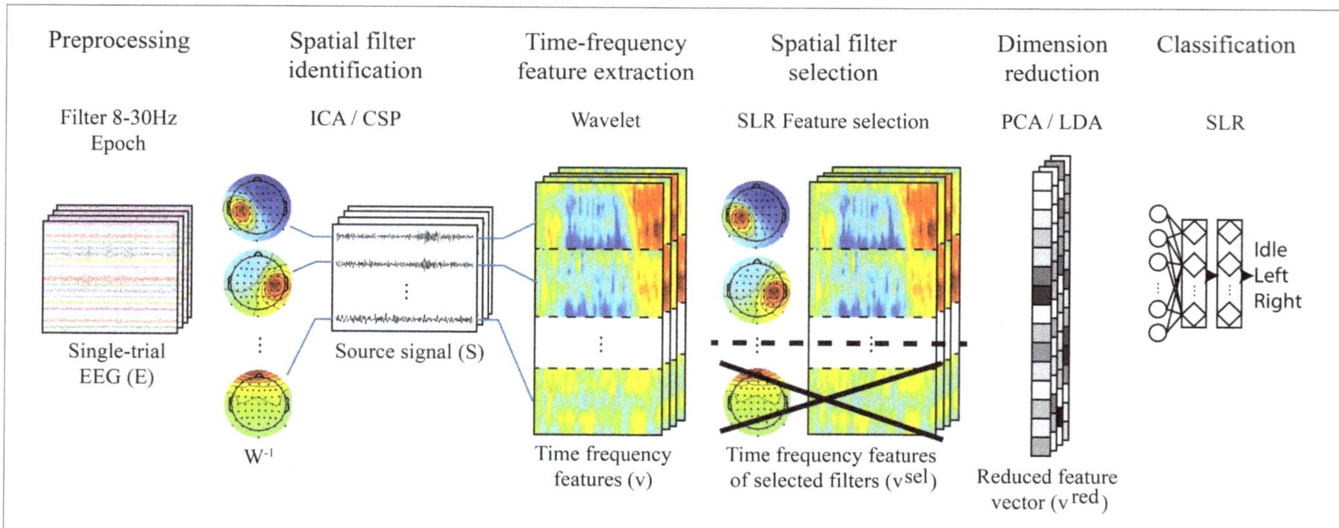

FIGURE 4 | Decoder training in a single fold of the cross-validation. In the *Unsupervised feature extraction*-based version, ICA and PCA are used, respectively, for spatial filter selection and dimension reduction, while CSP and LDA are, respectively, employed in the *Supervised feature extraction*-based one. Important to note that the transformation matrices of spatial filter identification, spatial filter selection and dimensionality reduction are computed only on the training set of each cross-validation fold. Moreover, the time-frequency features are vectorized in the algorithm, while in figure they are kept in matrix form for a visualization purpose: the horizontal axis represents the time, and the vertical axis represents the frequency.

$$\mathbf{S}_j = \mathbf{W}\mathbf{E}_j \tag{1}$$

where $\mathbf{E}_j$ represents the observed single-trial EEG signals, $\mathbf{W}$ the unmixing matrix, $\mathbf{S}_j$ the recovered single-trial sources and $j = 1 \ldots n$, where n is the number of training trials.

2.2.2.1. Independent Component Analysis (ICA). ICA is an unsupervised method that finds a linear transformation (W) of non-gaussian data ($\mathbf{E}$), so that the resulting components ($\mathbf{S}$) are as statistically independent as possible (Hyvärinen and Oja, 2000). Hence, the EEG signal is separated into Independent Components (ICs) accounting for different neural activities, but also stereotyped non-brain artifact signals including eye movements, line noise and muscle activities (Makeig et al., 2004). In this study, the logistic infomax ICA algorithm, implemented in the EEGLAB function *binica* (Delorme and Makeig, 2004), is executed on the preprocessed training set. This yields an unmixing matrix $\mathbf{W} \in \mathbb{R}^{s\times c}$ and source signals (independent components) $\mathbf{S}_j \in \mathbb{R}^{s\times t}$, where s is the number of sources, c the number of channels, t is the number of time samples and $j = 1 \ldots n$, where n is the number of training trials.

2.2.2.2. Common Spatial Patterns (CSP). CSP computes the unmixing matrix $\mathbf{W}$ to yield features whose variances are optimal for discriminating two classes of EEG measurements (Ramoser et al., 1998; Blankertz et al., 2008a) by solving the eigenvalue decomposition problem

$$\mathbf{\Sigma}_1 W = (\mathbf{\Sigma}_1 + \mathbf{\Sigma}_2)WD \tag{2}$$

where $\mathbf{\Sigma}_1$ and $\mathbf{\Sigma}_2$ represent the estimates of the covariance matrices of the EEG signal associated with two different tasks, the diagonal matrix $\mathbf{D}$ contains the eigenvalues of $\mathbf{\Sigma}_1$ and the column vectors of $\mathbf{W}^{-1}$ are the filters for the CSP projections. The best contrast is provided by those filters with the highest and lowest eigenvalues, therefore the common practice is to retain e eigenvectors from both ends of the eigenvalue spectrum (Blankertz et al., 2008a). CSP is applied in a One-vs-Rest (OvR) fashion, in order to cope with the multi-class nature of the problem, separately (Dornhege et al., 2004) for three different frequency bands 8–13 Hz (μ), 15–25 Hz (β), 8–30 Hz (μ and β), in the time segment starting 1 s after the cue (Blankertz et al., 2008b). Moreover, $e = 2$ eigenvectors from the top and from the bottom of the eigenvalue spectrum are retained. This procedure is performed only on the preprocessed training dataset, yielding the unmixing matrix $\mathbf{W} \in \mathbb{R}^{s\times c}$ and source signals $\mathbf{S}_j \in \mathbb{R}^{s\times t}$, where $s = 2 \times e \times 3$ (frequency bands)$\times 3$ (classes) is the number of sources (CSP projections), c is the number of channels, t is the number of time samples and $j = 1 \ldots n$, where n is the number of training trials.

It is important to note that, with both ICA and CSP, the unmixing matrix $\mathbf{W}$ is computed *only using the training set.*

2.2.3. Time-frequency analysis: the wavelet transform

In both the *Unsupervised* and *Supervised feature extraction*-based decoders, the Morlet Wavelet transform (Daubechies, 1990) is employed to extract time-frequency features, representing the subject-specific ERD/ERS patterns, from the source signals $\mathbf{S}$. For each trial, a wavelet coefficient matrix with 50 time samples and 20 frequency bins is computed for the i-th source signal. The resulting coefficients are squared to get the spectral power and the $10\log_{10}$ transformation is computed to obtain a final time-frequency representation ($\mathbf{c}_i$). Therefore, the feature vector of the j-th trial ($\mathbf{v}_j$) is obtained by the concatenation of the time-frequency coefficients $\mathbf{c}_i$ computed from the i-th source signal inside $\mathbf{S}_j$:

$$\mathbf{v}_j = \begin{bmatrix} \mathbf{c}_1 \\ \mathbf{c}_i \\ \vdots \\ \mathbf{c}_s \end{bmatrix}, \mathbf{c}_i = \begin{bmatrix} c_{11}, \ldots, c_{f1}, c_{12}, \ldots, c_{f2}, \ldots, c_{1t}, \ldots, c_{ft} \end{bmatrix}^{\top} \tag{3}$$

In the equations above, $\mathbf{v}_j$ represents the j-th feature vector, $j = 1 \ldots n$, where n is the number of training trials, $\mathbf{c}_i$ is the time-frequency coefficients vector of the i-th source, $i = 1 \ldots s$ where s is the number of sources in $\mathbf{S}_j$, t is the number of time samples and f is the number of frequency bins.

2.2.4. Spatial filter selection based on SLR

Not all the spatial filters that have been previously identified by ICA or CSP are related to the neural processes of the tapping task. In particular, ICA identifies a large number of independent components that account for artifacts and other neural sources, while CSP might return some spatial patterns that over-fit the training set. Therefore, in order to avoid over-fitting and to obtain results that are not influenced by artifacts, it is necessary to reduce the number of spatial filters to the ones that are strictly indispensable for the classification of the tapping task.

For this purpose, Sparse Logistic Regression (SLR) is used to select the most important spatial filters based on their time-frequency features. SLR is a Bayesian extension of logistic regression, which simultaneously performs feature selection and training of model parameters for classification. It utilizes automatic relevance determination (ARD) to determine the importance of each parameter while estimating its values. This process selects only a few parameters as important and prunes away others. The resulting model has a sparse representation with a small number of estimated parameters (Yamashita et al., 2008). In this work we apply the OvR version of the algorithm to cope with the multi-class problem. Moreover, prior to training, each feature of the training set is normalized using its mean across trials and scaled using the respective standard deviation. Furthermore, the mean and standard deviation of the training features are used to normalize also the feature vectors of the test set.

SLR can be used to assign scores to spatial filters based on the classification performance and selection recurrence of their time-frequency features. In the current study we were inspired by the method proposed by Yamashita et al. (2008), which selects features on the basis of their selection recurrence. Given the fact that our goal is not to select single features, but spatial filters which are, in turn, represented by a set of time-frequency features we had to modify the original algorithm. The revised method considers the recurrence of the group of time-frequency features belonging to each spatial filter. The basic idea is that spatial filters whose time-frequency features are repeatedly selected with good classification performance among a variety of training data sets could be important.

Specifically, the selection of spatial filters is implemented by estimating SLR weight parameters on 80% of the *training set* and evaluating the classification performance on the remaining 20% of the *training set*. This process is *repeated five times* so that each trial of the training set is used once to evaluate the performance. Therefore, we can define a score value for each i-th spatial filter ($i = 1 \ldots s$ where s is the number of sources in $\mathbf{S}_j$) based on the number of selected features that belong to it. More precisely, let $\overline{\theta}_j$ and p_j denote the estimated parameter vector and classification performance (percent) resulting from the j-th repetition of SLR ($j = 1 \ldots R$, where R is the number of SLR repetitions). Moreover, $\overline{\theta}_j(k) = 0$ if the k-th feature is not selected ($k = 1 \ldots |\overline{\theta}|$ where $|\overline{\theta}|$ is the length of the feature vector) . Then the score value (SC) for the i-th spatial filter (SF) is defined by:

$$SC_i = \sum_{j}^{R} \sum_{k \in SF_i}^{|\overline{\theta}|} I(\overline{\theta}_j(k) \neq 0) \times p_j \tag{4}$$

where $I(\cdot)$ denotes an indicator function that takes the value of 1 if the condition inside the brackets is satisfied, 0 otherwise. $R = 5$ is the number of SLR repetitions, $|\overline{\theta}|$ is the length of the feature vector and $\overline{\theta}_j(k)$ is the estimate of the k-th parameter belonging to the i-th spatial filter (SF), with respect to the j-th repetition. Once SC has been computed for all the spatial filters, we retain only those whose SC is above a given threshold. Specifically for selecting independent components the threshold is $\mu_{SC} + \sigma_{SC}$, while for CSP the threshold is simply μ_{SC}, where μ and σ represent respectively mean and standard deviation of the SC values. The reason for having two different thresholds is that ICA returns a large number of independent components, not related to the classification, that need to be removed, such as artifacts and other neural sources. On the other hand, being CSP a supervised method, it selects mainly spatial filters that are important for the classification, and we only remove the few ones that would cause over-fitting.

Supposing that the set D of selected filters contains $d < s$ components (s total number of sources in $\mathbf{S}_j$), the new feature vector $\mathbf{v}_j^{sel}$ is obtained by concatenating the time-frequency features of the selected filters $\mathbf{c}_{i \in D}$:

$$\mathbf{v}_j^{sel} = \begin{bmatrix} \mathbf{c}_1 \\ \mathbf{c}_i \\ \vdots \\ \mathbf{c}_d \end{bmatrix}, \mathbf{c}_{i \in D} = \left[c_{11}, \ldots, c_{f1}, c_{12}, \ldots, c_{f2}, \ldots, c_{1t}, \ldots, c_{ft} \right]^{\top} \tag{5}$$

In the equations above, $\mathbf{v}_j^{sel}$ represents the feature vector associated with the selected spatial filters of the j-th trial, $\mathbf{c}_{i \in D}$ the time-frequency coefficient vector of the i-th source belonging to the set of selected filters D, $j = 1 \ldots n$ where n is the number of training trials, $i = 1 \ldots d$ where d is the cardinality of D, t is the number of time samples and f is the number of frequency bins. Therefore, the j-th feature vector $\mathbf{v}_j^{sel}$ is composed by $l = d \times f \times t$ elements. Moreover, the spatial filter unmixing matrix takes the following form $\mathbf{W}^{sel} \in \mathbb{R}^{d \times c}$, where c is the number of channels and d the number of selected spatial filters. To note that the SLR-based spatial filter selection is performed *only on the training set*.

2.2.5. *Dimensionality reduction (PCA and LDA)*

Even though the spatial filter selection method reduces the number of sources, the dimensionality of the concatenated time-frequency feature vector is in the order of thousands elements. Moreover, *the time-frequency features are somewhat redundant, because the values of adjacent points in the spectrogram are highly correlated.* Therefore, it is important to perform dimensionality reduction. For this purpose, Principal Component Analysis (PCA) is employed in the *Unsupervised feature extraction*-based decoder, while Linear Discriminant Analysis (LDA) in the *Supervised feature extraction*-based one.

PCA and LDA are, respectively, the most popular unsupervised and supervised dimensionality reduction methods in literature (Wang and Paliwal, 2003) and they both reduce the features dimension by projecting the original feature vector into a new feature space through a linear transformation matrix. Nonetheless, they optimize the transformation matrix with different intentions: PCA optimizes the transformation matrix by finding the largest variations in the original unlabeled feature space, while LDA pursues the largest ratio of between-class variation and within-class variation when projecting the original labeled features to a subspace (Wang and Paliwal, 2003). In this study PCA is implemented by Singular Value Decomposition (SVD), while LDA is executed by means of the algorithm proposed by Cai et al. (2008). To note that prior to performing PCA or LDA the mean of the training set is subtracted, and that in the case of PCA the mean of the training set is also subtracted from the test set.

The dimensionality reduction step yields a linear transformation matrix $\mathbf{A} \in \mathbb{R}^{p \times l}$ that projects the original feature vector $\mathbf{v}_j^{sel} \in \mathbb{R}^l$ to the reduced vector $\mathbf{v}_j^{red} \in \mathbb{R}^p$, where l is the length of the original feature vector and p the number of projections (reduced features, $p < l$). When dimensionality reduction is performed by PCA, the number of retained principal components (p) is set so as to achieve 90% of variance (Jolliffe, 2002), bringing the length of the feature vector from the order of thousands to the order of hundreds elements. On the other hand, when using LDA, the number of projections $p = 2$ since the number of non-zero eigenvalues is bounded by $g - 1$, where g is the number of classes (Cai et al., 2008). Once again, it is important to note that, with both PCA and LDA, the projection matrix A is computed only using the training set.

2.2.6. *Classification*

Once the feature vectors of all the trials in the training dataset ($\mathbf{v}_j^{red}$) are obtained, it is possible to compute the ones of the test dataset ($\hat{\mathbf{v}}_k^{red}$), by the following steps:

1. to generate the source signal matrix of the k-th trial in the test set ($\mathbf{S}_k^{test}$), multiply the preprocessed k-th single-trial EEG of

the *test dataset* ($k = 1 \ldots m$, where m is the number of test trials) by the spatial filter unmixing matrix $\mathbf{W}^{sel}$, obtained on the training set by *spatial filter selection* (section 2.2.4);

2. to generate the test feature vectors $\hat{\mathbf{v}}_k^{sel}$, compute the time-frequency matrix for each trial k and source in $\mathbf{S}_k^{test}$;
3. to generate the reduced feature vector $\hat{\mathbf{v}}_k^{red}$, multiply $\hat{\mathbf{v}}_k^{sel}$ by the projection matrix $\mathbf{A}$, obtained on the training set by *dimensionality reduction* (section 2.2.5).

The reduced feature vectors of the training set $\mathbf{v}_j^{red}$ and the one of the test set $\hat{\mathbf{v}}_k^{red}$ are used, with the respective labels, to train and evaluate a SLR classifier (introduced in section 2.2.4). To note that the SLR classifier used to decode the finger tapping task is trained and tested on features and datasets that differ from to the ones used to select spatial filters in section 2.2.4.

2.3. PERFORMANCE ASSESSMENT

The main objective of this study is to verify that the decoding performance of the upper limb tasks is not affected by the lower limb periodic perturbation. To do so, we compare the performance of the finger tapping decoding under the two conditions *NoPert* and *Pert*. In other words, from a factorial point of view, the goal is to assess the main effect of leg perturbation on the decoding of finger tapping. Given the fact that the leg perturbation might influence each subject's performance in a different way, an intra-subject analysis is carried out.

Individually for each subject, the datasets of 9 out of 10 sessions are used as "training set," to train the decoder described in section 2.2, and the dataset of the remaining session is used as "test set." This procedure is repeated 10 times so as to use each session as test set once and only once , where a repetition is named "fold" and the whole operation is called 10-fold cross validation. Therefore, 5 out of 10 folds are characterized by a test set which belongs to the *NoPert* condition and the remaining 5 folds are characterized by a test set belonging to the *Pert* condition. In this way, the decoding performance of the test sets belonging to the *NoPert* condition is computed separately from the one of the *Pert* condition, in order to carry out a statistical comparison of the two.

Specifically, performance is evaluated by Cohen's Kappa (Cohen, 1960), also employed in the BCI Competitions (Tangermann et al., 2012):

$$k = \frac{Pr(a) - Pr(e)}{1 - Pr(e)} \tag{6}$$

where $Pr(a)$ is the proportion of observed agreements, and $Pr(e)$ is the proportion of agreements expected by chance. The range of possible values of Kappa is between -1 and 1, though it usually falls between 0 and 1. Perfect agreement between the true target labels and the predicted ones is represented by $k = 1$. Agreement no better than that expected by chance is indicated by $k = 0$. A negative kappa would indicate agreement worse than that expected by chance (Sim and Wright, 2005). An advantage of using the Kappa coefficient is the possibility to perform a Z-test to compare two classifications and determine if the accuracy level between the two is significantly different (Congalton et al., 1983, see Appendix for details).

3. RESULTS

3.1. DECODING PERFORMANCE

Table 1 represent the results obtained, respectively, by the *Unsupervised feature extraction*-based decoder and by the *Supervised feature extraction*-based one. The table contain the Kappa values for each subject, relative to the conditions *NoPert* and *Pert*, and the associated intra-subject comparison (Z-score). We observe that all the Kappa scores are above chance level ($K = 0$). Importantly, the comparisons between *NoPert* and *Pert* has always a Z-score <1.96, therefore, for every subject, the two conditions are not significantly different from a classification performance point of view.

3.2. FEATURE VISUALIZATION

In order to interpret the results, the features used in the decoding process are visualized separately for each subject. Specifically, we focus on the features of the *Unsupervised feature extraction*-based decoder, since ICA yields unmixing matrices ($\mathbf{W}$) that are similar along cross-validation folds. This means that ICA components can be clustered along folds, and for each cluster, topographies and time-frequency patterns can be averaged. Nonetheless, CSP patterns differ along cross-validation folds, given the supervised nature of CSP and the fact that the training set varies from fold to fold. Therefore, it is not possible to cluster and average the CSP features. For these reasons we decided to focus on the feature visualization of the *Unsupervised feature extraction*-method. Nonetheless, we report that, for each fold and subject, CSP filters and the associated ERD/ERS activations are compatible with the ones related to the *Unsupervised feature extraction* method.

3.2.1. Topographic maps

The spatial filters extracted after ICA and SLR spatial filter selection ($\mathbf{W}^{sel}$) are visualized in this section. In order to obtain a compact representation, they are clustered across folds, separately for each subject. Specifically, the rows of $\mathbf{W}^{sel}$ are clustered by means of hierarchical clustering, in such a way that only rows with a small Euclidean distance are grouped together. Moreover,

Table 1 | Intra-subject comparison of Kappa associated with *NoPert* and *Pert*, and the relative *Z*-score.

a. Unsupervised feature extraction				b. Supervised feature extraction			
Sbj	K(NoPert)	K(Pert)	Z-score	Sbj	K(NoPert)	K(Pert)	Z-score
S1	0.95	0.81	1.47	S1	0.97	0.85	1.23
S2	0.85	0.75	1.24	S2	0.79	0.67	1.47
S3	0.59	0.58	0.02	S3	0.58	0.48	1.16
S4	0.79	0.64	1.75	S4	0.63	0.67	0.42
S5	0.68	0.75	0.90	S5	0.76	0.76	0.02

Two conditions are significantly different ($\alpha = 0.05$) if Z-score is > 1.96. The table shows the results of the Unsupervised and Supervised feature extraction-based decoders. To note that chance level is $K = 0$.

for each cluster C we compute the selection ratio, representing how frequently a member of the cluster is selected along cross-validation folds: $r = |C| / k$, where $|C|$ represents the cardinality of C and k is the total number of cross-validation folds. In **Figure 5** the topographic maps of the average of each cluster and the respective selection ratio r are displayed separately for every subject. The figure shows that spatial filters with a selection ratio $r \geq 50\%$ represent, for every subject, either the activation of the left or right hemisphere. Moreover, it is important to note that the selected spatial filters cover areas of the EEG electrode space that are different from subject to subject.

3.2.2. *Time-frequency features*

In order to visualize the time-frequency features of the *Unsupervised feature extraction*-based decoder, the event-related spectral perturbation (ERSP, Grandchamp and Delorme, 2011) is employed:

$$ERSP(f, t) = 10log_{10}\left(\frac{ERS(f, t)}{\mu_B(f)}\right),$$

$$ERS(f, t) = \frac{1}{n}\sum_{k=1}^{n} |F_k(f, t)|^2 \qquad (7)$$

where *ERS* is the event related spectrum and is obtained by averaging across trials the time-frequency power estimate computed by wavelet (F), $\mu_B(f)$ is the mean spectral estimate at baseline, n is the total number of trials, $F_k(f, t)$ is the spectral estimate at frequency f and time point t for trial k.

The ERSP is computed separately for the test datasets of *NoPert* and *Pert*, for each subject and class (Idle, Left trapping, Right tapping). Thus, **Figure 6** is organized so that it is possible to compare the spectral perturbation associated with the two conditions (*NoPert*, *Pert*), while appreciating the features that characterize each class, individually for each subject. To note that only the ERSP of the spatial filters with a selection ratio $r = 100\%$, discussed in the previous section, are visualized. The ERSP visualization does not highlight differences in the ERD/ERS pattern between *NoPert* and *Pert* conditions. Moreover, we observe that the spectral perturbations are actually informative for the classification. In particular, the ERSP of the *Idle* class does not contain ERD/ERS, while the remaining two classes are characterized by strong spectral perturbations. Furthermore, we note subject-specific differences in the ERSP of the *Left* and *Right* classes as well. Subject 1 (S1) is characterized by a stronger beta ERS of the right hemisphere when left tapping is performed and by beta ERS of the left hemisphere in case of right tapping (contralateral activation); S2 displays a similar class-specific contralateral mu and beta ERS; for S3 we observe a stronger mu ERD of the left hemisphere when left tapping is executed (ipsilateral activation), compared to the mu ERD of the right hemisphere associated with the right tapping; for S4 we observe a stronger contralateral mu ERD and, lastly, for S5 we note a stronger contralateral beta ERS.

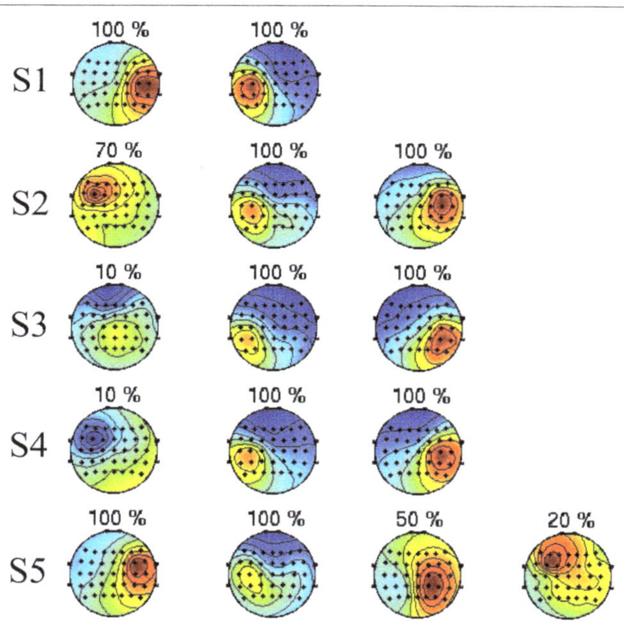

FIGURE 5 | Topographies of the automatically selected ICA components. Each row represents one subject, and each topographic map represents a cluster of ICA components obtained by hierarchical clustering along cross-validation folds. On top of each map there is the selection ratio r representing how frequently a member of the cluster is selected along folds. Spatial filters with a selection ratio $r \geq 50\%$ represent, for every subject, either the activation of the left or right hemisphere. Moreover, it is important to note that the selected spatial filters cover areas of the EEG electrode space that are different from subject to subject.

4. DISCUSSION

The aim of this study is to investigate the main effect of the leg afferent input, induced by a lower limb assistive robot, on the decoding performance of the sensorimotor hand area ERD/ERS. To do so, we devised an experiment to compare the finger tapping decoding performance under the conditions of leg perturbation (*Pert*) and no perturbation (*NoPert*). From the experimental results we find that the classification performance is always above chance ($K > 0$) and we do not observe intra-subject significant difference (Z-score <1.96, p-value >0.05) between the conditions *NoPert* and *Pert*.

To note that, in each cross-validation fold, a decoder is trained on both conditions. This is motivated by the fact that it is important to evaluate the performance on a common model. Training and testing a decoder separately for *NoPert* and *Pert* wouldn't allow for a sound comparison, since the underlying models would be different. Moreover, the datasets representing the two conditions might differ due to non-stationarities that are not related to the leg perturbations (e.g., electrode impedance variation, Wojcikiewicz et al., 2011). Training across both conditions should minimize the effect of those non-stationarities, while testing separately between *NoPert* and *Pert* should highlight the actual differences caused by leg perturbations.

In order to corroborate the interpretation of the quantitative analysis carried out so far, we visualize only the features of the *Unsupervised feature extraction*-based decoder in **Figures 5, 6**. This is motivated by the fact that spatial filters obtained by ICA are more stable along cross-validation folds. Therefore, they can be clustered and the ERSP of each cluster can be computed in a

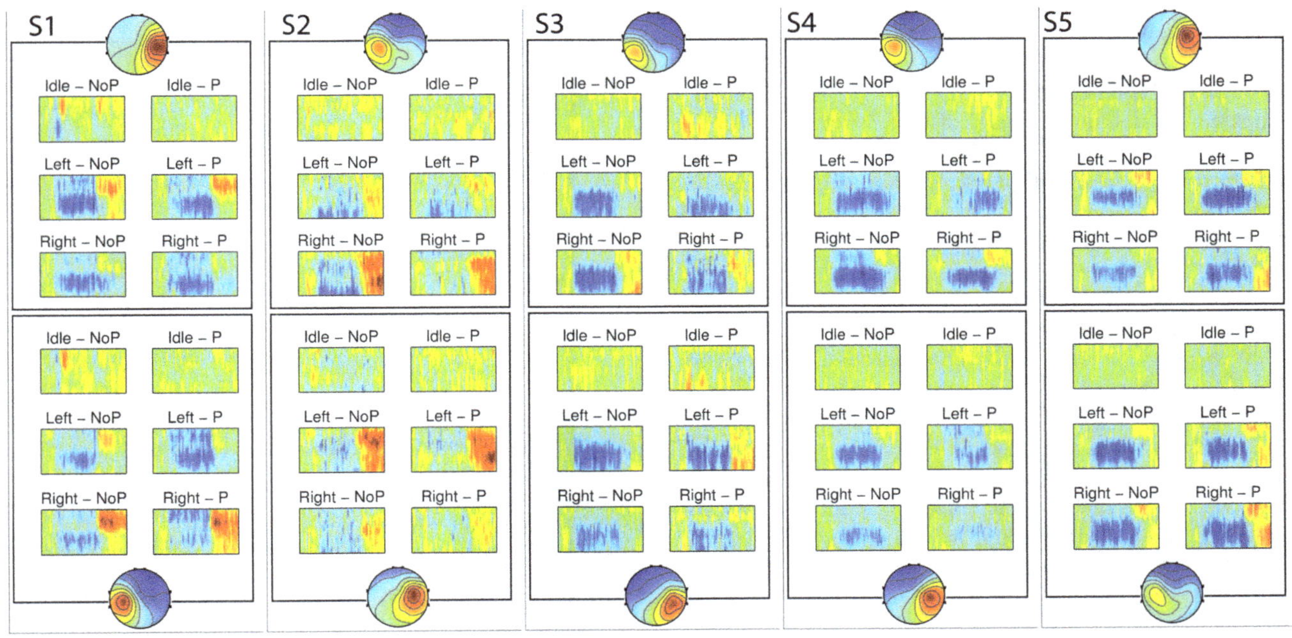

FIGURE 6 | ERSP visualization. In each ERSP image, the abscissa represents the time (−0.3 to +4.3 s), while the ordinate represents the frequency (from 8 to 30 Hz), the red color portrays power increase with respect to the baseline (dB), while the blue color power decrease (dB). For each subject, only the ERSP of the spatial filters with a selection ratio $r = 100\%$ are visualized. The figure is organized so that it is possible to compare the ERSP of *NoPert* (NoP) and *Pert* (P), while appreciating the features that characterize each class. To note that the ERD/ERS patterns are subjects-specific and informative for the classification. Moreover this representation do not highlight differences between the two conditions *NoPert* and *Pert*, confirming the quantitative results of the *Z*-test.

meaningful way. From this analysis we confirm that the spatial patterns with high selection ratio ($r \geq 50\%$) are compatible with the spatial mapping of the sensorimotor hand area ERD/ERS suggested by (Pfurtscheller and Lopes da Silva, 1999). Moreover, the fact that spatial topographies are different from subject to subject is in line with the thesis of Blankertz et al. (2008b), asserting that subject-specific spatial filters are important to enhance the decoding performance. Not only spatial patterns, but also the ERD/ERS patterns are highly subject-specific (Pfurtscheller and Neuper, 2006): compatibly with Pfurtscheller and Lopes da Silva (1999), for some subjects the discriminability between the three classes is to be inputed to strong post movement mu and/or beta ERS (S1, S2, and S5), while for other subjects we observe a predominance of mu ERD (S3 and S4). Importantly, the ERSP visualization does not highlight differences in the ERD/ERS pattern between *NoPert* and *Pert* conditions, which confirms the quantitative results of the *Z*-test.

One possible explanation to the fact that the ERD/ERS patterns associated with upper limb movements are not significantly changed by lower limb afferent input is that periodic lower limb passive movements do not produce EEG perturbation that are as significant as the ones of active movements. This is in line with other studies (Wagner et al., 2012; Jain et al., 2013) reporting a significant mu and beta desynchronization, at the primary motor cortex, associated with active periodic movements as opposed to passive periodic movements of the lower limbs. Nonetheless, in Müller-Putz et al. (2007) it is observed that for *non-periodic* passive and active movements, the beta ERD/ERS have similar levels of significance at the central sensorimotor and surrounding areas (electrodes Cz, C2, and Fcz). Therefore, it is possible that in the current study, being the leg perturbations periodic, they did not elicit ERD/ERS significant enough to interfere with the EEG perturbations associated with the upper limb task.

This paper focuses on one of the many aspects regarding the implementation of a brain-controlled assistive robot. Especially, it is important to highlight that, even though EEG topographies and ERD/ERS patterns are shared between actual movements and motor imagery (Pfurtscheller and Lopes da Silva, 1999; McFarland et al., 2000), the latter is characterized by a significantly smaller ERD/ERS magnitude (McFarland et al., 2000; Solis-Escalante et al., 2010). This raises the question, whether the EEG decoding of a motor imagery task might be affected by the leg afferent input. This issue will be investigated in future studies. Nonetheless, we need to stress the necessity of the current study, which establishes a "ground truth" understanding of the possible interference between the ERD/ERS of the sensorimotor area and the lower limb afferent input. In this context, the term "ground truth" is related to the fact that actual movements are observable by the experiment operator, or mechanically measurable, therefore we are certain that a motor command is elicited for every cue presented to the subject. On the other hand, motor imagery cannot be visually observed by the experiment operator, therefore, in case of misclassification it is impossible to say whether the subject failed to elicit motor imagery ERD/ERS or the leg perturbation actually inhibited it.

Moreover, it is important to note that finger movements are characterized by a significantly smaller EEG power perturbation as compared to hand movements (Pfurtscheller et al., 1998). This means that the finger tapping task is a good compromise in order to keep the spectral perturbation magnitude as close as possible to the one of motor imagery, while preserving the necessary property of mechanical measurability, or observability by the experiment operator.

Another issue, that must be addressed in future studies, regards the influence of a multi-DoF assistive robot on the ERD/ERS decoding. Especially, it remains an open question how the afferent input, induced by the passive movement of the whole lower limbs, affects the EEG decoding. An fMRI study by Newton et al. (2008) found a substantial overlap of the motor representations of ankle dorsiflexion, ankle plantarflexion and knee extension. This supports the notion that the afferent input induced by a multi-DoF robot should not differ significantly from the one induced by OneDOF robot. Nonetheless, further investigations are required to clarify this point.

Additionally, it is of interest whether reflex responses of the major leg muscles could influence the EEG patterns. For this purpose, in future experiments the electromyographic (EMG) signal will be recorded from the lower limbs. In this way, it would be possible to detect the onsets of possible reflex muscle activations at the leg, and further analyze the EEG signal based on this information.

Moreover, another concern regarding the application of our approach to a multi-DoF assistive robot is represented by the mechanical artifacts affecting the EEG signal. However, other researchers have shown that artifacts during walking (Gwin et al., 2010) and robotic-assisted treadmill walking (Wagner et al., 2012) can be significantly reduced by means of ICA, encouraging further studies with the multi-DoF assistive robot.

In conclusion, this study does not find a main effect of the leg afferent input, induced by a lower limb assistive robot, on the decoding performance of the sensorimotor area ERD/ERS. This establishes a solid ground for future experiments and studies aimed at controlling a multi-DoF assistive robot by motor imagery. A possible future application of such a Brain Robot Interface (BRI) system would be to modulate, by left or right motor imagery, the walking speed of an exoskeleton robot once it started moving.

ACKNOWLEDGMENTS

This research reflects the results of the "Brain Machine Interface Development" carried out under the auspeces of the Strategic Research Program for Brain Sciences by the Ministry of Education, Culture, Sports, Science, and Technology of Japan. Part of this research was supported by MIC-SCOPE and a contract with the Ministry of Internal Affairs and Communications entitled "Novel and innovative R&D making use of brain structures." This research was also partially supported by MEXT KAKENHI grant Number 23120004, JSPS KAKENHI Grant Number 24700203 and Strategic International Cooperative Program, Japan Science and Technology Agency (JST) and by JSPS and MIZS: Japan–Slovenia research Cooperative Program.

REFERENCES

Babiloni, C., Carducci, F., Cincotti, F., Rossini, P. M., Neuper, C., Pfurtscheller, G., et al. (1999). Human movement-related potentials vs desynchronization of EEG alpha rhythm: a high-resolution EEG study. *Neuroimage* 10, 658–665. doi: 10.1006/nimg.1999.0504

Babiloni, F., Cichocki, A., and Gao, S. (2007). Brain-computer interfaces: towards practical implementations and potential applications. *Comput. Intell. Neurosci.* 2007, 62637. doi: 10.1155/2007/62637

Blankertz, B., Losch, F., Krauledat, M., Dornhege, G., Curio, G., and Muller, K.-R. (2008a). The berlin brain–computer interface: accurate performance from first-session in BCI-naive subjects. *IEEE Trans. Biomed. Eng.* 55, 2452–2462. doi: 10.1109/TBME.2008.923152

Blankertz, B., Tomioka, R., Lemm, S., Kawanabe, M., and Muller, K.-R. (2008b). Optimizing spatial filters for robust EEG single-trial analysis. *IEEE Signal Process. Mag.* 25, 41–56. doi: 10.1109/MSP.2008.4408441

Cai, D., He, X., and Han, J. (2008). SRDA: an efficient algorithm for large-scale discriminant analysis. *IEEE Trans. Knowl. Data Eng.* 20, 1–12. doi: 10.1109/TKDE.2007.190669

Cassim, F., Monaca, C., Szurhaj, W., Bourriez, J. L., Defebvre, L., Derambure, P., et al. (2001). Does post-movement beta synchronization reflect an idling motor cortex? *Neuroreport* 12, 3859–3863. doi: 10.1097/00001756-200112040-00051

Cohen, J. (1960). A coefficient of agreement for nominal scales. *Educ. Psychol. Measur.* 20, 37–46. doi: 10.1177/001316446002000104

Congalton, R. G., Oderwald, R. G., and Mead, R. A. (1983). Assessing landsat classification accuracy using discrete multivariate analysis statistical techniques. *Photogramme. Eng. Remote Sens.* 49, 1671–1678.

Daly, J. J., and Wolpaw, J. R. (2008). Brain-computer interfaces in neurological rehabilitation. *Lancet Neurol.* 7, 1032–1043. doi: 10.1016/S1474-4422(08)70223-0

Daubechies, I. (1990). The wavelet transform, time-frequency localization and signal analysis. *IEEE Trans. Inform. Theor.* 36, 961–1005. doi: 10.1109/18.57199

Delorme, A., and Makeig, S. (2004). Eeglab: an open source toolbox for analysis of single-trial EEG dynamics including independent component analysis. *J. Neurosci. Methods* 134, 9–21. doi: 10.1016/j.jneumeth.2003.10.009

Dornhege, G., Blankertz, B., Curio, G., and Muller, K. (2004). Boosting bit rates in noninvasive EEG single-trial classifications by feature combination and multiclass paradigms. *IEEE Trans. Biomed. Eng.* 51, 993–1002. doi: 10.1109/TBME.2004.827088

Grandchamp, R., and Delorme, A. (2011). Single-trial normalization for event-related spectral decomposition reduces sensitivity to noisy trials. *Front. Psychol.* 2:236–236. doi: 10.3389/fpsyg.2011.00236

Guger, C., Ramoser, H., and Pfurtscheller, G. (2000). Real-time EEG analysis with subject-specific spatial patterns for a brain-computer interface (BCI). *IEEE Trans. Rehabil. Eng.* 8, 447–456. doi: 10.1109/86.895947

Gwin, J. T., Gramann, K., Makeig, S., and Ferris, D. P. (2010). Removal of movement artifact from high-density EEG recorded during walking and running. *J. Neurophysiol.* 103, 3526–3534. doi: 10.1152/jn.00105.2010

Huang, D., Qian, K., Fei, D.-Y., Jia, W., Chen, X., and Bai, O. (2012). Electroencephalography (EEG)-based brain-computer interface (BCI): a 2-d virtual wheelchair control based on event-related desynchronization/synchronization and state control. *IEEE Trans. Neural Syst. Rehabil. Eng.* 20, 379–388. doi: 10.1109/TNSRE.2012.2190299

Hyvärinen, A., and Oja, E. (2000). Independent component analysis: algorithms and applications. *Neural Netw.* 13, 411–430.

Jain, S., Gourab, K., Schindler-Ivens, S., and Schmit, B. D. (2013). EEG during pedaling: evidence for cortical control of locomotor tasks. *Clin. Neurophysiol.* 124, 379–390. doi: 10.1016/j.clinph.2012.08.021

Jolliffe, I. T. (2002). *Principal Component Analysis, 2nd Edn.* New York: Springer.

Makeig, S., Debener, S., Onton, J., and Delorme, A. (2004). Mining event-related brain dynamics. *Trends Cogn. Sci.* 8, 204–210. doi: 10.1016/j.tics.2004.03.008

McFarland, D. J., Miner, L. A., Vaughan, T. M., and Wolpaw, J. R. (2000). Mu and beta rhythm topographies during motor imagery and actual movements. *Brain Topogr.* 12, 177–186. doi: 10.1023/A:1023437823106

Müller, G. R., Neuper, C., Rupp, R., Keinrath, C., Gerner, H. J., and Pfurtscheller, G. (2003). Event-related beta EEG changes during wrist movements induced by functional electrical stimulation of forearm muscles in man. *Neurosci. Lett.* 340, 143–147. doi: 10.1016/S0304-3940(03)00019-3

Müller-Putz, G. R., Scherer, R., Pfurtscheller, G., Neuper, C., and Rupp, R. (2009). Non-invasive control of neuroprostheses for the upper extremity: temporal coding of brain patterns. *Conf. Proc. IEEE Eng. Med. Biol. Soc.* 2009, 3353–3356. doi: 10.1109/IEMBS.2009.5333185

Müller-Putz, G. R., Scherer, R., Pfurtscheller, G., and Rupp, R. (2005). EEG-based neuroprosthesis control: a step towards clinical practice. *Neurosci. Lett.* 382, 169–174. doi: 10.1016/j.neulet.2005.03.021

Müller-Putz, G. R., Scherer, R., Pfurtscheller, G., and Rupp, R. (2006). Brain-computer interfaces for control of neuroprostheses: from synchronous to asynchronous mode of operation. *Biomed. Tech. (Berl)* 51, 57–63. doi: 10.1515/BMT.2006.011

Müller-Putz, G. R., Zimmermann, D., Graimann, B., Nestinger, K., Korisek, G., and Pfurtscheller, G. (2007). Event-related beta EEG-changes during passive and attempted foot movements in paraplegic patients. *Brain Res.* 1137, 84–91. doi: 10.1016/j.brainres.2006.12.052

Mussa-Ivaldi, S. (2000). Neural engineering: real brains for real robots. *Nature* 408, 305–306. doi: 10.1038/35042668

Newton, J. M., Dong, Y., Hidler, J., Plummer-D'Amato, P., Marehbian, J., Albistegui-Dubois, R. M., et al. (2008). Reliable assessment of lower limb motor representations with fMRI: use of a novel MR compatible device for real-time monitoring of ankle, knee and hip torques. *Neuroimage* 43, 136–146. doi: 10.1016/j.neuroimage.2008.07.001

Noda, T., Sugimoto, N., Furukawa, J., Sato, M., Hyon, S., and Morimoto, J. (2012). "Brain-controlled exoskeleton robot for BMI rehabilitation," in *Proceedings of IEEE-RAS International Conference on Humanoid Robots* (Osaka). doi: 10.1109/HUMANOIDS.2012.6651494

Pfurtscheller, G., Guger, C., Müller, G., Krausz, G., and Neuper, C. (2000a). Brain oscillations control hand orthosis in a tetraplegic. *Neurosci. Lett.* 292, 211–214. doi: 10.1016/S0304-3940(00)01471-3

Pfurtscheller, G., and Lopes da Silva, F. H. (1999). Event-related EEG/MEG synchronization and desynchronization: basic principles. *Clin. Neurophysiol.* 110, 1842–1857. doi: 10.1016/S1388-2457(99)00141-8

Pfurtscheller, G., and Neuper, C. (1997). Motor imagery activates primary sensorimotor area in humans. *Neurosci. Lett.* 239, 65–68. doi: 10.1016/S0304-3940(97)00889-6

Pfurtscheller, G., and Neuper, C. (2006). Future prospects of ERD/ERS in the context of brain-computer interface (BCI) developments. *Prog. Brain Res.* 159, 433–437. doi: 10.1016/S0079-6123(06)59028-4

Pfurtscheller, G., Neuper, C., Guger, C., Harkam, W., Ramoser, H., Schlogl, A., et al. (2000b). Current trends in Graz brain-computer interface (BCI) research. *IEEE Trans. Rehabil. Eng.* 8, 216–219. doi: 10.1109/86.847821

Pfurtscheller, G., and Solis-Escalante, T. (2008). Could the beta rebound in the EEG be suitable to realize a brain switch? *Clin. Neurophysiol.* 120, 24–29. doi: 10.1016/j.clinph.2008.09.027

Pfurtscheller, G., Zalaudek, K., and Neuper, C. (1998). Event-related beta synchronization after wrist, finger and thumb movement. *Electroencephalogr. Clin. Neurophysiol.* 109, 154–160. doi: 10.1016/S0924-980X(97)00070-2

Ramoser, H., M§ller-Gerking, J., and Pfurtscheller, G. (1998). Optimal spatial filtering of single trial EEG during imagined hand movement. *IEEE Trans. Rehabil. Eng* 8, 441–446. doi: 10.1109/86.895946

Sim, J., and Wright, C. C. (2005). The kappa statistic in reliability studies: use, interpretation, and sample size requirements. *Phys. Ther.* 85, 257–268.

Solis-Escalante, T., Müller-Putz, G., Brunner, C., Kaiser, V., and Pfurtscheller, G. (2010). Analysis of sensorimotor rhythms for the implementation of a brain switch for healthy subjects. *Biomed. Signal Process. Control* 5, 15–20. doi: 10.1016/j.bspc.2009.09.002

Tangermann, M., Müller, K.-R., Aertsen, A., Birbaumer, N., Braun, C., Brunner, C., et al. (2012). Review of the BCI competition IV. *Front. Neurosci.* 6:55. doi: 10.3389/fnins.2012.00055

Tsui, C. S. L., Gan, J. Q., and Hu, H. (2011). A self-paced motor imagery based brain-computer interface for robotic wheelchair control. *Clin. EEG Neurosci.* 42, 225–229. doi: 10.1177/155005941104200407

Wagner, J., Solis-Escalante, T., Grieshofer, P., Neuper, C., Müller-Putz, G., and Scherer, R. (2012). Level of participation in robotic-assisted treadmill walking modulates midline sensorimotor EEG rhythms in able-bodied subjects. *Neuroimage* 63, 1203–1211. doi: 10.1016/j.neuroimage.2012.08.019

Wang, X., and Paliwal, K. K. (2003). Feature extraction and dimensionality reduction algorithms and their applications in vowel recognition. *Pattern Recogn.* 36, 2429–2439. doi: 10.1016/S0031-3203(03)00044-X

Wang, Y., Hong, B., Gao, X., and Gao, S. (2007). "Implementation of a brain-computer interface based on three states of motor imagery," in *Engineering in Medicine and Biology Society, 2007. EMBS 2007. 29th Annual International Conference of the IEEE* (IEEE), 5059–5062.

Wojcikiewicz, W., Vidaurre, C., and Kawanabe, M. (2011). "Stationary common spatial patterns: towards robust classification of non-stationary EEG signals," in *IEEE International Conference on Acoustics, Speech and Signal Processing (ICASSP), 2011* (Prague), 577–580. doi: 10.1109/ICASSP.2011.5946469

Wolpaw, J. R., Birbaumer, N., McFarland, D. J., Pfurtscheller, G., and Vaughan, T. M. (2002). Brain-computer interfaces for communication and control. *Clin. Neurophysiol.* 113, 767–791. doi: 10.1016/S1388-2457(02)00057-3

Wolpaw, J. R., McFarland, D. J., Vaughan, T. M., and Schalk, G. (2003). The wadsworth center brain-computer interface (BCI) research and development program. *IEEE Trans. Neural Syst. Rehabil. Eng.* 11, 204–207. doi: 10.1109/TNSRE.2003.814442

Yamashita, O., Sato, M. A., Yoshioka, T., Tong, F., and Kamitani, Y. (2008). Sparse estimation automatically selects voxels relevant for the decoding of fMRI activity patterns. *Neuroimage* 42, 1414–1429. doi: 10.1016/j.neuroimage.2008.05.050

Zhao, Q. B., Zhang, L. Q., and Cichocki, A. (2009). EEG-based asynchronous BCI control of a car in 3D virtual reality environments. *Chin. Sci. Bull.* 54, 78–87. doi: 10.1007/s11434-008-0547-3

A. APPENDIX

A.1 *Z*-TEST

Being k_N and k_P the Kappa scores, respectively, of the *NoPert* and *Pert* conditions, the Z-score of their difference can be computed as:

$$z_{NP} = \frac{|k_N - k_P|}{\sqrt{var(k_N) + var(k_P)}} \tag{A1}$$

where $var(k)$, the variance of k, can be computed according to the original formula in Congalton et al. (1983). Thus, two Kappa values are considered significantly different, with a significance level of p-value <0.05 if their Z-score is bigger than 1.96.

22

Donor/recipient enhancement of memory in rat hippocampus

Sam A. Deadwyler[1]*, Theodore W. Berger[2], Andrew J. Sweatt[1], Dong Song[2], Rosa H. M. Chan[2], Ioan Opris[1], Greg A. Gerhardt[3], Vasilis Z. Marmarelis[2] and Robert E. Hampson[1]

[1] *Department of Physiology and Pharmacology, Wake Forest School of Medicine, Winston-Salem, NC, USA*
[2] *Department of Biomedical Engineering, University of Southern California, Los Angeles, CA, USA*
[3] *Department of Neurobiology, Chandler Medical School, University of Kentucky, Lexington, KY, USA*

Edited by:
Mikhail Lebedev, Duke University, USA

Reviewed by:
Antonio Pereira, Federal University of Rio Grande do Norte, Brazil
Nelson A. M. Lemos, Edmond and Lily Safra International Institute of Neuroscience of Natal, Brazil
Mark O. West, Rutgers University, USA

****Correspondence:***
Sam A. Deadwyler, Department of Physiology and Pharmacology, Wake Forest University Health Sciences, Medical Center Blvd., Winston-Salem, NC 27157, USA
e-mail: sdeadwyl@wakehealth.edu

The critical role of the mammalian hippocampus in the formation, translation and retrieval of memory has been documented over many decades. There are many theories of how the hippocampus operates to encode events and a precise mechanism was recently identified in rats performing a short-term memory task which demonstrated that successful information encoding was promoted via specific patterns of activity generated within ensembles of hippocampal neurons. In the study presented here, these "representations" were extracted via a customized non-linear multi-input multi-output (MIMO) mathematical model which allowed prediction of successful performance on specific trials within the testing session. A unique feature of this characterization was demonstrated when successful information encoding patterns were derived online from well-trained "*donor*" animals during difficult long-delay trials and delivered via online electrical stimulation to synchronously tested naïve "*recipient*" animals never before exposed to the delay feature of the task. By transferring such model-derived trained (*donor*) animal hippocampal firing patterns via stimulation to coupled naïve *recipient* animals, their task performance was facilitated in a direct "*donor-recipient*" manner. This provides the basis for utilizing extracted appropriate neural information from one brain to induce, recover, or enhance memory related processing in the brain of another subject.

Keywords: memory-transfer, rodent, ensemble, non-linear model, electrical stimulation

INTRODUCTION

To understand the neural basis of memory, several features of the context in which the memories occur and are utilized, and the functional aspects of the brain areas involved, need to be identified and controlled (Hampson et al., 2008; Eichenbaum and Fortin, 2009). In prior studies we achieved both of these important contingencies as well as (1) overcoming possible alternative interpretations of the relationship between recorded hippocampal ensemble activity and the behavioral task in which short-term memory formation is necessary (Deadwyler and Hampson, 2006; Deadwyler et al., 2007), and (2) developing an effective mathematical/operational model for online prediction of CA1 hippocampal cell activity from simultaneously recorded input firing patterns from synaptically connected CA3 neurons (Song et al., 2009; Berger et al., 2011; Hampson et al., 2011). The combination of these approaches was made possible by the chronic recording of neural firing patterns in the above two major hippocampal subfields via specially designed mutineuron recording arrays that allowed simultaneous detection and analysis of behaviorally critical ensemble discharge patterns (Deadwyler and Hampson, 1997; Hampson et al., 1999, 2008). It has been shown that a non-linear multi-input/multi-output (MIMO) mathematical model provides the mean to translate the above ensemble activity into a format that allows predictions of CA1 firing patterns from CA3 activity required for successful task performance (Marmarelis, 2004; Zanos et al., 2008; Song et al., 2009).

In the following paper we demonstrate a critically important feature of the online extracted firing patterns of hippocampal ensembles by showing how alteration and facilitation of hippocampal function can be employed via direct connection with the same structure in a different "*donor*" animal performing the same task at the same time. A recent study (Pais-Viera et al., 2013) reported similar brain-to-brain transfer by directly stimulating motor cortex in the brain of a recipient rodent from a different animal. However, we report here the discovery that appropriate neural firing patterns which encode useable *memory* can be derived online from trained animals, and inserted via electrical stimulation of those same hippocampal regions to animals untrained to perform the memory extended requirement of the delayed-non-match-to-sample (DNMS) task. These findings confirm the functional significance of a previously identified "hippocampal prosthesis" (Berger et al., 2011) shown to repair and/or enhance damaged or disrupted memory processes in the same animal. However, the outcomes of the study described here also indicate ways of using brain systems from non-impaired subjects to impart functional information when and where it did not get formulated in affected subjects, via a *donor-recipient* paradigm.

METHODS

INFORMATION ENCODING BY HIPPOCAMPAL NEURAL ENSEMBLES DURING PERFORMANCE OF A DELAYED-NON-MATCH-TO-SAMPLE (DNMS) MEMORY TASK

Recording and analysis of hippocampal mutineuron activity over a number of years in rodents performing a DNMS memory task (cf. Hampson et al., 2008, 2011) provided the basis for application of a non-linear MIMO model to hippocampal neural ensemble firing patterns in the first demonstration of a memory prostheses in rodent brain (Berger et al., 2011; Hampson et al., 2012a,b). This extensively studied DNMS task requires rats to retain the position of a "Sample" lever that is presented and responded to (i.e., sample response: SR) at the start of the trial, over a temporal delay interval of variable duration (1–30 s) in order to make a "Non-match" response (NR) on the lever in the opposite position when both levers are presented simultaneously at the end of the delay (**Figure 1A**). During the delay period a nosepoke into a photocell on the wall opposite the levers is required to proceed to the Non-match phase. If there is no delay a single nosepoke produces both levers, for delays of increased duration a single nose poke is still the only requirement but animals make multiple nosepokes until the light terminates above the photocell as an indicator of delay termination and both levers are presented on the opposite wall (**Figure 1A**). **Figure 1D** (control) shows that DNMS performance accuracy decreases linearly as a direct function of the duration of the interposed delay interval.

NON-LINEAR MULTI-INPUT MULTI-OUTPUT (MIMO) MODEL DETECTION AND PREDICTION OF HIPPOCAMPAL ENSEMBLE MEMORY CODES

Electrophysiological recording during the DNMS task employs custom designed arrays of microwire (20 μm) electrodes implanted bilaterally in the hippocampus in each hemisphere to provide single neuron firing data from 8 pairs of aligned CA3-CA1 probes arranged at 200 μm intervals along the longitudinal axis in the dorsal hippocampus in rodent brain (**Figure 1B**). The neural correlates obtained from studies with these techniques in the DNMS task have been utilized in more than 2000 animals with respect to type and amount of behavioral training required for maximal performance in conjunction with extraction of distinct patterns of neural ensemble activity correlated with successful performance (Deadwyler and Hampson, 2006; Hampson et al., 2008, 2011). In recent studies the trial-by-trial nature of changes in ensemble firing patterns has been described in relation to non-linear fluctuations associated with successful task performance (**Figure 1C**), as well as applying the same non-linear model for reversing detrimental actions of drugs on performance (Song et al., 2009; Berger et al., 2011; Marmarelis et al., 2013).

This very precise MIMO non-linear mathematical model (**Figure 1C**) was employed to determine the "strength" of ensemble SR firing patterns or "codes" formulated specifically on successful (strong code) or error (weak code) DNMS trials (**Figures 1C,D**) across all delay durations. The application of this model (see *Supporting Material*) allowed prediction of CA1 neuron firing "output" patterns based on the "input" to the model (CA3 neuron firing) using Laguerre expansions of Volterra Kernels to determine the temporal relationships between spike occurrences recorded in these two areas during the task (Song et al., 2009, 2013; Berger et al., 2012). As shown previously the inputs to the MIMO model were CA3 cell discharges associated exclusively with outputs from simultaneously recorded postsynaptic CA1 cells connected via Schaeffer collateral monosynaptic connections (Witter and Amaral, 2004). Hence, as shown at the lower right in **Figure 1C**, the MIMO model analysis of CA3 and CA1 spike occurrences associated with critical DNMS task events provided the basis for online "detection" (CA3) and "prediction" of CA1 firing patterns associated with successful (strong code) vs. error (weak code) trials (Berger et al., 2011; Hampson et al., 2011). As a final verification that the MIMO model output could predict behaviorally relevant hippocampal encoded information, online calculations were utilized in a closed loop paradigm in which the detection of strong SR codes (**Figure 1C**) was used to adjust the difficulty of the same trial via increased or decreased delay duration. In accordance with the strength of SR codes (**Figure 1D**) performance was either above or below that on trials in which such SR codes were not present (Hampson et al., 2012a,b). This closed loop procedure served as the basis for the next phase in which strong SR code patterns were detected, mimicked and then administered as electrical stimulation, which is described next.

EXTERNAL INSERTION OF MIMO DERIVED FIRING PATTERNS VIA ELECTRICAL STIMULATION OF HIPPOCAMPAL CA1 NEURONS

The above successful application of the MIMO model provided the unique basis for activating CA1 cells if model derived inputs from CA3 neurons were no longer operative (Berger et al., 2011). This was accomplished by transforming the CA1 cell output pattern of the MIMO model into trains of electrical stimulation pulses (1.0 ms biphasic 20–100 μA) and delivering them in real time to the same CA1 electrode locations in the recording arrays via a multichannel stimulator (**Figure 2A**). CA1 stimulation patterns were therefore similar to the strong code SR firing patterns derived from each animal by the MIMO model from the same CA1 electrodes. Stimulation was delivered online via the inputs detected from CA3 electrodes on the same hippocampal array as shown in **Figure 2A** for hippocampal implants in both hemispheres. Intensities of stimulus pulses (20–100 μA) delivered to CA1 were adjusted to provide indications of extracellular current flow (i.e., local field potentials) at adjacent CA1 electrode locations on the same array (see below). MIMO generated strong code CA1 SR stimulation pulse trains were of 3.0 s duration and delivered within 50 ms of the detection of corresponding input patterns recorded in CA3 (see *Supporting Material*). Since both the pattern and time of application of the strong code CA1 SR stimulation were related directly to the MIMO model detection of corresponding CA3 input firing, it was also possible to deliver CA1 SR stimulation on trials in which "strong code" input patterns were not detected in CA3 recordings. This provided the means to facilitate performance above control levels by delivering strong code CA1 SR stimulation on trials that normally did not generate strong codes in CA3 or CA1 naturally (Berger et al., 2011; Hampson et al., 2012a,b).

The effectiveness of SR CA1 stimulation patterns is shown in **Figures 2B,C** as marked increases in DNMS task performance

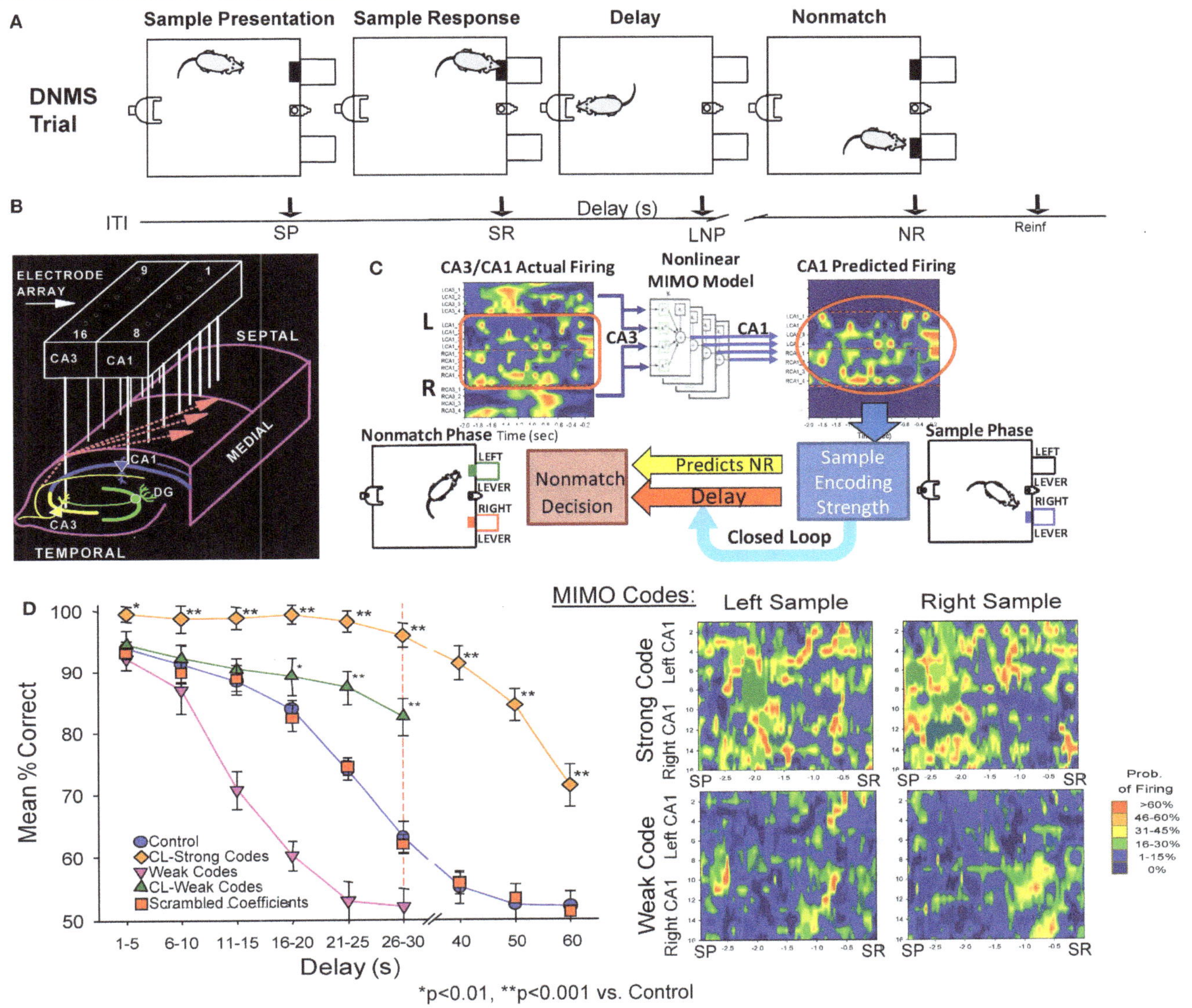

FIGURE 1 | Delayed non-match to sample (DNMS) task, MIMO model and associated hippocampal ensemble activity. (A) *DNMS Trial Diagram.* Sample lever presentation (SP) and Sample response (SR) are followed by a variable delay interval which required a nosepoke (NP) in a photocell on opposite wall. The Non-match phase began after delay timeout, with both levers presented simultaneously for reward contingent Non-match Response (NR) on the lever opposite the SR position. Correct non-match responses produced 0.2 ml of water delivered to the trough between the levers. Timeline below shows sequence of task phases: ITI–intertrial interval; SP–Sample Lever presentation; SR–Sample response; Delay–Delay interval; LNP–last required nosepoke during Delay; NR–Non-match (decision) response; Reinf.—Delivery of water reward. **(B)** Hippocampal recording array: two rows of 8 stainless steel 20 μm wires positioned longitudinally within hippocampus at 200 μm intervals for each electrode pair in CA3 and CA1 cell layers. Arrays were implanted bilaterally in both hippocampi providing a total of 32 indwelling chronic electrodes per animal. **(C)** Heatmap display (left) showing online array monitored hippocampal ensemble single neuron (actual firing) activity. Low-to-high (blue-to-red) firing rates are indicated at the separate CA3/CA1 locations on the array **(B)** during the occurrence of the SR (time 0.0 s). Schematic of non-linear MIMO model: Spike trains X_1–X_8 recorded from CA3 electrodes (CA3 input) on the hippocampal array (left) are input to the model and used to predict CA1 firing across the other 8 recording locations shown in the diagram on the right (1–8, predicted CA1) at the time of the SR. The schematic of the non-linear analysis used to construct the CA1 predicted outputs which illustrates estimation of the spatiotemporal relationship between each CA1 output (Y) and multiple CA3 inputs (X) modeled via Volterra kernels which are then combined to form the MIMO model for all CA1 locations (see Supplemental Material). The output of the model (right) is then employed to vary the delay interval of the DNMS task on the same trial in a closed loop manner as shown by the diagram below. Lower Right: MIMO Codes: Heatmap displays of MIMO model predicted CA1 firing in both hemispheres during the response on the Sample lever on individual trials during sample presentation (SP and response (SR) for trials both Left and Right sample lever presentation. Strong Codes: MIMO predicted CA1 sample lever firing on *successful trials.* Weak Codes: MIMO prediction of the same CA1 cell firing on *error trials.* Firing rates indicated by the scale bar at right. **(D)** MIMO mediated closed loop control of DNMS performance (mean ± s.e.m. % correct) summed over all animals, $n = 15$). Trials in which *strong (diamonds) and weak (triangles) SR codes* occurred are plotted as a function of length of delay, shown compared to Control performance on trials not sorted by code strength. Performance on trials with extended delays (40, 50, or 60 s, vertical dashed line) was significantly higher than on trials with the same delays (Control, 40–60 s) presented without

(Continued)

FIGURE 1 | Continued
MIMO Closed Loop regulation [$F_{(1,\ 401)} = 18.39$, $p < 0.001$, $^{*}p < 0.01$, $^{**}p < 0.001$, Closed Loop vs. Control trials]. DNMS (performance) for trials of 1–30 s delay (Control) is also shown compared to performance on trials in which only *weak SR codes* (Weak Codes) occurred [$F_{(1,\ 401)} = 11.81$, $p < 0.001$]. Performance on trials in which the MIMO model coefficients were randomly assigned (i.e., scrambled) to CA1 firing are also shown in the curve for scrambled coefficients (squares) as having no difference from Control performance.

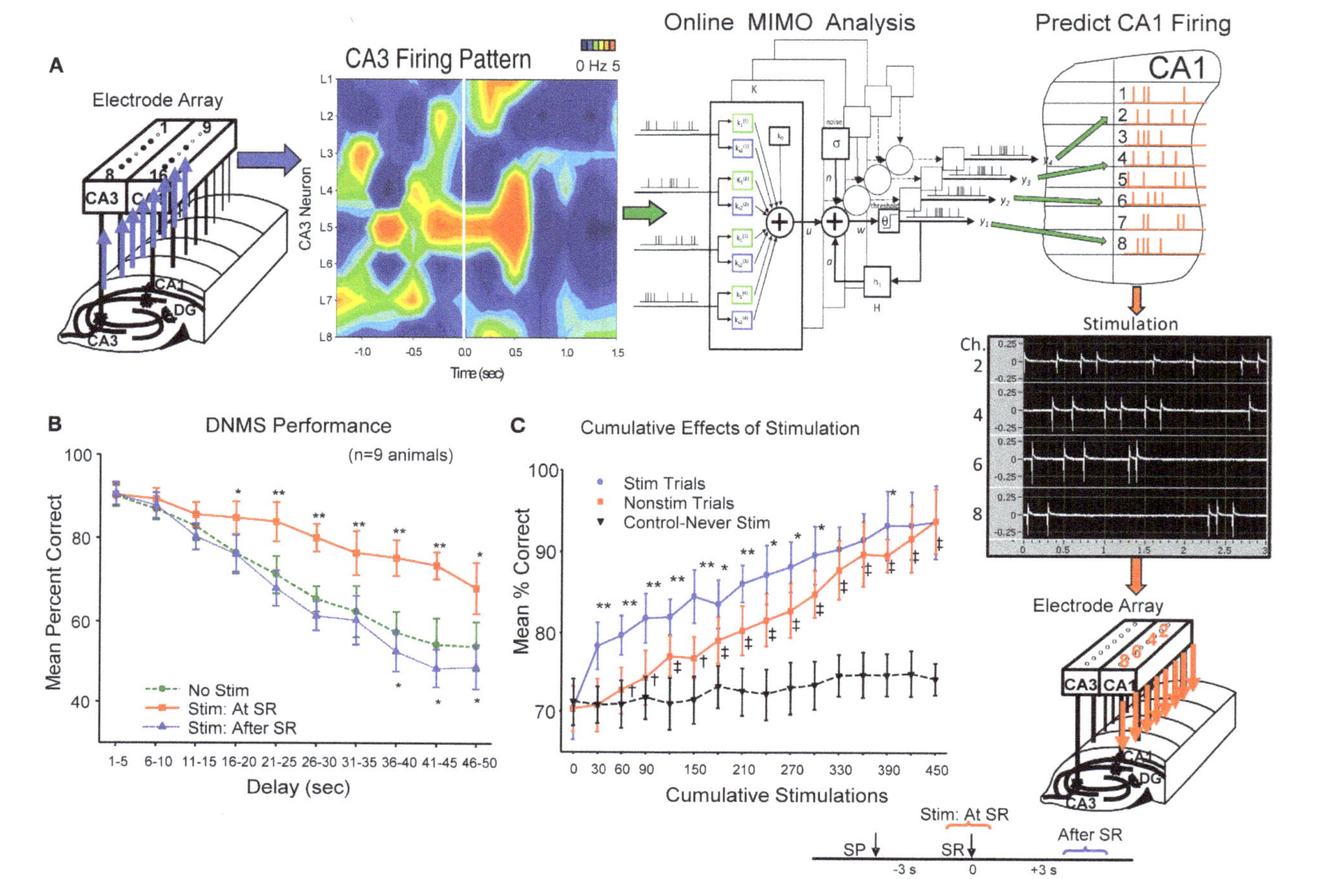

FIGURE 2 | Electrical stimulation utilizing MIMO predicted CA1 output patterns, facilitates DNMS performance. (A) Patterns of recorded CA3 cell firing in hippocampal array, shown as a heatmap (left), constitutes the input for online implementation of the MIMO model (center) to predict CA1 firing pattern (**Figure 1C**) indicated by red "tick" marks in hippocampal (CA1) layout (at right). This MIMO output pattern is fed to a programmable 8 channel stimulator (Supplemental Material) which delivers up to 3.0 s trains of bipolar electrical stimulation pulses (middle right) to the CA1 electrode locations showing the same firing pattern in each hemisphere. Stimulator output (photo display) is shown for 4 of the 8 channels to indicate different frequencies and intensities of stimulus trains delivered to separate CA1 locations (Supplemental Material). The time lag between CA3 recording, MIMO calculation and output of CA1 stimulation was approximately 50 ms. **(B)** DNMS performance graph of trained animals ($n = 9$) for delays of 1–60 s compares effects of 3.0 s stimulation delivered either: (1) at the time the SR occurred (Stim at SR) vs. No Stim [$F_{(1,\ 731)} = 11.50$, $p < 0.001$], or (2) delayed for 3.0 s after the SR was made (Stim after SR) vs. No Stim [$F_{(1,\ 731)} = 3.17$, n.s.] (see inset lower right). Asterisks ($^{*}p < 0.01$, $^{**}p < 0.001$) indicate significant difference in DNMS performance compared to control (No Stim.) trials (Berger et al., 2011). **(C)** Cumulative effects of MIMO generated SR stimulation over successive trials (Hampson et al., 2012a) shows progressive increase in overall mean (± s.e.m.) % correct performance in 30 trial blocks for animals ($n = 5$) receiving 25–30 SR stimulation trials (Stim Trials) per session for 15 sessions. Red curve (squares) shows overall performance on remaining trials within the same behavioral sessions in which no stimulation was delivered (No Stim). Inverted triangles (dotted line) shows performance over the same number of successive trials of equivalently trained animals ($n = 20$) that never received SR stimulation (Never Stim). Stim vs. Non-stim trials: $F_{(1,\ 145)} = 9.42$, $^{*}p < 0.01$, $^{**}p < 0.001$, Stim. vs. Never Stim: $F_{(1,\ 1349)} = 15.72$, $p < 0.001$, Non-stim vs. Never Stim. $F_{(1,\ 1349)} = 11.29$, $^{\dagger}p < 0.01$, $^{\ddagger}p < 0.001$.

on stimulation trials in comparison to trials in which no stimulation was delivered (No Stim). To control for other possible actions, the specificity of the CA1 stimulation pattern with respect to encoding of the SR was tested directly by delaying delivery of the same stimulation pattern to CA1 until 3.0 s after the SR which as shown in **Figure 2B** (Stim after SR) produced no changes in performance from control (No Stim) levels. Further verification was revealed by comparing trials in which SR CA1 stimulation was generated from different MIMO firing patterns with "scrambled" coefficients between neurons (**Figure 1D**) which actually impaired performance in some cases as shown in other studies (Hampson et al., 2012a). A final test of the similarity of the stimulation patterns to actual CA1 output firing patterns was assessed by repeating the procedure over several sessions and examining the trial-by-trial cumulative effects of continued exposure to MIMO predicted SR CA1 stimulation as shown in **Figure 2C** (Berger et al., 2011; Hampson et al., 2012b). These procedures verify that functional encoding of the SR could be imposed in subjects performing the DNMS task by matching the MIMO predicted CA1 firing pattern with stimulation pulses delivered within 50 ms to the same CA1 loci (**Figure 2A**), which provided encoding of lever position necessary to perform the task successfully across all interposed delay intervals.

A METHOD FOR TRANSFER OF MIMO SR STIMULATION FROM *DONOR* TO DELAY-NAÏVE *RECIPIENT* ANIMALS

The above MIMO model SR CA1 stimulation method served as the basis for testing a unique dual animal "*donor/recipient*" paradigm in which (1) a well-trained "*donor rat*" performed the DNMS task in one chamber at the same time as (2) a delay-naïve "*recipient rat*" was tested at the same time in a different chamber in a trial synchronized manner (**Figure 3A**). The "*recipient rat*" was not trained to perform the DNMS task over intervening delay intervals >1.0–3.0 s (red dotted delay phase in **Figure 3B**) which was the time it took to make the required nosepoke response on the opposite wall of the chamber to present the Non-match phase (**Figure 1A**). The imposition of trials with extended delay intervals during the session constituted the first exposure of *recipient rats* to the task requirement for retention of SR information across increased time intervals (8–16 s) in order to correctly select the opposite lever in the Non-match phase (Hampson et al., 2008). Performance in the Sample phase of the task was synchronized between animals by presentation of the Sample lever in the same position at the same time in both chambers to initiate the same trial simultaneously for both animals (**Figure 3B**). On synchronous trials in which the MIMO model applied to the *donor rat* CA3 firing patterns, generated a successful strong code SR CA1 pattern (**Figure 2A**), the stimulus pulses representing that MIMO strong SR code were routed instead to the corresponding CA1 electrodes in the *recipient rat* (**Figure 3A**) performing the SR at approximately the same time. For the naïve *recipient rat* following the delivery of the *donor rat* strong code SR CA1 stimulation pattern after the SR, an unfamiliar delay interval of 8, 12, or 16 s was introduced into the trial prior to onset of the Non-match phase. Since routing of SR CA1 stimulation to the *recipient rat* was determined by concurrent CA3 encoding strength in the hippocampus of the simultaneously performing *donor rat*, extended delay trials for the *recipient rat* occurred randomly within the paired sessions. As a control procedure, performance was compared on trials with the same delays administered to *recipient rats* by *donor rat* CA3 encoding strength on the same trial but without delivery of SR CA1 stimulation.

RESULTS

TRANSFER OF MEMORY TO DELAY-NAÏVE *RECIPIENT* ANIMALS BY DELIVERY OF MIMO STIMULATION FROM TRAINED *DONOR* ANIMALS

The employment of *donor rat* MIMO model generated SR CA1 stimulation was applied to test whether it was possible to facilitate performance in *delay-naïve recipient rats* untrained in the delay version of the DNMS task. Results in **Figure 4A** show the mean % correct performance of 5 different *recipient rats* subjected for the first time to 8, 12, and 16 s interpolated delays with MIMO derived SR CA1 stimulation patterns (Stim) delivered on half the trials from synchronously performing *donor rats*. *Donor rat* SR CA1 stimulation allowed *recipient rats* to perform significantly better than if they did not receive stimulation (No stim) and these levels are compared with their higher performance on trials in which no delay was interspersed (0.0 s). The overall performance of all *recipient* is shown in **Figure 4B** for recipient-stim and recipient-no stim trials in which highly significant improved performance is apparent across all delays. **Figure 4B** also shows that recipient-stim average performance was significantly below that of fully trained animals that did not receive SR stimulation at those same delays (trained subjects, $n = 23$).

The physiologically specific nature of the *donor rat* stimulation was further verified by the fact that performance was facilitated in a delay dependent manner (**Figures 4A,B**) in the same way that natural performance was affected by the duration of interposed delays during the trial. This was further verified by comparing the effects of MIMO stimulation patterns delivered by different *donor rats* to the same *recipient rat* within, as well as, across different behavioral sessions. **Figure 5A** shows the comparison of performance of the same *recipient rat* receiving SR stimulation from two different *donor rats* over similar interposed delay trials. **Figure 5A** shows the patterns of SR CA1 stimulation delivered by each *donor rat (donor rats 1 and 2)* on both left and right SR lever trials. Although there were slight differences with respect to the spatiotemporal delivery of CA1 stimulation pulses, the overall patterns related to the time of execution of the SR were highly similar. The graphs to the right in **Figure 5A** show the average performance of the same *recipient rat* on similar types of trials with stimulation and non-stimulated extended delays from the same two *donor rats*. It is clear that stimulation generated by both *donor* rats on different trials in the same session facilitated performance of the *recipient rat* in nearly identical fashion. **Figure 5B** summarizes the performance of all *recipient rats* ($n = 5$) over the 3 delay intervals for all *donor rat* ($n = 6$) stimulation (Stim) vs. non-stimulated (Non-Stim) trials compared to trials in which no delay was imposed (0 s).

Control manipulations performed to insure that *donor rat* SR stimulation was the basis for the improved performance of *recipient rats* included: (1) changing the *donor rat* stimulation patterns in different ways such as scrambling coefficients (**Figure 1A**), (2) delivering *donor rat* stimulation patterns at different times (i.e., 3.0 s) after the SR (**Figure 2B**), and (3) delivery of stimulation based on *recipient rat* MIMO-extracted SR CA1 patterns on the trials with interpolated delays determined by *donor rat* encoding patterns (not shown). None of the latter control procedures produced significant increases in *recipient rat* performance above that exhibited on trials with the same delays and no *donor rat* stimulation (**Figure 4** No Stim, **Figure 5B**).

NEURAL BASIS FOR MIMO STIMULATION ENHANCED MEMORY

A major factor that relates to the above demonstration of enhanced memory in the *donor* as well as *delay-naïve recipient rats*, is the actual neural basis for the enhancement invoked

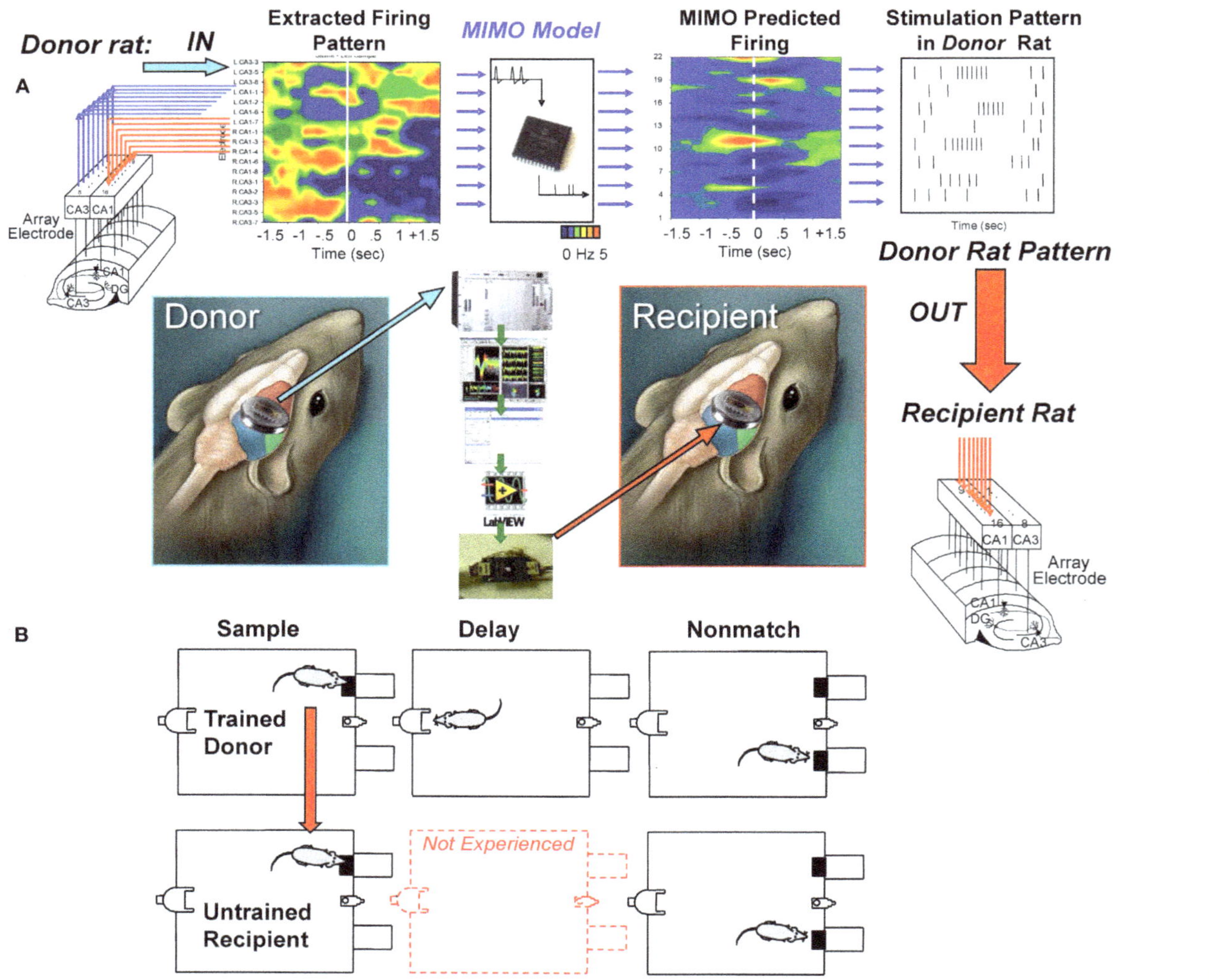

FIGURE 3 | Transference of successful MIMO coded ensemble firing patterns from trained *"donor"* rats to task-naïve *"recipient"* rats. **(A)** Recordings were obtained online from well-trained animals (i.e., *donor rats*) with validated effective MIMO SR CA1 stimulation patterns as shown in **Figure 2**. A second group of delay-naïve animals (*recipient rats*) were only trained to perform the operant responses in the DNMS task in sequence without exposure to variable and extended delay intervals interposed between the SR and NR task phases requiring completion of the nosepoke response on the opposite wall (red middle diagram). **(B)** *Donor-Recipient rat* "pairs" were recorded from and tested simultaneously in different chambers with DNMS trial execution synchronized by presentation of the sample lever in the same position at the same time. During performance of trials within the simultaneous sessions, *donor rat* hippocampal ensemble activity was monitored for presence of CA3 firing predictions of effective *strong SR code* CA1 stimulation patterns (**Figure 2**). When such *donor rat* strong code patterns occurred, the associated MIMO-predicted SR CA1 stimulation pattern was routed instead to the CA1 electrodes in the *recipient rat* hippocampus while performing the *SR* within 1–3 s after detection of *donor rat* strong SR code. Delay intervals of 8, 12, or 16s were then introduced on the same trial for the *recipient rat* which required the previously learned selection of the opposite lever in the Non-match phase of the task after timeout of the unfamiliar delay periods. All trials on which delays were imposed to *recipient rats* were determined when strong SR codes were generated by *donor rats*; hence occurrence of all delay trials during *recipient rat* sessions was essentially random and unpredictable.

by delivery of MIMO SR CA1 stimulation and also the type of changes that occur under normal conditions related to improved vs. impaired performance in the same subjects. The influence of administered MIMO CA1 stimulation on synaptic connectivity during the session was assessed using local field potentials (LFPs) recorded from each of the 8 CA1 locations generated by stimulating a single electrode location in CA3 on the same array (**Figure 6A**) with min-to-max voltage ranges. For these LFPs, it was possible to assess changes in identified voltage LFP components related to excitatory and inhibitory synaptic inputs (Hampson et al., 1989; Truccolo et al., 2002; Leung, 2011). CA1 LFPs were assessed before and after sessions in which MIMO stimulation was delivered and facilitated performance vs. sessions in which no stimulation was delivered. The most effective method of assessing such changes was to characterize differences in LFP waveforms by subtracting pre-session LFPs from post-session LFPs and comparing voltages (Post-Pre$_{diff}$) in 10 ms segments as shown in **Figure 6B**. The resulting Post-Pre$_{diff}$ waveforms reflect changes in particular components of the LFP generated from the same CA3 stimulation location related to both excitatory and

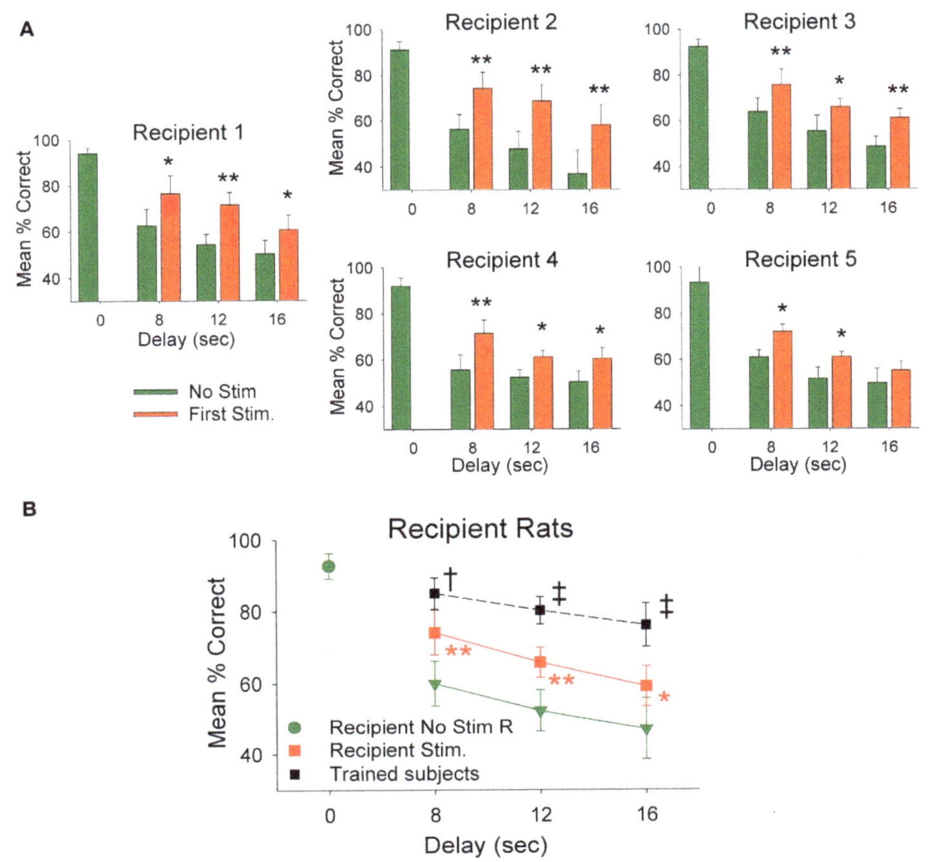

FIGURE 4 | *Recipient rat* performance on DNMS trials with unfamiliar superimposed delays facilitated by *donor rat* mediated SR stimulation. (A) Individual DNMS performance of five different *recipient rats* subjected to trials with 8, 12, and 16 s delays shown for trials in which no stimulation was delivered (No Stim) or on trials on which a simultaneously paired *donor rat* delivery of MIMO SR CA1 stimulation pattern was delivered (Stim). The similarity across each graph indicates generality of facilitated performance on imposed delay trials with delivery of *donor rat* MIMO generated CA1 SR stimulation. Asterisks $^{*}p < 0.01$, $^{**}p < 0.001$, Stim *donor rat* vs. No Stim. **(B)** Overall performance of *recipient rats* ($n = 5$) is shown as mean (±s.e.m.) % correct trials with no delays (green dot–0.0 s values) in comparison to trials with variable delays (8, 12, 16 s) without *donor rat* stimulation (green triangles-No Stim) delivered during the trial [$F_{(3,\ 279)} = 3.61$, $p < 0.001$]; and performance on trials with the same delays but including *donor rat* MIMO strong SR code stimulation (Recipient Stim, red squares) which significantly improved performance compared to No Stim trials [$F_{(1,\ 279)} = 9.82$, $p < 0.001$]. For comparison a plot of the average performance level of rats fully trained ($n = 20$) on the task at the same delays (Trained subjects) is shown (black squares) for comparison to *recipient rat* performance on stimulated trials [$F_{(1,\ 1349)} = 13.48$, $p = 0.001$, Trained subjects > *recipient rats*]. Symbols: $^{*}p < 0.01$, $^{**}p < 0.001$, $^{\dagger}p < 0.01$, $^{\ddagger}p = 0.001$.

inhibitory input over the same range of voltages, before and after behavioral sessions in which SR stimulation was, or was not, delivered.

Figure 6B shows the average of Post-Pre$_{diff}$ LFP waveforms for a single trained animal following SR stimulation (blue) vs. non-stimulation (red) sessions. It is clear that the LFP changes were related directly to both excitatory (40–80 ms) and inhibitory (90–175 ms) components of well-characterized LFPs recorded from the cell layer at each of the eight CA1 locations (Leung, 2011). The lack of as much change in Post-Pre$_{diff}$ LFP measures for non-stimulation (red curve) vs. SR stimulation (blue curve) sessions in **Figure 6B** reflects the increase in excitatory synaptic input to the same CA1 locations that received strong code SR CA1 stimulation patterns and facilitated performance during the behavioral sessions in the same animal. To demonstrate a more general feature of this effect, the dotted curve in **Figure 6B** reflects a further difference of the LFP Post-Pre$_{diff}$ values in terms of subtracted Stim session Post-Pre$_{diff}$ LFP waveforms from similar Non-stim session waveforms, i.e., Diff$_{stim}$—Diff$_{non-stim}$ LFP values. Thus, the dotted curve in **Figure 6B** reflects the average differences in LFPs across 5 individual animals calculated in the same manner as the two Post-Pre$_{diff}$ LFP difference curves (red and blue) but using Post-Pre$_{diff}$ LFPs instead to provide the resulting dotted curve average difference of LFP waveform for SR stim vs. non-stim sessions (i.e., Diff$_{stim}$—Diff$_{non-stim}$). Since this average difference (Diff$_{stim}$—Diff$_{non-stim}$) across all animals ($n = 5$) reflects alteration in the same LFP components as shown for individual waveforms in a single animal (red and blue Post-Pre$_{diff}$ LFPs), it is clear that synaptic processes mediating CA3-to-CA1 transmission were increased by MIMO stimulation delivery during the DNMS sessions in which performance within and between animals was facilitated (**Figures 4, 5**).

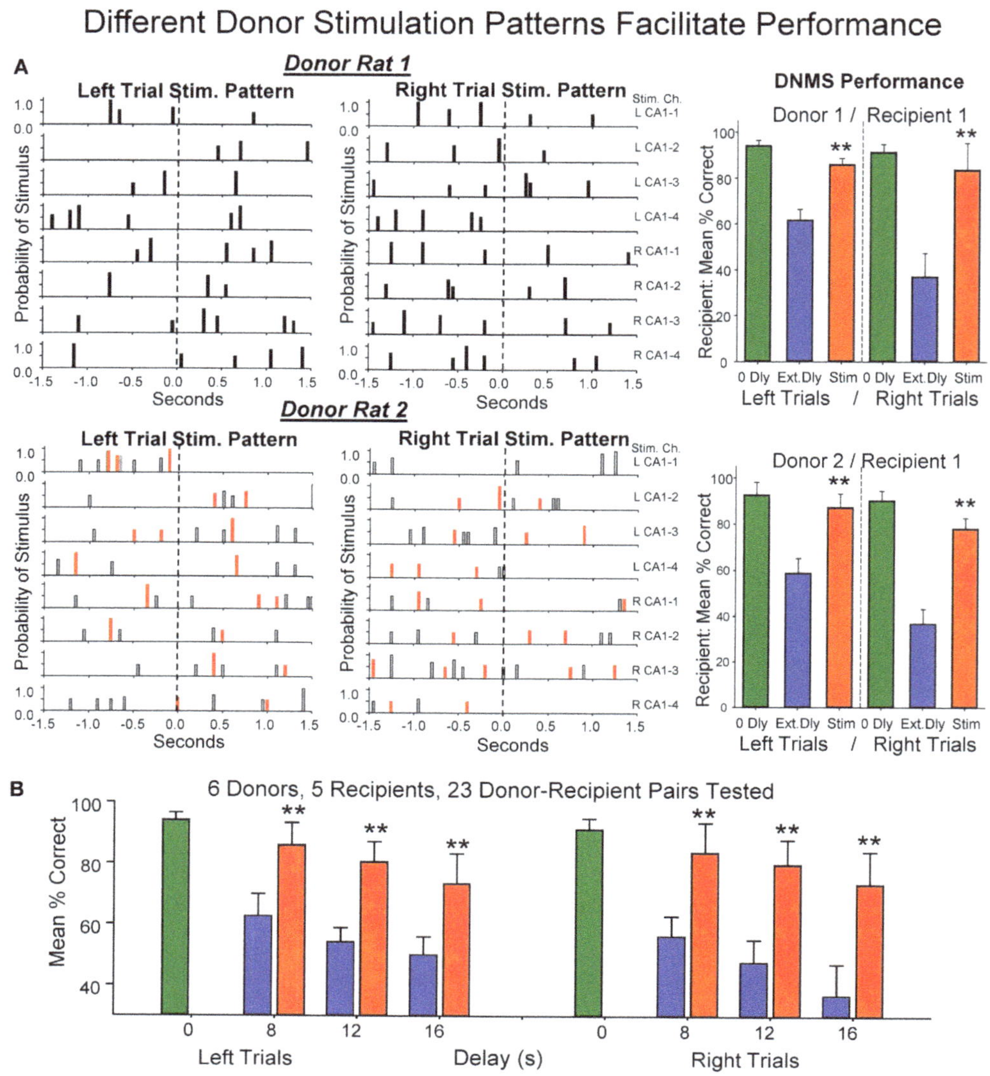

FIGURE 5 | Enhancement of performance of the same *recipient rat* by different *donor rats*. (A) Left: Delivered MIMO SR CA1 stimulation patterns showed for left and right lever trials from *Donor rat 1* (upper) and *Donor rat 2* (lower). Red marks in *Donor rat 2* patterns reflect occurrences of identical pulses delivered in *Donor rat 1* pattern (above) for direct comparison of the two SR Stimulation patterns delivered to the same *Recipient rat* on different trials. Right: Overall performance of the same *Recipient rat* for sessions in which SR Stimulation (Stim) on delay trials was contributed by *Donor rat 1* (upper) and *Donor rat 2* (lower) for left and right Sample lever trials summed over all delays (red) compared with delay trials in which SR stimulation was not delivered (blue). Green bars represent performance by the same *Recipient rat* on trials with no delay (0 Dly) presented in the same sessions as described above. **(B)** Lower plot shows overall average performance for all *Donor/Recipient* sessions ($n = 23$) for trials with Left and Right SR position and those which received *donor rat* SR stimulation (red) vs. no stimulation trials (blue) as a function of delay (0, 8, 12, 16 s). Plots include all *Donor/Recipient* pairs, 5 different *recipient rats* paired with one or more *donor rats* ($n = 6$). Asterisks (** $p < 0.001$) indicate significant difference compared to trials with no *donor rat* stimulation (No Stim).

DISCUSSION

DONOR/RECIPIENT RECOVERY OF HIPPOCAMPAL MEMORY: A MODEL FOR APPLICATION TO MEMORY DEFICITS

The above findings provide highly significant evidence that functional working memory can be enhanced by delivery of *donor rat* MIMO CA1 patterned electrical stimulation to the CA1 field in the hippocampus of *recipient rats*. This shows that information encoded by individual neural events in naïve *recipient rats* can be effectively altered by substitution of *donor rat* MIMO derived electrical stimulus patterns in the same manner as demonstrated in prior studies in which effective stimulus trains were generated by, and delivered to, the same animal (Berger et al., 2011; Hampson et al., 2012a). The demonstration of improved task performance in naïve *recipient rats* (**Figures 4, 5**), verifies that *donor rat* SR CA1 stimulation was capable of inducing the type of encoding process necessary when facilitated retention of information was required because of interposed unfamiliar delays of variable duration (**Figure 6**). The fact that MIMO stimulation

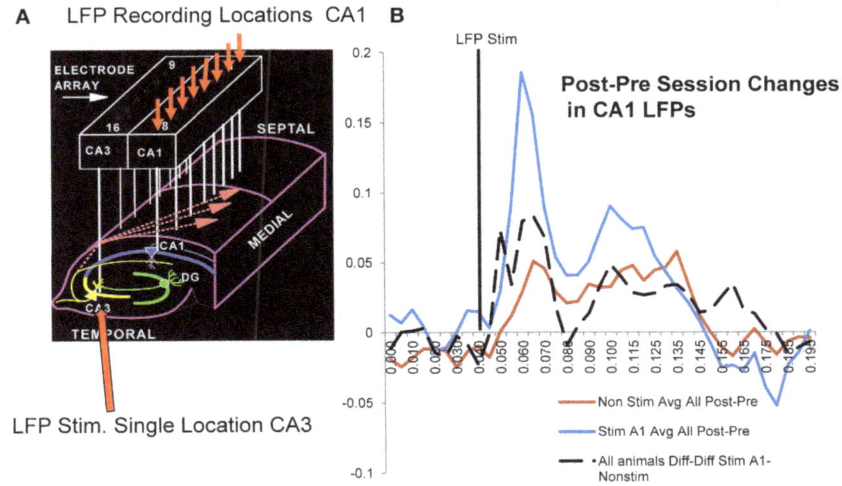

FIGURE 6 | Possible synaptic basis for facilitative *Donor/Recipient* MIMO SR stimulation. (A) Illustration of hippocampal synaptic connections between CA3 and CA1 cells in the same hippocampal region occupied by the same electrode array used to deliver SR Stimulation (**Figures 1–3**). Arrows show divergent projections from a single CA3 cell to multiple CA1 cells via Shaffer collateral connections used to determine changes in CA1 (small red arrows) local field potentials (LFPs) elicited by stimulation delivered to a single CA3 locus (large red arrow) before (Pre) and after (Post) behavioral sessions with MIMO SR Stimulation vs. non-stimulated sessions. **(B)** Average CA1 LFPs elicited by CA3 stimulation are plotted as differences (Post-Pre$_{diff}$) in voltage amplitude measured at the indicated time points (10 ms) of the LFP after stimulus pulse delivery (vertical black line). Red: Mean Post-Pre$_{diffs}$ in LFP amplitudes recorded prior to and following non-stimulation sessions for trained animals. Blue: Average Post-Pre$_{diffs}$ in LFP amplitude following sessions in which SR stimulation was delivered to facilitate performance. Positive Post-Pre$_{diffs}$ reflect average voltage changes related to increased CA1 LFP components after the behavioral session relative to voltages elicited by the same CA3 current intensities prior to the session. These Post-Pre$_{diffs}$ for sessions in which SR stimulation facilitated task performance (blue curve) are shown compared to Post-Pre$_{diffs}$ for those sessions in which stimulation was not delivered (red curve). Dotted: Diff-Diff shows average difference between CA1 LFP Post-Pre$_{diffs}$ for SR stim vs. non-stim sessions (Stim-Non-stim) measured in 6 of the *Donor rats* (all animals A1-non-stim).

can approximate normal ensemble firing involved in the encoding and retrieval of task-relevant information is consistent with other recent findings investigating relationships between multineuron firing in cortical ensembles and behavioral task requirements (Ross and Eichenbaum, 2006; Komorowski et al., 2009; Smith et al., 2009; Rouse et al., 2011). However, the demonstration that the patterns marked as effective and generated online in one animal, could be transferred via temporally matched electrical stimulation of similar CA1 regions in naïve *recipient* animals exposed to the same task contingencies, has not been shown previously. Although consistent in some ways with a recent "brain-to-brain transfer" experiment (Pais-Viera et al., 2013) in which sensorimotor cortical signals were used to influence behavioral choice in the recipient rodent, the results presented here differ significantly because in that experiment, stimulation was delivered at the time of the behavioral response, whereas in our study, the stimulation corresponded to the encoding phase of the task (SR) and was delivered up to 16 s prior to the behavioral response, confirming transfer of a *memory* code, and not simply induction of a motor response. In addition, the lack of enhancement or transfer when several control procedures were employed in the above memory transfer paradigm; i.e., temporal relation to SR, reduced stimulation intensity, closed-loop dependence, etc. (**Figures 1–5**), strongly supports the specificity of the transference of *donor rat* MIMO model derived SR information for hippocampal function to naïve *recipient rats* for task-relevant performance.

These results provide important insight for extending *donor/recipient* procedures to functions performed by other brain regions and other behavioral endpoints as shown recently (Pais-Viera et al., 2013), and eventually to similar circumstances involving humans (Boettiger and D'Esposito, 2005; Smith et al., 2009; Hasson et al., 2012). Once fabricated into a neural prosthesis for *recipients* this unique technology could (1) immediately enhance task-specific performance, (2) repair damaged or impaired task-dependent brain circuitry, and possibly even, (3) provide neural encoding of task-relevant information without prior training. The long history of investigation with hippocampal recording in the behavioral context employed, and prior collaboration perfecting application of the MIMO model to these recordings (Hampson et al., 2008, 2012a; Berger et al., 2012; Marmarelis et al., 2013; Song et al., 2013), as well as recent applications to the non-human primate hippocampus (Hampson et al., 2013) and prefrontal cortex (Hampson et al., 2012c; Opris et al., 2012), provided the insight necessary to extrapolate how *donor/recipient* memory transference could occur as demonstrated here. However, the fact that transferred patterns of electrical brain stimulation have significant functional impact and are capable of modifying performance via strategic online delivery provides another demonstration of *donor-recipient* brain compatibility (Pais-Viera et al., 2013), but this application to hippocampus for improving memory is the first demonstration specific to brain cognitive function. Such results not only provide important new insight into how hippocampal circuits can be operated to process memory-dependent information via external control, but also provide a basis for extending and/or perfecting similar *donor/recipient* type devices (Jarosiewicz et al., 2008;

Venkatraman and Carmena, 2011; Hasson et al., 2012) to enhance and/or replace memory deficiencies in humans.

ACKNOWLEDGMENTS

The authors appreciate the efforts of Vernell Collins, Rodrigo Espana, Lihong Shi, Chad Collins, George McLeod, Anushka Goonawardena. This work was supported by contracts to Sam A. Deadwyler and Theodore W. Berger from the DARPA REMIND Program (N66001-C-09-2080 and N66001-C-09-2081, COL. Geoff Ling, Program Manager), NSF EEC-0310723 (to Theodore W. Berger), NIDA DA07625 (to Sam A. Deadwyler).

REFERENCES

Berger, T. W., Hampson, R. E., Song, D., Goonawardena, A., Marmarelis, V. Z., and Deadwyler, S. A. (2011). A cortical neural prosthesis for restoring and enhancing memory. *J. Neural Eng.* 8, 046017. doi: 10.1088/1741-2560/8/4/046017

Berger, T. W., Song, D., Chan, R. H. M., Marmarelis, V. Z., LaCoss, J., Wills, J., et al. (2012). A hippocampal cognitive prosthesis: multi-input, multi-output nonlinear modeling and VLSI implementation. *Trans. Neural. Syst. Rehabil. Eng.* 20, 198–211. doi: 10.1109/TNSRE.2012.2189133

Boettiger, C. A., and D'Esposito, M. (2005). Frontal networks for learning and executing arbitrary stimulus-response associations. *J. Neurosci.* 25, 2723. doi: 10.1523/JNEUROSCI.3697-04.2005

Deadwyler, S. A., and Hampson, R. E. (1997). "The significance of neural ensemble codes during behavior and cognition," in *Annual Review of Neuroscience*, Vol. 20, eds W. M. Cowan, E. M. Shooter, C. F. Stevens, and R. F. Thompson (Palo Alto, CA: Annual Reviews, Inc), 217–244. doi: 10.1146/annurev.neuro.20.1.217

Deadwyler, S. A. and Hampson, R. E. (2006). Temporal coupling between subicular and hippocampal neurons underlies retention of trial-specific events. *Behav. Brain Res.* 174, 272–280. doi: 10.1016/j.bbr.2006.05.038

Deadwyler, S. A., Goonawardena, A. V., and Hampson, R. E. (2007). Short-term memory is modulated by the spontaneous release of endocannabinoids: evidence from hippocampal population codes. *Behav. Pharm.* 18, 571–580. doi: 10.1097/FBP.0b013e3282ee2adb

Eichenbaum, H., and Fortin, N. J. (2009). The neurobiology of memory based predictions. *Philos. Trans. R. Soc. Lond. B Biol. Sci.* 364, 1183. doi: 10.1098/rstb.2008.0306

Hasson, U., Ghazanfar, A. A., Galantucci, B., Garrod, S., and Keysers, C. (2012). Brain-to-brain coupling: a mechanism for creating and sharing a social world. *Trends Cogn. Sci.* 16, 114–121. doi: 10.1016/j.tics.2011.12.007

Hampson, R. E., Foster, T. C., and Deadwyler, S. A. (1989). Effects of delta-9-tetrahydrocannabinol on sensory evoked hippocampal activity in the rat: principal components analysis and sequential dependency. *J. Pharmacol. Exp. Ther.* 251, 870–877.

Hampson, R. E., Jarrard, L. E., and Deadwyler, S. A. (1999). Effects of ibotenate hippocampal and extrahippocampal destruction on delayed-match and –nonmatch-to-sample behavior in rats. *J. Neurosci.* 19, 1492–1507.

Hampson, R. E., Simeral, J. D., and Deadwyler, S. A. (2008). "Neural population recording in behaving animals: constituents of the neural code for behavior," in *Neural Population Encoding*, eds C. R Holscher and M. H. Munk (Cambridge: Cambridge University Press), 111–128.

Hampson, R. E., Sweatt, A. J., Goonawardena, A. V., Song, D., Chan, R. H., Marmarelis, V. Z., et al. (2011). Memory encoding in hippocampal ensembles is negatively influenced by cannabinoid CB1 receptors. *Behav. Pharmacol.* 22, 335–346. doi: 10.1097/FBP.0b013e3283473bfd

Hampson, R. E., Song, D., Chan, R. H. M., Sweatt, A. J., Fuqua, J., Gerhardt, G. A., et al. (2012a). A nonlinear model for hippocampal cognitive prostheses: memory facilitation by hippocampal ensemble stimulation. *Trans. Neural Syst. Rehabil. Eng.* 20,184–197. doi: 10.1109/TNSRE.2012.2189163

Hampson, R. E., Song, D., Chan, R. H. M., Sweatt, A. J., Riley, M. R., Goonawardena, A. V., et al. (2012b). Closing the loop for memory prostheses: detecting the role of hippocampal neural ensembles using nonlinear models. *Trans. Neural Syst. Rehabil. Eng.* 20, 510–525. doi: 10.1109/TNSRE.2012.2190942

Hampson, R. E., Gerhardt, G. A., Marmarelis, V. Z., Song, D., Opris, I., Santos, L., et al. (2012c). Facilitation and restoration of cognitive function in primate prefrontal cortex by a neuroprosthesis that utilizes minicolumn-specific neural firing. *J. Neural Eng.* 9, 056012. doi: 10.1088/1741-2560/9/5/056012

Hampson, R. E., Song, D., Opris, I., Santos, L. M., Gerhardt, G. A., Marmarelis, V. Z., et al. (2013). Facilitation of memory encoding in primate hippocampus by a neuroprosthesis that promotes task specific neural firing. *J. Neural Eng.* 10:066013. doi: 10.1088/1741-2560/10/6/066013

Jarosiewicz, B., Chase, S. M., Fraser, G. W., Velliste, M., Kass, R. E., and Schwartz, A. B. (2008). Functional network reorganization during learning in a brain-computer interface paradigm. *Proc. Natl. Acad. Sci. U.S.A.* 105, 19486. doi: 10.1073/pnas.0808113105

Komorowski, R. W., Manns, J. R., and Eichenbaum, H. (2009). Robust conjunctive item-place coding by hippocampal neurons parallels learning what happens where. *J. Neurosci.* 29, 9918. doi: 10.1523/JNEUROSCI.1378-09.2009

Leung, S. L. (2011). "Field potential generation and current source density analysis," in *Electrophysiological Recording Techniques*, eds R. P. Vertes and R. W. Stackman (New York, NY: Humana Press), 1–25. doi: 10.1007/978-1-60327-202-5_1

Marmarelis, V. Z. (2004). *Nonlinear Dynamic Modeling of Physiological Systems.* Hoboken, NJ: Wiley-IEEE Press. doi: 10.1002/9780471679370

Marmarelis, V. Z., Shin, D. C., Song, D., Hampson, R. E., Deadwyler, S. A., and Berger, T. W. (2013). Nonlinear modeling of dynamic interactions within neuronal ensembles using principal dynamic modes. *J. Comput. Neurosci.* 34, 73–87. doi: 10.1007/s10827-012-0407-7

Opris, I., Hampson, R. E., Gerhardt, G. A., Berger, T. W., and Deadwyler, S. A. (2012). Columnar processing in primate prefrontal cortex: evidence for executive control microcircuits. *J. Cogn. Neurosci.* 24, 2334–2347. doi: 10.1162/jocn_a_00307

Pais-Viera, M., Lebedev, M., Kunicki, C., Wang, J., and Nicolelis, M. A. L. (2013). A brain-to-brain interface for real-time sensorimotor information. *Sci. Rep.* 3, 1319. doi: 10.1038/srep01319

Ross, R. S., and Eichenbaum, H. (2006). Dynamics of hippocampal and cortical activation during consolidation of a nonspatial memory. *J. Neurosci.* 26, 4852. doi: 10.1523/JNEUROSCI.0659-06.2006

Rouse, A. G., Stanslaski, S. R., Cong, P., Jensen, R. M., Afshar, P., Ullestad, D., et al. (2011). A chronic generalized bi-directional brain–machine interface. *J. Neural Eng.* 8, 36018. doi: 10.1088/1741-2560/8/3/036018

Smith, N. J., Narayanan, N. S., and Laubach, M. (2009). Past performance is indicative of future returns. *Neuron* 63, 146. doi: 10.1016/j.neuron.2009.07.007

Song, D., Chan, R. H., Marmarelis, V. Z., Hampson, R. E., Deadwyler, S. A., and Berger, T. W. (2009). Nonlinear modeling of neural population dynamics for hippocampal prostheses. *Neural Netw.* 22, 1340–1351. doi: 10.1016/j.neunet.2009.05.004

Song, D., Wang, H., Tu, C. Y., Marmarelis, V. Z., Hampson, R. E., Deadwyler, S. A., et al. (2013). Identification of sparse neural functional connectivity using penalized likelihood estimation and basis functions. *J. Comput. Neurosci.* 35, 335–357. doi: 10.1007/s10827-013-0455-7

Truccolo, W. A., Ding, M., Knuth, K. H., Nakamura, R., and Bressler, S. L. (2002). Trial-totrial variability of cortical evoked responses: implications for the analysis of functional connectivity. *Clin. Neurophysiol.* 113, 206–226. doi: 10.1016/S1388-2457(01)00739-8

Venkatraman, S., and Carmena, J. M. (2011). Active sensing of target location encoded by cortical microstimulation. *IEEE Trans. Neural Syst. Rehabil. Eng.* 19, 317–324. doi: 10.1109/TNSRE.2011.2117441

Witter, M. P., and Amaral, D. G., (2004). "Hippocampal formation," in *The Rat Nervous System*, ed G. Paxinos (San Diego, CA: Academic Press), 635–704.

Zanos, T. P., Courellis, S. H., Berger, T. W., Hampson, R. E., Deadwyler, S. A., and Marmarelis, V. Z. (2008). Nonlinear modeling of causal interrelationships in neuronal ensembles. *IEEE Trans. Neural Syst. Rehabil. Eng.* 16, 336–352. doi: 10.1109/TNSRE.2008.926716

23

Volitional enhancement of firing synchrony and oscillation by neuronal operant conditioning: interaction with neurorehabilitation and brain-machine interface

***Yoshio Sakurai*[1]*, *Kichan Song*[1], *Shota Tachibana*[1] *and Susumu Takahashi*[2]**

[1] *Department of Psychology, Graduate School of Letters, Kyoto University, Kyoto, Japan*
[2] *Laboratory of Neural Circuitry, Graduate School of Brain Science, Doshisha University, Kizugawa, Japan*

Edited by:
Mikhail Lebedev, Duke University, USA

Reviewed by:
Mikhail Lebedev, Duke University, USA
Valerie Ego-Stengel, Centre national de la recherche scientifique, France

****Correspondence:***
Yoshio Sakurai, Department of Psychology, Graduate School of Letters, Kyoto University, Yoshida-honmachi, Sakyo-ku, Kyoto 606-8501, Japan
e-mail: ysakurai@bun.kyoto-u.ac.jp

In this review, we focus on neuronal operant conditioning in which increments in neuronal activities are directly rewarded without behaviors. We discuss the potential of this approach to elucidate neuronal plasticity for enhancing specific brain functions and its interaction with the progress in neurorehabilitation and brain-machine interfaces. The key to-be-conditioned activities that this paper emphasizes are synchronous and oscillatory firings of multiple neurons that reflect activities of cell assemblies. First, we introduce certain well-known studies on neuronal operant conditioning in which conditioned enhancements of neuronal firing were reported in animals and humans. These studies demonstrated the feasibility of volitional control over neuronal activity. Second, we refer to the recent studies on operant conditioning of synchrony and oscillation of neuronal activities. In particular, we introduce a recent study showing volitional enhancement of oscillatory activity in monkey motor cortex and our study showing selective enhancement of firing synchrony of neighboring neurons in rat hippocampus. Third, we discuss the reasons for emphasizing firing synchrony and oscillation in neuronal operant conditioning, the main reason being that they reflect the activities of cell assemblies, which have been suggested to be basic neuronal codes representing information in the brain. Finally, we discuss the interaction of neuronal operant conditioning with neurorehabilitation and brain-machine interface (BMI). We argue that synchrony and oscillation of neuronal firing are the key activities required for developing both reliable neurorehabilitation and high-performance BMI. Further, we conclude that research of neuronal operant conditioning, neurorehabilitation, BMI, and system neuroscience will produce findings applicable to these interrelated fields, and neuronal synchrony and oscillation can be a common important bridge among all of them.

Keywords: operant conditioning, synchrony, oscillation, neurorehabilitation, brain-machine interface

OPERANT CONDITIONING OF NEURONAL FIRING

When we require learning of volitional enhancement of a certain behavior, operant conditioning (Skinner, 1974; Reynolds, 1975) should be the first choice. The voluntary behavior immediately followed by reward, i.e., having contingency of reward, soon becomes more frequent, and humans and animals volitionally conduct the behavior more frequently to get more reward. Based on such methodology, an intriguing method of learning of volitional enhancement in neuronal firing has been developed and called neuronal operant conditioning, in which rewards are given for modulations of neuronal firing which are not linked to overt behaviors. Since Olds (1965) and Fetz (1969) published their pioneering research, conditioned enhancement of neuronal firing has been frequently reported in animals and humans. In particular, Fetz and collaborators (Fetz, 1969; Fetz and Finocchio, 1971; Fetz and Baker, 1973) had established the methodology of neuronal operant conditioning and reported that monkeys could control firing rates of individual neurons in the motor cortex (**Figure 1**). Following these pioneering and memorable experiments, several intriguing studies by Fetz and other researchers have been published.

Recently, for example, Kobayashi et al. (2010) has demonstrated a remarkable capacity of single neurons to be driven by volition by adapting to specific operant requirements. This experiment set variable relationships between levels of single-neuron activity in the monkey prefrontal cortex and rewarding outcomes. Prefrontal neurons changed firing rates according to the specific requirements for gaining reward, without the monkeys making a motor response, and indicated that neuronal firings constituted a volitional operant response enhanced by reward. The control task of the experiment suggested that these changes of firing were unlikely to reflect simple reward predictions. In humans, Cerf et al. (2010) demonstrated that subjects can regulate firing rates of single neurons in the medial temporal lobe (MTL) to

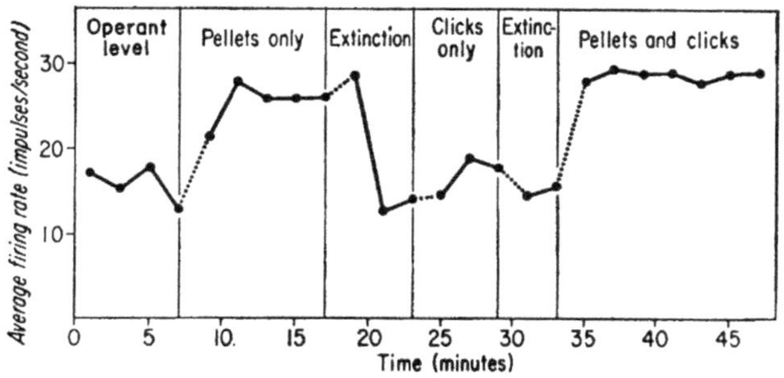

FIGURE 1 | Data showing firing rate of a motor cortex neuron of the monkey as a function of reinforcement schedule of neuronal operant conditioning. During operant level and extinction periods neither food nor click feedback was presented. During "Pellets only" period, the highest firing rates were reinforced with delivery of a food pellet without click feedback. During "Click only" period, a click was presented for each firing of the neuron; finally, both pellets and clicks were provided. (From Fetz, 1969, with permission).

obtain the rewarding outcome that visual images they liked to see became clearer on the computer screen in front of them. The study recorded from single neurons in patients implanted with intracranial electrodes for clinical reasons. The subjects looked at a hybrid superposition of two images representing familiar individuals, landmarks, objects, or animals and had to enhance one image at the expense of the other, competing one. Simultaneously, the firing of MTL neurons was decoded in real time to control the content of the hybrid, i.e., making one of the superposed images clearer than the other. The subjects reliably regulated the firing rate of these neurons, increasing the rate of some while simultaneously decreasing the rate of others. The subjects achieved this by focusing onto one image, which gradually became clearer on the computer screen, thereby overriding sensory input. On the basis of the firing of these MTL neurons, visual images in the subject's mind were visualized on an external display, which functioned as reward.

The most recent progress is reported by Arduin et al. (2013). They employed a strategy of accessing reward by controlling a prosthetic device with self-generated neuronal firing from a single neuron. They recorded multiple neurons from motor cortical areas in rats for controlling a linear actuator with a water bottle. To receive reward of water, the rats had to move the bottle until it reached a zone for drinking by raising and maintaining firing rate of each neuron above a high threshold. They defined the time the bottle took to reach the drinking zone after trial onset as time-to-reward. If the time-to-reward distribution during trials significantly differed from that during waiting periods, the single neuron was considered an operantly conditioned neuron (Opris et al., 2011b).

The firing rates of conditioned neurons increased instantaneously after a trial onset and the bottle entered the drinking zone within a very short time. The time-to-reward for the conditioned neurons soon decreased and exhibited significant difference compared to that for non-conditioned neurons. The majority of the conditioned neurons increased firing rates reliably and instantaneously after trial onset despite the absence of any temporal requisition. Furthermore, the conditioned neurons fired more frequently, instantaneously, and strongly than the neighboring neurons that were simultaneously recorded around the conditioned neurons (**Figure 2**). The authors concluded that only the operant-conditioned neurons possessing significantly increased firing rates take the lead as "master neurons", that exhibit most prominent volitionally driven modulations in a small neural network.

Such on-going progress of research into neuronal operant conditioning confirms the possibility of volitional enhancement of activity for specific individual neurons. However, possibility of chance reinforcement of a body movement rather than neuronal activity should always be checked. The question is whether operantly conditioned neuronal firing is directly controlled in certain central pathways or through an accidentally reinforced body movement which generates activity in the whole pathways leading to the muscles, including corollary discharge and proprioceptive and sensory feedbacks. Concerning involvement of the proprioceptive feedback, Wyler et al. (1979) reported that section of pyramidal tract and ventral rhizotomies disrupted operant conditioning of firing of precentral neurons and suggested that the precentral neurons were operantly controlled through the proprioceptive feedback from the peripheral mechanoreceptors. However, such lesions of nerve fibers could yield neuronal death and/or reorganization of neuronal networks, which may disrupt normal neuronal activity and/or potential for learning and conditioning. Intact brains and input-output pathways should be employed to answer the question of central pathways vs. body movements. Using the intact brains and pathways, several former and recent studies (Fetz and Finocchio, 1971; Koralek et al., 2012; Engelhard et al., 2013; Sakurai and Takahashi, 2013) reported the absence of specific body movements or muscle activity during the operant conditioning of neuronal firing. Although precise and detailed mechanisms that make neuronal operant conditioning possible are not clear yet, it is apparent that neuronal activity can be operantly conditioned without body movement and enhanced volitionally by setting direct contingency between changes of neuronal activity and delivery of reward.

OPERANT CONDITIONING OF FIRING SYNCHRONY AND OSCILLATION

The previous studies surely have confirmed robustness of operant conditioning of neuronal activity. Most of them, however, had a bias due to an exclusive focus on the firing rates of individual neurons of neocortices. Neuronal operant conditioning should be used to explore the extent to which synchronous activity in neurons can be volitionally enhanced. Synchronous neuronal activity reflects functional connectivity among multiple neurons and had not been the target of neuronal operant conditioning, though the brain functions can be considered to be realized by activities not of individual neurons but of ensembles of populations of neurons interrelated with each other. Therefore, enhancement of neuronal activity related to brain functions could be realized more reliably by operant conditioning of such ensemble activity of neuronal populations typically reflected by synchronized firing of multiple neurons.

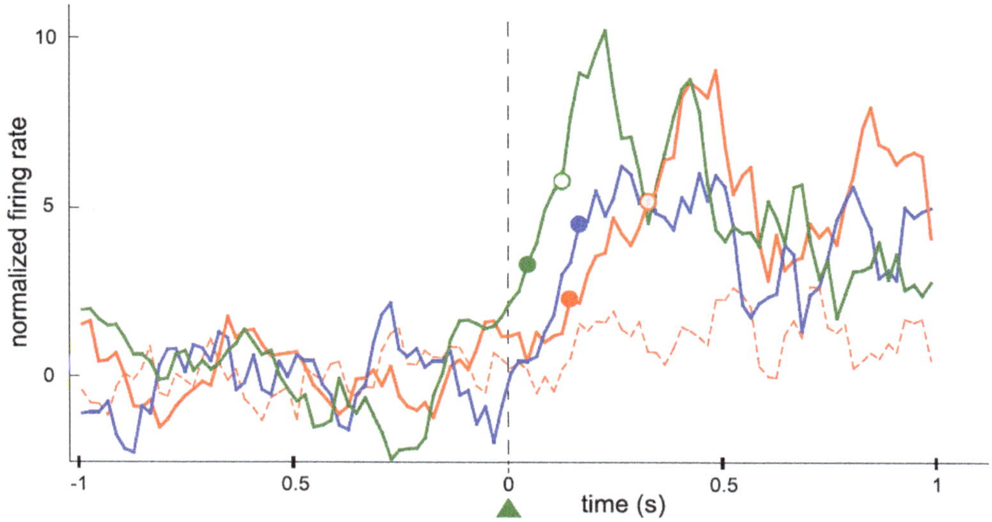

FIGURE 2 | Data showing differences in the rank of activation between conditioned neurons and simultaneously recorded neighboring neurons. Firing rate of motor cortex neurons in the rat was operantly conditioned. This presents perievent time histogram of neuronal activity normalized and centered on trial onset, for four neurons simultaneously recorded during the same session (green: the conditioned neuron; blue: a previously conditioned neuron; red: two neighboring neurons never conditioned). Filled and empty circles of different colors represent the latency of the neurons until their firings exceeded the thresholds at 2 and 5 standard deviations (SD), respectively. One of the neurons (red dashed line) did not have a measurable latency for that recording session. The latency of the blue neuron could only be defined for the 2 SD threshold. Additional (n = 20) neurons that were simultaneously recorded during that recording session have not been included for sake of clarity. Bin size: 20 ms; each value is the z-transform of the firing rate integrated over a sliding window of 100 ms. Latencies were calculated using a 20 ms bin scale. (From Arduin et al., 2013, with permission).

Engelhard et al. (2013) has recently reported that periodically synchronized activity, i.e., oscillatory activity, of motor cortical neurons can be enhanced by operant conditioning. The study has succeeded to train monkeys to increase motor cortex low-gamma waves of local field potential (LFP) (**Figure 3**). Single-neuron firing was recorded, and the enhancement of operantly conditioned oscillatory waves was accompanied by a correlated increase in the synchrony of the entrained neurons. This relation of LFP and neuronal firing can be explained by the fact that LFPs are produced by postsynaptic potentials, and periodicity in neuronal firing would be associated with periodicity in LFPs. They also documented the spatial extent of neurons entrained with the operantly conditioned oscillatory activity. Over the extent of 4 × 4 mm electrode grids, enhanced gamma power in the LFP and phase locking of neuronal firings occurred in a broad range (approximately 500 μm), and depth of entrained modulation decreased as a function of distance from the operant conditioning sites of electrodes. The study also confirmed that the enhancement of oscillatory activity was not associated with any observed movements or increases in muscle activity. From these findings, the authors argue that the findings link volitional control of LFP oscillations and neuronal-firing synchrony.

The low-gamma oscillations have been found in many different brain areas and are considered to be associated with different functions such as attention, perception, cognition, and computation (Herrmann et al., 2010) and to play as neural synchrony both within (Salinas and Sejnowski, 2001) and between (Siegel et al., 2012) brain areas. Therefore, the results of Engelhard et al. (2013) are ground breaking, whereby monkeys demonstrated the ability to directly modulate and enhance specific patterns of synchrony of many neurons in somewhat broad ranges, which may be related to several motor functions of the brain.

On the other hand, it is desirable to directly demonstrate operant enhancement of firing synchrony among individual neurons located closely in restricted smaller ranges. For such experiments, precise separation of extracellular firing from closely neighboring neurons in real time is required. It had been difficult, however, for traditional spike-sorting techniques (Lewicki, 1994; Fee et al., 1996), primarily because spike waveforms overlap on a common electrode when nearby neurons fire coincidently. To address this problem, we (Takahashi et al., 2003a,b) developed a unique method of spike-sorting using independent component analysis (ICA; Comon, 1994) with a specific multielectrode (Takahashi and Sakurai, 2005, 2007, 2009a,b). The method allows sorting of the firings of closely neighboring neurons in real time and the detection of firing synchrony. Using this technique, we have recently reported that synchronized firing of closely neighboring neurons in rat hippocampus can be enhanced by neuronal operant conditioning (Sakurai and Takahashi, 2013).

We trained rats to engage in a free-operant task in which nose-poke behavior was rewarded in session 1, and firing rates and synchrony of multiple neighboring neurons above preset criteria were rewarded in sessions 2 and 3, respectively. Placing contingency of reward on firing synchrony in session 3 resulted in selective enhancement of firing synchrony of the hippocampal neurons (**Figure 4**). Control experiments revealed that the enhancement of firing synchrony was not attributable to increments of behaviors

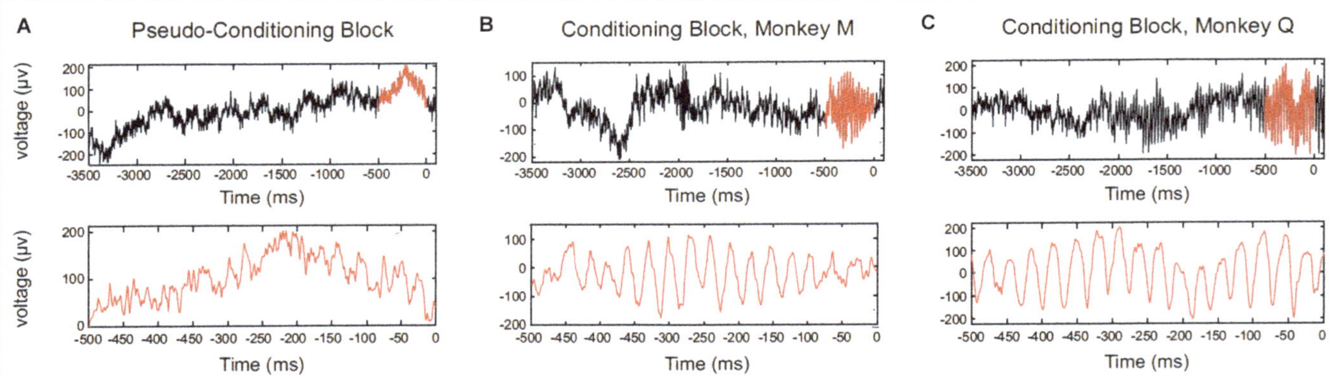

FIGURE 3 | Data showing single-trial examples of LFP aligned to reward delivery (0). Oscillatory firing of motor cortical neurons of the monkey was operantly conditioned. **(A)** Data for monkey M (session #20). Upper panel shows a raw LFP trace in the pseudoconditioning block. The 500 ms period before reward is highlighted in red. Lower panel is an expanded view of the 500 ms period before reward. **(B)** The same as in **(A)**, but for a trial in the conditioning block. **(C)** The same as in **(A)**, but for a trial in the conditioning block, monkey Q (session #17). (From Engelhard et al., 2013, with permission).

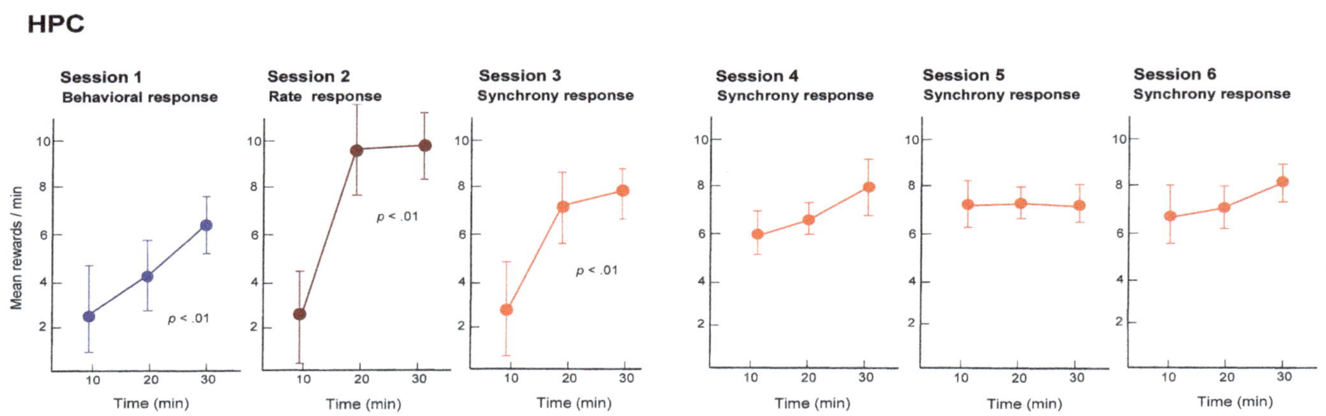

FIGURE 4 | Mean quantities of pellets, reward in the operant conditioning, delivered by behavior (session 1), firing rate above preset criteria (session 2) and firing synchrony above preset criteria (sessions 3–6) during each 30 min conditioning session. Neuronal firing rate and synchrony were obtained from a group of neighboring neurons in the hippocampal CA1 of the rat and operantly conditioned. In sessions 1–3, means were calculated for three periods (10–20, 21–30 and 31–40 min) of each session. Data recorded for the first 10 min of each session are not presented because the first 10 min were used to perform behavioral shaping (session 1) and selection of criteria for the neuronal activities (sessions 2 and 3). In sessions 4–6, means were calculated for periods of 0–10, 11–20 and 21–30 min of each session because criterion selection had been conducted in session 3 and was thus unnecessary. (From Sakurai and Takahashi, 2013, with permission).

or excitation caused by reward delivery. Analysis of the firing rates and synchrony of individual neurons and neuron pairs during the conditioning revealed that the firing rates and synchrony of some but not all neurons and neuron pairs increased in each group of neighboring neurons (**Figures 5, 6**). No firing enhancement was observed in any neurons and neuron pairs recorded by closely placed electrodes not used for the conditioning. From all these findings, we conclude that neuronal operant conditioning can lead to volitional enhancement of firing synchrony in a small group of neurons in a small restricted area in the hippocampus.

In that study, operant conditioning of firing synchrony was obtained in the hippocampus but not in the motor cortex. One explanation might be that the hippocampus has the high level of plasticity causing learning-related changes of firing synchrony among the neurons (e.g., Sakurai, 1996a, 2002). This explanation, however, does not exclude the possibility of motor cortical neurons to be conditioned in their firing synchrony. The hippocampal synchrony functions could be revealed at small timescales such as the bin (2–4 ms) used for the operant conditioning in our study (Sakurai and Takahashi, 2013), whereas in the motor cortex synchrony could be best functional at longer timescales such as that of low gamma oscillations. This assumption is apparently supported by the result of Engelhard et al. (2013) introduced above.

It should be noted that, as Fetz (2013) suggested, synchronous neuronal firing was detected not only as lasting and periodic, e.g., oscillations, but also as temporal and episodic. For example, Riehle et al. (1997) has reported that such temporally short and episodic synchrony of firing of motor cortical neurons can be detected during some specific behavior. Such synchrony was termed "unitary event" which appeared consistently at particular times in relation to an expected cue at times unrelated to sensory

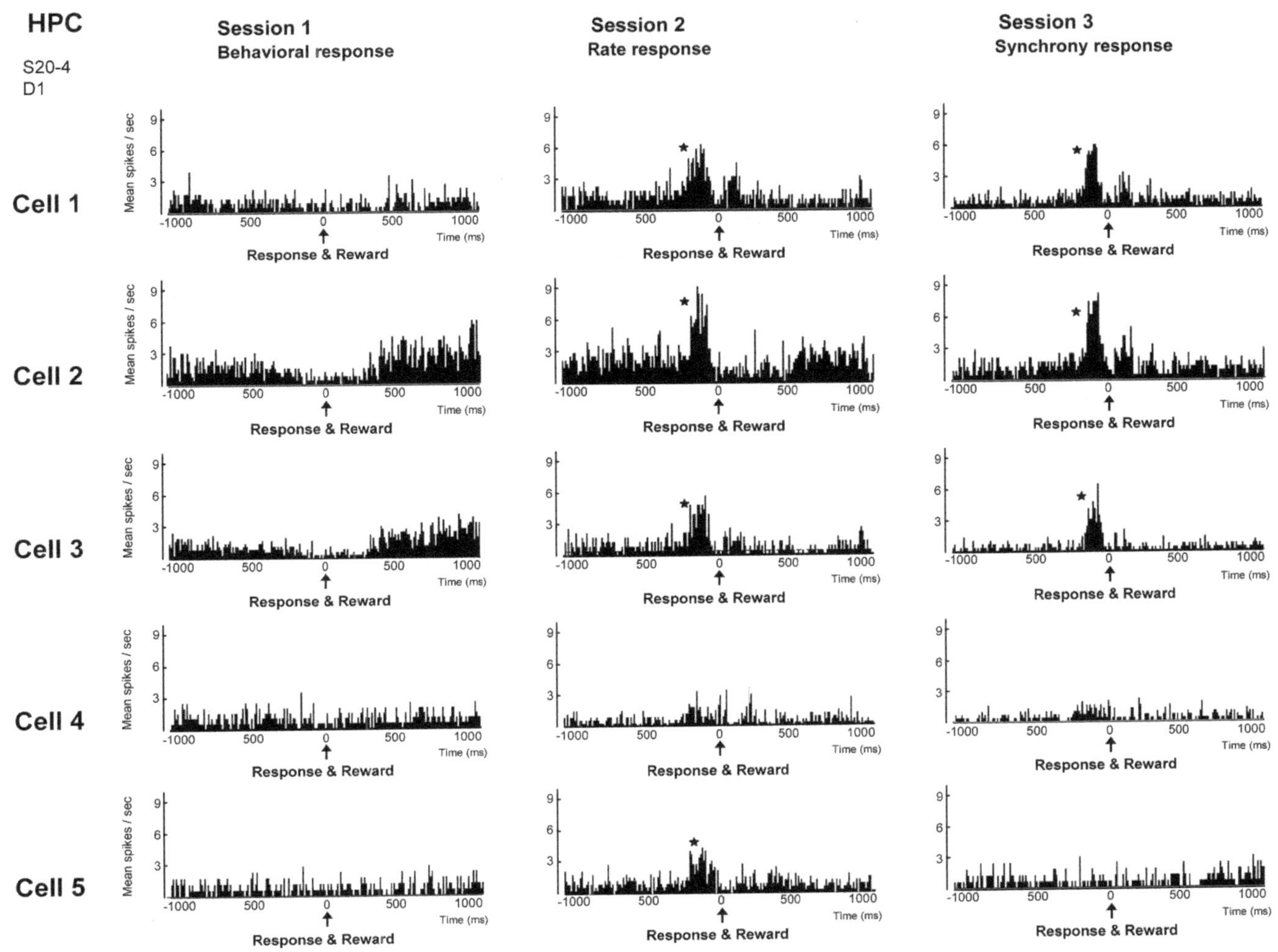

FIGURE 5 | Firing-rate histograms of five individual neurons comprising a group of neighboring neurons in the hippocampal CA1 in sessions 1–3. The center (0) of each histogram means the time when behavior (session 1), firing rate above preset criteria (session 2) and firing synchrony above preset criteria (session 3) immediately followed by reward delivery were conducted. A bin is 10 ms and an asterisk indicates a significant increment of firing (confidence limit, $p < 0.005$). (From Sakurai and Takahashi, 2013, with permission).

or motor events. Such episodic synchrony of firing should be a target of neuronal operant conditioning. Schmied et al. (1993) reported that humans could be operantly conditioned to increase some episodic synchrony of groups of motor cortical neurons. However, because synchronized firings can be caused by common synaptic inputs, such demonstration may be essentially equivalent to demonstrating enhancement of firing of the common input neurons. In contrast, periodic synchrony of firing represents a rhythmic phenomenon involving a different mechanism generating more prolonged circuit resonance (Fetz, 2013).

WHY SYNCHRONY AND OSCILLATION?—VIEW ON "CELL ASSEMBLY"

As described above, operant conditioning of oscillation and synchrony of multiple neurons can be indispensable to enhancing brain functions because they are realized by ensemble activities of populations of neurons that are functionally connected with each other. Such a functional population of neurons has been proposed to be "cell assembly" (Hebb, 1949), postulated to act as a functional unit that represents information in the working brain and underlie perception, learning, and memory for adaptive behavior (Eichenbaum, 1993; Sakurai, 1996b, 1999; Harris, 2005; Opris et al., 2013). The original concept of cell assembly was a theoretical notion and it could have value and be substantial when it accounts for experimentally observed phenomena. The experimental observations showing major properties of the cell assembly are, as Sakurai (1999) suggested, the task-related functional overlapping of individual neurons (Sakurai, 1994) and the task-dependent dynamics of the functional connectivity among the neurons (Sakurai, 1993). In particular, the latter phenomena, reflected as dynamically changing synchrony of firing of multiple neurons, has often been reported and regarded as the popular operational definition or indirect evidence of the activity of cell assemblies (Sakurai, 1996a, 2002; Riehle et al., 1997; Engel

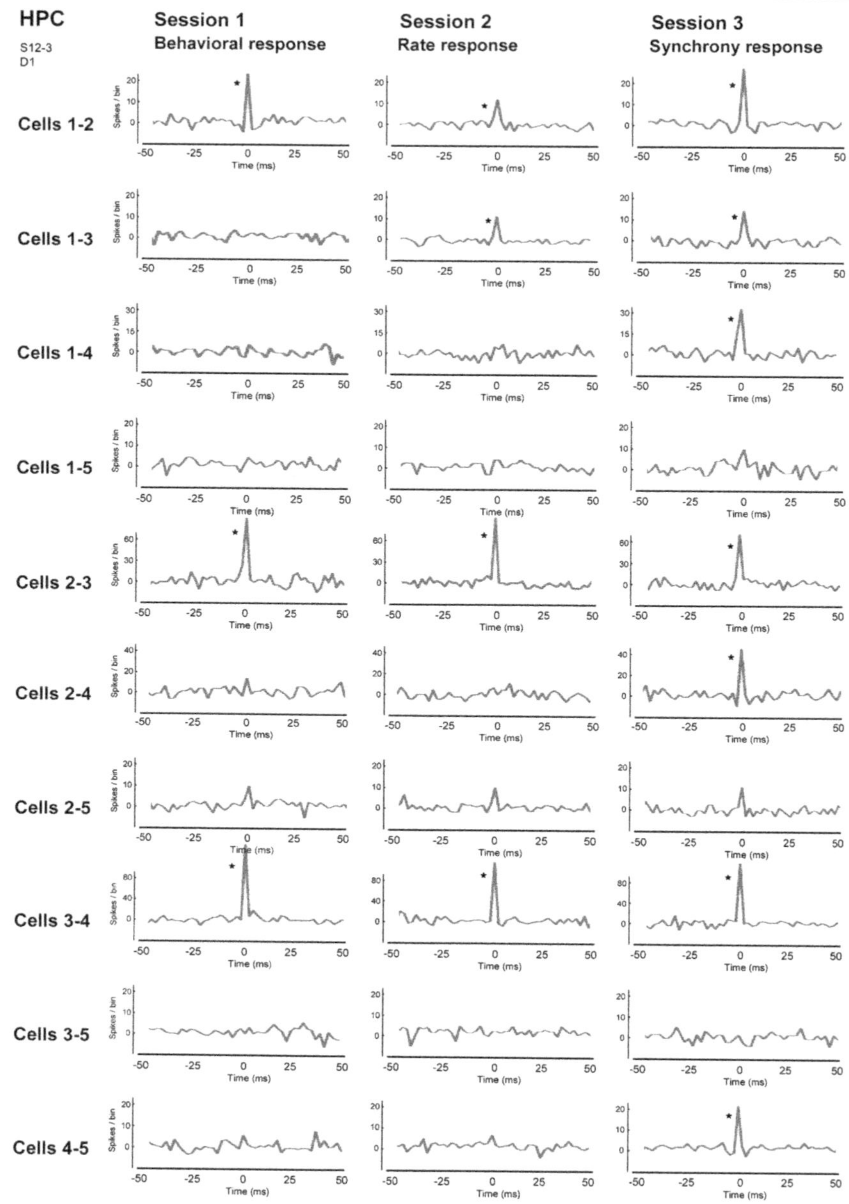

FIGURE 6 | Correlograms of all neuron pairs of five neighboring neurons in the hippocampal CA1 in sessions 1–3. The center (0) of each correlogram means the time when two neurons fired simultaneously, i.e., achieved firing synchrony. A bin is 2 ms and an asterisk indicates a significant increment in firing synchrony (confidence limit, $p < 0.005$). (From Sakurai and Takahashi, 2013, with permission).

et al., 2001). Therefore, the target activity of neuronal operant conditioning should include not only firing rates but also firing synchrony of multiple neurons, as reported in Engelhard et al. (2013) and Sakurai and Takahashi (2013).

However, operant conditioning of the activity of cell assemblies is not an easy task because the ranges in the patterns of activation of cell assemblies, i.e., sizes of cell assemblies, have been postulated to be diverse (Sakurai et al., 2013). A cell assembly could be comprised of a small number of localized neurons or a large number of broadly distributed neurons (Eichenbaum, 1993). Therefore, neurons in the neocortices and the limbic structures, particularly the hippocampus, are expected to show various forms of firing synchrony, which represent dynamic and diverse representation by cell assemblies, in various behavioral tasks. Actually, several former studies have reported the task- and behavior-dependent dynamic synchrony of neurons in the wide ranges (Abeles et al., 1993; Vaadia et al., 1995; Seidemann et al., 1996; Engel et al., 2001; Opris et al., 2011a, 2012a,b) and the local ranges (Funahashi and Inoue, 2000; Constantinidis et al., 2001; Sakurai and Takahashi, 2008). We have reported task-dependent sharp synchrony of firing among the neighboring neurons, reflecting the small and localized cell assemblies, in the monkey prefrontal cortex, but at the same time, we have also found dynamically changing broad synchrony of firing among the distant neurons (Sakurai and Takahashi, 2006). The sizes of cell assemblies are certainly diverse and dependent on information representation and processing in behavioral tasks.

The diversity in the sizes of cell assemblies should be considered when neuronal operant conditioning is applied to enhance synchronized neuronal activity. Our study (Sakurai and Takahashi, 2013) has operantly enhanced firing synchrony of the small and localized groups of neighboring neurons, using the specific electrode and the spike sorting, in the rat hippocampus. Such synchronized firing among close neurons has been shown to be valid for some information processes. For example, Fujisawa et al. (2008) has reported clear synchrony of firing among neighboring neurons in the rat prefrontal cortex. The authors focused on the sharp peaks in cross-correlograms between pyramidal neurons and interneurons with millisecond time lags that were consistent with monosynaptic delays. The temporal relationships of the activities of neurons were examined during a working memory task. Numerous monosynaptic pairs between the pyramidal neurons and interneurons dynamically varied their peaks in the cross-correlograms across various phases of the task beyond the statistical accounting for the effects of covarying the firing rates of the neurons. This indicates that functional interplay among the close neurons linked by monosynaptic connections is working during the behavioral task. This finding was consistent with those of previous studies that have observed variance in the short-term synchrony between neuronal pairs as a function of behavioral performance and learning (Constantinidis et al., 2002; Baeg et al., 2007; Opris et al., 2011a, 2012a).

On the other hand, the study of Engelhard et al. (2013), introduced above, can be considered to have succeeded to operantly enhance activity of broader cell assemblies reflected by oscillatory low-gamma waves of LFP, because the oscillatory LFPs are produced by synchronized postsynaptic potentials of many neurons in broader ranges. Oscillatory activity in the motor cortex has been observed in many experiments and led various hypotheses about its possible functions, such as motor preparation and attention to aspects of movement (Murthy and Fetz, 1996; Donoghue et al., 1998). Oscillatory activity has also been documented most thoroughly in the visual system, where many experiments have suggested that the widespread periodicity is involved in top-down processing (Engel et al., 2001) and plays a role in long-range interactions between different cortical regions (Siegel et al., 2012).

Discussion is still ongoing about the actual functional role of oscillatory and synchronous activities. But with neuronal operant conditioning, as Fetz (2013) suggested, those activities become the independent variable in the experiments, and their effects on behavior are more compelling evidence of their functions. Actually, Keizer et al. (2010) has shown that volitionally increased gamma oscillation at occipital and frontal sites in humans surely improved performance on cognitive tests of sensory binding and memory. This result supports the notion that various information processes are generated by oscillatory activity in the motor and sensory cortices.

In addition to the findings of oscillation, synchrony of firings among individual neurons in broader ranges has been reported. Pipa and Munk (2011) trained monkeys to perform a short-term visual memory task and simultaneously recorded multi-neuronal activity from the prefrontal cortex with electrodes that were arranged in a square-shaped 4 × 4 grid with a distance between the nearest neighbors of 500 μm. The authors found firing synchrony of neurons with high temporal precision across the electrode sites. The frequency of synchrony was modulated depending on the behavioral performance and the specific stimuli that were presented. In particular, during the delay period, larger groups of up to 7 electrode sites showed performance-dependent modulation of the synchronous firings. These findings indicate dynamic activity of broad populations of distributed neurons that underlie the higher temporal organization of information being processed for the task performance.

Recent technological advances have made it possible to record from larger neuronal populations. New principal component analysis (PCA) methods (Peyrache et al., 2009; Lopes-dos-Santos et al., 2011) are suitable for detecting larger cell assemblies that are constructed from larger number of distributed neurons. However, classical methods, such as cross-correlation analyses, have merit in detection of detailed structures of functional connectivity between neighboring neurons. A combination of the new methods of PCA and the classical methods may be ideal in detecting diverse synchrony of neuronal activity and useful to selectively enhance activities of cell assemblies with different sizes.

RELEVANCE TO NEUROREHABILITATION AND BRAIN-MACHINE INTERFACE

NEUROREHABILITATION

Neuronal operant conditioning can elucidate the potential of neuronal plasticity (Dobkin, 2007) induced by conditioning of neuronal activity including synchronous and oscillatory activities. Such elucidation contributes to progress in the development of neurorehabilitation methods (Raskin, 2011), the majority of which attempt artificial enhancement of neuronal activity to compensate for loss of brain motor functions. A turning point of neuronal operant conditioning to be applicable may be the fact that it does not require selection of functionally specific neurons for the conditioning. It would not be possible to condition and enhance inherent motor neurons for compensation of motor functions because most motor-function losses are accompanied by loss of inherent motor neurons. Therefore, neuronal operant conditioning should have the potential to enhance any neuron and hopefully any brain region unrelated to the target functions to be compensated. This could be related to the theory of multipotentiality of the brain (John, 1980). That theory suggests that any neuron and region may contribute to the mediation of a diversity of functions and that many neurons and regions contribute to every function, but it does not imply that different neurons and regions are functionally equivalent or that different functions depends equally on diverse neurons and regions.

Actually in our study (Sakurai and Takahashi, 2013), the neurons showing rapid enhancement in firing rates and synchrony during the neuronal operant conditioning had been selected randomly and originally manifested no behavior-related activity responsible for motor responses. This finding indicates that neurons not initially involved in behavioral performance can be enhanced by the conditioning and subsequently utilized to compensate for loss of motor functions responsible for behavior. Such an indication had previously emerged from the findings of Moritz et al. (2008), who observed that monkeys could learn to use task-unrelated neurons to control an external device if they were provided with operant control training.

Besides the notion of non-selectivity of neurons, it is again noted that conditioning of oscillatory and synchronous activities are expected to lead to more effective neurorehabilitation. Synchronous oscillations in motor cortical neurons have been observed in many behavioral experiments, leading to hypotheses about its possible function. For example, it has been reported to occur during an instructed delay period prior to movement and then disappear during the overt movement, suggesting a role in motor preparation (Donoghue et al., 1998). Oscillations have also been observed to appear during a maintained precision grip (Baker et al., 1999) and free exploratory hand movements (Murthy and Fetz, 1996). It should be emphasized that these oscillations entrained both task-related and unrelated neurons equally, and coherent oscillations occurred over widespread cortical areas, including both hemispheres, but correlations between different cortical sites did not depend on the site's relation to the task (Fetz, 2013). Consequently, inducing such oscillatory activity by operant conditioning could thus enhance several motor-related functions.

In addition to the motor-related functions, synchrony and oscillations are considered to be associated with attention, perception, cognition, and computation (Fries, 2009; Herrmann et al., 2010) and active both within (Salinas and Sejnowski, 2001) and between (Siegel et al., 2012; Terada et al., 2013) brain locations, as described previously. These indicate the possibility of enhancing such higher functions by conditioning of synchrony and oscillations of firing. An issue to be addressed is whether any neuron can be available for the conditioning to enhance the higher functions in the sensory and higher brain regions, as motor functions in the motor-related regions. Addressing this issue involves testing the validity of the view of multipotentiality of the brain (John, 1980) briefly introduced above.

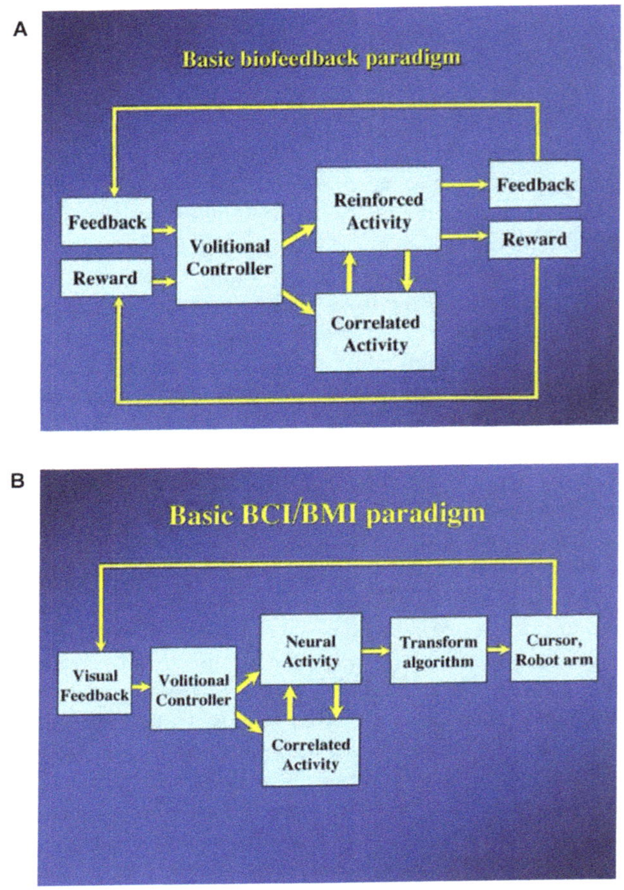

FIGURE 7 | (A) Basic components of neuronal operant conditioning (biofeedback) paradigm. Feedback and reward are contingent on the reinforced activity and provided to the brain of the "volitional controller". The correlated activity consists of additional neural or physiological activity either causally or adventitiously associated with the reinforced activity. (From Fetz, 2007, with permission). **(B)** Basic components of the brain–computer interface (BCI) or brain-machine interface (BMI) paradigms. Essential components are identical to those of the neuronal operant conditioning, except that feedback (usually visual) is provided by the controlled device or cursor, and a more sophisticated transform algorithm is typically used to convert neural activity to the requisite control signals. (From Fetz, 2007, with permission).

BRAIN-MACHINE INTERFACE

As Fetz (2007) suggested, the basic paradigm for neuronal operant conditioning (neural biofeedback) is essentially identical to the paradigm for brain-machine interface (BMI) (**Figure 7**). BMI is for neuroprosthetic control of external devices by neuronal activity instead of behavior (Berger et al., 2008; Hatsopoulos and Donoghue, 2009; Nicolelis and Lebedev, 2009; Andersen et al., 2010; Green and Kalaska, 2011). Neuronal operant learning can elucidate the possibility of volitional control of neuronal activity and contribute to the development of BMI. One difference is the transform algorithm converting neural activity to the control signals operating the external device to get reward. Though this interposes an intermediate stage that may complicate the relationship between neural activity and device control, the final outcome is identical with that of neuronal operant conditioning, i.e., getting reward. The device control in BMI finally results in getting of reward and sometimes, particularly in humans, being able to control the device itself functions as reward. This leads to the conclusion that the basic strategy—volitional activity associated with getting reward is enhanced by reinforcement feedback—is identical between BMI and neuronal operant conditioning. **Figure 8** summarizes the common and different stages in BMI and neuronal operant conditioning.

Although the development of invasive BMI is promising (Lebedev and Nicolelis, 2006), currently available BMIs are limited in terms of accuracy and the facility with which they can be controlled. The most significant factor to which these limits may be attributable may be changes in the plasticity of neuronal activities and functions induced by the use of BMI (Zacksenhouse et al., 2007; Ganguly et al., 2011). In most BMI experiments based on the decoding approach, conversion of neuronal signals is aided by appropriate transform algorithms to generate the adequate

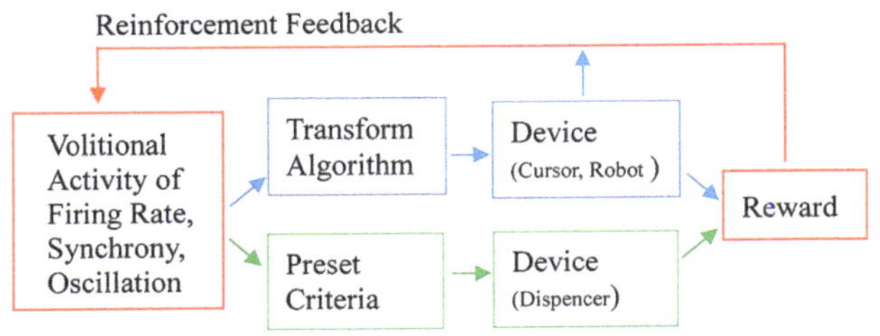

FIGURE 8 | An integrated view of basic components of neuronal operant conditioning (Figure 7A) and BMI (Figure 7B) paradigms. The different stages are shown in blue and green parts, the former for BMI and the latter for neuronal operant conditioning, and the common stages are shown in red parts. See the text for detail.

control parameters. However, the conversion parameters obtained for one set of trials provided increasingly poor predictions of future responses, indicating a source of drift over tens of minutes. Therefore, accurate device control under BMI conditions depends significantly on the degree to which the neuronal activity can be volitionally modulated even for experiments not based on neuronal operant conditioning. Research on such volitional modulation of neuronal activity can be conducted by investigating neuronal operant conditioning, which contributes to realization of a higher performing BMI. The other significant factor affecting the limited performance of the current BMIs may be the bias on firing rate or amplitude of neuronal activity as the source signals. As emphasized in the present paper, synchronous and oscillatory activities have the potential to be neuronal signals constantly representing valid information in the brain. Research for volitional modulation of neuronal synchrony and oscillation by neuronal operant conditioning may contribute much to development of a higher performing BMI.

The issue of neuron selectivity and multipotentiality in the study of neuronal operant conditioning is also a significant issue in BMI studies. Many BMI studies first obtain an optimal basis for brain control by recording the neural activity associated with real limb movement from precentral motor cortex and deriving appropriate transform algorithms (Chapin et al., 1999; Taylor et al., 2002; Carmena et al., 2003; Hochberg et al., 2006; Koike et al., 2006; Choi et al., 2009). However, several other studies demonstrated the ability to extract movement predictions from neurons in postcentral as well as precentral cortical areas (Wessberg et al., 2000; Carmena et al., 2003). Precentral motor neurons could provide the accurate predictions of force and displacement even in small numbers (Koike et al., 2006; Choi et al., 2009), but many neurons from other areas also had potential to provide significant predictions (Wessberg et al., 2000; Carmena et al., 2003). The prediction accuracy increased with the number of neurons included, even when the included neurons were randomly selected and not related to motor movement in nature (Wessberg et al., 2000; Carmena et al., 2003).

Neuronal plasticity, which is inherent in BMI experiments, is not always an obstacle but can be actively applied to induce changes in neuronal connections for functional compensation. For example, Mavoori et al. (2005) investigated the operation of a small computer chip in conjunction with wire electrodes implanted in monkey motor cortex. This "neurochip", useful for invasive BMI, can convert firings of a cortical neuron not to control signals for external devices but to stimuli directly delivered to other neurons and regions to appropriately modify the neural activity in these regions. Jackson et al. (2006) configured the neurochip as action potentials recorded at one site triggered synchronous stimulation at the neighboring site in the monkey motor cortex. Continuous operation for a day or more resulted in long-term changes in the output effects evoked from the recording site and the changes remained stable for more than a week of testing after the conditioning had terminated. Such conditioning effects were related to time-dependent plasticity and obtained only when the delays between neuronal firings and stimuli were less than 50 ms, indicating that firing synchrony could be involved as an effective factor in such plastic changes.

Finally, we introduce the recent findings that learning to operate BMI induces synchronous and oscillatory activity in other brain regions related to specific functions. Koralek et al. (2012) investigated the role of corticostriatal plasticity, usually involved in learning physical skills, in abstract skill learning using BMI. The authors trained rats to learn to control the pitch of an auditory cursor to reach one of two targets by modulating firing activity in the motor cortex independently of physical movement. During the learning of BMI, alteration of activity was observed in striatal neurons, with more neurons modulating activity in relation to the progress in learning to reach the targets. Concurrently, strong correlations, reflected in oscillatory coupling, between the neuronal activity in the motor cortex and the striatum emerged. This suggests that corticostriatal plasticity and oscillatory interaction underlying physical skill learning is also necessary for abstract skill learning using BMI and that neuroprosthetic movements capitalize on the neural circuitry involved in natural motor learning. Most recently, Koralek et al. (2013) also reported that coherence of activity between motor cortex and striatum during learning of the BMI task is selectively increased in neurons controlling behavioral output relative to adjacent neurons. The temporal offset of these oscillatory interactions aligned closely with corticostriatal conduction delays, demonstrating highly precise timing. Firings from either region were followed by a consistent phase in the other region, suggesting that network feedback reinforces the coherent activity. The authors conclude that temporally precise coherence develops during learning specifically in motor output-related neuronal populations and oscillatory activity serves to synchronize widespread brain networks to produce adequate behavior. This confirms that selective temporal coordination between neurons leading to development of cell assemblies is fundamental in learning to control behavior. Koralek et al. (2012, 2013) reliably indicate that research using BMI can be research of system neuroscience and can provide significant data to reveal normal brain functions and their mechanisms.

In conclusion, research into neuronal operant conditioning, neurorehabilitation, BMI, and system neuroscience will produce findings applicable to all these interrelated fields, and synchrony and oscillation of neuronal activity can be a common key bridge interrelating these disciplines.

ACKNOWLEDGMENTS

This work was supported by JST Core Research for Evolution Science and Technology (CREST) program and JSPS KAKENHI grant Nos. 24223004 and 24243069 (Yoshio Sakurai) and 24300148 and 25560435 (Susumu Takahashi).

REFERENCES

Abeles, M., Bergman, H., Margalit, E., and Vaadia, E. (1993). Spatiotemporal firing patterns in the frontal cortex of behaving monkeys. *J. Neurophysiol.* 70, 1629–1638.

Andersen, R. A., Hwang, E. J., and Mulliken, G. H. (2010). Cognitive neural prosthetics. *Annu. Rev. Psychol.* 61, 169–190. doi: 10.1146/annurev.psych.093008.100503

Arduin, P., Fregnac, Y., Shulz, D. E., and Ego-Stengel, V. (2013). "Master" neurons induced by operant conditioning in rat motor cortex during a brain-machine interface task. *J. Neurosci.* 33, 8308–8320. doi: 10.1523/JNEUROSCI.2744-12.2013

Baeg, E. H., Kim, Y. B., Ghim, J. W., Kim, J. J., and Jung, M. W. (2007). Learning-induced enduring changes in functional connectivity among prefrontal cortical neurons. *J. Neurosci.* 27, 909–918. doi: 10.1523/jneurosci.4759-06.2007

Baker, S. N., Kilner, J. M., Pinches, E. M., and Lemon, R. N. (1999). The role of synchrony and oscillations in the motor output. *Exp. Brain Res.* 128, 109–117. doi: 10.1007/s002210050825

Berger, T. W., Chapin, J. K., Gerhardt, G. A., McFarland, D. J., Principe, J. C., Soussou, W. V., et al. (2008). *Brain-Computer Interfaces.* New York: Springer.

Carmena, J. M., Lebedev, M. A., Crist, R. E., O'Doherty, J. E., Santucci, D. M., Dimitrov, D. F., et al. (2003). Learning to control a brain-machine interface for reaching and grasping by primates. *PLoS Biol.* 1:E42. doi: 10.1371/journal.pbio.0000042

Cerf, M., Thiruvengadam, N., Mormonn, F., Kraskov, A., Quiroga, R. Q., Koch, C., et al. (2010). On-line, voluntary control of human temporal lobe neurons. *Nature* 467, 1104–1108. doi: 10.1038/nature09510

Chapin, J. K., Moxon, K. A., Markowitz, R. S., and Nicolelis, M. A. (1999). Real-time control of a robot arm using simultaneously recorded neurons in the motor cortex. *Nat. Neurosci.* 2, 664–670. doi: 10.1038/10223

Choi, K., Hirose, H., Sakurai, Y., Iijima, T., and Koike, Y. (2009). Prediction of arm trajectory from the neural activities of the primary motor cortex with modular connectionist architecture. *Neural Netw.* 22, 1214–1223. doi: 10.1016/j.neunet.2009.09.003

Comon, P. (1994). Independent component analysis, a new concept? *Signal Process.* 36, 287–314. doi: 10.1016/0165-1684(94)90029-9

Constantinidis, C., Franowicz, M. N., and Goldman-Rakic, P. S. (2001). Coding specificity in cortical microcircuits: a multiple-electrode analysis of primate prefrontal cortex. *J. Neurosci.* 21, 3646–3655.

Constantinidis, C., Williams, G. V., and Goldman-Rakic, P. S. (2002). A role for inhibition in shaping the temporal flow of information in prefrontal cortex. *Nat. Neurosci.* 5, 175–180. doi: 10.1038/nn799

Dobkin, B. H. (2007). Brain-computer interface technology as a tool to augment plasticity and outcomes for neurological rehabilitation. *J. Physiol.* 597, 637–642. doi: 10.1113/jphysiol.2006.123067

Donoghue, J. P., Sanes, J. N., Hatsopoulos, N. G., and Gaál, G. (1998). Neural discharge and local field potential oscillations in primate motor cortex during voluntary movements. *J. Neurophysiol.* 79, 159–173.

Eichenbaum, H. (1993). Thinking about brain cell assemblies. *Science* 261, 993–994. doi: 10.1126/science.8351525

Engel, A. K., Fiees, P., and Singer, W. (2001). Dynamic predictions: oscillations and synchrony in top-down processing. *Nat. Rev. Neurosci.* 2, 704–716. doi: 10.1038/35094565

Engelhard, B., Ozeri, N., Israel, Z., Bergman, H., and Vaadia, E. (2013). Inducing gamma oscillations and precise spike synchrony by operant conditioning via brain-machine interface. *Neuron* 77, 361–375. doi: 10.1016/j.neuron.2012.11.015

Fee, M., Mitra, P., and Kleinfeld, D. (1996). Variability of extracellular spike waveforms of cortical neurons. *J. Neurophysiol.* 76, 3823–3833.

Fetz, E. E. (1969). Operant conditioning of cortical unit activity. *Science* 163, 955–958. doi: 10.1126/science.163.3870.955

Fetz, E. E. (2007). Volitional control of neural activity: implications for brain-computer interfaces. *J. Physiol.* 579, 571–579. doi: 10.1113/jphysiol.2006.127142

Fetz, E. E. (2013). Volitional control of cortical oscillations and synchrony. *Neuron* 77, 216–218. doi: 10.1016/j.neuron.2013.01.003

Fetz, E. E., and Baker, M. A. (1973). Operantly conditioned patterns on precentral unit activity and correlated responses in adjacent cells and contralateral muscles. *J. Neurophysiol.* 36, 179–204.

Fetz, E. E., and Finocchio, D. V. (1971). Operant conditioning of specific patterns of neural and muscular activity. *Science* 174, 431–435. doi: 10.1126/science.174.4007.431

Fries, P. (2009). Neuronal gamma-band synchronization as a fundamental process in cortical computation. *Annu. Rev. Neurosci.* 32, 209–224. doi: 10.1146/annurev.neuro.051508.135603

Fujisawa, S., Amarasingham, A., Harrison, M. T., and Buzsaki, G. (2008). Behavior-dependent short-term assembly dynamics in the medial prefrontal cortex. *Nat. Neurosci.* 11, 823–833. doi: 10.1038/nn.2134

Funahashi, S., and Inoue, M. (2000). Neuronal interactions related to working memory processes in the primate prefrontal cortex revealed by cross-correlation analysis. *Cereb. Cortex* 10, 535–551. doi: 10.1093/cercor/10.6.535

Ganguly, K., Domitrov, D. F., Wallis, J. D., and Carmena, J. M. (2011). Reversible large-scale modification of cortical networks during neuroprosthetic control. *Nat. Neurosci.* 14, 662–667. doi: 10.1038/nn.2797

Green, A. M., and Kalaska, J. F. (2011). Learning to move machines with the mind. *Trends Neurosci.* 34, 61–75. doi: 10.1016/j.tins.2010.11.003

Harris, K. D. (2005). Neural signatures of cell assembly organization. *Nat. Rev. Neurosci.* 6, 399–407. doi: 10.1038/nrn1669

Hatsopoulos, N. G., and Donoghue, J. P. (2009). The science of neural interface systems. *Annu. Rev. Neurosci.* 32, 249–266. doi: 10.1146/annurev.neuro.051508.135241

Hebb, D. O. (1949). *The Organization of Behavior—A Neuropsychological Theory.* New York: Wiley.

Herrmann, C. S., Frund, I., and Lenz, D. (2010). Human gamma-band activity: a review on cognitive and behavioral correlates and network models. *Neurosci. Biobehav. Rev.* 34, 981–992. doi: 10.1016/j.neubiorev.2009.09.001

Hochberg, L. R., Serruya, M. D., Friehs, G. M., Mukand, J. A., Saleh, M., Caplan, A. H., et al. (2006). Neuronal ensemble control of prosthetic devices by a human with tetraplegia. *Nature* 442, 164–171. doi: 10.1038/nature04970

Jackson, A., Mavoori, J., and Fetz, E. E. (2006). Long-term motor cortex plasticity induced by an electronic neural implant. *Nature* 444, 56–60. doi: 10.1038/nature05226

John, E. R. (1980). "Multipotentiality: a statistical theory of brain function–evidence and implications" in *The Psychobiology of Consciousness*, ed D. Richard (New York: Springer), 129–146.

Keizer, A. W., Verment, R. S., and Hommel, B. (2010). Enhancing cognitive control through neurofeedback: a role of gamma-band activity in managing episodic retrieval. *Neuroimage* 49, 3404–3413. doi: 10.1016/j.neuroimage.2009.11.023

Kobayashi, S., Schultz, W., and Sakagami, M. (2010). Operant conditioning of primate prefrontal neurons. *J. Neurophysiol.* 103, 1843–1855. doi: 10.1152/jn.00173.2009

Koike, Y., Hirose, H., Sakurai, Y., and Iijima, T. (2006). Prediction of arm trajectory from a small number of neuron activities in the primary motor cortex. *Neurosci. Res.* 56, 146–153. doi: 10.1016/j.neures.2006.02.012

Koralek, A. C., Costa, R. M., and Carmena, J. M. (2013). Temporally precise cell-specific coherence develops in corticostriatal networks during learning. *Neuron* 79, 865–872. doi: 10.1016/j.neuron.2013.06.047

Koralek, A. C., Jin, X., Long, J. D. II., Costa, R. M., and Carmena, J. M. (2012). Corticostriatal plasticity is necessary for learning intentional neuroprosthetic skills. *Nature* 483, 331–335. doi: 10.1038/nature10845

Lebedev, M. A., and Nicolelis, M. A. L. (2006). Brain-machine interfaces: past, present and future. *Trends Neurosci.* 29, 536–546. doi: 10.1016/j.tins.2006.07.004

Lewicki, M. (1994). Bayesian modelling and classification of neural signals. *Neural Comput.* 6, 1005–1030. doi: 10.1162/neco.1994.6.5.1005

Lopes-dos-Santos, V., Conde-Ocazionez, S., Nicolelis, M. L., Ribeiro, S. T., and Tort, A. B. L. (2011). Neuronal assembly detection and cell membership specification by principal component analysis. *PLoS One* 6:e20996. doi: 10.1371/journal.pone.0020996

Mavoori, J., Jackson, A., Diorio, C., and Fetz, E. (2005). An autonomous implantable computer for neural recording and stimulation in unrestrained primates. *J. Neurosci. Meth.* 148, 71–77. doi: 10.1016/j.jneumeth.2005.04.017

Moritz, C. T., Perimutter, S. I., and Fetz, E. E. (2008). Direct control of paralysed muscles by cortical neurons. *Nature* 456, 639–642. doi: 10.1038/nature 07418

Murthy, V. N., and Fetz, E. E. (1996). Oscillatory activity in sensorimotor cortex of awake monkeys: synchronization of local field potentials and relation to behaviour. *J. Neurophysiol.* 76, 3949–3967.

Nicolelis, M. A. L., and Lebedev, M. A. (2009). Principles of neural ensemble physiology underlying the operation of brain-machine interfaces. *Nat. Rev. Neurosci.* 10, 530–540. doi: 10.1038/nrn2653

Olds, J. (1965). Operant conditioning of single unit responses. *Excerpta. Med. Int. Cong. Ser.* 87, 372–380.

Opris, I., Fuqua, J. L., Huettl, P. F., Gerhardt, G. A., Berger, T. W., Hampson, R. E., et al. (2012a). Closing the loop in primate prefrontal cortex: inter-laminar processing. *Front. Neural Circuits* 6:88. doi: 10.3389/fncir.2012. 00088

Opris, I., Hampson, R. E., Gerhardt, G. A., Berger, T. W., and Deadwyler, S. A. (2012b). Columnar processing in primate pFC: evidence for executive control microcircuits. *J. Cog. Neurosci.* 24, 2334–2347. doi: 10.1162/jocn_a_00307

Opris, I., Hampson, R. E., Stanford, T. R., Gerhardt, G. A., and Deadwyler, S. A. (2011a). Neural activity in frontal cortical cell layers: evidence for columnar sensorimotor processing. *J. Cog. Neursci.* 23, 1507–1521. doi: 10.1162/jocn.2010. 21534

Opris, I., Lebedev, M., and Nelson, R. (2011b). Motor planning under unpredictable reward: modulations of movement vigor and primate striatum activity. *Front. Neurosci.* 5:61. doi: 10.3389/fnins.2011.00061

Opris, I., Santos, L., Gerhardt, G. A., Song, D., Berger, T. W., Hampson, R. E., et al. (2013). Prefrontal cortical microcircuits bind perception to executive control. *Sci. Rep.* 3:2285. doi: 10.1038/srep02285

Peyrache, A., Khamassi, M., Benchenane, K., Wiener, S. I., and Battaglia, F. P. (2009). Replay of rule-learning related neural patterns in the prefrontal cortex during sleep. *Nat. Neurosci.* 12, 919–926. doi: 10.1038/nn.2337

Pipa, G., and Munk, M. H. (2011). Higher order spike synchrony in prefrontal cortex during visual memory. *Front. Comput. Neurosci.* 5:23. doi: 10.3389/fncom. 2011.00023

Raskin, S. A. (2011). *Neuroplasticity and Rehabilitation.* New York: Guilford.

Reynolds, G. S. (1975). *A Primer of Operant Conditioning.* Glenview: Scott Foresman.

Riehle, A., Grün, S., Diesmann, M., and Aertsen, A. (1997). Spike synchronization and rate modulation differentially involved in motor cortical function. *Science* 278, 1950–1953. doi: 10.1126/science.278.5345.1950

Sakurai, Y. (1993). Dependence of functional synaptic connections of hippocampal and neocortical neurons on types of memory. *Neurosci. Lett.* 158, 181–184. doi: 10.1016/0304-3940(93)90259-n

Sakurai, Y. (1994). Involvement of auditory cortical and hippocampal neurons in auditory working memory and reference memory in the rat. *J. Neurosci.* 14, 2606–2623.

Sakurai, Y. (1996a). Hippocampal and neocortical cell assemblies encode memory processes for different types of stimuli in the rat. *J. Neurosci.* 16, 2809–2819.

Sakurai, Y. (1996b). Population coding by cell assemblies—what it really is in the brain. *Neurosci. Res.* 26, 1–16. doi: 10.1016/0168-0102(96)01075-9

Sakurai, Y. (1999). How do cell assemblies encode information in the brain? *Neurosci. Biobehav. Rev.* 23, 785–796. doi: 10.1016/s0149-7634(99)00017-2

Sakurai, Y. (2002). Coding of auditory temporal and pitch information by hippocampal individual cells and cell assemblies in the rat. *Neurosci.* 115, 1153–1163. doi: 10.1016/s0306-4522(02)00509-2

Sakurai, Y., and Takahashi, S. (2006). Dynamic synchrony of firing in the monkey prefrontal cortex during working memory tasks. *J. Neurosci.* 26, 10141–10153. doi: 10.1523/jneurosci.2423-06.2006

Sakurai, Y., and Takahashi, S. (2008). Dynamic synchrony of local cell assembly. *Rev. Neurosci.* 19, 425–440. doi 10.1515/revneuro.2008.19.6.425

Sakurai, Y., and Takahashi, S. (2013). Conditioned enhancement of firing rates and synchrony of hippocampal neurons and firing rates of motor cortical neurons in rats. *Eur. J. Neurosci.* 37, 623–639. doi: 10.1111/ejn.12070

Sakurai, Y., Nakazono, T., Ishino, S., Terada, S., Yamaguchi, K., and Takahashi, S. (2013). Diverse synchrony of firing reflects diverse cell-assembly coding in the prefrontal cortex. *J. Physiol. Paris* 107, 459–470. doi: 10.1016/j.jphysparis.2013. 05.004

Salinas, E., and Sejnowski, T. J. (2001). Correlated neuronal activity and the flow of neural information. *Nat. Rev. Neurosci.* 2, 539–550. doi: 10.1038/35086012

Schmied, A., Ivarsson, C., and Fetz, E. E. (1993). Short-term synchronization of motor units in human extensor digitorum communis muscle: relation to contractile properties and voluntary control. *Exp. Brain Res.* 97, 159–172. doi: 10.1007/bf00228826

Seidemann, E., Meilijson, I., Abeles, M., Bergman, H., and Vaadia, E. (1996). Simultaneously recorded single units in the frontal cortex go through a sequence of discrete and stable states in monkeys performing a delayed localization task. *J. Neurosci.* 16, 752–768.

Siegel, M., Donner, T. H., and Engel, A. K. (2012). Spectral fingerprints of large-scale neuronal interactions. *Nat. Rev. Neurosci.* 13, 121–134. doi: 10. 1038/nrn3137

Skinner, B. F. (1974). *About Behaviorism.* New York: Alfred A. Knopf.

Takahashi, S., and Sakurai, Y. (2005). Real-time and automatic sorting of multineuronal activity for sub-millisecond interactions in vivo. *Neurosci.* 134, 301–315. doi: 10.1016/j.neuroscience.2005.03.031

Takahashi, S., and Sakurai, Y. (2007). Coding of spatial information by soma and dendrite of pyramidal cells in the hippocampal CA1 of behaving rats. *Eur. J. Neurosci.* 26, 2033–2045. doi: 10.1111/j.1460-9568.2007.05827.x

Takahashi, S., and Sakurai, Y. (2009a). Information in small neuronal ensemble activity in the hippocampal CA1 during delayed non-matching to sample performance in rats. *BMC Neurosci.* 10:115. doi: 10.1186/1471-2202-10-115

Takahashi, S., and Sakurai, Y. (2009b). Sub-millisecond firing synchrony of closely neighboring pyramidal neurons in hippocampal CA1 of rats during delayed non-matching to sample task. *Front. Neural Circuits* 3:9. doi: 10.3389/neuro.04. 009.2009

Takahashi, S., Anzai, Y., and Sakurai, Y. (2003a). Automatic sorting for multi-neuronal activity recorded with tetrodes in the presence of overlapping spikes. *J. Neurophysiol.* 89, 2245–2258. doi: 10.1152/jn.00827.2002

Takahashi, S., Anzai, Y., and Sakurai, Y. (2003b). New approach to spike sorting for multi-neuronal activities recorded with a tetrode—how ICA can be practical. *Neurosci. Res.* 46, 265–272. doi: 10.1016/s0168-0102(03)00103-2

Taylor, D. M., Tillery, S. I., and Schwartz, A. B. (2002). Direct cortical control of 3D neuroprosthetic devices. *Science* 296, 1829–1832. doi: 10.1126/science.107 0291

Terada, S., Takahashi, S., and Sakurai, Y. (2013). Oscillatory interaction between amygdala and hippocampus coordinates behavioral modulation based on reward expectation. *Front. Behav. Neurosci.* 7:177. doi: 10.3389/fnbeh.2013. 00177

Vaadia, E., Haalman, I., Abeles, M., Bergman, H., Prut, Y., Slovin, H., et al. (1995). Dynamics of neuronal interactions in monkey cortex in relation to behavioural events. *Nature* 373, 515–518. doi: 10.1038/373515a0

Wessberg, J., Stambaugh, C. R., Kralik, J. D., Beck, P. D., Laubach, M., Chapin, J. K., et al. (2000). Real-time prediction of hand trajectory by ensembles of cortical neurons in primates. *Nature* 408, 361–365. doi: 10.1038/35042582

Wyler, A. R., Burchiel, K. J., and Robbins, C. A. (1979). Operant control of precentral neurons in monkeys: evidence against open loop control. *Brain Res.* 171, 29–39.

Zacksenhouse, M., Lebedev, M. A., Carmena, J. M., O'Doherty, J. E., Henriquez, C., and Nicolelis, M. A. L. (2007). Cortical modulations increase in early sessions with brain-machine interface. *PLoS One* 2:e629. doi: 10.1371/journal.pone. 0000619

24

Cognitive enhancement kept within contexts: neuroethics and informed public policy

John R. Shook[1], Lucia Galvagni[2] and James Giordano[3,4]*

[1] Philosophy Department and Graduate School of Education, University at Buffalo, Buffalo, NY, USA
[2] Bruno Kessler Foundation, Trento, Italy
[3] Neuroethics Studies Program, Pellegrino Center for Clinical Bioethics and Department of Neurology, Georgetown University Medical Center, Washington, DC, USA
[4] Human Science Center, Ludwig-Maximilians Universität, Munich, Germany

Edited by:
Manuel Casanova, University of Louisville, USA

Reviewed by:
Gary N. Garcia-Molina, Philips Research North America, USA
Markus Christen, University of Zurich, Switzerland

***Correspondence:**
James Giordano, Neuroethics Studies Program, Pellegrino Center for Clinical Bioethics and Department of Neurology, Georgetown University Medical Center, 4000 Reservoir Road, Washington, DC 20057, USA
e-mail: jg353@georgetown.edu

Neurothics has far greater responsibilities than merely noting potential human enhancements arriving from novel brain-centered biotechnologies and tracking their implications for ethics and civic life. Neuroethics must utilize the best cognitive and neuroscientific knowledge to shape incisive discussions about what could possibly count as enhancement in the first place, and what should count as genuinely "cognitive" enhancement. Where cognitive processing and the mental life is concerned, the lived context of psychological performance is paramount. Starting with an enhancement to the mental abilities of an individual, only performances on real-world exercises can determine what has actually been cognitively improved. And what can concretely counts as some specific sort of cognitive improvement is largely determined by the classificatory frameworks of cultures, not brain scans or laboratory experiments. Additionally, where the public must ultimately evaluate and judge the worthiness of individual performance enhancements, we mustn't presume that public approval towards enhancers will somehow automatically arrive without due regard to civic ideals such as the common good or social justice. In the absence of any nuanced appreciation for the control which performance contexts and public contexts exert over what "cognitive" enhancements could actually be, enthusiastic promoters of cognitive enhancement can all too easily depict safe and effective brain modifications as surely good for us and for society. These enthusiasts are not unaware of oft-heard observations about serious hurdles for reliable enhancement from neurophysiological modifications. Yet those observations are far more common than penetrating investigations into the implications to those hurdles for a sound public understanding of cognitive enhancement, and a wise policy review over cognitive enhancement. We offer some crucial recommendations for undertaking such investigations, so that cognitive enhancers that truly deserve public approval can be better identified.

Keywords: ethics, neuroethics, cognitive science, neuroscience, cognitive enhancement, culture, public policy

In its disciplinary stance and practice, neuroethics acknowledges the most sufficiently confirmed theories of the neural and cognitive sciences as (provisionally) accurate in an overriding manner. Indeed, neuroethics should not ignore or set aside such theories if/when these prove to be inconvenient for, or incompatible with, practical applications, principled values, private intuitions, or popular common sense. Nor should these theories be muted when neuroethical engagement of real-world issues, questions and problems are needed. The actual functions of the brain, as best as can be described at present, is—and must remain—fundamental to any and all neuroethical discourse and deliberations.

In light of this, we argue that neuroethical inquiries into cognitive enhancement should establish the crucial role for context, especially socio-cultural contexts to conceptions of the "cognitive", so as to better define the realities of neuroethical debates about cognitive performance enhancement (and enhancers). We write in support of investigations into putative neuro-enhancers which adopt the theoretical stance that hoped-for improvements cannot be evaluated in isolation from human activities that provide the meaningful context to any alteration in performance. At key points of our argument we appeal to empirical studies examining performance alterations, to exemplify our concern for due attentiveness to real-world situational conduct as possible enhancers are tested and utilized. Where relevant contexts to neuroscientific inquiry and information utilized for normative purposes are taken seriously, the work of formulating and guiding neuroethical quandaries would be appreciably strengthened.

With our argument for this role of context established, we then outline crucial policy considerations regarding neuro-cognitive enhancement, and raise some warnings about over-eager advocacy for enhancement. While remaining cautiously optimistic toward opportunities for cognitive enhancement, we insist upon fostering public understanding of the issues, and upon development of sound public policy. In this way we join the ranks of other neuroethicists who have voiced similar views and concerns (Illes and Bird, 2006; Levy, 2011; Farah, 2012; Gunson, 2012; Fitz et al., 2014; Maslen et al., 2014b; Racine et al., 2014).

As a discipline and set of practices, neuroethics must utilize the best cognitive and neuroscientific knowledge to shape incisive discussions about what could possibly count as enhancement in the first place, and what should count as genuinely "cognitive" enhancement. Where cognitive processing and mental life is concerned, the lived context of psychological performance is paramount. In the absence of any nuanced appreciation for the control which performance contexts and public contexts exert over what "cognitive" enhancement could actually be, enthusiastic promoters of cognitive enhancement can all too easily depict brain modifications as being good for individuals and for society. Such claims are not unaware of serious hurdles—hurdles noted in oft-heard observations and express concerns—that may impede enhancement derived from neurophysiological modifications. Yet those observations are far more common than penetrating investigations into the implications that such hurdles may evoke—both for the sound public understanding of cognitive enhancement, and for wisely informing policy to guide and govern cognitive enhancement. To wit, we offer what we maintain to be crucial recommendations for undertaking such investigations, so as to better identify cognitive enhancers that truly deserve public approval and policy support.

Civics and general ethics can be idealistic, but neuroethics should not be unrealistic, and must be liberated from ethical theorizing done in ignorance of the most contemporary understanding of the structure and function of the brain. In this way, neuroethics must strive to comprehend the genuine basis of conceptions of self, society, and morality, and rely on changes or replacements to those conceptions when and where scientifically warranted (Shook and Giordano, 2014).

ENHANCEMENT STANDARDS

Bioethicist Thomas Murray identifies two primary meanings to the term "enhancement": first, "to advance, augment, elevate, heighten, increase"; and second, "to increase the worth or value of." (Murray, 2007) In both definitions, context is axiomatic. Numerous scholars have similarly noted the "metric" and "normative" dimensions of this term. For an organism such as a human being, enhancement implies opportunities to improve capacities or abilities—features that can be simultaneously measurable and valuable, and possibly moral, as well. Structure and function cooperate and even interfuse, even as they have distinct implications for ethicality, and this can confuse discussions of enhancement, in general, and of "cognitive enhancement" more specifically.

Hence, it is important to ask whether a particular modification is responsible for altered performance of a specified task. If it is, then that physiological modification is a *performance modifier*, and if that change is regarded as positive relative to some normative standard, then we can refer to it as a *performance improver*. Furthermore, if we call a particular activity an "intellectual" task, then we are really talking about an *intellectual enhancement* for performing that task. This physiological modification may be labeled as an "intellectual enhancement" in an easy, colloquial manner of speaking, although at this point in the description, a scientific understanding of the brain or intellectual capacities is not yet involved.

In light of that science, however, it can no longer be enough to simply track cognitive functions and the resulting performance on particular tasks to verify enhancers. An alteration to a physiological process associated with cognition can be measured and compared against some organic standard. Has enhancement occurred? It is still too soon to say; a pre-set physiological standard is never simply a "given" normative standard. Detecting a physiological alteration within an individual requires an individual-relative standard against which to measure that alteration, to be sure. But what may be expected from one person needn't expected from others. Setting someone's neurological functioning as the standard for any human brain's "normal" functioning, so that a baseline for cognitive functioning can be established in preparation for detecting cognitive improvement done to anyone, is quite another normative decision. One that normality standard is put in place, then actual cognitive function (for the processing and integration of various types of sensations, memories, emotions, subconscious valuations, and so on) can be estimated and compared against some standard of normality. Even after this has been done, it still may be premature to say whether or not the evoked changes represent an enhancement; reliable cognitive performance (for one's overall management of life activities and achievements) must be judged in light of some *ethical* standard. Just as human-normal performance can't be reduced to any single individual's functioning, ethically responsible enhancement cannot be reduced to any superiority over what has been conventionally set as generically normal for "average" humans.

Standards at the three levels of individual physiology, human-generic normality, and sensible ethicality all compete for prominence where definitions of "enhancement" are concerned. Furthermore, it doesn't help that the complexities of the nervous system can permit odd scenarios in which an increase in physiological function(s) might diminish cognitive ability; and diminishing a specific type of cognitive function might be conducive to optimizing a person's actions or general well-being (Earp et al., 2014). Rigidly demanding only one standard, or one direction by that standard, with which to dictate enhancement is a stubborn path to take, and one that we assert any rational approach to neuroethical analysis and discourse should avoid.

Letting the concept or term "enhancement" stand for any non-therapeutic benefits conferred by an intervention is a common way to avoid taking any (if not all three) standards seriously. Does enhancement begin when a medical treatment exceeds the usual dosage or typical extent of repair? Perhaps enhancement refers to those instances where treatment yields physiological functioning beyond the normal range. Or, enhancement might entail evoking superior performance that lends distinct advantages to life. Arguing over these options overlooks the mistake that enhancement can begin where therapy ends. It is a mistake that is easy to make.

Therapeutic medicine simplifies its standards because it takes all of humanity to be its proper field of work; a good treatment for a health deficiency generically helps any patient suffering from that problem. So long as the reference class remains "humanity," then a physiological "average" functioning can be equated with generic normality, and there would only be "disease treatments" (aiming towards normality) and "enhancement treatments" (aiming beyond normality). However, patients aren't so generic in the real world. Broad culture and local society are contexts that always exert influence.

For example, what can count as normality and abnormality within a particular culture might not obtain for all of humanity too. But, if that culture's influence (viz.—power) is sufficiently strong, clinicians, patients, publics and governing bodies might not necessarily notice, or care (or feel empowered to act even if they did). Furthermore, any social group within that culture could come to regard itself as the proper reference class, expressly if that group enjoys some status and/or privilege. When that social group requests medical treatment, it is set in terms of what counts as "group normal" rather than just "culturally normal" or "normal for humanity." For example, when middle-aged privileged men take their reference class as "adult men like us", they surely aren't thinking about "all human males on the planet between the ages of 18 and 80." Nor are they taking their reference class to be people very much like them, such as "successful men between 45 and 65." Instead, what counts as "normality" is the reference class that these men desire to be, perhaps something like "healthy guys in their 30s-50s." So, in effect they want what counts as "subgroup optimal." Growing approval among a subgroup about using a drug or device off-label lends credence towards that intervention's status as an "enhancer", even if that subgroup expects more than just intellectual performance (Hildt et al., 2014; Wade et al., 2014). Interventions can transition from enhancers back to treatments, as well. If a culture's medicine proves willing, then treatment for achieving subgroup optimality could be labeled as medical "therapy", rather than enhancement.

Neuroethics must take close notice of: (1) the kinds of standards applied for determining enhancement; (2) the chosen reference class serving as the background against which enhancement would stand out; and (3) the selection of "normality" or "optimality" as the envisioned goal to enhancement. Medicine's traditional focus on generic remedies for universal application to all humanity is not the best (or perhaps even a viable) framework for identifying and classifying enhancements. Cultural inheritance, group socialization, personal values, and physiological factors are each and all necessarily involved when defining and addressing enhancement. The advent of "personalized" medicine aiming towards the individualization of diagnostics and treatments should raise awareness across neuroethics that specifics will matter to ever greater degrees in the future.

ENHANCING COGNITION IN CONTEXT

The temptation to regard cognition as an entirely neurophysiological matter, amenable to objective study, definition, and measurement, isn't just a symptom of overreaching reductionism or scientism. Frustration with too much context can set in for anyone reconciled to cognition's reliance on brain functioning. If cognition is, in some sense, objectively present as subjects undergo experimental study, then it could be objectively modified. Researchers would be able to determine when and how cognition is improved when compared against some preset standard of cognitive ability. Serious attention to cognitive enhancement came to the fore as a consequence of experimental facilitation of cognitive ability, with due caution leveraged against exaggerated claims of capability, meaning and utility. (Metzinger and Hildt, 2011; Sahakian and Morein-Zamir, 2011; Sandberg, 2011; Chatterjee, 2013; Cohen Kadosh, 2013; Hildt and Franke, 2013). Hard lessons learned from pharmaceutical studies apply to any sort of performance effects produced by alteration of brain structure and function (Luber, 2014).

Neuroethical attention must be paid to wider contexts of neurological manipulation, beyond the fairly objective and narrow ways that cognitive performances can be adjusted in desired directions. Determining if a neurological intervention can actually produce a desired enhancement is one thing; ascertaining that some sort of adjustment is truly cognitive (in the expected manner) is quite another, and these distinctions deserve priority. Imitating medicine's quest for therapies that have universal utility for anyone suffering from a generic health problem is no longer a wise undertaking for the application of 21st century biomedical advancements. As well, we maintain that it is equally unwise to promote enhancements as if they could be universally beneficial for generic cognitive improvements to anyone's intellectual performances. Indeed, we argue that there may not be such a thing as a "generic enhancement to cognitive performance." A major reason for this involves cultural contexts. Two people from two different cultures, or even two people from two subgroups of the same culture, may not necessarily agree on what is cognitively adjusted by some alteration of neurological function. Thus, neuroethical inquiry cannot avoid an interpretative circle: some group of people ascribe a "function" to a cognitive process in service of a task that is considered to be "normal"—but this is a social imposition of normality on a neurophysiological process. In this way, performance, not neurophysiology in isolation, decides functionality, and what counts as "normal".

For illustration, consider an analogy: suppose a practical way to increase muscle mass (without deleterious side effects) is offered as a general "athletic enhancer" that could be used by anyone. Athleticism depends on one's musculature, surely, so given this rationalization, more muscle should enable more athleticism. But muscle mass alone does not equate with athletic ability (or in some cases even potential ability!) For example, one can take anabolic-androgenic steroids (AAS) to augment muscle mass. As matter of fact, these very likely will lend something of an "edge" to (important) dispositions and characteristics necessary for improved athletic performance (i.e.,—muscle size and strength; Llewellyn, 2010). However, the underlying premise is that the agent is increasing specific qualities of muscle (e.g.,—diameter of muscle fibers, contractile force, etc.) that have been shown to be operative in a number of athletic events.

Herein though, are important caveats. While an AAS may yield mass and strength gains, these are only preparatory for "training effects", because an athlete must still train for a particular sport. AAS can facilitate that training, but if training is conducted improperly, less success at a sport is a likely result. Furthermore, different physiological agents can elicit distinct effects. Some will enable gains in muscle mass but not necessarily facilitate definition; others will be more lipolytic, and produce lean, muscular density, but will not greatly increase mass, and so forth. Also, AAS does little for aerobic endurance *per se*, just as an endurance-facilitating agent (such as erythropoietin, EPO) does little for mass or strength. (consult Llewellyn, 2010). The adage is: The right agent for the right effect.

These points account for the ample evidence—and practical wisdom—indicating that if one wants to become proficient in a particular sport, then it is necessary to vigorously train in that sport. There are generic athletic training exercises, but each sport must evaluate their utility. For example, cross training can lend overall benefits to components of athleticism, but it doesn't necessarily permit direct performance gains peculiar to each sport. Only after specific kinds of athletic performances, and the individual athletes performing them, are identified and targeted, would an intervention be intelligently developed and employed to exert positive effect(s) within selected contexts. Expanding upon this example of sports performance, we may expect that most types of neurological interventions intended for the enhancement of performances displaying much complexity may only work best in conjunction with cognitive training regimens. Not only must any trials confirming a modification for cognitive improvement involve successful routine practice under controlled conditions, only implementing that modification in conjunction with strenuous performance training result in the practical enhancements to performances actually valued outside of any laboratory.

More generally, it is naïve to suppose that a compensatory adjustment, much less an enhancing adjustment, could be generically assigned validity across all of humanity. Even best-case scenarios must remain stubbornly diffuse. Calling a performance test a "cognitive performance test" and observing that individuals who are subjected to intervention "x" perform better doesn't mean that some purely cognitive functioning has been isolated and targeted as the improved factor. Fortunately, careful research is hardly so naïve, as recent exemplars have noted (Pringle et al., 2013). The lesson is that no one pondering cognitive enhancement should assume that higher cognition can occur in some "pure" forms, no matter how specific the task. To begin with, multiple affective and motor processes are interfused with the functional components that are operative in executive control. In turn, executive control is interfused with every sophisticated practice acquired during childhood and adolescence. This is especially the case when dealing with higher cognition manifesting in social and moral behaviors (Shook, 2012; Specker et al., 2014).

Enculturalization takes advantage of advanced executive control for instilling specialized task performances, such as learning mathematics and logic. It is no paradox that the more cognitively abstract the task, the more it has a cultural rather than a purely biological basis; hence such tasks are very much subject to the vagaries of cultural history and practice. Something as simple as conceptualizing number and amount has been shown to be culturally variant (Núñez, 2011). Similarly, memory performance has been shown to be culture-dependent and -influenced (Gutchess et al., 2011; Hewer and Roberts, 2012). Cultures contribute to cognition as much as cognition contributes to culture (Han and Pöppel, 2011; Ishii, 2013; Kim and Sasaki, 2014). Even context is contextual as far as cognition is concerned, since the developing sensitivity towards, and responsiveness to, environing interpersonal context displays cultural variability (Imada et al., 2013).

The contextual factors raised here are not posed to endorse a thorough relativism or dismissive eliminativism about potential enhancers. Cognitive enhancement can be quite real, when and where it is created. To be sure, confirmable cognitive enhancements can be achieved because improved cognitive (i.e.,—intellectual and/or emotional) performances by selected and trained participants can be measured under controlled conditions. Generally speaking, under sufficiently similar conditions, similarly altered people having enough in common will perform similarly, all other things being equal. What more could be expected from science?

ENHANCEMENT IN PUBLIC CONTEXTS

Desires to "improve the human condition" conjure proposals for a proverbial "rising tide" of neuroscientific and neurotechnological modifications that will "raise all boats"—and brains. But when realistically looking ahead, unavoidable questions loom: How much can humans be enhanced without deforming or destroying aspects of the social or natural world on which life relies? and, Will human character and moral progress be sustained if hopes for enhancement become realized? Some have supported a duty to urge enhancers and even intervene with required enhancement, once we can apply a safe and effective intervention. However, our comprehension of long-term consequences is limited, and encouraging (what may be long-lasting) modifications without ensuring equally durable individual welfare is reckless (Rossi et al., 2013).

Shall the position of the responsible individual prevail instead? Letting individuals choose for themselves is no less reckless. Even when individual benefits can be guaranteed, it must be asked: who should receive them? The answer, "All who can benefit," is no answer at all, because it will not be the case that everyone will have the same, or even similar, access at the same time. Differential access is inevitable in a world of finite time and resources. Such differential access is *prima facie* unjust, as those who already possess certain traits, attributes, and/or resources will likely and quickly get even more. Hence, essential concerns for distributive justice arise from the position of society at large. The distribution of improved health and lifestyle status, and even improved moral status, will always be a social concern (Buchanan, 2011; Douglas, 2013).

Worries over distribution cannot—nor should not—be easily dispelled. Those with the least assets are those most unlikely to get access to state-of-the-art scientific and technological interventions. It is unrealistic to assume that some massive shift in the social architectonics of medical resource allocation will occur so as to allow neuroscience and neurotechnology to close the gap between those who "have" and those who "have not." Given this reality, does everyone really want a society where the people getting the most enhancement(s) are precisely those enjoying great wealth? The prospect of cognitive enhancement surely highlights this worry: intelligence does what character directs, and the kinds of characters getting so wealthy in a society may not be the people to be trusted with even more intelligence—and power. Proponents of unlimited access to enhancement simply point the way toward an unbalanced distributive scheme. Contests between rival distribution methods can be debated in ethics, but they get adjudicated in politics.

Hence, entering the realm of politics becomes unavoidable. The politics surrounding access to enhancement will be intense. Of equal importance is the temptation to use brain science within agendas of political power to control fundamentally biological aspects of individuals' and communities' existence (invoking what Foucault referred to as biopolitics; see Foucault, 2008; Anderson et al., 2012). Bioethical and neuroethical analyses cannot avoid addressing science as a public good; ethics as a search for the good and the right; and politics as the participation of citizens in decisions about the guidance of public order. As public debate over the impact(s) of enhancement interventions accelerates, the search for principled guidelines has ensued, and neuroethics has become ever more involved (Bostrom and Sandberg, 2009).

Irrespective of whether enhancement is regarded as a bountiful cornucopia or a ticking bomb, the differing contexts of enhancement radically transform its biopolitical status. Recall from a previous section our attention to the choice among physiology, normality, and ethical standards for identifying what counts as enhancement. Experimental medical research focusing upon physiological alterations (typically) emphasizes interventions for those who are the most unhealthy. Policy tends to approve funding for basic research if and when it could soon help those with the most severe, and/or epidemiologically extensive, health conditions. These prioritizations wouldn't work in the realm of enhancement for three reasons. First, a traditional approach to funding and engaging research would tend to leave most enhancements on the theoretical drawing board. Second, while there may be desires for expensive advanced research into fundamental neurological mechanisms that can be targeted for cognitive performance enhancement, unless these approaches can be ascribed to incur some "therapeutic" benefit against an identified disease, disorder or (medical) condition, financial and administrative support for broad scale research and translation of outcomes and products would tend to be lacking. Third, while there may be a viable—and perhaps growing—market for certain cognitive performance enhancements, it is difficult to generate the funding necessary to support and sustain exploratory research required for translation to safe commercial technologies (unless developed and marketed as "non-medical" products such as toys and games, which then raises the specter of inapt and/or unsound development, distribution and use; see, for example, Giordano and DuRousseau, 2011; and Plischke et al., 2011).

A related issue is the contemporary medical endorsement of interventions that restore or sustain "normality." Explicitly and implicitly this position conforms to socio-cultural requirements that all people should seek and exhibit "normal" functioning, rather than (what is regarded to be) abnormal or anti-social conduct that deviates from socially established standards. What posture should be assumed when (a) certain people seek optimal functioning in pursuit of what they personally deem as the apex of the good life, and/or (b) society sets requirements that individuals in special roles (such as physicians, pilots, peace officers, or warfighters) must attain some level of optimal functioning? (Giordano et al., 2013; Goold and Maslen, 2014) Medicine's laudable work in service of living a good life isn't automatically extendable to living a great life, or to achieving great performance in a socially-sanctioned service. Justifications for specialized enhancements for enabling idiosyncratic lifestyles or for extraordinary public service will not necessarily be obtained in and from medical principles.

A second set of examples arise from our earlier discussion of the cultural relativism inherent to the precise identification of cognitive improvements. Medicine's due caution with clinical application, watching carefully for deleterious health and lifestyle side-effects, relies upon cultural consensus about what constitutes "normal" performance in daily life (Gini et al., 2010). Those seeking significant enhancements, by contrast, won't be interested in conforming to cultural norms about ordinary performance, and medicine may not be able to restrain them. When the recipient of an enhancement is achieving extraordinary performance levels and feeling empowered to transgress cultural expectations in the name of greatness (despite the risks), what social institution or cultural tradition can and will reign-in their pursuits?

Evidently, society turns to law for such proscriptions. Yet, here it becomes necessary to ask how restrictions of, and prohibitions against certain types and extents of enhancement will be determined. Targeting concrete neurological modifications for legal bans (i.e.,—imitating medical bans of performance enhancing substances for professional athletes, and/or scheduling certain drugs) has the merit of objective verification. But this only spurs those seeking improved types of cognitive performance to find alternative physiological methods not yet banned or detectable, and the chase is begun anew.

POLICY PRIORITIES AND THE ROLE OF NEUROETHICS

Frustration over excessive contextualization is a perennial complaint. Simplifying matters can seem attractive when modest advances require prompt address and short-term priorities are within reach. Simplification would be possible if the construct and term "enhancement" satisfied defined and pragmatic scientific and ethical criteria. That way, any continued debate would be centered on those improvements that were already deemed to be fairly good for people in general, so far as could be scientifically and ethically determined. Warnings are certainly in order that current enhancement interventions rarely prove to be wholly effective or without deleterious effects. Unsurprisingly, wide agreement among scientific, ethics, and policy communities can be found on the view that enhancing interventions shouldn't be counterproductive or harmful to overall health.

However, we posit that practical risk-benefit analyses aren't entirely sufficient. Detailed ethical scrutiny is required before any such practical improvements can be classified as good enhancers. It is wise to demand that putatively enhancing interventions do not diminish self-control or autonomy, degrade personal growth or self-worth, or diminish life-management and social skills (de Melo-Martín, 2010; Allhoff et al., 2011). These demands can be reasonably placed upon envisioned enhancements, even if they aren't applied so stringently to proven medical therapies. Improvements towards health are usually consistent with personal empowerment, and the consequences of restoring normal functioning are largely understood. By contrast, the longer term effects of experimental enhancements, especially cognitive performance enhancements, on the psychological self and internal self-conceptions and motivations are among the least predictable and understood aspects of this issue. Ethics is rightly concerned about the vital capacities for autonomy, dignity, and morality. All the same, as we have noted, setting high standards for cognitive performance enhancing interventions need not cast dark suspicions upon the persistent search for, and studies of enhancements. A number of scholars have advocated for practical and ethical standards while endorsing the pursuit of enhancement (including Buchanan, 2011; Glannon, 2011; Giordano, 2012; Heinrichs, 2012; Clark, 2014; Maslen et al., 2014a). In short, the goal is to develop helpful interventions able to meet these high standards.

If such normative thresholds are maintained, public and regulatory approval could be a helpfully expedited matter. But approval may not be automatic. Labeling an intervention as an "enhancement" once it makes individual lives demonstrably better can't be the final hurdle before regulatory approval (Giordano and DuRousseau, 2011). One further—and arguably major factor—that cannot be omitted is the wider public context. We believe that this is where the broadest and deepest deliberations over the wisdom of enhancement should occur. We are forced to ponder what shall be done when sound public priorities cannot automatically approve genuinely ethical enhancements.

Policy principles should be well informed, ethical, and just. When some reliable enhancements are deemed safe and effective, and seem capable of promoting the good life, why wouldn't they be approved through policy and law? Here, it is important to appreciate that sincere advocacy of genuine individual enhancers could still be under-informed, potentially unethical, and possibly unjust. In those cases, public wisdom should lean against approval.

In this regard, two issues must remain distinct: First, it must be asked, and determined, if an intervention is a genuine enhancer. Second, if it is, then it must be asked if this enhancer is something that sound policy can approve and sanction. The criteria by which an enhancement is deemed conducive for the "good life" cannot be the same criteria that are used to determine whether to approve it. In the open space of public deliberation, it must be possible that sound policy can proscribe or prevent something that is presently understood to be reliably conducive to the "good life".

Here we avoid assumptions that knowing what is conducive to the good life for each person constitutes knowing what is ethical and wise. We also avoid the position that knowledge about what is conducive to the "good life" for everyone constitutes knowing what is ethical and wise. Rather, we posit an alternative stance. We argue that (1) well-informed policy would use more information than just the scientific facts about a performance enhancer promoting the "good life"; (2) ethical policy would use other ethical criteria beside simple promotion of the "good life" (individually or collectively); and (3) just policy may prefer a stable and well-ordered society that isn't advancing the individual or collective "good life" quite as fast as could be technologically possible (or imagined by technophiles).

Gazing upon the stance we propose, eager advocates of enhancement might ask why objective scientific facts couldn't or shouldn't lead the way, especially when cognitive performance enhancement seems so modest, practical, and generically useful? In doing so, they appear to endorse the general ethical guideline that:

> *A sound policy decision will always approve what, in light of ascertainable scientific facts, can be expected to be an enhancement to an individual that is conducive to what "our society" regards as the "good life."*

This guideline does not represent our position; we deem it unwise and replete with confusions, and when it appears to be doing the real work behind hasty encouragements of cognitive performance enhancement, we deplore it. Whether this is the actual view of any bioethicist or neuroethicist, or just a caricature for academic target practice, we cannot really say, because few scholars have explicated their meta-ethical presumptions. We do assert, however, that this stance is inadequate to meet the urgent complexities and contextualities inherent to authentic human life as we all must actually live it. In fact, there is little that is genuinely neuroethical in it. Our call for a neuroethics that takes context seriously, especially where cognitive performance enhancement is the issue, isn't merely fodder for academic debate.

Sarewitz and Karas (2012) outline several different approaches that can be adopted in order to make choices and decisions about cognitive enhancing technologies. Among those, our view aligns with the "optimistic" approach, via engagement of a managed technological optimism that best represents our position as relevant to ethical decision-making processes and public policies in this field. We endorse continued research into cognitive performance enhancements. We also call for the need to optimize definitions of any/all concepts and terms, and to equally define the contexts in which any cognitive task optimization can/would occur. Only from that point can one be optimistic that a progressive, non-static concept of the human and human function will be realistically entertained and enhanced, both practically and ethically. This position takes a pluralistic, democratic approach towards options of emergent (rather than merely proscriptive) governance, and the final section of this essay points to ways that neuroethics can play a supportive role.

We posit that a contextualized neuroethical outlook allows for better-informed approaches, utilizing all relevant interdisciplinary input, for considering what therapies and enhancements could be. It permits neuroethical deliberation to rise above local conventionality and a single social ethos, to instead survey the rich cultural diversity of human self-understandings and dynamic cognitive capacities. And, it encourages neuroethics to render verdicts against destabilizing and unjust procedures in policy debates that rashly extend medical models beyond their proper functioning.

This neuroethics isn't proscriptive, nor does it seek to uniformly obstruct enhancement. In its naturalistic basis, it establishes grounds to view the human as engaging biology (through intellectual and physical tools) to optimize survival and flourishing in changing ecologies. And in its appreciation for the human as a bio-psychosocial organism it engenders an interdisciplinary approach (conjoining anthropology, sociology, economics, and political science) to depict and address ethical issues within the contexts in which human activities are conducted. Thus, in the spirit of cognitive enhancement itself, neuroethics as a discipline—and in its methods, approaches, and practices—should embody and enable greater human self-understanding, and improve our public deliberations over the many dimensions of life that we treasure.

ACKNOWLEDGMENTS

This work was supported in part by the Bruno Kessler Foundation, Trento, Italy (Lucia Galvagni); William H. and Ruth Crane Schaefer Endowment (James Giordano), and funding from the Pellegrino Center for Clinical Bioethics, Georgetown University Medical Center (Lucia Galvagni, James Giordano).

REFERENCES

Allhoff, F., Lin, P., and Steinberg, J. (2011). Ethics of human enhancement: an executive summary. *Sci. Eng. Ethics* 17, 201–212. doi: 10.1007/s11948-009-9191-9

Anderson, M., Fitz, N., and Howlader, D. (2012). "Neurotechnology research and the world stage: ethics, biopower and policy," in *Neurotechnology: Premises, Potential and Problems*, ed J. Giordano (Boca Raton, FL: CRC Press), 287–300.

Bostrom, N., and Sandberg, A. (2009). Cognitive enhancement: methods, ethics, regulatory challenges. *Sci. Eng. Ethics* 15, 311–341. doi: 10.1007/s11948-009-9142-5

Buchanan, A. (2011). *Beyond Humanity? The Ethics of Biomedical Enhancement.* Oxford: Oxford University Press.

Chatterjee, A. (2013). "The ethics of neuroenhancement," in *Ethical and Legal Issues in Neurology: Handbook of Clinical Neurology* (vol. 118), eds J. Bernat and R. Beresford (Amsterdam: Elsevier), 323–334.

Clark, V. P. (2014). The ethical, moral and pragmatic rationale for brain augmentation. *Front. Syst. Neurosci.* 8:130. doi: 10.3389/fnsys.2014.00130

Cohen Kadosh, R. ed. (2013). *The Stimulated Brain: Cognitive Enhancement Using Non- Invasive Brain Stimulation.* Amsterdam: Elsevier.

de Melo-Martín, I. (2010). Defending human enhancement technologies: unveiling normativity. *J. Med. Ethics* 36, 483–487. doi: 10.1136/jme.2010.036095

Douglas, T. (2013). Human enhancement and the supra-personal moral status. *Philos. Stud.* 162, 473–497. doi: 10.1007/s11098-011-9778-2

Earp, B., Sandberg, A., Kahane, G., and Savulescu, J. (2014). When is diminishment a form of enhancement? Rethinking the enhancement debate in biomedical ethics. *Front. Syst. Neurosci.* 8:12. doi: 10.3389/fnsys.2014.00012

Farah, M. J. (2012). Neuroethics: the ethical, legal and societal impact of neuroscience. *Annu. Rev. Psychol.* 63, 571–591. doi: 10.1146/annurev.psych.093008.100438

Fitz, N., Nadler, R., Manogaran, P., Chong, E., and Reiner, P. (2014). Public attitudes toward cognitive enhancement. *Neuroethics* 7, 173–188. doi: 10.1007/s12152-013-9190-z

Foucault, M. (2008). *The Birth of Biopolitics: Lectures at the Collège de France, 1978–79.* Basingstoke, UK and New York: Palgrave Macmillan.

Gini, A., Rossi, P. J., and Giordano, J. (2010). Considering enhancement (and/or treatment): on the need to regard contingency and develop dialectic evaluation-a commentary on singh and kelleher. *AJOB Neurosci.* 1, 25–27. doi: 10.1080/21507740903504392

Giordano, J. (2012). "Neurotechnology as demiurgical force: avoiding icarus' folly," in *Neurotechnology: Premises, Potential and Problems*, ed J. Giordano (Boca Raton: CRC Press), 1–14.

Giordano, J., and DuRousseau, D. (2011). Toward right and good use of brain-machine interfacing neurotechnologies: ethical issues and implications for guidelines and policy. *Cognit. Technol.* 15, 5–10.

Giordano, J., Howlader, D., and Shook, J. (2013). Enablement: a neuroethical and legal course between the scylla of treatment and charybdis of enhancement (abstract). *AJOB Neurosci.* 4:69.

Glannon, W. (2011). *Brain, Body and Mind: Neuroethics with a Human Face.* Oxford: Oxford University Press.

Goold, I., and Maslen, H. (2014). Must the surgeon take the pill? Negligence duty in the context of cognitive enhancement. *Mod. Law Rev.* 77, 60–86. doi: 10.1111/1468-2230.12056

Gunson, D. (2012). "Cognitive enhancement, analogical reasoning and social justice," in *Neurotechnology: Premises, Potential and Problems*, ed J. Giordano (Boca Raton, FL: CRC Press), 243–267.

Gutchess, A., Schwartz, A., and Boduroglu, A. (2011). "The influence of culture on memory," in *Proceedings of the International Workshop on Human-Computer Interaction, Lectures Notes in Computer Science*, eds D. Schmorrow and C. Fidopiastis (Dordrecht: Springer), 67–76.

Han, S., and Pöppel, E. ed. (2011). *Culture and Neural Frames of Cognition and Communication.* Dordrecht: Springer.

Heinrichs, J. (2012). The promises and perils of non-invasive brain stimulation. *Int. J. Law Psychiatry* 35, 121–129. doi: 10.1016/j.ijlp.2011.12.006

Hewer, C. J., and Roberts, R. (2012). History, culture and cognition: towards a dynamic model of social memory. *Cult. Psychol.* 18, 167–183. doi: 10.1177/1354067x11434836

Hildt, E., and Franke, A. ed. (2013). *Cognitive Enhancement: An Interdisciplinary Perspective.* Dordrecht: Springer.

Hildt, E., Lieb, K., and Franke, A. (2014). Life context of pharmacological academic performance enhancement among university students—a qualitative approach. *BMC Med. Ethics* 15:23. doi: 10.1186/1472-6939-15-23

Illes, J., and Bird, S. (2006). Neuroethics: a modern context for ethics in neuroscience. *Trends Neurosci.* 29, 511–517. doi: 10.1016/j.tins.2006.07.002

Imada, T., Carlson, S., and Itakura, S. (2013). East-West cultural differences in contextsensitivity are evident in early childhood. *Dev. Sci.* 16, 198–208. doi: 10.1111/desc.12016

Ishii, K. (2013). Culture and the mode of thought: a review. *Asian J. Soc. Psychol.* 16, 123–132. doi: 10.1111/ajsp.12011

Kim, H., and Sasaki, J. Y. (2014). Cultural neuroscience: biology of the mind in cultural context. *Annu. Rev. Psychol.* 65, 487–514. doi: 10.1146/annurev-psych-010213-115040

Levy, N. (2011). Neuroethics: a new way of doing ethics. *AJOB Neurosci.* 2, 3–9. doi: 10.1080/21507740.2011.557683

Llewellyn, W. (2010). *Anabolics.* 10th Edn. Jupiter, FL: Molecular Nutrition Press.

Luber, B. (2014). Neuroenhancement by noninvasive brain stimulation is not a net zero-sum proposition. *Front. Syst. Neurosci.* 8:127. doi: 10.3389/fnsys.2014.00127

Maslen, H., Douglas, T., Cohen Kadosh, R., Levy, N., and Savulescu, J. (2014a). The regulation of cognitive enhancement devices: extending the medical model. *J. Law Biosci.* 1, 68–93. doi: 10.1093/jlb/lst003

Maslen, H., Faulmüller, N., and Savulescu, J. (2014b). Pharmacological cognitive enhancement—how future neuroscientific research could advance ethical debate. *Front. Syst. Neurosci.* 8:107. doi: 10.3389/fnsys.2014.00107

Metzinger, T., and Hildt, E. (2011). "Cognitive enhancement," in *Oxford Handbook of Neuroethics*, eds J. Illes and B. Sahakian (Oxford: Oxford University Press), 245–264.

Murray, T. (2007). "Enhancement," in *Oxford Handbook of Bioethics*, ed B. Steinbock (Oxford: Oxford University Press), 491–515.

Núñez, R. (2011). No innate number line in the human brain. *J. Cross. Cult. Psychol.* 42, 651–668. doi: 10.1177/0022022111406097

Plischke, H., Du Rousseau, D., and Giordano, J. (2011). EEG-based neurofeedback: the promise of neurotechnology and need for neuroethically-informed guidelines and policies. *Ethics Biol. Eng. Med.* 4, 7–18. doi: 10.1615/EthicsBiologyEngMed.2012004853

Pringle, A., Browning, M., Parsons, E., Cowen, P., and Harmer, C. (2013). Early markers of cognitive enhancement: developing an implicit measure of cognitive performance. *Psychopharmacology (Berl)* 230, 631–638. doi: 10.1007/s00213-013-3186-6

Racine, E., Martin Rubio, T., Chandler, J., Forlini, C., and Lucke, J. (2014). The value and pitfalls of speculation about science and technology in bioethics: the case of cognitive enhancement. *Med. Health Care Philos.* 17, 325–337. doi: 10.1007/s11019-013-9539-4

Rossi, P. J., Okun, M., and Giordano, J. (2013). Translational imperatives in deep brain stimulation research: addressing neuroethical issues of consequences and continuity of clinical care. *AJOB Neurosci.* 5, 46–48. doi: 10.1080/21507740.2013.863248

Sahakian, B., and Morein-Zamir, S. (2011). Neuroethical issues in cognitive enhancement. *J. Psychopharmacol.* 25, 197–204. doi: 10.1177/0269881109106926

Sandberg, A. (2011). "Cognition enhancement: upgrading the brain," in *Enhancing Human Capacities*, eds J. Savulescu, R. ter Meulen and G. Kahane (Malden, MA: Wiley-Blackwell), 71–91.

Sarewitz, D., and Karas, T. (2012). "Policy implications of technologies for cognitive enhancement," in *Neurotechnology: Premises, Potential and Problems*, ed J. Giordano (Boca Raton, FL: CRC Press), 267–285.

Shook, J. R. (2012). Neuroethics and the possible types of moral enhancement. *AJOB Neurosci.* 3, 3–14. doi: 10.1080/21507740.2012.712602

Shook, J. R., and Giordano, J. (2014). A principled and cosmopolitan neuroethics: considerations for international relevance. *Philos. Ethics Humanit. Med.* 9:1. doi: 10.1186/1747-5341-9-1

Specker, J., Focquaert, F., Raus, K., Sterckx, S., and Schermer, M. (2014). The ethical desirability of moral bioenhancement: a review of reasons. *BMC Med. Ethics* 15:67. doi: 10.1186/1472-6939-15-67

Wade, L., Forlini, C., and Racine, E. (2014). Generating genius: how an Alzheimer's drug became considered a "cognitive enhancer" for healthy individuals. *BMC Med. Ethics* 15:37. doi: 10.1186/1472-6939-15-37

Permissions

All chapters in this book were first published in ABFFFC, by Frontiers; hereby published with permission under the Creative Commons Attribution License or equivalent. Every chapter published in this book has been scrutinized by our experts. Their significance has been extensively debated. The topics covered herein carry significant findings which will fuel the growth of the discipline. They may even be implemented as practical applications or may be referred to as a beginning point for another development.

The contributors of this book come from diverse backgrounds, making this book a truly international effort. This book will bring forth new frontiers with its revolutionizing research information and detailed analysis of the nascent developments around the world.

We would like to thank all the contributing authors for lending their expertise to make the book truly unique. They have played a crucial role in the development of this book. Without their invaluable contributions this book wouldn't have been possible. They have made vital efforts to compile up to date information on the varied aspects of this subject to make this book a valuable addition to the collection of many professionals and students.

This book was conceptualized with the vision of imparting up-to-date information and advanced data in this field. To ensure the same, a matchless editorial board was set up. Every individual on the board went through rigorous rounds of assessment to prove their worth. After which they invested a large part of their time researching and compiling the most relevant data for our readers.

The editorial board has been involved in producing this book since its inception. They have spent rigorous hours researching and exploring the diverse topics which have resulted in the successful publishing of this book. They have passed on their knowledge of decades through this book. To expedite this challenging task, the publisher supported the team at every step. A small team of assistant editors was also appointed to further simplify the editing procedure and attain best results for the readers.

Apart from the editorial board, the designing team has also invested a significant amount of their time in understanding the subject and creating the most relevant covers. They scrutinized every image to scout for the most suitable representation of the subject and create an appropriate cover for the book.

The publishing team has been an ardent support to the editorial, designing and production team. Their endless efforts to recruit the best for this project, has resulted in the accomplishment of this book. They are a veteran in the field of academics and their pool of knowledge is as vast as their experience in printing. Their expertise and guidance has proved useful at every step. Their uncompromising quality standards have made this book an exceptional effort. Their encouragement from time to time has been an inspiration for everyone.

The publisher and the editorial board hope that this book will prove to be a valuable piece of knowledge for researchers, students, practitioners and scholars across the globe.

List of Contributors

Brian D. Earp and Julian Savulescu
Faculty of Philosophy, Oxford Uehiro Centre for Practical Ethics, University of Oxford, Oxford, UK
Faculty of Philosophy, Institute for Science and Ethics, University of Oxford, Oxford, UK
Faculty of Philosophy, Oxford Centre for Neuroethics, University of Oxford, Oxford, UK

Anders Sandberg
Faculty of Philosophy, Oxford Uehiro Centre for Practical Ethics, University of Oxford, Oxford, UK
Faculty of Philosophy, Future of Humanity Institute, University of Oxford, Oxford, UK

Guy Kahane
Faculty of Philosophy, Oxford Uehiro Centre for Practical Ethics, University of Oxford, Oxford, UK
Faculty of Philosophy, Oxford Centre for Neuroethics, University of Oxford, Oxford, UK

Singh Deepeshwar, Suhas Ashok Vinchurkar, Naveen Kalkuni Visweswaraiah and Hongasandra RamaRao Nagendra
ANVESANA Research Laboratory, Department of Yoga and Life Sciences, Swami Vivekananda Yoga Research Foundation, Bangalore, Karnataka, India

Jared C. Horvath, Olivia Carter and Jason D. Forte
Psychological Sciences, University of Melbourne, Melbourne, VIC, Australia

Alexander V. Lebedev and Françoise J. Siepel
Department of Psychiatry, Centre for Age-Related Medicine, Stavanger University Hospital, Stavanger, Norway

Eric Westman, Aleksandra Lebedeva and Joana B. Pereira
Department of Neurobiology, Care Sciences and Society, Karolinska Institutet, Stockholm, Sweden

Andrew Simmons
Department of Neuroimaging, Institute of Psychiatry, King's College London, London, UK
NIHR Biomedical Research Centre for Mental Health and Biomedical Research Unit for Dementia, London, UK

Dag Aarsland
Department of Psychiatry, Centre for Age-Related Medicine, Stavanger University Hospital, Stavanger, Norway
Department of Neurobiology, Care Sciences and Society, Karolinska Institutet, Stockholm, Sweden

Cyrus K. Foroughi, Eric J. Blumberg and Raja Parasuraman
Department of Psychology, Arch Lab, George Mason University, Fairfax, VA, USA

Zheng Li
State Key Laboratory of Cognitive Neuroscience and Learning and IDG/McGovern Institute for Brain Research, Beijing Normal University, Beijing, China
Center for Collaboration and Innovation in Brain and Learning Sciences, Beijing Normal University, Beijing, China

Martijn E. Wokke
Amsterdam Brain and Cognition, University of Amsterdam, Amsterdam, Netherlands
Consciousness, Cognition and Computation Group, Department of Psychology, Université Libre de Bruxelles, Brussels, Belgium

Lotte J. Talsma and Marlies E. Vissers
Amsterdam Brain and Cognition, University of Amsterdam, Amsterdam, Netherlands
Department of Psychology, University of Amsterdam, Amsterdam, Netherlands

Adam C. Oei and Michael D. Patterson
Division of Psychology, School of Humanities and Social Sciences, Nanyang Technological University, Singapore, Singapore

Djamila Bennabi, Solène Pedron, Yvan Peterschmitt and Vincent Van Waes
EA 481 Laboratory of Integrative and Clinical Neuroscience, University of Franche-Comté/SFR FED 4234, Besançon, France

Emmanuel Haffen and Julie Monnin
EA 481 Laboratory of Integrative and Clinical Neuroscience, University of Franche-Comté/SFR FED 4234, Besançon, France
INSERM CIC-IT 808 Clinical Investigation Centre for Innovative Technology, University Hospital of Besançon, Besançon, France

Estate M. Sokhadze and Manuel F. Casanova
Department of Psychiatry and Behavioral Sciences, University of Louisville, Louisville, KY, USA

Ayman S. El-Baz
Department of Bioengineering, University of Louisville, Louisville, KY, USA

Lonnie L. Sears
Department of Pediatrics, University of Louisville, Louisville, KY, USA

Ioan Opris
Department of Physiology and Pharmacology, Wake Forest University, Winston-Salem, NC, USA

Gary Lynch
Department of Psychiatry and Human Behavior, University of California, Irvine, CA, USA
Department of Anatomy and Neurobiology, University of California, Irvine, CA, USA

Conor D. Cox and Christine M. Gall
Department of Anatomy and Neurobiology, University of California, Irvine, CA, USA

Emmanuel Mandonnet
Department of Neurosurgery, Hôpital Lariboisière, Paris, France
Department of Neurosurgery, Université Paris Diderot, Paris, France
IMNC, UMR 8165, Orsay, France

Hugues Duffau
Department of Neurosurgery, Gui de Chauliac Hospital, Montpellier University Medical Center, Montpellier, France
Team "Plasticity of Central Nervous System, Stem Cells and Glial Tumors," INSERM U1051, Institute for Neuroscience of Montpellier, Montpellier University Medical Center, Montpellier, France

Mikhail I. Rabinovich
BioCircuits Institute, University of California San Diego, La Jolla, CA, USA

Yury Sokolov and Robert Kozma
Department of Mathematical Sciences, University of Memphis, Memphis, TN, USA

Daniel E. Callan
Center for Information and Neural Networks (CiNet), National Institute of Information and Communications Technology (NICT), Osaka University, Osaka, Japan
Multisensory Cognition and Computation Laboratory Universal Communication Research Institute, National Institute of Information and Communications Technology, Kyoto, Japan

Kimberly J. Schelle
Department of Industrial Design, Eindhoven University of Technology, Eindhoven, Netherlands

Gautier Durantin
Centre Aéronautique et Spatial, Institut Supérieur de l'Aéronautique et de l'Espace, Université de Toulouse, Toulouse, France

Cengiz Terzibas
Multisensory Cognition and Computation Laboratory Universal Communication Research Institute, National Institute of Information and Communications Technology, Kyoto, Japan

Nadira Faulmüller
Department of Experimental Psychology, University of Oxford, Oxford, UK
Department of Values, Technology and Innovation, Delft University of Technology, Delft, Netherlands

Lucius Caviola and Miles Hewstone
Department of Experimental Psychology, University of Oxford, Oxford, UK
Department of Values, Technology and Innovation, Delft University of Technology, Delft, Netherlands

Maryam Alimardani and Hiroshi Ishiguro
Department of System Innovation, Graduate school of Engineering science, Osaka University, Osaka, Japan
Advanced Telecommunications Research Institute International, Kyoto, Japan

Shuichi Nishio
Advanced Telecommunications Research Institute International, Kyoto, Japan

Leslie C. Jellen
Department of Genetics, Genomics, and Informatics, University of Tennessee Health Science Center, Memphis, TN, USA

Alexander Aliper
Aging Research, Insilico Medicine, Emerging Technology Center, Johns Hopkins University Eastern, Baltimore, MD, USA

Anton Buzdin
Personalized Medicine, Pathway Pharmaceuticals Ltd, Wan Chai, Hong Kong

Alex Zhavoronkov
Aging Research, Insilico Medicine, Emerging Technology Center, Johns Hopkins University Eastern, Baltimore, MD, USA
Research, Biogerontology Research Foundation, Truro, UK

Ivan N. Pigarev
Institute for Information Transmission Problems (Kharkevich Institute), Russian Academy of Sciences, Moscow, Russia

Marina L. Pigareva
Institute of Higher Nervous Activity and Neurophysiology, Russian Academy of Sciences, Moscow, Russia

Yvonne Höller and Eugen Trinka
Department of Neurology, Christian Doppler Medical Centre and Centre for Cognitive Neuroscience, Paracelsus Medical University, Salzburg, Austria

Dasuni S. Alwis and Ramesh Rajan
Department of Physiology, Monash University, Clayton, VIC, Australia

Giuseppe Lisi
ATR Computational Neuroscience Laboratories, Department of Brain Robot Interface, ATR, Kyoto, Japan
Mathematical Informatics Laboratory, Department of Information Science, Nara Institute of Science and Technology, Nara, Japan

Tomoyuki Noda and Jun Morimoto
ATR Computational Neuroscience Laboratories, Department of Brain Robot Interface, ATR, Kyoto, Japan

Sam A. Deadwyler, Andrew J. Sweatt, Ioan Opris and Robert E. Hampson
Department of Physiology and Pharmacology, Wake Forest School of Medicine, Winston-Salem, NC, USA

Theodore W. Berger, Dong Song, Rosa H. M. Chan and Vasilis Z. Marmarelis
Department of Biomedical Engineering, University of Southern California, Los Angeles, CA, USA

Greg A. Gerhardt
Department of Neurobiology, Chandler Medical School, University of Kentucky, Lexington, KY, USA

Yoshio Sakurai, Kichan Song and Shota Tachibana
Department of Psychology, Graduate School of Letters, Kyoto University, Kyoto, Japan

Susumu Takahashi
Laboratory of Neural Circuitry, Graduate School of Brain Science, Doshisha University, Kizugawa, Japan

John R. Shook
Philosophy Department and Graduate School of Education, University at Buffalo, Buffalo, NY, USA

Lucia Galvagni
Bruno Kessler Foundation, Trento, Italy

James Giordano
Neuroethics Studies Program, Pellegrino Center for Clinical Bioethics and Department of Neurology, Georgetown University Medical Center, Washington, DC, USA
Human Science Center, Ludwig-Maximilians Universität, Munich, Germany

Index

www.ingramcontent.com/pod-product-compliance
Lightning Source LLC
LaVergne TN
LVHW080926210926
848485LV00004B/738